GYNECOLOGIC RADIATION ONCOLOGY

A Practical Guide

Patricia J. Eifel, MD
Professor, Section of Gynecology
Department of Radiation Oncology
The University of Texas MD Anderson Cancer Center
Houston, Texas

Ann H. Klopp, MD, PhD
Associate Professor, Section of Gynecology
Department of Radiation Oncology
The University of Texas MD Anderson Cancer Center
Houston, Texas

Wolters Kluwer

Philadelphia • Baltimore • New York • London
Buenos Aires • Hong Kong • Sydney • Tokyo

Executive Editor: Rebecca Gaertner
Senior Product Development Editor: Emilie Moyer
Editorial Assistant: Brian Convery
Production Project Manager: David Saltzberg
Design Coordinator: Teresa Mallon
Illustration Coordinator: Jennifer Clements
Manufacturing Coordinator: Beth Welsh
Marketing Manager: Rachel Mante Leung
Prepress Vendor: SPi Global

9 8 7 6 5 4 3 2 1

Printed in China

Library of Congress Cataloging-in-Publication Data
Names: Eifel, Patricia, author. | Klopp, Ann H., author.
Title: Gynecologic radiation oncology : a practical guide / by Patricia J. Eifel, Ann H. Klopp.
Description: Philadelphia : Wolters Kluwer, [2017] | Includes bibliographical references and index.
Identifiers: LCCN 2016009430 | ISBN 9781451192650
Subjects: | MESH: Genital Neoplasms, Female—radiotherapy
Classification: LCC RC280.G5 | NLM WP 145 | DDC 616.99/465—dc23 LC record available at https://lccn.loc.gov/2016009430

LWW.com

RRS1606

To our husbands, Dr. James Belli and David Klopp, whose unwavering support and patience made this project possible.
Also, to our patients, whose lives and stories have become a part of us and of this book.
We thank them for trusting us to care for them, for inspiring us, and for teaching us so much.

PREFACE

The radiation treatment of gynecologic cancers can be challenging but also extremely rewarding. Specialized knowledge, skill, attention to detail, and close multidisciplinary collaboration are required to design and deliver highly successful treatments. However, those treatments are very often curative, and the satisfaction derived from knowing that a woman with locoregionally advanced gynecologic cancer has been successfully treated and gone on to lead a normal life is unmatched. We have been fortunate to be able to devote most of our careers to the study and treatment of these patients. During the years of our tenure at MD Anderson, approximately 10,000 patients have been treated on the gynecologic radiation oncology service; we have treated more than 1,500 gynecologic cancer patients with IMRT and have performed more than 5,000 intracavitary and interstitial brachytherapy procedures. The better part of our academic careers has been spent collating these experiences, analyzing and reporting outcomes, studying the findings of other investigators, and searching for ways to understand and improve the treatment of these diseases.

Our experiences and those of other dedicated gynecologic radiation oncologists have led to the publication of thousands of manuscripts, review articles, and textbook chapters. However, although peer-reviewed manuscripts and general textbooks can provide valuable insights about specific topics and useful surveys of relevant literature, they tend not to be ideal vehicles for describing the techniques, methods, and difficult deliberations that characterize the day-to-day practice of gynecologic radiation oncology. Also, the content of these scattered resources is not always readily accessible when it is needed in the course of daily practice.

With this book, our primary goal was to address practical aspects of gynecologic radiation oncology—how to evaluate the role of radiation therapy in various clinical settings; how to explain the rationale for treatment recommendations to referring physicians and patients; when and how to apply various external beam and brachytherapy techniques to address specific clinical problems; and how to monitor and manage patients during and after treatment. Although we have not attempted to exhaustively catalogue the gynecologic radiation oncology literature, we have cited references that we have found particularly helpful in our clinical decision making, emphasizing important clinical trials, meta-analyses of relevant data, and high-quality review articles. Throughout this book, and particularly in Chapter 2, we have tried to explain not only the insights gained from the clinical literature but also the opportunities for misinterpretation, suggesting how trial results can be more accurately applied to everyday clinical practice.

The concepts discussed in *Gynecologic Radiation Oncology* have been illustrated with more than 700 figures and tables. Using these aids and the accompanying text, we have sought to describe in detail each aspect of radiation oncology practice from the initial patient evaluation and treatment recommendation, through the process of radiation treatment planning and delivery, to the posttreatment monitoring of patients for recurrence and treatment-related side effects. Because the multidisciplinary and technical aspects of gynecologic radiation oncology tend to apply to gynecologic cancers of various types and sites of origin, the principles of tumor biology, multidisciplinary management, clinical evaluation, radiation therapy treatment planning and delivery, and symptom management are discussed in general terms in Chapters 1 to 9 of this book. Subsequent chapters focus more specifically on the features of individual disease sites and on the bases for site-specific management decisions. With this structure, we have minimized repetition of broadly relevant content; however, to help readers navigate the text, we have extensively cross-referenced the material contained in individual chapters. To further unify these concepts and to demonstrate how they can be applied in real clinical situations, we have included 54 case studies that are cited throughout the text; these are found at the end of the relevant disease site chapters, with each group of case studies preceded by a summary of the cases and a list of abbreviations.

The contents of this book have been informed not only by our direct clinical experiences, research, and knowledge of the literature but also by years of discussions with colleagues, visits to radiation oncology departments, and attempts to answer questions fielded from practicing radiation oncologists. These experiences have given us some sense of the variations in clinical practice and of the issues that clinicians find particularly challenging in their care of gynecologic cancer patients. With this book, we have tried to suggest some practical approaches to common clinical problems. However, although our experience has given us some answers, it has also made us very aware of the many unknowns in our field. We recognize that some of the topics addressed in this book are controversial. However, clinical decisions must be made even in the face of controversy. We have done our best to explain the rationales behind our current approaches to the management of gynecologic cancers. However, others will disagree, and our own views will undoubtedly evolve as new information emerges. In the meantime, we hope that all of our readers find something in this book that will help them to care for their patients. We also welcome your feedback and encourage you to write us with your comments about the content and character of this book.

Patricia Eifel
Ann Klopp

ACKNOWLEDGMENTS

We are grateful for the many colleagues, too numerous to count, who have provided support and encouragement during our careers and during the development of this book. Several individuals deserve special thanks for their specific contributions to this work.

First, we want to thank our colleagues in radiation oncology, who provided valuable sounding boards throughout the progress of this project. In particular, we thank our departed colleague, Kian Ang, whose practical text on the radiation therapy of head and neck cancers was an early inspiration for this book. We thank Dr. Luis Delclos and Dr. Anuja Jhingran, whose dedicated patient care and innovative ideas have enriched our gynecologic radiation oncology practice, and we thank our gynecologic oncology colleagues, whose skill, knowledge, and dedication to multidisciplinary collaboration have helped to shape our understanding of the field. We also give special thanks to Gillian Thomas for her valuable input during the formative stages of this book.

Many members of our department made important contributions to this book. We give particular thanks to members of our medical dosimetry group, including, James Kanke, Kelly Perrin, Lehendrick Turner, Pamela Castillo, Paula Berner, Mandy Cunningham, and others who helped us to navigate our treatment planning systems and who created the comparative treatment plans for Chapter 6. We also want to thank Michael Kantor for always being available to troubleshoot problems as we attempted to use our treatment planning systems to create illustrations that were informative and free of clutter.

Particular thanks go to Dr. Gaiane Rauch of our diagnostic imaging department, who lent us her expertise in gynecologic tomographic imaging, carefully reviewing for accuracy each of the vascular contours, labels, and annotations for the illustrations in Chapter 5.

We also thank Jordan Pietz for his beautiful illustrations depicting pelvic examination technique and Stephanie Deming and Michael Worley for their thoughtful, detailed copy editing of the text.

Finally, we want to express our gratitude to the team at Wolters Kluwer, particularly Jonathan Pine, who supported the initial concept, and Julie Goolsby and Emilie Moyer, who guided us through the editorial process and kept us on track throughout this marathon effort.

CONTENTS

PART I

PRINCIPLES OF GYNECOLOGIC ONCOLOGY

CHAPTER 1

Pathology, Molecular Biology, and Etiology of Gynecologic Cancers

INTRODUCTION

Radiation treatment recommendations for gynecologic cancers are guided primarily by the site of origin and the morphology of the primary tumor. Morphologically, similar gynecologic cancers from different sites of origin tend to share molecular features and demonstrate similar patterns of spread. However, even among morphologically similar cancers, the site of origin plays a critical role in the method and ease of initial cancer detection, the prognosis, and the patterns of regional spread (Chapter 5).

In recent years, research has greatly expanded our understanding of the molecular correlates of prognosis. Although the practical uses of this knowledge have focused primarily on refinements to diagnostic criteria, there is reason to hope that these findings will eventually contribute to the development of new, more effective treatments. In addition, better understanding of the roles of human papillomavirus (HPV) infection and heredity in the etiology of gynecologic cancers is leading to successful strategies for prevention of many cancers.

CORRELATES BETWEEN MORPHOLOGY AND BIOLOGIC BEHAVIOR

Most gynecologic cancers fall into three major groups: carcinomas, sarcomas, and germ cell tumors. Among gynecologic cancers, carcinomas are much more common than other types of cancers.

Carcinomas arise from the squamous or glandular epithelial linings of the vulva, vagina, cervix, uterus, fallopian tubes, or ovaries and account for the vast majority of gynecologic cancers that are treated with radiation. Squamous carcinomas predominate in structures that are normally lined by squamous epithelium (vulva, vagina, and cervix), while adenocarcinomas predominate in structures that are lined with glandular epithelium (uterus, fallopian tubes, and ovaries). However, adenocarcinomas can also arise from glandular elements of lower genital tract structures, and areas of squamous differentiation can be a prominent feature in endometrial and, occasionally, ovarian cancers.

Carcinosarcomas are defined by the presence of both a malignant epithelial and a mesenchymal component; these tumors can originate throughout the female genital tract but are most commonly found in the endometrium and ovary.

Sarcomas are derived from the mesenchymal components of female genital tract structures. The most common of which are leiomyosarcomas, which are derived from smooth muscle of the uterus and other structures, and endometrial stromal sarcomas, which are derived from endometrial stroma. Rarely, cancers are derived from hormone-secreting ovarian stroma; these include granulosa cell tumors, which are derived from the sex cord and are comparable to testicular Sertoli cell tumors, and thecomas, which are derived from gonadal stroma and are comparable to Leydig cell tumors of the testis. Tumors that contain a mixture of granulosa cell tumor and thecoma are called Sertoli–Leydig cell tumors.

Germ cell tumors in females arise from the ovary and include teratomas, dysgerminomas, yolk sac tumors (also called endodermal sinus tumors), embryonal carcinomas, and choriocarcinomas. Germ cell tumors are rarely treated with radiation, as they generally have a favorable prognosis with surgery alone (teratomas) or are highly chemotherapy sensitive (choriocarcinomas, dysgerminomas).

Müllerian Adenocarcinomas

Most gynecologic adenocarcinomas arise from cells that had their origin in the embryologic müllerian duct (Chapter 5). The shared developmental origin of these müllerian carcinomas explains the shared behavioral and biologic characteristics of müllerian adenocarcinomas arising in various sites. Grade is an important prognostic factor for all types of adenocarcinoma.

Subtypes of Müllerian Adenocarcinoma

There are four major subtypes of müllerian adenocarcinoma:

- *Endometrioid carcinomas* resemble normal endometrial glands in their differentiated state. The grade of endometrioid carcinomas is based on the percentage of the tumor area that has a solid growth pattern and tends to be correlated with the degree of nuclear atypia.
- *Mucinous carcinomas* resemble normal endocervical glandular epithelium. Many cervical adenocarcinomas have mucinous features.[1]
- *Serous carcinomas* resemble fallopian tube epithelium. They tend to have a papillary architectural pattern, but grade is based on cytologic features. Adnexal serous carcinomas can range from very low-grade lesions of uncertain malignant potential (so-called borderline tumors) to very pleomorphic, high-grade cancers. Serous carcinomas of any grade metastasize to peritoneal surfaces more frequently than other müllerian variants do. High- and low-grade serous carcinomas arise from the ovary, while uterine serous carcinomas are virtually always high-grade cancers.
- *Clear cell carcinomas* have glycogen-rich cytoplasm, which gives them the characteristic appearance of cleared cytoplasm. Although clear cell carcinomas are believed to be of müllerian origin, their precise origins are uncertain.[2]

Variants of müllerian adenocarcinoma arise throughout the gynecologic tract with varying frequency; however, they tend to occur more frequently in the tissues that share their differentiated features, for example, endometrioid carcinomas in the endometrium, serous carcinomas in the ovary or fallopian tube, and endocervical-type mucinous carcinomas in the cervix.

Type I and Type II Histologic Variants of Endometrial and Ovarian Cancer

Endometrial and ovarian cancers demonstrate greater morphologic variability than do cancers at other gynecologic sites, and all subtypes of müllerian adenocarcinoma play a major role. Endometrial and ovarian cancers have sometimes been grouped according to their likelihood of demonstrating aggressive behavior.

Endometrial cancers are frequently divided according to their morphologic features and aggressiveness into type I and type II cancers. Type I cancers, which include endometrioid and the relatively rare mucinous carcinomas, typically present at an early stage and have a relatively favorable prognosis. Type I cancers are thought to frequently develop as a consequence of excess estrogen exposure, which triggers proliferation in the estrogen-responsive endometrial cells. A higher lifetime risk of estrogen exposure is seen in women with early menarche, fewer pregnancies, exogenous estrogen exposure, or obesity, which increases estrogen exposure through aromatization of androgens from peripheral adipose tissues. Type I endometrial cancers classically arise in a proliferative endometrium with complex hyperplasia, supporting the suggestion that estrogen exposure fosters the development of these cancers. Other risk factors for type I endometrial cancer include hypertension, diabetes, anovulation, and polycystic ovarian syndrome. Type II cancers, which include serous carcinomas, clear cell carcinomas, and in some descriptions, carcinosarcomas, are more aggressive. Type II cancers typically arise in an atrophic endometrium in older patients than the ones in which the type I variants arise.

Ovarian cancers have similarly been divided into type I and type II tumors.[3] According to this classification, type I tumors include low-grade serous, low-grade endometrioid, clear cell, and mucinous carcinomas—subtypes that are more likely to present at an early stage and have a more indolent course. Type II tumors include high-grade serous and high-grade endometrioid subtypes, which are more likely to present at an advanced stage and have an aggressive course.

The various subtypes of müllerian adenocarcinoma are frequently admixed; in these cases, prognosis is usually dictated by the type II or highest grade lesion.

The gynecologic origins of müllerian adenocarcinomas can be traced by detecting the expression of PAX8. This transcriptional factor drives the development of müllerian tumors and is persistently expressed in many müllerian adenocarcinomas of gynecologic origin. Immunohistochemical staining for PAX8 can be used to determine the primary tumor site in the case of a metastatic tumor of unknown primary site.[4]

Squamous Carcinomas

Gynecologic squamous carcinomas arise predominantly from the squamous epithelium that lines the vulva, vagina, and cervix; most cancers involving lower genital tract sites are squamous. Although the cytologic grade of squamous carcinomas varies, grade is at most weakly correlated with prognosis. Squamous carcinomas of gynecologic origin, as well as squamous cancers arising at other mucosal sites, such as the head and neck, tend to behave more predictably than cancers of other histologic subtypes, first invading locally and then disseminating to regional lymph nodes before distant sites. HPV plays a critical role in the development of many gynecologic squamous carcinomas.

MOLECULAR BIOLOGY OF GYNECOLOGIC CANCERS

Methods of Molecular Characterization

Immunohistochemical techniques have played a critical role in advancing our understanding of the molecular features of gynecologic cancers. Immunohistochemical tests involve incubation of a labeled antibody on fixed, paraffin-embedded sections. The staining intensity is scored qualitatively, and generally only a single marker can be tested at a time. Because immunohistochemical studies are performed on fixed, paraffin-embedded tissue, these markers were most readily incorporated into practice. Many immunohistochemical markers with diagnostic, predictive, and prognostic potential in gynecologic cancer have been identified, but few have been developed into clinically useful tools.

More recently, techniques to comprehensively survey gene expression, copy number, and mutations (genomics) and protein expression (proteomics) have become more feasible. These techniques survey the entire landscape of a tumor rather than focusing on a single gene or protein. As a result, these studies can be used to simultaneously evaluate the functionality of hundreds of pathways. As the number of biologically targeted agents expands, the hope is that treatments can be tailored to the molecular profile of each patient's tumor. This approach holds great promise but remains investigational and is employed primarily in patients with advanced and recurrent disease. To date, molecular features have not proven to reliably identify which patients with gynecologic cancers will benefit from radiation therapy, but this is an active area of investigation that is likely to bring changes to clinical practice in the next decade.

Correlation of Molecular Markers with Morphology and Prognosis

Several molecular features of gynecologic cancers have been found to correlate with morphology. For example, in type I endometrial cancer, molecular analysis frequently detects mismatch repair deficiencies with areas of repeating DNA sequences, called microsatellite instability; mutations in genes such as *PTEN*, *KRAS*, *CDH1*, and *CTNNB1* are also common. In contrast, in type II endometrial cancer, mutations in *TP53*, *ERBB2*, and *TERT* are more common.

Type II, high-grade ovarian cancers have a higher rate of mutations in *TP53* and greater genomic instability than type I cancers. Type II ovarian cancers are also more likely to have disruption of *BRCA* gene function because of genetic or epigenetic changes.[3]

Molecular features have also been correlated with prognosis. The Cancer Genome Atlas recently reported a comprehensive analysis of molecular changes in endometrial cancers. The authors performed whole-genome sequencing, gene expression, methylation, and copy number analyses on 373 endometrial cancers.[5] Tumors were classified into four groups on the basis of features identified in the analysis. Of perhaps greatest interest was a small subgroup of tumors that had mutations in the catalytic subunit of DNA polymerase epsilon (POLE). These tumors were associated with an extremely favorable prognosis despite a high-grade, often serous, morphology; they were also characterized by tumor-infiltrating T cells and a high rate of mutations throughout the genome.[5,6] The Cancer Genome Atlas analysis also identified a poor-prognosis group of tumors with a high rate of increases in the number of copies of genes. These tumors had frequent mutations in *TP53* and included serous tumors, as well as 25% of grade 3 endometrioid cancers. In the future, these molecular subtypes may find clinical utility in the management of endometrial cancer.

Hormone Receptor Expression

Endometrial and ovarian cancers often express estrogen receptor (ER) and progesterone receptor (PR) on the cell surface, and evaluation of these receptors can be useful in determining the role of hormonal therapy. In general, signaling through the ER stimulates tumor cell proliferation, while signaling through the PR suppresses tumor cell proliferation. As a result, antiestrogen therapy has been investigated for patients with ER-positive tumors, and progestin analogs have been studied for patients with PR-positive tumors.

ER and PR are frequently expressed on well-differentiated and early-stage endometrial cancers.[7] For patients with recurrent or advanced ER- and/or PR-positive endometrial cancer, treatment with megestrol acetate with or without tamoxifen can be considered. However, response rates are low even with combined therapy.[8] Although use of antiestrogens, such as tamoxifen, has a strong biologic rationale, studies investigating the use of tamoxifen in endometrial and ovarian cancer have not been encouraging. Hormonal therapy appears to have limited benefit in high-grade ovarian cancers but have shown efficacy in the management of low-grade endometrial cancers that are more likely to be ER/PR positive and have more indolent clinical course.[9,10]

Women with squamous cancers who have experienced premature menopause are often given estrogen replacement therapy to treat vasomotor symptoms, but exogenous estrogen is often not recommended for women with endometrial or ovarian cancers because of concern that estrogen exposure could stimulate growth of residual tumor cells, thus increasing the risk of endometrial cancer recurrence in endometrial cancer survivors. However, the available literature in women with a history of endometrial cancer suggests that there is no evidence of higher rates of recurrence in women treated with estrogen replacement therapy.[10]

ROLE OF HPV IN GYNECOLOGIC CANCERS

HPV is detectable in nearly all cervical cancers, ~75% of vaginal cancers and 50% of vulvar cancers of both squamous and adenocarcinoma histology. Morphologically, HPV-positive carcinomas are not distinguishable from HPV-negative carcinomas, although HPV-positive vulvar cancers are frequently associated with characteristic basaloid or warty vulvar intraepithelial neoplasia (VIN).

HPV infection is the most common sexually transmitted infection; 20% of women aged 20 to 24 years test positive for high-risk subtypes associated with cervical, vaginal, and vulvar cancer.[4] For 90% of women, the infection is asymptomatic and is cleared completely. However, for a small percentage of exposed individuals, the infection persists. Expression of the viral proteins E6 and E7 can then disrupt function of the critical tumor suppressor genes *TP53* and *RB1*, leading to dysplasia. In the cervix, vagina, and vulva, this can lead to the development of an intraepithelial squamous lesion (cervical, vaginal, or vulvar intraepithelial neoplasia). Low-grade dysplastic lesions often regress spontaneously and can be carefully observed, whereas higher-grade lesions are ablated with or resected using various site-specific methods. In higher-grade lesions, HPV is often integrated into host DNA. The process of integration may disrupt the function of tumor suppressor genes or activate oncogenes, which facilitates the formation of malignant lesions. The process of development of a persistent viral infection, development of an intraepithelial lesion, and progression to invasive cancer may take years or even decades.[11]

Although invasive cervical cancers continue to express viral proteins, infectious viral particles are not released. Concerned partners and patients with HPV-associated cancers can be assured that there is no risk of HPV transmission from the cancer and that because the HPV infection was probably acquired years or even decades before the cancer was diagnosed, the presence of an HPV-related cancer does not suggest that either the patient or her partner was recently exposed to HPV.

Non–HPV-associated squamous cancers of the vagina and vulva have unique molecular and epidemiologic features. They typically occur in women in their seventh and eighth decades and are more likely to occur in smokers and in women with a history of lichen sclerosis of the vulva. *TP53* mutations are more common in women with non–HPV-associated vulvar and vaginal cancers than in women with HPV-positive vulvar and vaginal cancer in which p53 function is disrupted by the virally encoded E6 protein.[12]

HPV and Prognosis

In patients with oropharyngeal cancer, HPV status has been shown to be a favorable prognostic factor associated with higher rates of survival following radiation therapy.[13] Ongoing studies are designed to test whether radiation dose reduction is feasible in HPV-positive head and neck cancer. Cervical cancers are virtually all HPV positive. Data suggest that HPV-positive vulvar cancers tend to occur in younger women. However, initial studies of the impact of HPV status on vulvar cancer outcomes have reported mixed results regarding the prognostic implications of HPV status.[14,15]

Prevention of HPV-Associated Cancers

The risk factors for developing HPV-associated cancer are primarily related to exposure to HPV; these include early coitarche, higher number of sexual partners, other sexually transmitted diseases, and impaired immune function. HPV testing performed routinely in combination with a Pap test can more accurately identify women at higher risk for malignancy who need further investigation or more frequent surveillance. The current recommendation from the U.S. Preventive Services Task Force is to screen for HPV in combination with cytology for women between 30 and 65 years of age. HPV positivity is so common in women younger than 30 that routine screening is not recommended.

Vaccination against HPV has been proven to be highly effective at preventing HPV-associated lesions in women who have not previously been exposed to HPV. In large randomized trials, vaccination against HPV reduced by 98% the proportion of women subsequently diagnosed with cervical intraepithelial neoplasia grade 2 or 3, adenocarcinoma in situ, or cervical cancer related to HPV-16 or HPV-18 in women with no prior exposure to HPV.[16] The two approved HPV vaccines, Gardasil and Cervarix, deliver viral-like particles composed of a viral capsid protein, which is essential for viral entry. The vaccine is DNA free and thus carries no risk of infection. Because the vaccine generates an immune response to a capsid protein critical for viral entry into host cells, it prevents initial infection but does not impact recognition of tumor antigens. As a result, the vaccine has no role in the treatment of HPV-related cancers.

Because these vaccines are designed to prevent initial infection, they are recommended for girls between the ages of 11 and 12 to prevent HPV infection before coitarche. The vaccine produces lasting immunity, extending for at least 5 years and likely significantly longer.[17] Despite the efficacy of the vaccine, rates of vaccination remain relatively low. In the United States in 2013, 57.3% of adolescent girls and 34.6% of adolescent boys had received the HPV vaccine.[18]

HEREDITARY CANCER SYNDROMES

A list of heritable syndromes associated with gynecologic cancers is described in **Table 1.1**.

Lynch Syndrome

Lynch syndrome is an autosomal dominant disorder sometimes referred to as hereditary nonpolyposis colorectal cancer. Mutations in DNA mismatch repair genes *MLH1*, *MSH2*, *MSH6*, and *PMS2* lead to an increased risk of endometrial, colon, gastric, and ovarian cancer. Evidence for these mutations can be found by testing tumor tissue immunohistochemically to confirm the absence of proteins encoded by any of the four genes that are mutated in Lynch syndrome. If the tumor analysis shows loss of expression of these mismatch repair genes, patients can be referred to a genetic counselor for discussion of testing for germline mutations. At MD Anderson, tumor testing for evidence of Lynch syndrome is performed routinely in all patients with colon and endometrial cancers.[19]

TABLE 1.1 Hereditary Cancer Syndromes Associated with Gynecologic Cancers

Syndrome	Genes affected	Gene function	Percentage of cancers linked to syndrome	Family characteristics that should prompt screening	Interventions for individuals with syndrome
Lynch	*MLH1*, *MSH2*, *MSH6*, and *PMS2*	DNA mismatch repair	40%–50% of endometrial cancers 60%–80% of colon cancers	At least three relatives with any Lynch syndrome-associated cancer (colorectal cancer or cancer of the endometrium, small bowel, ureter, or renal pelvis) One relative a first-degree relative of the other two At least two successive generations affected At least one individual diagnosed before age 50 y	Colonoscopy annually; endometrial biopsy annually after age 30–35 y; hysterectomy after childbearing
HBOC	*BRCA1* and *BRCA2*	Repair of DNA double-strand breaks	≈10% of ovarian cancers	Any of the following: Female breast cancer diagnosed before age 50 y TNBC diagnosed before age 60 y Male breast cancer Ashkenazi Jewish ancestry, particularly if the proband has been diagnosed with any HBOC-associated cancer	Screening with CA-125 and transvaginal ultrasonography annually; salpingo-oophorectomy after 40 y or when childbearing is complete
Li-Fraumeni	*TP53*	Cell cycle arrest in response to DNA damage	<1% of endometrial and ovarian cancers	Proband with sarcoma diagnosed before age 45 y First-degree relative with any cancer diagnosed before age 45 y First- or second-degree relative with any cancer diagnosed before age 45 y or a sarcoma diagnosed at any age	No ovarian-specific recommendations, but whole-body magnetic resonance imaging may be considered
Cowden	*PTEN*	Phosphatase that regulates cell growth	<1% of endometrial cancers	Combination of benign lesion syndromes and cancer history	Education regarding endometrial cancer and prompt response to uterine bleeding Consider annual endometrial biopsies and transvaginal ultrasonography beginning at age 30–35 y

HBOC, hereditary breast and ovarian cancer; TNBC, triple negative breast cancer.

BRCA-Associated Ovarian Cancer

Approximately 10% of patients with ovarian cancer have an inherited predisposition to developing ovarian cancer. The most common causes are the breast cancer susceptibility genes *BRCA1* and *BRCA2*.[20] The *BRCA* genes are involved in repair of double-strand DNA breaks, which are produced by agents such as platinum and radiation. Women with ovarian cancer with *BRCA* mutations have a more protracted course and a longer median survival than women with non–*BRCA*-associated ovarian cancer.[21] Women with *BRCA* mutations are more likely than women without such mutations to respond to platinum agents and also to poly(ADP-ribose) polymerase inhibitors. It is not known whether *BRCA* mutation status impacts the role of radiation therapy in treatment. Women with mutations in *BRCA* are also at an elevated risk of developing uterine serous cancers.[22]

Risk Reduction Strategies

Several criteria have been proposed to identify patients without endometrial cancer who should be screened for Lynch syndrome on the basis of family history, including the Amsterdam and Bethesda criteria.[19] In a woman diagnosed with Lynch syndrome, the risk of endometrial and colon cancer can be reduced significantly with screening and prophylactic hysterectomy following childbearing. Recommendations include annual endometrial biopsy with total abdominal hysterectomy and bilateral salpingo-oophorectomy performed between the ages of 35 and 40 years or after childbearing is complete[23] and colonoscopy performed every 1 to 2 years between the ages of 25 and 40 years and annually thereafter.

Efforts to detect ovarian cancers early have focused on screening for serum biomarkers combined with ultrasound imaging. The best serum biomarker, CA-125, is elevated in 50% to 90% of women with ovarian cancer but is also elevated in many other conditions. The Prostate, Lung, Colorectal and Ovarian Cancer Screening Trial tested the impact of annual screening with CA-125 and transvaginal ultrasonography in 78,216 women aged 55 to 74 years.[24] The number of ovarian cancers diagnosed was slightly higher (5.7 vs. 4.7 per 10,000 person-years) in the screened arm, but this did not translate to an improvement in ovarian cancer mortality, and surgeries performed to investigate positive findings led to complications. As a result, screening is not routinely recommended for women at average risk. Women with *BRCA* mutations are recommended to undergo CA-125 testing and transvaginal ultrasonography starting at age 35 years or 5 to 10 years earlier than the earliest age of first diagnosis of ovarian cancer in the family. After childbearing is complete, oophorectomy is recommended for women with a *BRCA* mutation.

Pathologic analysis of fallopian tubes removed from women with *BRCA* mutations revealed the presence of premalignant lesions within the epithelium of the fallopian tubes.[3,25,26] This important observation led to the hypothesis that ovarian cancers may originate from the epithelium of the fallopian tube and subsequently implant and grow in the ovaries. The observation that there is a reduced risk of ovarian cancer in women who have undergone tubal ligation supports this hypothesis.[26] This has led to current investigations into whether salpingectomy can reduce the risk of ovarian cancer without the need for premenopausal oophorectomy, which is known to increase cardiovascular mortality.[27]

References

1. Zaino RJ. Glandular lesions of the uterine cervix. *Mod Pathol.* 2000;13:261–274.
2. Alduaij A, Hansen K, Karim TA, et al. Clear cell carcinomas of the mullerian system: does the pathogenesis vary depending on their nuclear grade and their association with endometriosis? An immunohistochemical analysis. *Pathol Res Int.* 2012;2012:674–748.
3. Kurman RJ, Shih IeM. Molecular pathogenesis and extraovarian origin of epithelial ovarian cancer—shifting the paradigm. *Hum Pathol.* 2011;42:918–931.
4. Ozcan A, Liles N, Coffey D, et al. PAX2 and PAX8 expression in primary and metastatic mullerian epithelial tumors: a comprehensive comparison. *Am J Surg Pathol.* 2011;35:1837–1847.
5. Cancer Genome Atlas Research Network; Kandoth C, Schultz N, et al. Integrated genomic characterization of endometrial carcinoma. *Nature.* 2013;497:67–73.
6. Hussein YR, Weigelt B, Levine DA, et al. Clinicopathological analysis of endometrial carcinomas harboring somatic POLE exonuclease domain mutations. *Mod Pathol.* 2015;28:505–514.
7. McCarty KS Jr, Barton TK, Fetter BF, et al. Correlation of estrogen and progesterone receptors with histologic differentiation in endometrial adenocarcinoma. *Am J Pathol.* 1979;96:171–183.
8. Fiorica JV, Brunetto VL, Hanjani P, et al. Phase II trial of alternating courses of megestrol acetate and tamoxifen in advanced endometrial carcinoma: a Gynecologic Oncology Group study. *Gynecol Oncol.* 2004;92:10–14.
9. Gershenson DM. The life and times of low-grade serous carcinoma of the ovary. *Am Soc Clin Oncol Educ Book.* 2013. doi: 10.1200/EdBook_AM.2013.33.e195.
10. Shim SH, Lee SJ, Kim SN. Effects of hormone replacement therapy on the rate of recurrence in endometrial cancer survivors: a meta-analysis. *Eur J Cancer.* 2014;50:1628–1637.
11. Dunne EF, Unger ER, Sternberg M, et al. Prevalence of HPV infection among females in the United States. *JAMA.* 2007;297:813–819.
12. Choschzick M, Hantaredja W, Tennstedt P, et al. Role of TP53 mutations in vulvar carcinomas. *Int J Gynecol Pathol.* 2011;30:497–504.
13. Fakhry C, Westra WH, Li S, et al. Improved survival of patients with human papillomavirus-positive head and neck squamous cell carcinoma in a prospective clinical trial. *J Natl Cancer Inst.* 2008;100:261–269.
14. Monk BJ, Burger RA, Lin F, et al. Prognostic significance of human papillomavirus DNA in vulvar carcinoma. *Obstet Gynecol.* 1995; 85:709–715.
15. Alonso I, Fuste V, del Pino M, et al. Does human papillomavirus infection imply a different prognosis in vulvar squamous cell carcinoma? *Gynecol Oncol.* 2011;122:509–514.
16. Group FIS. Quadrivalent vaccine against human papillomavirus to prevent high-grade cervical lesions. *N Engl J Med.* 2007;356: 1915–1927.
17. Harper DM, Franco EL, Wheeler CM, et al. Sustained efficacy up to 4.5 years of a bivalent L1 virus-like particle vaccine against human papillomavirus types 16 and 18: follow-up from a randomised control trial. *Lancet.* 2006;367:1247–1255.
18. Stokley S, Jeyarajah J, Yankey D, et al. Human papillomavirus vaccination coverage among adolescents, 2007–2013, and postlicensure vaccine safety monitoring, 2006–2014—United States. *MMWR Morb Mortal Wkly Rep.* 2014;63:620–624.
19. Umar A, Boland CR, Terdiman JP, et al. Revised Bethesda Guidelines for hereditary nonpolyposis colorectal cancer (Lynch syndrome) and microsatellite instability. *J Natl Cancer Inst.* 2004;96:261–268.
20. Russo A, Calo V, Bruno L, et al. Hereditary ovarian cancer. *Crit Rev Oncol Hematol.* 2009;69:28–44.
21. Rubin SC, Benjamin I, Behbakht K, et al. Clinical and pathological features of ovarian cancer in women with germline mutations of BRCA1. *N Engl J Med.* 1996;335:1413–1416.
22. Pennington KP, Walsh T, Lee M, et al. BRCA1, TP53, and CHEK2 germline mutations in uterine serous carcinoma. *Cancer.* 2013;119:332–338.
23. Schmeler KM, Lynch HT, Chen LM, et al. Prophylactic surgery to reduce the risk of gynecologic cancers in the Lynch syndrome. *N Engl J Med.* 2006;354:261–269.

24. Buys SS, Partridge E, Black A, et al. Effect of screening on ovarian cancer mortality: the Prostate, Lung, Colorectal and Ovarian (PLCO) Cancer Screening Randomized Controlled Trial. *JAMA.* 2011;305:2295–2303.
25. Shaw PA, Rouzbahman M, Pizer ES, et al. Candidate serous cancer precursors in fallopian tube epithelium of BRCA1/2 mutation carriers. *Mod Pathol.* 2009;22:1133–1138.
26. Hankinson SE, Hunter DJ, Colditz GA, et al. Tubal ligation, hysterectomy, and risk of ovarian cancer. A prospective study. *JAMA.* 1993;270:2813–2818.
27. Parker WH, Broder MS, Chang E, et al. Ovarian conservation at the time of hysterectomy and long-term health outcomes in the nurses' health study. *Obstet Gynecol.* 2009;113:1027–1037.

CHAPTER 2

Interpretation of Clinical Research Results as They Apply to Daily Practice

INTRODUCTION

Investigators have been evaluating the role of radiation therapy in the management of gynecologic cancers for more than 100 years. However, despite an extensive body of literature and, in some cases, decades of focused study, many key questions and controversies remain unresolved.

Clinical application of the gynecologic radiation oncology literature can be particularly challenging for several reasons, including:

- *Inconsistent methods that have been used to describe and classify tumors.* Variations, ambiguities, and misapplications of tumor descriptors have often made it difficult to generalize the results of studies to other settings.
- *Complex, rapidly evolving treatment methods.* Variations in method and technique may limit the relevance of results to different clinical settings.
- *Cancers that either are rare or have low event rates.* Small numbers of patients limit the statistical power of many retrospective studies and make it difficult to design and complete adequately powered prospective trials.
- *Widely varying disease presentations within individual studies.* Studies that have very heterogeneous study populations can yield overall conclusions that overestimate or underestimate the benefit of specific treatments to distinct subsets.

No matter how high the quality of the underlying study, relative risks, survival rates, and complication probabilities can never tell us with certainty which treatment will most benefit any individual patient. Nevertheless, a thorough understanding of the literature, including the strengths and weaknesses of relevant studies, can increase the likelihood that clinicians will choose an effective approach and reduce the probability that they will select an ineffective or potentially harmful treatment.

Of course, a thorough discussion of problems in clinical data interpretation is beyond the scope of this book. Specific strengths and weaknesses of key studies are discussed in context in the site-specific chapters (Chapters 10 to 14). The purpose of this chapter is to highlight a few of the most important factors that should be considered when reading and evaluating the validity of the gynecologic oncology literature. Ambiguities caused by inconsistent nomenclature and poorly defined end points can occur in all types of clinical research; in the next two sections, these sources of error are discussed with specific examples from the gynecologic oncology literature. Subsequent sections will discuss some common sources of error in specific types of clinical research.

AMBIGUITIES CAUSED BY INCONSISTENT NOMENCLATURE

The relevance of any study's results to specific daily practice situations hinges upon clinicians' ability to relate the characteristics of study patients to those of patients entering their clinics. To make this possible, publications must describe all relevant patient, tumor, and treatment characteristics in unambiguous terms that can be easily understood and applied after the results are disseminated. Failure to do this can lead to misunderstanding and misapplication of the study's results. In this section, we have discussed some of the ways in which ambiguous nomenclature has compromised the generalizability of gynecologic oncology studies.

Inconsistencies in the Use and Interpretation of Staging Systems

Most studies of gynecologic cancer treatment use FIGO stage as a criterion for eligibility. However, although FIGO stage categories are usually at least roughly correlated with outcome, they are generally very imprecise measures of recurrence risk. Inconsistent application of staging systems and evolving category descriptions can also be important sources of miscommunication. The following factors have limited the utility of FIGO staging systems as guides for determining prognosis and treatment.

Failure to Consider Important Prognostic Factors

Most FIGO staging systems consider only a few of the important prognostic variables. As a result, stage categories often include definable subgroups with widely varying prognoses. For example, stage IB2 can describe a 4.1-cm cervical cancer with negative nodes or a massive 8-cm cancer with gross para-aortic lymphadenopathy. Stage alone rarely provides sufficient information about the composition of study populations.

Ambiguous Category Descriptions

In some cases, stage categories depend on highly subjective assessments of disease extent. Wide variations in clinicians' thresholds for deciding that a patient has, for example, parametrial or pelvic wall involvement from cervical cancers (Chapter 10) or submucosal involvement of vaginal cancers (Chapter 11) can lead to very large differences in the baseline risk profiles of study patients labeled with the corresponding stages. These variations confound comparisons between similarly staged patients treated in different settings.

Misapplication of FIGO Rules for Staging

Although FIGO has published specific rules for the staging of gynecologic cancers, these are rarely reproduced when the staging systems are quoted in secondary sources. Ignorance of FIGO rules frequently leads to erroneous stage assignments. For example, although FIGO rules do not allow most results of CT, MRI, or PET to influence the stage of cervical or vaginal cancers, this admonition is often ignored. As a result, patients who have extrapelvic metastases diagnosed by these methods may be inappropriately assigned an advanced stage; this error influences the apparent survival rates of patients with all stages. Misapplication of surgical staging criteria to nonsurgical patients is another common source of error (Chapter 10).

Variations in the Extent of Surgical Staging

Although current endometrial and vulvar staging systems are based in part on the findings of lymphadenectomy, many patients have only limited node dissections or even none at all. This variability causes uncertainties about the composition of study populations and is an important source of stage migration. Adding to this is the recent advent of sentinel node mapping, which allows the detection of very small metastases that are typically undetectable with standard histologic processing methods. Although the surgical staging systems for endometrial and vulvar cancer are technically not applicable to patients treated with initial radiation or chemotherapy, stage categories are routinely applied to such patients even though key features used in the staging system cannot be evaluated without initial surgery.

Problems Caused by Evolving Staging Systems

Modifications of the FIGO staging systems have, over time, been important causes of ambiguity and stage migration. Major changes in the endometrial (Table 13.1), vulvar (Table 12.1), and cervical (Chapter 10) staging systems have caused historical discontinuities in the language used to describe cancers. For example, since 1993, there have been two major revisions of the vulvar staging system (Table 12.1). Although most studies traverse at least one of these transitions, investigators frequently fail to explain how they have ensured that stage assignments were applied consistently throughout their study. Also, unless clinicians are aware of the timing and nature of changes in the methods used to classify patients, they can easily draw erroneous conclusions from older studies that described patients using a previous staging method.

For all of these reasons, FIGO stage alone is never a sufficient method for characterizing the makeup of study populations. Detailed descriptions of the morphologic and histologic features that influence treatment outcomes can greatly improve clinicians' confidence in the comparability of staging methods and therefore in the applicability of study results to their patients. The generalizability of studies that describe cancers in terms of tumor stage without clearly stating how, when, and with what rules stage was assigned and without providing other measures of disease extent should be considered suspect.

Inconsistent Interpretation of Histologic Findings

All gynecologic cancers are classified according to their histologic appearance. For cancers that are treated with initial surgery, histologic measures of disease extent, including tumor size, depth of stromal infiltration, lymph–vascular space invasion, surgical margin status, and other features, are used to guide recommendations regarding adjuvant treatment. Although clinicians often assume that the terms used to define these features are universally understood and consistently applied, there is considerable evidence that pathologists vary widely in their interpretations of findings. This can hamper accurate application of study findings in several ways.

Evolving Histologic Criteria

Pathologists' criteria for assigning grade and for diagnosing other measures of biologic aggressiveness evolve as research refines their understanding of clinicopathologic correlations. Because the recognition and adoption of these shifting definitions tend to be gradual, the meaning of key terminology is easily obscured. For example, for at least two decades before FIGO's 1988 revised recommendations for grading of endometrial cancer (Table 13.2), academic pathologists had already been changing their grading criteria, shifting toward relatively lower-grade assignments for endometrioid cancers and higher-grade assignments for aggressive histologic variants. Hendrickson et al.,[1] in their 1982 reexamination of histologic material from 361 patients diagnosed with endometrial cancer between 1959 and 1978, found that 99 (27%) no longer even met their criteria for the diagnosis of cancer; many other lesions were reclassified as lower or higher grade than was specified in the original pathology reports. It is likely that reexamination of most early prospective studies would reveal similar findings. Even after revised methods were codified by FIGO in 1988, pathologists' applications of FIGO recommendations were gradual and often inconsistent.

Shifts in nomenclature compromise historical comparisons in ways that can be very difficult to detect. When terms are applied inconsistently, multivariate analyses may not be valid and can easily lead to erroneous conclusions, particularly if evolving treatment strategies parallel changes in histologic criteria.[2]

Retrospective reviews that are based on vintage pathology reports and obsolete language may be impossible to interpret in contemporary terms. Investigators should always carefully consider whether older terminology will be correctly understood in a modern context; if not, histologic material should, if possible, be reexamined and classified using contemporary criteria.

Inconsistencies in Contemporary Application of Histologic Terminology

Variations in pathologists' use of key terminology can lead to misinterpretation of research results and inappropriate treatment in several ways:

- *Histologic criteria are frequently used to determine eligibility and to estimate event rates for patients entered on multi-institutional trials.* However, these estimates will be inaccurate if principal investigators base their calculations on diagnostic criteria that are not followed by pathologists in contributing institutions. The degree to which this can affect otherwise high-quality trials is illustrated by the PORTEC studies of endometrial cancer (Chapter 13).[3,4] Histologic grade, a determinant of eligibility for these trials, was obtained from the original reports generated by local community pathologists. After the trials were completed and initial results reported, expert review of the material revealed that local pathologists had overestimated the cancer grades in 40% of cases. As a result, the study populations had much lower than expected baseline risks for recurrence. Unknown diagnostic errors undoubtedly affect many other studies that have not had central pathology review. Investigators should always state whether expert pathologists reviewed the histologic diagnoses underpinning their study. If not, the generalizability of the results should be viewed with skepticism.
- *The results of research studies, even when based on expert pathology review, may be applied incorrectly by practicing clinicians if local decisions depend on the reports of less expert pathologists.* Expert review of diagnoses made by general pathologists has revealed frequent discrepancies and even major errors in diagnosis.[5] Close multidisciplinary collaboration and appropriate consultation with expert pathologists may improve diagnostic precision and increase the likelihood that study results will be replicated in other settings (Chapter 3).

Other Sources of Ambiguity

Diagnostic Methods

Wherever possible, authors should describe the criteria used to reach clinical diagnoses. For example, what diagnostic methods were used to identify patients with lymph node involvement? If tomographic imaging methods were used, what size or other criteria were used to make the diagnosis of probable involvement? How did the authors handle equivocal findings? How many cases were confirmed histologically and how were these selected?

Categorization of Continuous Variables

In some cases, the handling of continuous variables (e.g., laboratory results, tumor size, patient age, BMI) can have a major effect on the final result and conclusions. If numerical variables have a continuous relationship to the study end point, they should be summarized and analyzed in that form. However, this is rarely the case. A variety of methods have been used to categorize continuous variables.[6] Investigators commonly choose the median or quartiles to define study groups. These methods may reveal correlations but typically reduce the power of variables to define risk. For example, cervical tumor diameter is commonly treated as a dichotomous variable. Virtually any cutoff point will demonstrate a positive correlation between tumor size and disease recurrence. However, this method obscures additional prognostic information obtained through more detailed subdivision according to size.[7] Another approach is to focus on patients whose values are considered clinically significant by the investigator. However, other investigators and readers may not agree with the authors' determination of clinical significance.

For large studies, statistical methods should be used to define categories with cutoff points that most completely describe the relationship between the study variable and end points. For smaller studies, cutoff points that have been validated using larger data sets of patients with similar diagnoses can be used and referenced.

Summary

The language of clinical staging, diagnostic imaging, and histologic description forms the basis for all communications between researchers and practitioners. The quality of those communications and the applicability of trial results depend critically upon the precision of that language. Adequate description of clinical variables also allows readers to evaluate the degree to which selection bias has influenced the findings of a study.

For these reasons, clinical reports should always attempt to provide:

- Tabulated descriptions of the clinical characteristics of the overall study group and of subgroups compared in the study.
- The version of the staging system used (with a citation).
- The source of clinical findings. Who performed the exams and how were the data recorded? How were conflicting descriptions resolved?
- Whether and how stage was reassigned if some patients were initially staged using an outdated staging system.
- A detailed description of the diagnostic methods used to evaluate important clinical variables such as lymph node involvement, tumor size and extent, and others.
- A specific description of the source of histologic diagnoses. Was the diagnosis obtained from multiple sources, from a single pathologist or group of pathologists that reviewed the material at diagnosis, or from a reexamination of the material performed specifically for the authors' study? In many cases, inclusion of a gynecologic pathologist as coauthor can be particularly helpful.
- If the authors chose to categorize continuous variables (e.g., tumor size), how were the cut points chosen and validated?
- A description of missing data elements and how they were handled in the final analysis.
- A detailed discussion of possible inconsistencies in the nomenclature used in the study. This is particularly important when historical comparison groups are used.

Authors and readers of the clinical literature should never underestimate the importance of clear terminology and expert application of diagnostic criteria. Improvements in the clarity of diagnostic terms and greater attention to the specialized expertise of diagnosticians could undoubtedly yield major improvements in the generalizability of trial results and the outcome of patients.

EVALUATING THE NATURE AND VALIDITY OF TRIAL END POINTS

The NCI Dictionary of Cancer Terms defines a clinical trial end point as "an event or outcome that can be measured objectively to determine whether the intervention being studied is beneficial." Trial results may be misinterpreted if:

- The study end point(s) are not clearly defined.
- A large number of patients are lost to follow-up before the end point is reached.
- The end point is not measured objectively.
- The relationship between the end point and treatment benefit is misinterpreted.

A number of factors lead investigators to select specific trial end points. Although overall survival is often considered the most important end point for gynecologic cancer trials, other end points may shed greater light on the cause of failure. In some cases, "surrogate" end points that have shorter event horizons than overall survival are used to determine whether a treatment is beneficial; although surrogate end points can give an answer more quickly, they may not be true indicators of benefit, particularly if their relationship to the primary end point has not been adequately validated. End points commonly used to evaluate gynecologic cancer treatments and possible pitfalls that arise from their use include the following:

Overall Survival

This end point, which requires only an assessment of patients' survival, is often considered to be the best measure of treatment effectiveness. However, for most potentially curable gynecologic cancers, 5 years or more is needed to obtain mature survival data. This is a long time to wait for an answer; in low-resource settings, it is also a long time to maintain continual follow-up of study patients.

The ability to accurately and reliably record deaths also varies greatly with the trial setting; socioeconomic standards, migration patterns, customary practices regarding end-of-life care, national methods of record keeping, access to death records, and other factors affect access to survival data. For example, in Norway, which has low rates of emigration and a robust tumor registry system that is tied to national identification numbers, patients are very rarely lost to follow-up before their death. On the other hand, in many developing countries, 30% or more of patients may be lost to follow-up in the first year after treatment. In the United States, the death of most citizens and legal residents is eventually recorded in the Social Security Death Index. However, there is typically a 4- to 6-month delay before death information appears in the Index, a factor that can have a profound effect on preliminary data analyses. Also, patients who lack a Social Security number (illegal residents and individuals with temporary visas) may be difficult or impossible to track down after they stop coming to the hospital for treatment. At the very least, cases that are censored before reaching the study end point decrease the power to detect differences; if these losses are nonrandom, they can lead investigators to erroneous conclusions.

Relapse-free Survival (RFS) and Disease-free Survival (DFS)

According to the NCI Dictionary of Cancer Terms, RFS and DFS may be used interchangeably to describe the length of time after primary treatment that a patient survives without any signs or symptoms of cancer. Any cancer recurrence and death from any cause are scored as events.

RFS has been very popular in gynecologic oncology trials, primarily because it has a shorter event horizon than overall survival. A major disadvantage of this end point is its dependence on the method used to detect recurrence. Studies that use more frequent assessments and sensitive detection methods will tend to report relatively short RFS rates. Also, equally effective treatments (in terms of overall survival) may have recurrences detected at different times, either because the pattern of recurrence differs between compared treatments (e.g., pelvic RT vs. chemotherapy) or because one treatment (e.g., adjuvant chemotherapy) delays the appearance of residual disease but does not prevent recurrence.

It is also important to recognize that successful salvage treatments do not influence RFS rates. In rare cases, this can lead to erroneous conclusions about the efficacy of treatment. See the discussion of GOG-122 (Chapter 13, Fig. 13.4) for a possible example.

Disease-specific Survival (DSS)

Events are scored at the time of death, but noncancer deaths are censored. We have used this end point as a means of illustrating the effect of disease on long-term survival. However, DSS can be misleading if there is a high rate of early intercurrent death (e.g., if the study population is very elderly) or if a significant number of patients have died of unknown causes. Investigators that use this end point should always clearly describe the nature and number of censored deaths. In our retrospective studies of cervical and vaginal cancer, deaths of unknown causes occurring <5 years after treatment are scored as treatment-related deaths in calculations of DSS.

Time to Recurrence

Events are scored at the time of recurrence; deaths that occur without evidence of recurrent disease are censored. To have any meaning, this end point requires very complete follow-up with very few deaths from unknown causes.

Time to Pelvic Disease Recurrence and Other Assessments of Failure Pattern

Gynecologic radiation oncologists are particularly interested in understanding whether recurrences have occurred within the field of irradiation (an indication of inadequate radiation dose), marginal to the radiated field (an indication of inadequate radiation volume), or extraregionally (usually in sites that could not be addressed with radiation therapy). The rate of pelvic recurrence is frequently interpreted as a measure of the effectiveness of radiation. However, these assessments must be viewed with caution for several reasons. Some investigators record pelvic recurrences only if they are the first site of recurrence; this was a particular problem before high-quality tomographic imaging because distant metastases were typically much easier to detect than deep pelvic relapses. However, because the timing of pelvic recurrence is heavily influenced by the sensitivity of the detection method, we recommend that all intrapelvic recurrences be recorded and reported whether they are detected before or after relapse at other sites. In addition, the methods used to detect pelvic recurrence should be described, including frequency of exams and imaging.

Another cause of confusion is the fact that recurrences labeled as "iliac" are often coded as pelvic recurrences even if they are superior to the upper border of the treatment field. See Chapter 5 for more discussion of this subject.

Summary

Ambiguous end points and incomplete data are important sources of miscommunication. Investigators can reassure readers about the integrity of their data by providing:

- Clear descriptions of all end points, including the criteria used to censor data.
- The median follow-up duration of all patients and of surviving patients (with quartiles and ranges).
- The frequency and methods of posttreatment evaluation.
- The number of patients lost to follow-up and when.
- The number of patients living with active disease, particularly if these lack recent follow-up.
- The number of patients whose cause of death is unknown.
- The relationship between postradiation locoregional relapses and radiation fields.
- The number of patients who received potentially curative salvage treatment and their outcomes.

Studies that fail to provide these details should be viewed with caution.

OBSERVATIONAL STUDIES

Because there are very few high-quality randomized trials to guide the radiation treatment of gynecologic cancers, treatment decisions are frequently based on data acquired from observational, usually retrospective analyses of clinical data.

Evaluation and Management of Bias

The greatest threats to the validity of studies arise from systematic errors caused by various sources of bias (**Table 2.1**).[8] Studies that attempt to retrospectively compare the efficacy of different treatments are particularly prone to confounding bias because treatments are nearly always allocated on the basis of risk. Although carefully designed observational studies can yield important information about disease processes and potentially valuable insights about treatment efficacy, investigators and readers must always be vigilant for possible sources of uncontrolled bias. The gynecologic oncology literature is particularly prone to this type of error for all of the reasons discussed earlier in this chapter.

If the important risk factors have been described in a thorough and consistent fashion, it may be possible to reduce the influence of bias on the comparison of interest by using

TABLE 2.1 Forms of Bias That Threaten the Validity of Clinical Trials

Type of bias	Definition	Comments
Confounding bias	Systematic differences between baseline characteristics that influence both the allocation and outcomes of treatments	Confounding risk factors are commonly used to select treatments. Confounding by indication can occur from patient- or physician-directed treatment selection.
Selection bias (bias in the selection of patients for study)	Occurs when the association between treatment and outcome of study patients differs from that of excluded, potentially eligible patients	Includes inappropriate selection of controls in a case–control study, differential loss to follow-up for groups being compared, and inclusion or exclusion of specific groups for study.
Performance bias	Systematic differences in the care provided to participants; protocol deviation	Examples include contamination of the control group with the experimental treatment or intervention, unbalanced provision of additional interventions or cointerventions, and inadequate blinding of providers and participants.
Detection bias	Systematic differences in outcomes assessment among groups being compared	Includes misclassification of the covariates or outcomes because of variable definitions and timings, inconsistent or faulty diagnostic measures, recall from memory, and others.
Reporting bias	Systematic differences between reported and unreported findings	Differential reporting of outcomes or harms and incomplete reporting of study findings.

Adapted from Viswanathan M, Berkman ND, Dryden DM, et al. Assessing Risk of Bias and Confounding in Observational Studies of Interventions or Exposures: Further Development of the RTI Item Bank. Rockville, MD: Agency for Healthcare Research and Quality (US); 2013.

multivariate Cox regression analysis. However, the study cohort must also be large enough to sustain a stable regression model. The rule of thumb that requires 10 events per predictor variable can be difficult to achieve in studies of gynecologic cancers that have many risk factors and, often, relatively low event rates. *For this reason, a small cohort with many potential sources of confounding bias is rarely a worthwhile subject for study of treatment comparisons.* Readers should be particularly wary of treatment comparison studies that have fewer than five events per variable or that have failed to include all of the important prognostic factors in the analysis.

Some investigators have attempted to reduce the role of bias by comparing patients treated in different institutions using different techniques or by comparing a recent cohort with a historical comparison group. Such studies can provide valuable insights but can have sources of hidden bias. In particular, if the methods of staging, histologic diagnosis, or other rules of nomenclature differ between two groups of differently treated patients, erroneous conclusions can arise when the cohorts are analyzed using multivariate regression methods.[2]

The Role of Belief Bias

Another factor that can influence interpretation of data is the so-called belief-bias effect. Research suggests that subjects are more likely to rate a deductive argument as valid if the suggested conclusion fits with their beliefs; this is particularly true if the data do not logically lead to a conclusive answer (**Fig. 2.1**).[9] Because many of the methods used to treat gynecologic neoplasms are based on more or less inconclusive data, there is substantial room for belief bias to play a role in our interpretation of the literature. Because it is unlikely that any of us are immune to this form of bias, it is important to be vigilant and self-aware as we interpret our own and others' data. One way to test whether belief bias has influenced our receptiveness to a research conclusion is to ask whether we would retain faith in the validity of the analysis if it had suggested an opposite result that ran counter to our beliefs.

Are Observational Studies Ever Free of Bias?

There are some situations in which observational studies are largely free of bias. For example, if archived material is used to study the prognostic importance of a previously unknown biologic marker, the results are unlikely to be affected by treatment selection bias. The prognostically powerful DNA polymerase epsilon (POLE) marker for high-grade but low-risk endometrial cancers (Chapter 1) is an excellent example of such a finding. However, before one can dismiss the possibility that confounding bias has influenced the results of this type of study, it must be proven that the new predictive factor is not closely tied to a known predictor that was used to select treatments.

Interestingly, anecdotal reports can also be powerful sources of information if they can serve as proof of principle. For example, while collecting data for a large retrospective study, we came across a patient treated 15 years prior for supraclavicular node recurrence from cervical cancer. Her treatment, node excision followed by radiation (30 Gy in

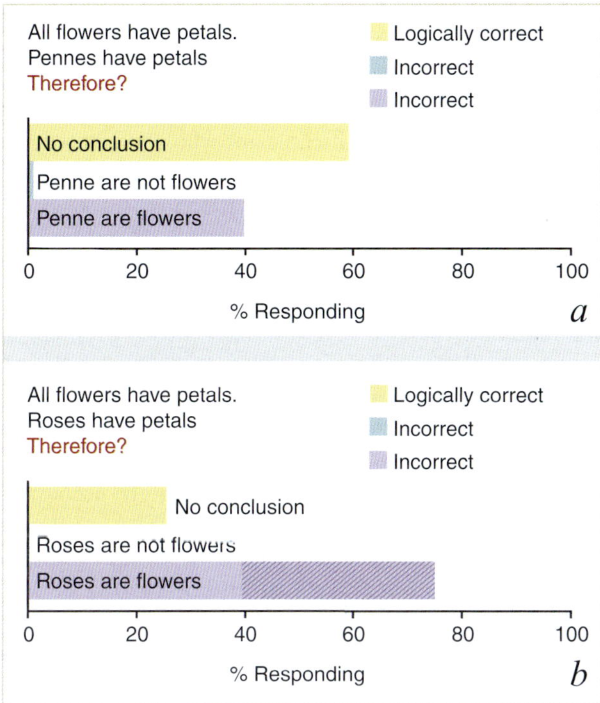

FIGURE 2.1 In their study of the belief-bias effect, Markovits and Nantel[9] gave subjects a series of problems in the form of syllogisms. For each problem, subjects were asked to give the conclusions that followed logically from the premises or, if no conclusion could be logically and unequivocally derived from the premises, to state "none." Some subjects were given problems that either had a believable but incorrect conclusion (determinate form) or, as in the example above (*b*), had a conclusion that was believable but that did not conclusively follow from the premises (indeterminate form). Other subjects received the same problems but with the terms substituted with neutral terms as in (*a*). In the above example, the magnitude of the belief-bias effect is reflected in the greater number of incorrect answers given when one of the conclusions was believable (*b, crosshatch*) rather than neutral. The belief-bias effect was greatest when the premises (i.e., the data) were inconclusive. (From Markovits H, Nantel G. The belief-bias effect in the production and evaluation of logical conclusions. *Mem Cognit.* 1989;17:11–17.)

10 fractions), was thought to be palliative but turned out to be curative. This case began a shift in our view of the curability of extensive regional metastasis from cervical cancer, eventually leading to successful up-front treatments such as that described in CS 10.10.

Evaluation of the Suitability of Potential Study Cohorts

Investigators can save a great deal of time and can reduce their risk of eventually publishing a misleading study by carefully evaluating their proposed retrospective study cohort for potential sources of bias. The following steps are recommended:

- *Critically evaluate prior studies and reviews concerning the subject of interest and catalogue the known and potential sources of bias.* What were the grounds for criticism of previous studies? As the proposed new cohort is characterized, it should be evaluated to determine whether it is likely to be the source of valid, new insights.
- *Define the study population.* Because exclusions are a potential source of selection bias, they should be carefully recorded and described in the final publication.
- *Determine whether information on all relevant prognostic factors is available for the entire cohort.* Omission of critical prognostic factors that may correlate with treatment variables of interest will limit the ability to draw valid conclusions from the proposed study. This is a particular challenge with studies using publicly available data sets, such as SEER, that do not include critical clinical variables.
- *Evaluate sample records from the proposed study cohort to determine the quality of the information about patient, tumor, and treatment characteristics.* For large series, we have found it worthwhile to first collect data from 10 to 20 cases during each decade of study. This provides worthwhile information about the quality of documentation and the evolution of diagnostic and treatment methods. Because missing data and inconsistently defined data degrade the value of multivariate regression analyses, cohorts that are not well characterized tend to be poor subjects for study.
- *Estimate the size of the study cohort, the quality of follow up, and the event rate.* Will it be possible to answer the question of interest with this cohort? If not, it may be time to abandon the project.

THE BENEFITS AND LIMITATIONS OF RANDOMIZED TRIALS

The prospective randomized trial is generally viewed as the gold standard of clinical research, yielding the highest attainable level of evidence. The allocation of treatments by random sampling breaks the link between prescription and prognosis, eliminating an important source of bias. Focused, well-designed, carefully conducted randomized trials can yield evidence that leads to important improvements in clinical practice. However, large prospective randomized trials are difficult to launch, expensive, and often fraught with problems that can limit their utility.

Since the early 1970s, many issues relevant to gynecologic radiation oncology practice have been addressed in prospective randomized trials. However, only a few questions posed by investigators regarding the influence of radiation therapy on survival have been answered with a reasonably high degree of confidence, and even these questions have not been fully resolved:

- *The benefit of chemoradiation for locoregionally advanced cervical cancer.* In 1999, after more than 20 years of study and many inconclusive trials, convincing data from several trials finally led to a major change in practice. However, some clinicians still question the value of concurrent chemotherapy for stage III and stage IVA disease[10] (Chapter 10).

- *The benefit of adjuvant RT for node-positive vulvar cancer.* Although GOG-37 convinced many practitioners of the value of adjuvant RT, erroneous interpretation of recurrence patterns and delayed publication of the mature trial results contributed to variable penetration of the study's findings into some practices (Chapter 12).[11,12]
- *The lack of benefit of external beam RT for patients with low intermediate-risk endometrial cancer.* The findings of randomized trials have demonstrated conclusively that external pelvic RT is not of sufficient benefit for patients with low-grade, minimally invasive endometrial cancer to justify the side effects of treatment. However, in its 2016 published guidelines for management of endometrial cancer, the European Society of Gynecologic Oncology concluded that the recommendation not to treat patients with low-risk disease was the only one of 31 guidelines regarding adjuvant treatment that could be scored as a strong (grade A) recommendation backed by level 1 evidence.[13]

Flaws in the design, conduct, and interpretation of gynecologic oncology trials have often led to inconclusive results or even erroneous conclusions about the effectiveness of treatment. Specific limitations of key trials are discussed in disease site chapters. However, some of the more common problems include the following:

Inadequate Randomization Methods

An unpredictable allocation sequence that is concealed from providers is required to prevent bias from influencing a trial. Although most large multi-institutional trials follow these guidelines, reports of some trials either have failed to describe their method of allocation or have failed to use recommended methods. For example, two frequently quoted "randomized" trials comparing the outcome of patients treated with high-dose rate (HDR) versus low-dose rate (LDR) brachytherapy for cervical cancer[14,15] used nonrandom (alternating) allocation methods and failed to conceal the sequences from the treating physicians; in at least one of the studies,[15] patients were shifted to the HDR arm when LDR was unavailable. Such methods leave the trials open to confounding bias.

Inadequate Statistical Power

Many of the randomized trials quoted in this text (and even more of those that are not mentioned) were, at least in retrospect, too small to reach definitive conclusions about treatment efficacy. A number of factors can lead to underpowered trials. In some cases, investigators open trials without adequately considering the number of patients necessary to answer their question. This practice raises ethical concerns that should be carefully considered before patients are committed to a trial that has little chance of yielding a valid conclusion.[16]

Inaccurate sample size calculations are another common cause of underpowered trials. Investigators frequently overestimate the rate of disease-related events. In some cases, stage migration caused by increasingly precise diagnostic methods causes patients with apparently similar stage disease to have a lower baseline risk than the historical series used to estimate the required sample size. Trials may also have lower than expected event rates if clinicians who contribute to the trial preferentially decide not to enter eligible patients who have relatively high-risk profiles.

Statistical power may also be lost if large numbers of patients are noncompliant with the treatment protocol or posttreatment follow-up requirements. Poor compliance with radiation therapy standards has been a problem for many gynecologic oncology trials. Inadequate follow-up is a particular problem in trials that include patients from medically underserved communities; for this reason, poor compliance has compromised many cervical cancer trials. Trials that are designed without adequately accounting for compliance failures are likely to yield false-positive or false-negative results. Imbalances in the compliance rates for competing arms of a study can also be a source of selection bias.

A serious consequence of underpowered studies is the tendency for investigators and readers to confuse "no significant evidence of benefit" with "no benefit." All trial outcome results should be reported in terms of relative risks with confidence intervals. *An investigational treatment should be described as lacking benefit only if the trial has sufficient power to demonstrate equivalence or inferiority to the control arm.*

Heterogeneity within the Study Population

Because most gynecologic cancers are relatively uncommon, investigators may try to increase the projected accrual rate of a trial by broadening the eligibility criteria. This practice commonly yields a study with patients having widely differing baseline risks for the outcome of interest. Failure to stratify such trials according to known confounders can lead to imbalances in the baseline risks of comparison groups. Adjusting for such imbalances *post hoc* raises concerns that bias influenced the decision and methods used to apply the correction. GOG-122 (Chapter 10) is an excellent example of a randomized trial that achieved a significant difference in the primary end point only after a controversial adjustment was made for an imbalance in the stages of patients in the trial.

Broad eligibility criteria can also obscure the importance of treatments that are effective only for a subset of the study cohort. In many clinical trials, the distribution of risk is skewed, with most of the recurrences occurring in a small group of patients having multiple risk factors. For the majority of patients whose baseline risk of recurrence is low, even a small absolute risk of treatment-related harm will counterbalance the reduction in recurrence risk; this will typically result in a negative trial even if a potentially identifiable group of high-risk patients benefitted from the investigational treatment (**Fig. 2.2**).[17] GOG-99 (Fig. 13.5) and other studies of intermediate-risk endometrial cancer (Chapter 13) are excellent examples of the phenomenon described in **Figure 2.2**.

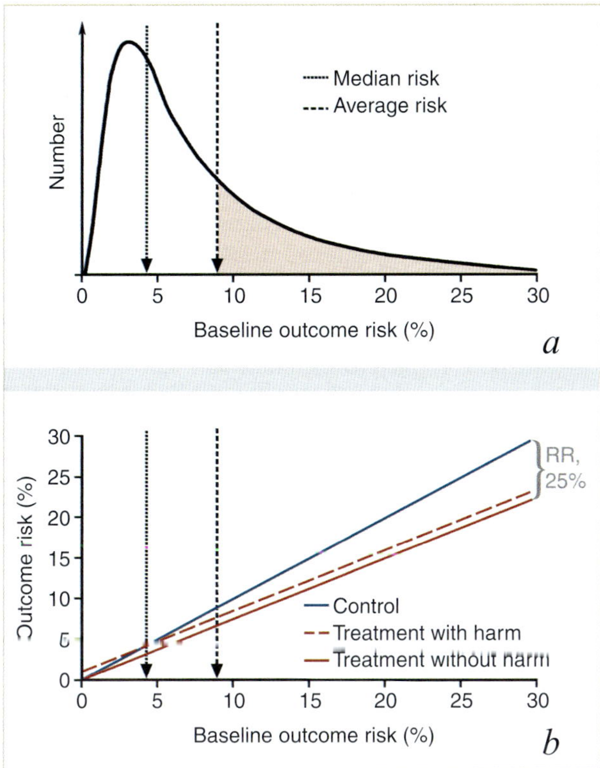

FIGURE 2.2 Many trials include patients with widely varying risks for the outcome of interest. In this example, the distribution of risk is skewed, as is the case if a relatively small group of patients with multiple risk factors account for most of the adverse outcomes (*a*). Only about one-quarter of the patients (*shaded*) have a greater than average risk. In *b*, an investigational treatment has reduced the relative risk (RR) by a constant of 25%, resulting in increasing absolute benefits as the baseline risk increases (*b*). In this scenario, however, a 1% risk of treatment-related harm will result in a net harm for all patients who have a baseline risk of <4% (50% of the patients). The average baseline risk will determine whether the trial's summary results are positive overall. However, the overall results may not reflect the trade-offs between the risks and benefits for individual patients in the trial. (Adapted from Kent DM, Hayward RA. Limitations of applying summary results of clinical trials to individual patients: the need for risk stratification. *JAMA.* 2007;298:1209–1212.) (RR, relative risk.)

Evolving Treatment Standards

The methods used to evaluate and treat gynecologic cancers are some of the most challenging and rapidly changing in radiation oncology practice. As technologic advances are integrated into standard practice, the relevance of trials that lacked those techniques may be questioned. However, as is illustrated throughout this book, many of the brachytherapy and external beam techniques used to treat gynecologic cancers are highly specialized and technically difficult. Poor radiation technique has been a frequent criticism of gynecologic oncology trials and a reason for clinicians in large academic centers to question the generalizability of findings to their specialized practices. On the other hand, small or medically underserved communities may not have the same access to skillfully applied advanced radiotherapy techniques, expert diagnostic services, or high-quality supportive care as do participants in clinical trials; this limits the relevance and penetration of the findings of some trials to community practice settings. By holding themselves to the highest standards of clinical care and research conduct, investigators have the greatest chance to improve cure rates of patients with gynecologic cancers. However, a part of their mission should always be to communicate their methods and confirm the reproducibility of published outcomes in the broader community.

META-ANALYSIS

Meta-analysis is a method for aggregating and analyzing results of data pooled from multiple trials that have addressed a common question. In recent years, many studies have applied meta-analysis to gynecologic oncology problems. Meta-analysis may be used:

- To address important clinical questions with greater statistical power than has been achieved with individual trials.
- To resolve apparently conflicting results of clinical trials.
- To learn which treatments are optimal for different types of patients entered in clinical trials.

Some meta-analyses are performed using individual patient data obtained from the trials of interest, whereas others use summary data (odds ratios) of individual trials to create an overall odds ratio. To our knowledge, only two questions relevant to gynecologic radiation oncology have been addressed in meta-analyses using individual patient data from randomized trials; these related to the benefit of concurrent[18] or neoadjuvant[19] chemotherapy combined with radiation for treatment of cervical cancer (Chapter 10, Fig. 10.4). Most other studies have aggregated summary data from randomized trials. However, some investigators have applied meta-analysis to reviews of retrospective data, and at least one study used data from surveys that queried physicians about their (undocumented) survival rates for HDR or LDR brachytherapy, respectively.[20,21]

At its best, meta-analysis is a powerful tool that can add to our confidence in the benefit of certain treatments. However, it can also be problematic. A detailed discussion of this topic is well beyond the scope of this book. However, some of the issues that should be considered when reviewing meta-analyses include the following:

- *The quality of the underlying data.* To paraphrase an early critique of meta-analysis, tons of garbage probably cannot yield a single diamond.[6] Meta-analyses of biased retrospective studies will never yield a trustworthy conclusion.
- *Flaws in the underlying trials that may be perpetuated in analyses of pooled data.* Meta-analysis of summary data from studies of pelvic radiation therapy for intermediate-risk endometrial cancer concluded that pelvic radiation was of no benefit. However, the pooling of results did not overcome the inherent problem that many patients in these trials had low-risk disease.[22] The pooled aggregated

results were likely just as susceptible as the individual trials to the problem shown in Figures 2.2 and 13.5.

- *Heterogeneity*. Analysts generally perform tests for heterogeneity—evidence that one class of trials with a certain feature yields a different result than do other classes. However, these methods do not detect important variations that affect only one or two trials. For example, in the large meta-analysis of concurrent chemoradiation for cervical cancer, the authors reported an odds ratio for "non–platinum-based" chemotherapy that was similar to that for platinum-based regimens.[18] This does not mean that all nonplatinum regimens were effective. Sixty-eight percent of the patients treated with non–platinum-based chemotherapy were from two studies of concurrent mitomycin and 5-fluorouracil; the odds ratios and sizes of these trials dominated the contributions of smaller studies of bleomycin or epirubicin.
- *Analyses that include relatively few studies with one large study dominating the results*. It is probably worthwhile to be wary of such situations. For example, in a 2014 analysis of chemotherapy versus RT for treatment of stage III and IV endometrial cancer, two-thirds of the patients originated from GOG-122; flaws in that trial would have heavily influenced the results of the meta-analysis (Chapter 13).[23]

BIG DATA: OUTCOMES ANALYSIS

Although many types of studies evaluate outcomes, this term is often used to refer to studies based on large databases or patient registries. These studies are very appealing for studies of gynecologic cancers because of the large number of patients represented in the databases and the opportunity to evaluate methods and outcomes of treatment outside the rarified environments of large academic institutions and randomized trials.

In the United States, most such studies have been based on two large cancer registries, the Surveillance, Epidemiology, and End Results (SEER) database, which is sponsored by the National Cancer Institute, and the National Cancer Database (NCDB), which is sponsored by the American College of Surgeons and the American Cancer Society. Both databases depend on nationally standardized data transmission format specifications coordinated by the North American Association of Central Cancer Registries and there is considerable overlap in the patients represented; however, these efforts are not closely coordinated and there are some important differences in the populations represented and in certain features of data collection. More recently, an increasing number of investigators have used insurance claims databases, such as the SEER-Medicare database or MarketScan, an employment-based health care claims database, to investigate gynecologic oncology questions.

Some very valuable results have come from gynecologic oncology studies based on these large databases. However, outcomes research studies are some of the most difficult to perform, critique, and interpret for a number of reasons, including the following:

- It is usually impossible to eliminate important sources of confounding bias because many of the important risk factors used to select treatment are not recorded or have been inconsistently recorded in the databases.
- Patients can move in and out of these data sets because of geographic migration (SEER, NCDB), age group (SEER-Medicare), or insurance coverage (MarketScan). This is less of a problem in some countries (e.g., Norway, Canada) that have databases tied to a comprehensive national health care system.
- It can be extremely difficult to rule out coding errors as a source of erroneous results. For example, both the NCDB and SEER implemented major revisions of their coding manuals in 2003. These changes resulted in some significant shifts in the apparent distributions of patients by stage[24] and other factors, highlighting the dependence of variables on the interpretation of tumor registrars. An example of the possible influence of inconsistent coding methods on the apparent incidence of brachytherapy utilization is shown in Figure 2.3.[25,26]

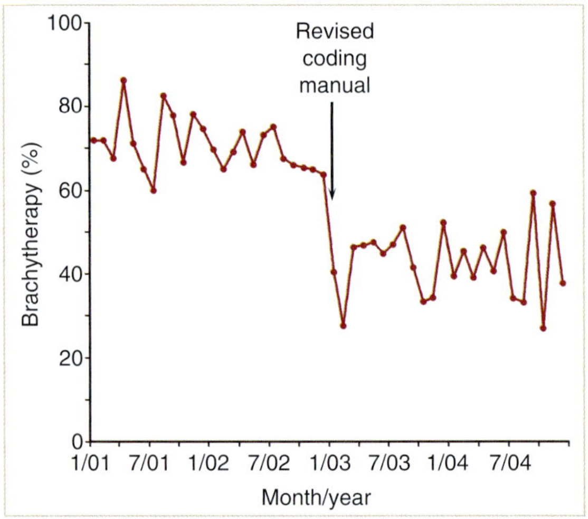

FIGURE 2.3 In 2014, Han et al.[25] reported that a marked decline had occurred in the rate of brachytherapy utilization in SEER patients treated for cervical cancer between 2000 and 2010. The authors hypothesized that this may have reflected a change in practice caused by physicians replacing brachytherapy with IMRT boosts. In a responding letter, Smith and Eifel[26] proposed an alternative hypothesis based on more detailed, month-by-month analysis of brachytherapy utilization in an SEER cohort similar to that described by Han et al. The analysis by Smith and Eifel revealed a precipitous decline in reports of brachytherapy use between January and March 2003, a 2-month period that followed immediately on the heels of implementation of a major revision in the SEER coding manual. Smith and Eifel hypothesized that the increased complexity of the new brachytherapy coding instructions may have led to underreporting of brachytherapy utilization in the SEER database. (From Smith GL, Eifel PJ. Trends in the utilization of brachytherapy in cervical cancer in the United States. In regard to Han et al. *Int J Radiat Oncol Biol Phys.* 2014;88:459–460.)

- Underreporting of radiation therapy delivery seems to be a significant problem.[27,28] Patients who receive combined external beam radiation and brachytherapy may pose particularly difficult coding challenges because treatments are often performed in two different facilities, both of which may differ from the SEER or NCDB registry site.
- Even when radiotherapy has been coded, key data elements including radiation dose, fractionation, and treatment duration may be missing or incorrectly coded. Complex IMRT treatments that may involve integrated boosts to multiple targets pose particular challenges for registry coding.
- The methodology used to mine large data sets is complex and requires involvement of both an experienced analyst and an investigator with in-depth knowledge of the specific research area. For many reasons, including those described above, even experienced analysts given the same data set can arrive at differing conclusions (**Fig. 2.4**).[29]

Registry data sets are repositories of vast stores of information but should be used with great caution and an acceptance of the fact that some questions are not suitable for study in this way.

SUMMARY

Dedicated researchers have made great progress through incremental improvements in our understanding of gynecologic oncology disease processes and their treatments.

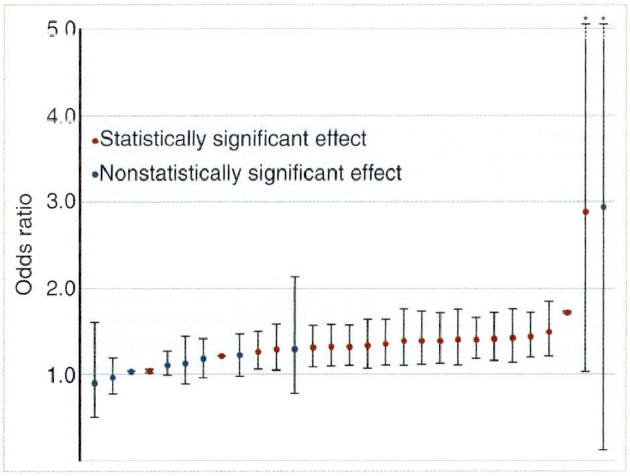

FIGURE 2.4 For this study, Silberzahn and Uhlmann recruited 29 independent teams of analysts to evaluate the same data set to answer the following question: Are soccer referees more likely to give red cards to dark skin-toned players than to light skin-toned players? The analysts, who were not prescribed any specific analytic approach, used various methods to reach their final answers. This figure shows the point estimates and 95% confidence intervals for the results calculated by each team of analysts. Asterisks represent truncated upper bounds for the last two estimates. Note that although all were working with the same large data set, the teams' conclusions varied widely. (From Silberzahn R, Uhlmann EL. Crowdsourced research: many hands make tight work. *Nature*. 2015;526:189–191.)

However, there is a great deal of work left for future generations of clinical researchers. Careful attention to the limitations of previous work can help us to improve the value of future studies and, ultimately, the outcomes of our patients.

References

1. Hendrickson M, Ross J, Eifel PJ, et al. Adenocarcinoma of the endometrium: analysis of 256 cases with carcinoma limited to the uterine corpus. Pathology review and analysis of prognostic variables. *Gynecol Oncol.* 1982;13:373–392.
2. Eifel PJ, Hendrickson M. Stage I endometrial carcinoma: the importance of pathologic review in retrospective analyses. *Int J Radiat Oncol Biol Phys.* 1990;18:1271–1273.
3. Creutzberg CL, Nout RA, Lybeert ML, et al. Fifteen-year radiotherapy outcomes of the randomized PORTEC-1 trial for endometrial carcinoma. *Int J Radiat Oncol Biol Phys.* 2011;81:e631–e638.
4. Nout RA, Smit VT, Putter H, et al. Vaginal brachytherapy versus pelvic external beam radiotherapy for patients with endometrial cancer of high-intermediate risk (PORTEC-2): an open-label, non-inferiority, randomised trial. *Lancet.* 2010;375:816–823.
5. Scholten AN, Smit VT, Beerman H, et al. Prognostic significance and interobserver variability of histologic grading systems for endometrial carcinoma. *Cancer.* 2004;100:764–772.
6. Spilker B. *Guide to Clinical Trials.* New York: Raven Press, Ltd.; 1991.
7. Eifel PJ, Morris M, Wharton JT, et al. The influence of tumor size and morphology on the outcome of patients with FIGO stage IB squamous cell carcinoma of the uterine cervix. *Int J Radiat Oncol Biol Phys.* 1994;29:9–16.
8. Viswanathan M, Berkman ND, Dryden DM, et al. *Assessing Risk of Bias and Confounding in Observational Studies of Interventions or Exposures: Further Development of the RTI Item Bank.* Rockville, MD: Agency for Healthcare Research and Quality (US); 2013.
9. Markovits H, Nantel G. The belief-bias effect in the production and evaluation of logical conclusions. *Mem Cognit.* 1989;17:11–17.
10. Eifel PJ. Concurrent chemotherapy and radiation: a major advance for women with cervical cancer. *J Clin Oncol.* 1999;17:1334–1335.
11. Kunos C, Simpkins F, Gibbons H, et al. Radiation therapy compared with pelvic node resection for node-positive vulvar cancer: a randomized controlled trial. *Obstet Gynecol.* 2009;114:537–546.
12. Mahner S, Jueckstock J, Hilpert F, et al. Adjuvant therapy in lymph node–positive vulvar cancer: the AGO-CaRE-1 study. *J Natl Cancer Inst.* 2015;107:dju426.
13. Colombo N, Creutzberg C, Amant F, et al. ESMO-ESGO-ESTRO Consensus Conference on Endometrial Cancer: diagnosis, treatment and follow-updagger. *Ann Oncol.* 2016;27:16–41.
14. Patel FD, Sharma SC, Negi PS, et al. Low dose rate vs. high dose rate brachytherapy in the treatment of carcinoma of the uterine cervix: a clinical trial. *Int J Radiat Oncol Biol Phys.* 1994;28:335–341.
15. Shigematsu Y, Nishiyama K, Masaki N, et al. Treatment of carcinoma of the uterine cervix by remotely controlled afterloading intracavitary radiotherapy with high-dose rate: a comparative study with a low-dose rate system. *Int J Radiat Oncol Biol Phys.* 1983;9:351–356.
16. Halpern SD, Karlawish JH, Berlin JA. The continuing unethical conduct of underpowered clinical trials. *JAMA.* 2002;288:358–362.
17. Kent DM, Hayward RA. Limitations of applying summary results of clinical trials to individual patients: the need for risk stratification. *JAMA.* 2007;298:1209–1212.

18. Green J, Kirwan J, Tierney J, et al. Concomitant chemotherapy and radiation therapy for cancer of the uterine cervix. *Cochrane Database Syst Rev.* 2005:CD002225.
19. Neoadjuvant Chemotherapy for Cervical Cancer Meta-Analysis Collaboration. Neoadjuvant chemotherapy for locally advanced cervix cancer. *Cochrane Database Syst Rev.* 2004:CD001774.
20. Eifel PJ. High-dose-rate brachytherapy for carcinoma of the cervix: high tech or high risk? *Int J Radiat Oncol Biol Phys.* 1992;24:383–386; discussion 387–388.
21. Orton CG, Seyedsadr M, Somnay A. Comparison of high and low dose rate remote afterloading for cervix cancer and the importance of fractionation. *Int J Radiat Oncol Biol Phys.* 1991;21:1425–1434.
22. Eifel PJ. The role of adjuvant radiation therapy for stage I endometrial cancer: does meta-analysis reveal the answer? *J Natl Cancer Inst.* 2012;104:1615–1616.
23. Galaal K, Al Moundhri M, Bryant A, et al. Adjuvant chemotherapy for advanced endometrial cancer. *Cochrane Database Syst Rev.* 2014;5:CD010681.
24. Wu XC, Yu Q, Andrews PA, et al. Comparisons of directly coded SEER Summary Stage 2000 and Collaborative Staging Derived SEER Summary Stage 2000. *J Registry Manag.* 2010;37:137–140.
25. Han K, Milosevic M, Fyles A, et al. Trends in the utilization of brachytherapy in cervical cancer in the United States. *Int J Radiat Oncol Biol Phys.* 2013;87:111–119.
26. Smith GL, Eifel PJ. Trends in the utilization of brachytherapy in cervical cancer in the United States. In regard to Han et al. *Int J Radiat Oncol Biol Phys.* 2014;88:459–460.
27. Jagsi R, Abrahamse P, Hawley ST, et al. Underascertainment of radiotherapy receipt in Surveillance, Epidemiology, and End Results registry data. *Cancer.* 2012;118:333–341.
28. Walker GV, Giordano SH, Williams M, et al. Muddy water? Variation in reporting receipt of breast cancer radiation therapy by population-based tumor registries. *Int J Radiat Oncol Biol Phys.* 2013;86:686–693.
29. Silberzahn R, Uhlmann EL. Crowdsourced research: many hands make tight work. *Nature.* 2015;526:189–191.

CHAPTER 3

Principles of Multidisciplinary Management

INTRODUCTION

Successful treatment of gynecologic cancers depends heavily on the effectiveness of multidisciplinary collaboration. The increasing use of chemotherapy to treat gynecologic cancers and technologic advances in surgery and radiation therapy (RT) methods have increased the number and complexity of treatment options. In every phase of care—diagnosis and evaluation, treatment planning, treatment implementation, and surveillance—a team of providers must collaborate and communicate with each other, with the patient, and with the patient's primary care providers to provide the highest quality of cancer care. To effectively discuss the pros and cons of various therapeutic options, providers must have specialized expertise in the management of gynecologic cancers and must also understand the basic principles governing each discipline's interventions.

The first section of this chapter describes key components and characteristics of an effective multidisciplinary gynecologic oncology care team. Subsequent sections review general principles that influence the selection of single-modality and multiple-modality treatments and some of the specific surgical procedures and chemotherapies that are commonly used in combination with or as an alternative to RT. Specific applications of these principles are discussed in Chapters 10 to 16 and illustrated in the case studies accompanying those chapters.

THE MULTIDISCIPLINARY TEAM

Despite an increasing body of literature emphasizing the importance of teamwork and collaboration in the delivery of high-quality health care, very little research has focused on the specific characteristics of an effective multidisciplinary gynecologic oncology care team. However, there is ample evidence that poor teamwork and ineffective communication lead to treatment delays, errors, frustrated providers, and dissatisfied patients.[1–3] There is also general agreement that the presence of a highly functioning multidisciplinary team improves the quality of care.

In general terms, a multidisciplinary team can be defined as "a group of people with various expertises, responsible for individual decisions, who hold a common purpose and meet together to communicate, share and consolidate knowledge from which plans are made."[4] The ways in which specialized expertise, communication and knowledge transfer, and collaborative planning are facilitated and applied to achieve the team's common purpose influence the quality of decision making, treatment delivery, supportive care, and posttreatment management.

Members of the Team

The membership of an individual patient's multidisciplinary gynecologic oncology care team depends on the specific diagnosis and phase of care.[5] However, a care team is most effective if it is built around a group of key individuals with specialized expertise and defined roles and with established relationships and lines of communication. A truly collaborative environment can only flourish if the members of the team have confidence in each other's knowledge and skills. Key members of the multidisciplinary gynecologic oncology care team include the following:

- *The surgeon.* In North America, gynecologic oncologists are board-certified specialists who have 3 to 4 years of postresidency training specific to the surgical and chemotherapeutic management of gynecologic cancers. Gynecologic oncologists are typically at the hub of gynecologic cancer patient care and generally have close access to other subspecialists, including dedicated gynecologic pathologists and diagnostic imagers. For this reason, biopsies and imaging studies obtained by a gynecologic oncologist are more likely to yield high-quality cancer-specific information than are studies obtained by a family physician or general gynecologist. Also, several studies have demonstrated that patients whose initial surgery is performed by a gynecologic oncologist are less likely to have inappropriate or failed procedures and tend to have better outcomes than patients whose initial surgery is performed by a nonspecialized surgeon.[6,7]

- *The radiation oncologist.* Because fewer than 10% of new radiation oncology patients have gynecologic cancers, very few radiation oncologists can dedicate all or even most of their practice to the management of these cancers. There may be some point below which the number of gynecologic cases seen by a radiation oncologist is too small to provide an adequate base of experience, particularly experience with the more uncommon cancers and specialized techniques. When the frequency of gynecologic cases is low, radiation oncologists may also find it difficult to build relationships with other members of the multidisciplinary team. For this reason, it is recommended that radiation oncology practices identify one or two individuals who can commit significant effort to this subspecialty area. Whenever possible, complex cases should be referred to large centers with radiation oncologists who subspecialize in gynecologic cancer and are well integrated into multidisciplinary gynecologic oncology care teams.
- *The chemotherapy provider.* Depending on the practice setting, chemotherapy may be prescribed and managed by a gynecologic oncologist or by a medical oncologist. Because gynecologic cancers are uncommon and because many patients with such cancers have chemotherapy given by a gynecologic oncologist, medical oncology practices may treat only very small numbers of gynecologic cancers. When chemotherapy is given by a medical oncologist, close collaboration between the radiation oncologist, gynecologic oncologist, and medical oncologist is particularly important to achieve appropriate coordination of combined-modality regimens.
- *The pathologist.* The importance of expert pathology review of cancer specimens cannot be overemphasized. Critical prognostic information about surgical margin status, sites of lymph node involvement, and other tumor features can easily be lost if surgical specimens are handled incorrectly. Misdiagnosis and under- and overdiagnosis of histologic risk factors by inexpert pathologists have undoubtedly caused clinicians to give inappropriate treatments and to fail to give necessary treatments to patients with gynecologic cancers (Chapter 2).[8]
- *The diagnostic imager.* Multidisciplinary decision making and radiation oncology practice are heavily dependent on accurate and complete diagnostic imaging interpretation. The use of optimized techniques can markedly improve the utility of gynecologic diagnostic imaging modalities (Chapter 4). Specialized understanding of the behaviors of gynecologic cancers and their treatment typically leads to diagnostic reports that are more accurate and informative.
- *The primary care provider.* The importance of the primary care provider's specialized expertise—namely, his or her knowledge of the patient and the patient's precancer health care history—should not be underestimated. Communication between oncology and primary care providers is essential to provide continuity throughout the phases of cancer treatment and follow-up, to identify and manage comorbid conditions that may affect cancer treatment, and to coordinate supportive care.[9]
- *Nurses.* Nurses play a vital role in patient care and communication within the multidisciplinary team. Radiation oncology nursing is becoming a well-recognized nursing subspecialty. Gynecologic radiation oncology nursing requires special skills, particularly related to the nursing of brachytherapy patients.
- *Social workers.* Gynecologic cancer patients are frequently burdened by a host of social problems that can compromise the quality and continuity of their care. A skilled social worker who can facilitate access to social services and who understands the nature and imperatives of gynecologic cancer treatments can provide critical assistance to patients who are trying to complete complex treatments while juggling financial, family, and personal concerns. Early involvement of social services can reduce missed appointments and treatment delays, improving the quality of treatment and the quality of the patient's experience.
- *Other consulting specialists.* Gynecologic cancer treatments are complex, and patients often benefit from consultation with other specialized providers. Most patients benefit from consultation with a dietician. A pain management consultant can help to optimize pain control. Depending on the patient's individual needs, interventional radiology, gastroenterology, urology, anesthesiology, audiology, and other consultants may be needed to optimize management (Chapter 7). Although these providers are not always part of the patient's primary care team, it is helpful for the primary care team members to have well-established working relationships with consultants who understand the specific needs of patients with gynecologic cancers treated with radiation.

Ideally, all primary members of the multidisciplinary gynecologic oncology care team should have gynecologic cancer as a major focus of their practice. However, this may not always be possible. In the United States, patients are often treated in small, nonacademic private care centers by providers who have limited expertise in management of uncommon gynecologic cancers. Studies have shown that patients with rare, complex problems such as locally advanced cervical cancer are less likely to complete all the elements of treatment in a timely manner if they are treated in small, nonacademic centers.[10,11]

Many factors contribute to such disparities, but the risk of suboptimal care can be lessened if generalist providers understand their limits and those of other team members, are willing to seek specialized opinions to supplement their knowledge, and have a low threshold for referral of patients to providers with specialized skills. However, even specialists with the most advanced training in gynecologic cancer management can fail to provide optimal care if they lack a robust system for communication between members of the multidisciplinary team.

Communication among Team Members

The correlation between characteristics of the multidisciplinary team and patients' survival or disease recurrence rates has never been studied directly. However, poor communication between providers and between providers and patients undoubtedly leads to diagnostic and scheduling errors that impair the process of care in ways that are known to affect outcomes. Providers who fail to share information and opinions or who deliver mixed messages erode trust and promote patients' anxiety. In the context of gynecologic radiation oncology, consequences of poor communication include the following:

- Failure of key providers to make appropriate referrals for RT
- Delayed or protracted RT
- Poor coordination of chemotherapy and RT resulting in missed or improperly scheduled treatments
- Inaccurate radiation target delineation because of inaccurate or missing diagnostic information
- Suboptimal management of tumor or treatment sequelae
- Patients who are frustrated by unmet informational needs and inconsistent messages about the goals and expectations of treatment

The members of a robust multidisciplinary team communicate with each other frequently in a variety of ways. The methods and nature of the interactions may vary according to the practice setting but should be designed to enhance the team as a whole and to meet the specific needs of individual patients.

Communication that Enhances the Team as a Whole

A multidisciplinary team with an effective communication strategy will have mechanisms in place that enhance the overall multidisciplinary care environment by

- Providing continuing education about the nature and needs of each member's specialty and possible indications for various treatments
- Enabling members to discuss treatment guidelines and implementation of new research findings
- Providing a forum for discussion of adverse outcomes and quality improvement measures

Tumor boards are the classic forum for addressing these needs. These multidisciplinary meetings have been used and accepted as an established part of cancer management for decades.[12] Among the American College of Surgeons requirements for accreditation of cancer programs is that the program must have a multidisciplinary cancer conference with prospective review of cases and discussion of management decisions. At their best, tumor boards serve a critical role, bringing members of the team face-to-face to address real diagnostic and therapeutic problems.

However, the degree to which tumor boards meet ongoing needs of the multidisciplinary gynecologic oncology care team depends on many factors, including the agenda of the meetings, expertise of the attendees, number of attendees, and frequency of the meetings. General tumor boards tend to be less effective than specialized tumor boards, particularly for patients with gynecologic cancers, who account for only a small proportion of the cancer patients seen in a hospital or network.[12] Monthly or biweekly tumor boards are less useful than weekly meetings for planning the treatment of individual patients but can still serve an important function by bringing specialists and other members of the team face-to-face to discuss shared management problems.

Communication that Enhances Individual Patient Care

A robust multidisciplinary gynecologic oncology care team will have in place solid lines of communication that enable team members to:

- Develop coordinated, consensus-driven treatment plans for each patient
- Share all clinical findings and test results
- Provide all involved team members with frequent updates about the progress of patients' ongoing treatments
- Disseminate information about ongoing patient needs and concerns
- Communicate with patients in a consistent and effective manner
- Develop and implement a coordinated plan for long-term follow-up

The most effective communication probably occurs when team members are in the same location, which permits face-to-face discussion between multiple team members and the patient. This is particularly true for management of complex gynecologic oncology problems. Clinicians working together in multidisciplinary clinics can readily compare and achieve consensus about physical examination findings, discuss the patient's proposed treatment plan in concert, and coordinate recommendations, thereby reducing the risk of delivering mixed messages.

A shared electronic medical record system also greatly facilitates communication of a patient's past treatment history, test results, and clinical findings and the status of ongoing treatments.

When collocation of team members is not possible, the treatment plan must be developed and carried out using a virtual team strategy.[5] In this situation, it is particularly important that the content of individual patient visits be documented in detail and shared with team members. If members of the team do not have open access to portions of a patient's medical record, they must develop another reliable, rapid method of information sharing. Patient care that is delivered using a virtual team model depends heavily on the use of staff and clinic coordinators to ensure that paths of communication are open and effective. However, physicians are ultimately responsible for assuring that potential communication barriers do not prevent them from obtaining effective shared access to the patient's medical information.

Nothing can replace direct communication between key providers. An ambiguous pathology report should always be clarified by direct communication with the pathologist and, if necessary, should be sent for review by an outside expert. Ambiguous or equivocal diagnostic imaging findings should always be clarified by email, telephone, or joint review of the images together with the diagnostic imager. Key physician providers should always communicate directly before the initial treatment plan is finalized and at major decision points in patients' care.

External Factors Influencing Team Function

A variety of factors can all have major influences on the cohesiveness and effectiveness of multidisciplinary care, including demographic characteristics of the community, competition within the medical marketplace, reimbursement mechanisms and rates, and the quality of the information technology infrastructure. Radiation oncologists have a responsibility to advocate for systems and infrastructure that enhance multidisciplinary collaboration.

CHOOSING AND SEQUENCING LOCOREGIONAL TREATMENTS

The locoregional management of gynecologic cancers is discussed by disease site in Chapters 10 to 15. However, there are some general principles that guide decision making, particularly for lower genital tract and endometrial cancers. An understanding of these commonalities can help to put the management of individual cases in a broader context. Many factors, including the experience and skill set of individual team members, may influence decisions about the roles and application of surgery, RT, and chemotherapy. Close collaboration in an environment of mutual respect is essential to the treatment planning process.

Choosing between Surgery and RT for Initial Treatment

To determine whether the initial treatment should be surgical resection or RT, several questions should be considered once distant metastases have been ruled out:

- *Is there a high probability that treatment with surgery alone will be sufficient to cure the patient?* If the answer is yes, and if the morbidity of the necessary operation is expected to be low, surgery is usually the preferred treatment. However, if there is a high likelihood that adjuvant treatment will be required, the risks and benefits of combined-modality treatment versus definitive RT should be weighed carefully through multidisciplinary discussion.
- *Can the primary tumor be resected with clear margins?* If not, primary RT is usually preferred over surgery. There is little evidence that subtotal tumor "debulking" improves the ability to achieve local control with radiation or chemoradiation—the dose of radiation required to sterilize positive surgical margins (usually at least 60 Gy) is often similar to that required to treat unresected gross disease. Furthermore, an extensive operation in which tumor is peeled off adjacent bowel or bladder can compromise the local vascular supply, worsening the adverse effects of high-dose RT.
- *Would definitive surgical resection compromise critical organ function?* The fact that the reproductive organs are adjacent to critical structures means that definitive surgical resection frequently cannot be achieved without removing or damaging critical organs. In most cases, definitive RT is preferred over ultraradical surgical procedures that sacrifice bowel or bladder function.
- *Could surgical resection compromise the ability to deliver an adequate dose of radiation to the target volume?* Removal of the uterus or upper vagina limits brachytherapy options, often making it difficult to safely deliver high-dose RT to a site of residual disease at a resection margin.
- *Is the patient medically fit?* If the risk of major postoperative morbidity or mortality is high, this risk may outweigh any potential advantages of initial surgery over primary RT.
- *What is the risk of major perioperative complications that could delay necessary postoperative RT?* For reasons discussed below, delays of more than 6 weeks between surgery and RT may reduce the effectiveness of postoperative RT. This is an important consideration in the management of locally advanced vulvar cancer; extensive resections in this area are frequently complicated by wound separations and infections that delay adjuvant treatment; these may in turn increase the risk of recurrence and contribute to late scarring and fibrosis.

Although the above considerations are relevant to treatment planning for all gynecologic cancers, the anatomic relationships between the reproductive organs and adjacent structures mean that certain treatments are used more often than others to treat cancers at specific sites. Because the serosally covered uterine fundus is anatomically separated from adjacent structures, even very large cancers confined to the body of the uterus can usually be removed with hysterectomy, which is the standard initial treatment in most cases.

In contrast, because most of the vagina is within 5 mm of bladder, urethra, or rectum, most cancers that primarily or secondarily involve the vagina are treated with RT because definitive surgical resection of even very small cancers would usually require a partial or total exenteration. The optimal treatment for cervical and vulvar cancers depends on the location of the lesion and the likelihood that it can be completely resected without damaging critical structures.

Types of Hysterectomy and Associated Complications

Most gynecologic cancers involve either the fundus or cervix of the uterus. Because the uterus is no longer critical once childbearing is complete, hysterectomy is the treatment of choice for many uterine and cervical cancers. Although a simple hysterectomy is sufficient for treatment of most endometrial and some very early cervical cancers, most cancers that involve the cervix are treated with more radical procedures that include resection of varying amounts of paracervical tissue. Technical variations in the procedures termed "radical hysterectomy" have led to several attempts to classify hysterectomies according to the extent of the paracervical resection (Table 3.1).[13] More radical procedures are generally used in patients with locally advanced (stage IB2 or greater) cancers.

The most common long-term complication of radical hysterectomy is bladder dysfunction (atony or incontinence) caused by partial disruption of the autonomic nerve supply to the bladder. Disruption of autonomic nerves can also cause chronic constipation. The severity of complications of hysterectomy is related to the radicality of the procedure, particularly the extent of the vaginal resection.[14] For this reason, it is inappropriate to compare the incidence of major complications from surgical versus radiation treatment of cervical cancer unless the comparison groups have tumors of similar size, stage, and extent of vaginal involvement.

The classical radical hysterectomy described by Meigs in the 1950s is an extensive procedure, somewhere between type III and type IV hysterectomy as described by the European Organisation for Research and Treatment of Cancer (EORTC) Gynecological Cancer Group (Table 3.1), that involves removal of at least the proximal half of the vagina and paravaginal tissues.[13] It should be noted that removal of the ovaries is not part of a radical hysterectomy per se. Lymphadenectomy is nearly always performed with a radical hysterectomy but is discussed separately later in this chapter. The classic radical hysterectomy, designed to enable excision of relatively large cancers, is associated with a high incidence of bladder atony (often requiring long-term self-catheterization), incontinence, and chronic constipation. With subsequent improvements in RT,

TABLE 3.1 Types of Hysterectomy

Classification system		
EORTC-GCG	**Querleu and Morrow**	**Description**
Type I	Type A	*Simple or extrafascial hysterectomy* Ureters visualized or palpated but not dissected Uterine artery and supporting ligaments transected immediately adjacent to the uterus Minimal vagina (<10 mm) removed
Type II	Type B	*Modified radical hysterectomy* Limited dissection of the ureters Partial removal of the paracervical-supporting ligaments At least 1–2 cm of vagina removed
Type III	Type C	*Radical hysterectomy* Ureters completely mobilized Complete transection of the parametria (cardinal ligaments) Removal of the uterosacral ligaments to the rectum Removal of the vesicouterine ligaments to the bladder Proximal third of the vagina or 1–2 cm from tumor removed
Type IV	—	*Extended radical hysterectomy* Type III plus removal of three-fourths of the vagina and paravaginal tissue
	Type D	Resection of the entire paracervix to the pelvic sidewall together with resection of the hypogastric vessels with or without adjacent fascia or muscle
Type V	—	*Partial exenteration* Removal of the terminal ureter or a portion of the bladder with the uterus and parametria

EORTC-GCG, European Organisation for Research and Treatment of Cancer Gynecological Cancer Group.

From Verleye L, Vergote I, Reed N, et al. Quality assurance for radical hysterectomy for cervical cancer: the view of the European Organization for Research and Treatment of Cancer–Gynecological Cancer Group (EORTC-GCG). Ann Oncol. 2009;20:1631–1638.

including the development of megavoltage RT beams, larger tumors were referred for RT, and the use of classical radical hysterectomy declined in many practices.

Today, most of the procedures performed for treatment of early-stage cervical cancer are modified radical (type II) hysterectomies. When this more limited procedure is performed with nerve-sparing techniques, the incidence of severe complications is low.

Today, some patients with small cervical cancers who wish to retain fertility are treated with a radical trachelectomy, as discussed in Chapter 10.

Indications for RT after Primary Tumor Resection

The decision whether to recommend irradiation of the primary tumor site after surgical resection of gynecologic cancers is based on the answers to several questions:

- What are the probabilities of local recurrence with and without adjuvant RT?
- What proportion of patients will develop distant disease despite local control?
- What is the likelihood that a local recurrence can be successfully treated if it does occur?
- What are the predicted short- and long-term adverse effects of adjuvant RT?
- If surgical salvage treatment were necessary, what adverse effects would the surgery have?

Taken together, these questions address the fundamental question that governs all cancer treatments: Do the benefits of treatment outweigh the risks?

In general, postoperative RT is used in patients with positive surgical margins and in patients with negative margins but features associated with a high risk of recurrence.

Positive Surgical Margins

For patients who have positive resection margins after primary surgical treatment, the risk of local recurrence is likely close to 100%, and postoperative RT is recommended in nearly all cases. There is little evidence that chemotherapy alone is sufficient to prevent operative bed recurrence of most gynecologic cancers. Positive margins usually occur because an anatomic barrier limited the surgeon's resection; for this reason, re-excision is typically not possible without risking critical organ dysfunction. When re-excision is performed, the radiation oncologist should always communicate with the surgeon afterward to learn whether the surgeon is confident that the re-excision removed the region of residual disease.

Negative Surgical Margins with Local High-Risk Features

For every disease site discussed in this book, a subset of patients can be defined who have a significant risk of local recurrence despite having negative surgical margins. The specific risk factors for local recurrence differ somewhat from one disease site to another, but large tumor size, lymphovascular space invasion, adenocarcinoma histology, and high tumor grade are nearly always on the list of risk factors.

It is interesting to speculate about the reasons why some subgroups have such a high risk of local recurrence even in the face of widely negative surgical margins. Several mechanisms have been suggested:

- *Colonization of individual tumor cells in the operative bed.* Most gynecologic cancers are open to the mucosal or skin surface and therefore are potentially open to the region of the operative bed. In their 2005 review, Höckel and Dornhofer[15] made a compelling argument that free-floating tumor cells may be attracted by the microenvironment of healing wounds and then encouraged in their growth by cytokines, growth factors, and wound-associated angiogenesis (**Fig. 3.1**). Empirical evidence also suggests that implantation of tumor cells is a cause of many local recurrences. The apical vaginal incision is the most common site of posthysterectomy recurrence of endometrial and cervical cancers. Isolated recurrences have also been reported in laparoscopic surgery port sites (**CS 13.9**),[16] abdominal wound incisions, episiotomy scars,[17] and, rarely, in the needle tracks from fine needle aspiration.[18] The relatively high cure rates for apical vaginal incision and other scar recurrences argue against hematogenous spread as a mechanism of metastasis to these sites.
- *Lymphangitic spread.* Although some local recurrences of gynecologic cancers may result from lymphangitic spread, most local recurrences have a localized distribution, different from the diffuse recurrence patterns seen in cancers known to disseminate via lymphangitic spread—for example, inflammatory breast cancer and pulmonary lymphangitic carcinomatosis. Vaginal recurrences can occur even when the primary tumor had no evidence of lymphovascular invasion. Also, the relatively high salvage rates for some recurrences that arise in the vicinity of surgical scars argue against lymphangitic spread as a common mechanism.
- *New primary cancers.* Some late recurrences, particularly in patients treated for human papillomavirus–related carcinomas, most likely represent new primary cancers. However, the development of new primary cancers cannot explain the disproportionately high incidence of local recurrences in the first few years after operation compared to later years.[19]

For most gynecologic cancers, postoperative RT has been demonstrated to improve local control for patients with high-risk features. For the reasons discussed in Chapter 2 and in Chapters 10 to 15, the impact of postoperative RT on survival has been more difficult to quantify.

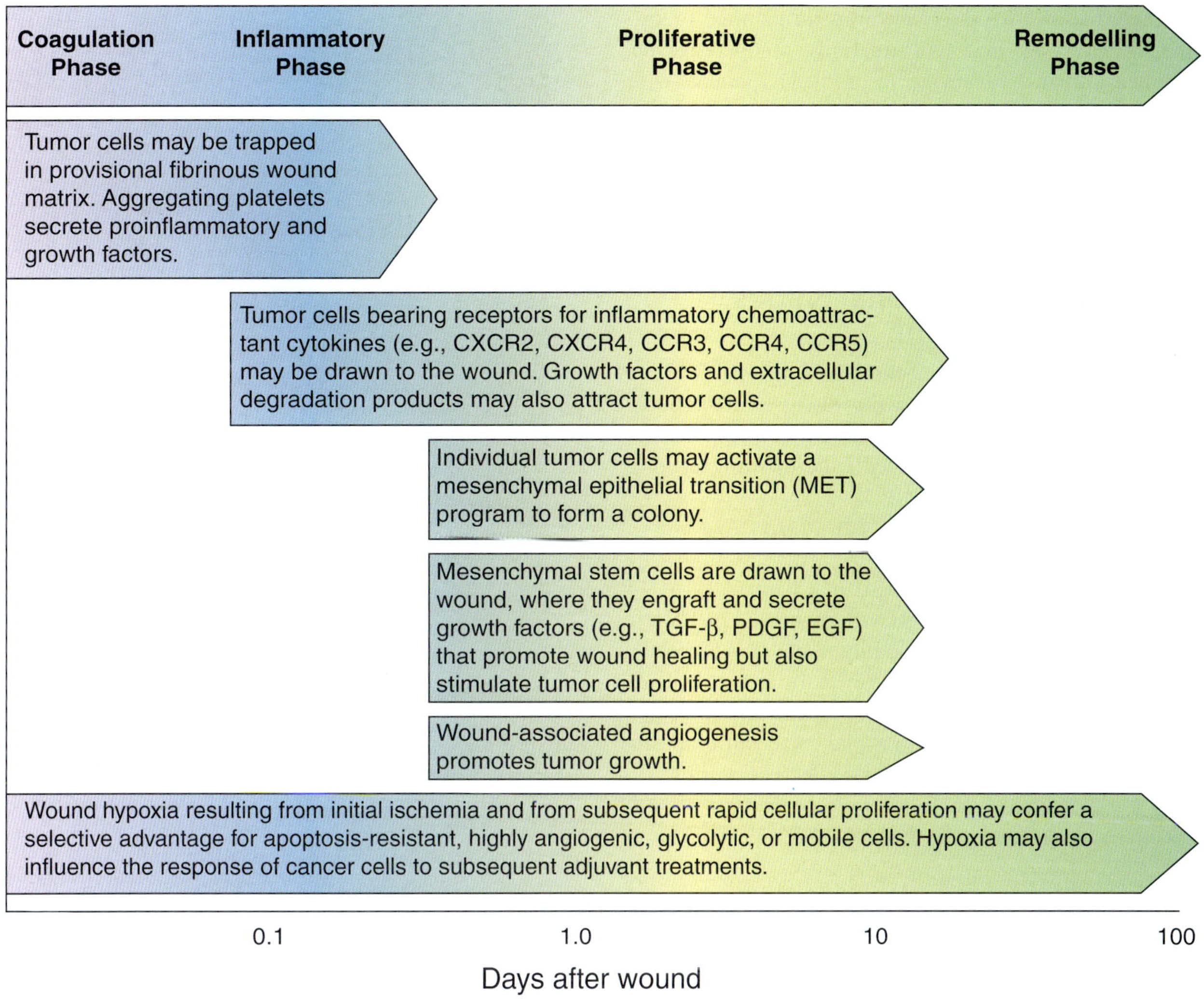

FIGURE 3.1 Cytokines and other factors associated with the four phases of wound healing may also promote survival and proliferation of cancer cells remaining in the region after surgical resection. This may explain some tumor recurrences that occur despite apparently negative surgical margins. (TGF, transforming growth factor; PDGF, platelet-derived growth factor; EGF, epidermal growth factor.) (Adapted from Hockel M, Dornhofer N. The hydra phenomenon of cancer: why tumors recur locally after microscopically complete resection. *Cancer Res.* 2005;65:2997–3002.)

Preoperative RT for Locally Advanced Disease

Preoperative RT (with or without concurrent chemotherapy) has been advocated in a number of settings, with interest waxing and waning over the years. The theoretical goal of this approach has usually been to shrink the primary tumor to improve the operability of advanced lesions and to sterilize peripheral microscopic disease to reduce postoperative recurrences.

Preoperative RT has several disadvantages that apply regardless of disease site:

- In general, the dose of RT must be reduced to about 75% of the optimal definitive RT dose if adjuvant surgery is planned. Even with this reduced dose, the rate of major postoperative complications is usually higher than that observed after treatment with surgery alone.
- It is usually recommended that surgery be performed no sooner than 4 to 6 weeks after external beam RT to allow acute postradiation inflammatory reactions to subside. However, if at that point it is determined that definitive surgery cannot be performed or if surgery is performed but leaves positive resection margins, few if any organ-sparing treatment options will be available.
- Preoperative RT obscures potentially important information about histologic risk factors.
- There are no level 1 data for any site demonstrating superiority of preoperative RT over definitive RT or surgery followed by adjuvant RT. The only direct comparison between preoperative RT and definitive RT was a randomized trial in patients with stage IB2 cervical cancer that showed no advantage of the combination of preoperative RT and adjuvant hysterectomy over RT alone.[20]

For these reasons, we rarely recommend planned preoperative RT. However, in a few situations, preoperative RT may confer a distinct advantage. In particular, patients with cancers that extensively involve both the cervix, which is most effectively treated with radiation, and the uterine fundus, which is more effectively treated with hysterectomy, may benefit from a combined approach. See Chapters 10, 12, and 13 for more detailed site-specific discussions of preoperative RT.

Management of Regional Nodes: Surgery or Radiation?

The relative roles of lymphadenectomy and regional RT have been debated for each of the disease sites discussed in this book. The issues and controversies are remarkably consistent across disease sites and include those outlined in the following sections.

Are Patients Who Have Regional Metastases Curable?

The data and case studies discussed in Chapters 10 to 15 provide ample proof that patients with regionally metastatic cancers arising in any gynecologic tumor site are potentially curable. However, in all cases, the chance for a cure depends on accurate evaluation of the disease extent and multidisciplinary collaboration to devise a plan that will eradicate regional metastases with as few adverse effects as possible.

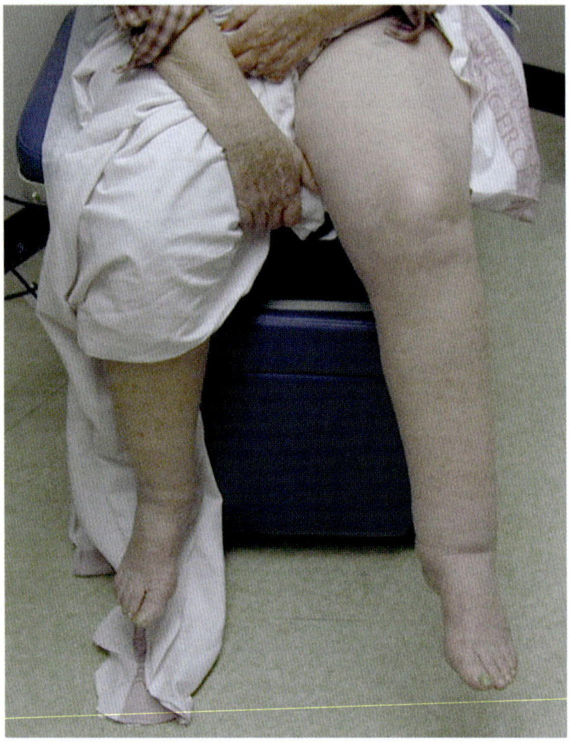

FIGURE 3.2 Left lower-extremity lymphedema in a patient treated with radical vulvectomy and inguinal node dissection.

Is Lymphadenectomy Therapeutic, or Is It Strictly Diagnostic?

In most cases, the primary purpose of lymphadenectomy is to diagnose regional metastasis, which facilitates triage of patients for adjuvant treatment. In terms of diagnostic accuracy, no imaging study comes close to a thorough histologic examination of the primary echelon nodes. However, the sensitivity of lymphadenectomy generally depends on the number and location of the nodes removed and on the handling of the specimen by the examining pathologist.

For most primary tumor sites, there are examples of patients with nodal metastases who have been cured with surgery alone; thus, it appears that lymphadenectomy can, at least occasionally, be curative. However, in all of these reports, the surgery performed was radical lymphadenectomy, with its attendant adverse effects (discussed below). The only level 1 evidence on the role of lymphadenectomy comes from two randomized trials that failed to demonstrate any overall survival benefit from pelvic lymphadenectomy in patients with endometrial cancer (Chapter 13).[21,22]

What Are the Potential Complications of Lymphadenectomy?

The addition of lymphadenectomy to primary cancer surgery lengthens the duration of the surgical procedure and increases the incidence of intraoperative and perioperative complications. The longer-term complications of radical lymphadenectomy are strongly correlated with the extent of the dissection and include the following:

- *Lymphedema.* Secondary lower-extremity lymphedema (**Fig. 3.2**) is caused by disruption of lymphatic drainage, usually by tumor or surgical trauma. Patients with lymphedema complain of heaviness, pain, skin changes, and altered body image. Edematous tissues are prone to secondary infections, which in some cases can be life threatening (**CS 12.9**). The reported incidence of lymphedema in patients undergoing lymphadenectomy for gynecologic cancers averages about 20% but ranges from 10% to 60% depending on the type of surgery performed and the method used to measure this complication.[23] Although the symptoms of lymphedema usually begin within 6 months to 1 year of surgery, they can arise many years later, particularly if the leg is traumatized or becomes infected. Adjuvant RT appears to increase the risk of postsurgical lymphedema. However, in our experience, symptomatic secondary lymphedema after RT alone is rare and is usually a sign of disease recurrence. Secondary lymphedema is generally incurable, although pressure stockings or pneumatic compression can decrease the symptoms. Patients who present acutely with lower extremity edema should always be evaluated to rule out pelvic tumor recurrence or deep vein thrombosis.
- *Lymphocyst formation.* A lymphocyst (also known as a lymphocele) is a collection of lymph fluid occurring after operations that disturb the normal lymphatic flow. Reported incidences vary with the type of surgery and the method of screening. Small lymphocysts are very common after pelvic or inguinal lymphadenectomy, are usually asymptomatic, and require no treatment.[24,25] Large lymphocysts (**Fig. 3.3**) can cause pain, become infected, and contribute to other secondary complications, including deep venous thrombosis,

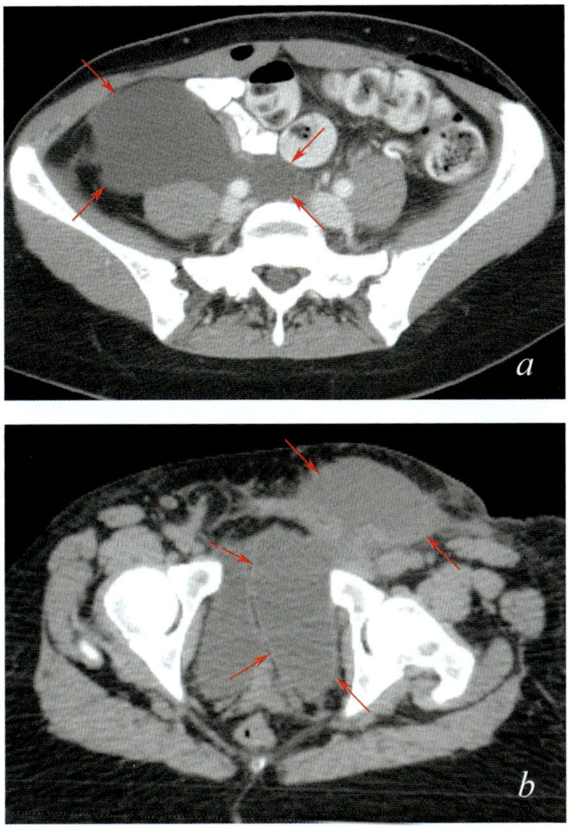

FIGURE 3.3 Two cases of massive lymphocysts that developed after diagnostic lymph node dissection in a patient with cervical cancer (*a*) and in a patient who underwent inguinal and distal anterior iliac node dissection for regional metastases from vulvar cancer (*b*). Although lymphocysts of this size are uncommon, they can be a cause of pain, secondary complications, and treatment delays.

ileus, and lymphedema. The usual treatment is percutaneous drainage. Lymphocysts can delay adjuvant RT, particularly if they become infected. Furthermore, displacement of structures due to lymphocysts and fluctuations in the size of lymphocysts can complicate radiation treatment planning.

- *Neurologic complications.* Injury to branches of the lumbosacral plexus during pelvic node dissection can cause sensory or motor changes, most commonly numbness or hyperesthesias. These symptoms usually resolve spontaneously but can, in rare cases, persist.[26]

Given these potential complications, if lymphadenectomy will not improve the likelihood of regional disease control either directly or by revealing the need for adjuvant treatments that improve regional control, the morbidity of the procedure is not justified.

Can RT Alone Control Subclinical Nodal Metastases?

Most studies suggest that subclinical nodal metastases from carcinomas can almost always be controlled with 45 to 50 Gy if image guidance has been used to verify that the target is being comprehensively treated with adequate margins and if all suspicious nodes receive at least 60 Gy. Studies that suggest that 45 to 50 Gy is not sufficient to control subclinical nodal disease generally have not met these requirements.[27]

Does Pre-RT Debulking of Gross Lymphadenopathy Improve Regional Control Rates?

Although it is tempting to remove gross disease before giving adjuvant RT, the benefits of debulking do not always justify the risks, for the following reasons:

- When nodes are no larger than 2 cm and care is taken to identify and treat all sites of gross disease to at least 60 Gy, recurrence is rare. In recent years, intensity-modulated RT has facilitated safe delivery of such doses for most cases of gross regional disease.
- Although there may be some benefit from resecting larger nodes if they are well encapsulated, debulking procedures that leave residual gross disease probably do not improve the chance of local control. Large nodes frequently have extracapsular disease extension; in such cases, experience suggests that the dose required to prevent postoperative recurrence is nearly as great as the dose required to control gross disease. In addition, because treatment of the entire operative bed is recommended for cases of extracapsular extension, the radiation target volume may be substantially increased after lymph node debulking (Fig. 6.8). For this reason, we often recommend definitive RT even for nodes that are larger than 2 cm, particularly if the relationship of tumor to adjacent vessels suggests that complete resection is unlikely.
- Postoperative complications, which are more frequent after removal of bulky or extensive nodal disease, can delay necessary adjuvant treatment. Postoperative delays provide an opportunity for accelerated repopulation of residual tumor for the reasons discussed in **Figure 3.1**.
- Late complications, including lymphedema, fibrosis, and pain, tend to be more frequent and more severe for combined regional treatment than for RT alone.

The choice of treatment for known or suspected regional metastases must also take into account the treatment options for the primary tumor site. If the primary tumor site is known to require primary or adjuvant RT, lymphadenectomy should be performed only if it will result in a greater likelihood of regional control than RT alone. If the primary tumor site is likely to be treatable with surgery alone but there is a significant risk of nodal metastases, surgical evaluation of the nodes is usually indicated, regardless of whether the primary tumor site is in the cervix, vulva, or endometrium.

The advent of sentinel node evaluation promises a major change in the overall management of regional nodes. Already considered by many to be a standard approach for patients with vulvar cancer (Chapter 12), sentinel node evaluation may provide an accurate means of triaging patients for adjuvant treatment of endometrial cancer without the serious adverse effects of radical pelvic and paraaortic lymphadenectomy (Chapter 13). Its possible role in the management of early cervical cancer has yet to be established.

EFFICACY AND SEQUENCING OF COMBINED CHEMOTHERAPY AND RT

Until the late 1990s, there were no gynecologic cancers for which the combination of chemotherapy and RT was considered standard; until that time, chemoradiation was generally recommended only for patients who were being treated in a clinical trial. In contrast, today, chemoradiation is used to treat most cervical cancers and many vulvar, vaginal, and endometrial cancers.

This change followed at least 40 years during which clinicians evaluated various combinations of chemotherapy and RT. Although most of the focus has been on the use of chemotherapy delivered concurrently with RT or neoadjuvant chemotherapy, recently, there has been a surge in interest in the possible value of post-RT adjuvant chemotherapy. Observational studies and randomized trials that have evaluated the combination of chemotherapy and RT for individual disease sites are discussed in detail in Chapters 10 to 15.

In this section, we will discuss the evidence, including evidence from potentially relevant nongynecologic tumor sites, and theoretical arguments supporting the use of various combinations of chemotherapy and RT. This broad view is important because level 1 evidence supporting combined treatment is only available for a few specific clinical situations. For some of the more uncommon clinical situations, randomized trials will probably never be feasible, and wise decisions about multidisciplinary management will have to be based on extrapolation from potentially applicable data from other cancers.

Because most of the patients we treat for gynecologic malignancies will receive or have received chemotherapy, it is important to understand and recognize the toxic effects of chemotherapy. **Table 3.2** provides a brief summary of some of the more frequently used drugs and their toxic effects.[28]

Evidence from Studies of Gynecologic Cancers

Any discussion of chemoradiation for gynecologic cancers must begin with the powerful evidence of benefit from trials of concurrent cisplatin-based chemoradiation for locoregionally advanced cervical cancer (Chapter 10, Fig. 10.2).[29] The results of these trials have been remarkably consistent, demonstrating reductions in the risks of death, local recurrence, and distant metastasis of up to 50% when concurrent chemotherapy was added to RT. Although most trials studied cisplatin-based regimens, several studies suggest that mitomycin C combined with 5-fluorouracil may also be effective. Population-based studies have also indicated that concurrent chemotherapy benefits patients with locally advanced cervical cancers,[30] vulvar cancer,[31] and vaginal cancers.[32]

In contrast, although up to 60% of patients with previously untreated cervical cancer have at least a partial response to cisplatin-based chemotherapy, trials that have evaluated neoadjuvant chemotherapy before RT have been disappointing. A large meta-analysis using individual patient data from 18 randomized trials showed no overall survival benefit from cisplatin-based neoadjuvant chemotherapy[33](Fig. 10.4). The only suggestion of benefit came from three trials from a single institution that used a relatively short course of neoadjuvant chemotherapy. This result has not yet been repeated elsewhere. The compiled results from trials that had a somewhat more prolonged course of pre-RT chemotherapy actually demonstrated a net harm from neoadjuvant chemotherapy (Fig. 10.4).

The only other setting in which sequential chemotherapy and RT has been studied is in patients treated with RT with or without chemotherapy after hysterectomy for high intermediate-risk or high-risk stage I to III endometrial cancer. Reporting the pooled data from two trials, Hogberg et al.[34] reported better progression-free survival ($p = 0.01$) with combined RT and chemotherapy (the latter given either before or after RT) than with RT only. The overall survival comparison did not reach statistical significance but favored combined treatment ($p = 0.07$). To date, there has been no comparison of concurrent chemoradiation versus concurrent chemoradiation followed by adjuvant chemotherapy for any gynecologic cancer site, although there are several ongoing trials addressing which approach is better.

Evidence from Studies of Nongynecologic Cancers

Although the level 1 data on the combination of chemotherapy and RT for patients with gynecologic cancers are limited to the trials described above, there is a large body of relevant evidence from trials conducted in other disease sites that are treated with definitive RT. The stories told by these trials and the cervical cancer trials are remarkably consistent. In most cases, concurrent chemotherapy has been demonstrated to be the most effective approach, and sequential chemotherapy has been either ineffective or less effective than concurrent treatment.

- *Head and neck cancers.* Because of the mucosal origin of head and neck cancers, the association of many such cancers with human papillomavirus infection, and the large number of trials in head and neck cancer, findings in head and neck cancer may be the most relevant to gynecologic cancer. A 2009 meta-analysis included pooled individual patient data on 16,485 patients from 87 trials.[35] The analysis demonstrated a highly significant recurrence-free survival benefit from concurrent chemoradiation versus RT alone (HR = 0.81 [95% CI, 0.78 to 0.86]) but no advantage from the addition of neoadjuvant chemotherapy before RT (HR = 0.99 [95% CI, 0.93 to 1.05]) or from the addition of adjuvant chemotherapy after RT (HR = 0.99 [95% CI, 0.89 to 1.10]). Results were similar for overall survival. A subsequent meta-analysis that compared neoadjuvant chemotherapy followed by chemoradiation versus chemoradiation alone found no significant differences in overall survival, locoregional recurrence, or relapse-free survival but did find a substantially higher rate of grade 3 or greater hematologic complications in patients treated with neoadjuvant chemotherapy.[36]

TABLE 3.2 Mechanism of Action, Route of Elimination, Indications for Use, and Toxic Effects of Some Drugs Commonly Used in the Treatment of Gynecologic Malignancies

Drug	Mechanism; elimination	Indications	Toxic effects[a]					
			Hematologic	Gastrointestinal	Alopecia	Neurologic	Renal	Other
Cisplatin	Formation of DNA adducts; eliminated via glomerular and tubular excretion	Radiosensitization; neoadjuvant CT; recurrent or metastatic squamous cancers; germ cell tumors	Cumulative; ANC nadir variable, usually at 2–3 wk; anemia primarily mediated through renal toxic effects	Nausea/vomiting	Rare	High-frequency hearing loss; peripheral neuropathy	Glomerular, tubular injury; decreased Mg, K	
Carboplatin	Formation of DNA adducts; eliminated via glomerular filtration	Ovarian cancer; recurrent or metastatic cancers	Affects all lineages; thrombocytopenia much more severe than with cisplatin	Nausea/vomiting (less than with cisplatin); diarrhea	Uncommon	Peripheral neuropathy (less than with cisplatin)	Uncommon (compared with cisplatin)	
Paclitaxel	Microtubular stabilization; metabolized by the liver	Ovarian cancer; recurrent or metastatic cancers; radiosensitization	Neutropenia, nadir at 8–11 d	Nausea/vomiting; mucositis	Always	Peripheral, mostly sensory neuropathy (dose limiting; worse when combined with cisplatin)	Minimal excretion of unchanged drug	Headache; fatigue; hypersensitivity; cardiac arrhythmias
Docetaxel	Microtubular stabilization; metabolized by the liver	Ovarian cancer; recurrent or metastatic cancers	Neutropenia	Mucositis	Always	Similar to paclitaxel but less severe	Minimal excretion of unchanged drug	Hypersensitivity; fluid retention
Liposomal doxorubicin	Binds DNA and inhibits nucleic acid synthesis; biliary excretion	Recurrent, metastatic cancers	Myelosuppression (less than with standard doxorubicin)	Nausea (mild to moderate); diarrhea; mucositis	Sometimes	Headache, fatigue		Hand and foot syndrome; hypersensitivity; cardiomyopathy
Topotecan	Inhibits topoisomerase I and produces single-strand DNA breaks; hepatic metabolism and renal excretion	Recurrent or metastatic cancers	Dose-limiting myelosuppression; neutropenia greater than thrombocytopenia	Nausea (mild); mucositis; constipation	Sometimes	Paresthesias, neuropathy		
Gemcitabine	Active metabolite inhibits ribonucleotide reductase, blocks DNA, polymerase, and other mechanisms	Radiosensitization; recurrent or metastatic cancers	Myelosuppression, particularly thrombocytopenia	Nausea/vomiting; stomatitis; changes in bowel habits	Sometimes	Headache; somnolence	Hemolytic uremic syndrome; hematuria; proteinuria	Transaminitis; hyperbilirubinemia; asthenia and flu-like symptoms (common); hypersensitivity

(*Continued*)

TABLE 3.2 Mechanism of Action, Route of Elimination, Indications for Use, and Toxic Effects of Some Drugs Commonly Used in the Treatment of Gynecologic Malignancies (*Continued*)

Drug	Mechanism; elimination	Indications	Toxic effects[a]					
			Hematologic	**Gastrointestinal**	**Alopecia**	**Neurologic**	**Renal**	**Other**
Mitomycin C	Alkylating agent and formation of DNA adducts; metabolized by the liver	Radiosensitization	Leukopenia, thrombocytopenia, nadir at 4–5 wk; hemolytic uremic syndrome can occur months later	Nausea/vomiting; anorexia	Sometimes		Hemolytic uremic syndrome (endothelial damage)	Venoocclusive liver disease; interstitial pneumonitis
Bleomycin	DNA single-strand breaks; renal excretion	Neoadjuvant CT; germ cell tumors	Myelosuppression (mild)	Nausea (mild); anorexia	Sometimes			Interstitial pneumonitis; rash; hyperpigmentation
5-Fluorouracil	Inhibition of DNA synthesis through depletion of thymidine; metabolized by the liver (short half-life)	Radiosensitization, usually combined with cisplatin or mitomycin C	Myelosuppression, nadir at 9–14 d	Watery diarrhea, may be severe; stomatitis; mucositis	Sometimes	Cerebellar syndrome		Hepatotoxicity; dermatitis; keratitis; photosensitivity; cardiac ischemia (rare); others

[a]Listed are some of the more common side effects of the drugs listed; see the manufacturers' information for more complete listing of drug-related toxic effects.

ANC, absolute neutrophil count; CT, chemotherapy.

From DuPont J, Sovak M, Benjamin I, et al. Chemotherapeutic agents used in the treatment of gynecologic malignancies. In: Rubin SC, ed. Chemotherapy of Gynecologic Cancers: Society of Gynecologic Oncologists Handbook. Philadelphia, PA: Lippincott Williams & Wilkins; 2004:17–88.

- *Lung cancer*. Meta-analyses of trials conducted in patients with locally advanced non–small cell lung cancer have demonstrated cisplatin-based chemoradiation to be superior to RT alone (HR = 0.71) and superior to neoadjuvant chemotherapy followed by RT (HR = 0.74) and have found that the addition of adjuvant chemotherapy after chemoradiation has no value (HR = 0.94).[37] Most of the analyzed trials used platinum-based chemotherapy regimens.

- *Anal cancer*. Randomized trials in patients with anal cancer demonstrated that concurrent chemoradiation with 5-fluorouracil and mitomycin C improved colostomy-free survival over RT alone or chemoradiation with 5-fluorouracil only.[38] Although one trial suggested that mitomycin C and 5-fluorouracil were superior to cisplatin and 5-fluorouracil, a second randomized trial showed no difference between the two regimens.[38] Another randomized trial that investigated the addition of neoadjuvant cisplatin and 5-fluorouracil to chemoradiation showed no added benefit from neoadjuvant chemotherapy.[38]

Why Is Neoadjuvant Chemotherapy Not More Effective, and When Might It Be of Benefit?

The initial responses that are frequently observed with neoadjuvant chemotherapy are so compelling that clinicians still find this approach tempting despite a vast quantity of evidence demonstrating that it has relatively little benefit in terms of local control and survival. There are several possible explanations for the modest benefit of neoadjuvant chemotherapy[39]:

- Only one or two logs of cell kill are required to produce a partial or even complete clinical response. For gross tumors, which typically are composed of 10^8 cells or more, this degree of cell killing may be less clinically relevant than the observed response suggests.

- Neoadjuvant chemotherapy may select for chemoresistant clones that are also resistant to radiation.

- Neoadjuvant chemotherapy may induce drug resistance, decreasing the effectiveness of subsequent chemotherapy.

- Toxic effects of neoadjuvant chemotherapy may decrease bone marrow reserve and the patient's tolerance of subsequent treatments. Decreases in the deliverable dose of concurrent chemotherapy, toxicity-related treatment breaks, and reduced patient compliance can all reduce the overall effectiveness of treatment.

- Interdigitation of chemotherapy between surgery and RT protracts the interval between surgery and RT, which may allow proliferation of resistant clonogens within the operative bed, reducing the efficacy of standard-dose external beam or vaginal brachytherapy.

For these reasons, we rarely recommend delivery of chemotherapy before curative RT for patients who have gross disease or who are at high risk for local recurrence after surgery; this is particularly true for patients with lower genital tract cancers. Sequential chemotherapy and RT have not been compared with concurrent chemoradiation for patients with high-risk endometrial cancer; however, on theoretical grounds, we generally recommend concurrent chemoradiation with or without post-RT adjuvant chemotherapy for many of the reasons described above. In addition, we believe that the sandwich approach of chemotherapy–RT–chemotherapy may not take full advantage of the possible systemic benefit of chemotherapy because the midcourse interruption of chemotherapy may allow accelerated proliferation of resistant extraregional clonogens.

However, although pre-RT neoadjuvant chemotherapy appears to have only a limited survival benefit for most patients, neoadjuvant chemotherapy may be useful in certain situations as response to this treatment tends to predict patients who are more likely to have a good outcome with organ-sparing treatment approaches. In patients with head and neck cancer, response to neoadjuvant chemotherapy has been used to triage patients with advanced laryngeal cancer to treatment with organ-sparing chemoradiation versus laryngectomy. In patients with cervical cancer, neoadjuvant chemotherapy is being studied as a method for identifying patients with stage IB disease who may be candidates for fertility-sparing trachelectomy (Chapter 10). On the other end of the spectrum, we have occasionally treated patients who have particularly massive locoregional disease with several courses of up-front chemotherapy with the plan to proceed to definitive RT only if there is a good response to chemotherapy. However, the drawback of this approach is that we are often asked to treat with radiation even if the disease has responded poorly to chemotherapy; at that point, the effectiveness of chemotherapy as a sensitizer may be diminished for the reasons described above. Case study 15.1 and Figure 16.3 are good examples of the issues that arise in this situation and a good illustration of why we usually avoid neoadjuvant chemotherapy.

SUMMARY

Many factors must be considered to optimize the risk–benefit ratio for patients who have potentially curable gynecologic cancers. We have provided our perspectives regarding the overall arguments in favor of various treatment approaches, but many of the issues and questions raised in this chapter remain topics of sometimes-heated controversy. Ultimately, the most important determinant of high-quality care is a highly functioning multidisciplinary team whose members respect and communicate with each other, with referring physicians, and with the patient to achieve a consensus-driven, maximally effective management plan.

References

1. Taplin SH, Clauser S, Rodgers AB, et al. Interfaces across the cancer continuum offer opportunities to improve the process of care. *J Natl Cancer Inst Monogr.* 2010;2010:104–110.
2. Walsh J, Young JM, Harrison JD, et al. What is important in cancer care coordination? A qualitative investigation. *Eur J Cancer Care (Engl).* 2011;20:220–227.
3. Zapka J, Taplin SH, Price RA, et al. Factors in quality care—the case of follow-up to abnormal cancer screening tests—problems in the steps and interfaces of care. *J Natl Cancer Inst Monogr.* 2010;2010:58–71.
4. Brill NI. *Team-Work: Working Together in the Human Services.* Philadelphia, PA: Lippincott; 1976.
5. Fennell ML, Das IP, Clauser S, et al. The organization of multidisciplinary care teams: modeling internal and external influences on cancer care quality. *J Natl Cancer Inst Monogr.* 2010; 2010:72–80.
6. Ramanathan SA, Baratiny G, Stocks NP, et al. General practitioner referral patterns for women with gynaecological symptoms: a randomised incomplete block study design. *Med J Aust.* 2011;195:602–606.
7. Chan JK, Sherman AE, Kapp DS, et al. Influence of gynecologic oncologists on the survival of patients with endometrial cancer. *J Clin Oncol.* 2011;29:832–838.
8. Kwon JS, Francis JA, Qiu F, et al. When is a pathology review indicated in endometrial cancer? *Obstet Gynecol.* 2007; 110:1224–1230.
9. Sussman J, Baldwin LM. The interface of primary and oncology specialty care: from diagnosis through primary treatment. *J Natl Cancer Inst Monogr.* 2010;2010:18–24.
10. Eifel PJ, Ho A, Khalid N, et al. Patterns of radiation therapy practice for patients treated for intact cervical cancer in 2005 to 2007: a quality research in radiation oncology study. *Int J Radiat Oncol Biol Phys.* 2014;89:249–256.
11. Smith GL, Jiang J, Giordano SH, et al. Trends in the quality of treatment for patients with intact cervical cancer in the United States, 1999 through 2011. *Int J Radiat Oncol Biol Phys.* 2015;92:260–267.
12. Keating NL, Landrum MB, Lamont EB, et al. Tumor boards and the quality of cancer care. *J Natl Cancer Inst.* 2013;105:113–121.
13. Verleye L, Vergote I, Reed N, et al. Quality assurance for radical hysterectomy for cervical cancer: the view of the European Organization for Research and Treatment of Cancer–Gynecological Cancer Group (EORTC-GCG). *Ann Oncol.* 2009; 20:1631–1638.
14. Zullo MA, Manci N, Angioli R, et al. Vesical dysfunctions after radical hysterectomy for cervical cancer: a critical review. *Crit Rev Oncol Hematol.* 2003;48:287–293.
15. Höckel M, Dornhofer N. The hydra phenomenon of cancer: why tumors recur locally after microscopically complete resection. *Cancer Res.* 2005;65:2997–3002.
16. Grant JD, Garg AK, Gopal R, et al. Isolated port-site metastases after minimally invasive hysterectomy for endometrial cancer: outcomes of patients treated with radiotherapy. *Int J Gynecol Cancer.* 2015;25:869–874.
17. Copeland LJ, Saul PB, Sneige N. Cervical adenocarcinoma: tumor implantation in the episiotomy sites of two patients. *Gynecol Oncol.* 1987;28:230–235.
18. Ripley D, Levenback C, Eifel P, et al. Adenocarcinoma of the cervix in a renal transplant patient. *Gynecol Oncol.* 1995; 59:151–155.
19. Eifel PJ, Jhingran A, Brown J, et al. Time course and outcome of central recurrence after radiation therapy for carcinoma of the cervix. *Int J Gynecol Cancer.* 2006;16:1106–1111.
20. Keys HM, Bundy BN, Stehman FB, et al. Radiation therapy with and without extrafascial hysterectomy for bulky stage IB cervical carcinoma: a randomized trial of the Gynecologic Oncology Group. *Gynecol Oncol.* 2003;89:343–353.
21. Benedetti Panici P, Basile S, Maneschi F, et al. Systematic pelvic lymphadenectomy vs. no lymphadenectomy in early-stage endometrial carcinoma: randomized clinical trial. *J Natl Cancer Inst.* 2008;100:1707–1716.
22. Kitchener H, Swart AM, Qian Q, et al. Efficacy of systematic pelvic lymphadenectomy in endometrial cancer (MRC ASTEC trial): a randomised study. *Lancet.* 2009;373:125–136.
23. Cormier JN, Askew RL, Mungovan KS, et al. Lymphedema beyond breast cancer: a systematic review and meta-analysis of cancer-related secondary lymphedema. *Cancer.* 2010;116:5138–5149.
24. Achouri A, Huchon C, Bats AS, et al. Complications of lymphadenectomy for gynecologic cancer. *Eur J Surg Oncol.* 2013; 39:81–86.
25. Kondo E, Tabata T, Shiozaki T, et al. Large or persistent lymphocyst increases the risk of lymphedema, lymphangitis, and deep vein thrombosis after retroperitoneal lymphadenectomy for gynecologic malignancy. *Arch Gynecol Obstet.* 2013;288: 587–593.
26. Biglia N, Librino A, Ottino MC, et al. Lower limb lymphedema and neurological complications after lymphadenectomy for gynecological cancer. *Int J Gynecol Cancer.* 2015;25:521–525.
27. Stehman FB, Bundy BN, Thomas G, et al. Groin dissection versus groin radiation in carcinoma of the vulva: a Gynecologic Oncology Group study. *Int J Radiat Oncol Biol Phys.* 1992;24:389–396.
28. DuPont J, Sovak M, Benjamin I, et al. Chemotherapeutic agents used in the treatment of gynecologic malignancies. In: Rubin SC, ed. *Chemotherapy of Gynecologic Cancers: Society of Gynecologic Oncologists Handbook.* Philadelphia, PA: Lippincott Williams & Wilkins; 2004:17–88.
29. Green J, Kirwan J, Tierney J, et al. Concomitant chemotherapy and radiation therapy for cancer of the uterine cervix. *Cochrane Database Syst Rev.* 2005:CD002225.
30. Pearcey R, Miao Q, Kong W, et al. Impact of adoption of chemoradiotherapy on the outcome of cervical cancer in Ontario: results of a population-based cohort study. *J Clin Oncol.* 2007; 25:2383–2388.
31. Gill BS, Bernard ME, Lin JF, et al. Impact of adjuvant chemotherapy with radiation for node-positive vulvar cancer: a National Cancer Data Base (NCDB) analysis. *Gynecol Oncol.* 2015; 137:365–372.
32. Rajagopalan MS, Xu KM, Lin JF, et al. Adoption and impact of concurrent chemoradiation therapy for vaginal cancer: a National Cancer Data Base (NCDB) study. *Gynecol Oncol.* 2014;135:495–502.
33. Neoadjuvant Chemotherapy for Cervical Cancer Meta-Analysis Collaboration. Neoadjuvant chemotherapy for locally advanced cervix cancer. *Cochrane Database Syst Rev.* 2004:CD001774.
34. Hogberg T, Signorelli M, de Oliveira CF, et al. Sequential adjuvant chemotherapy and radiotherapy in endometrial cancer—results from two randomised studies. *Eur J Cancer.* 2010;46:2422–2431.
35. Pignon JP, le Maitre A, Maillard E, et al. Meta-analysis of chemotherapy in head and neck cancer (MACH-NC): an update on 93 randomised trials and 17,346 patients. *Radiother Oncol.* 2009;92:4–14.

36. Zhang L, Jiang N, Shi Y, et al. Induction chemotherapy with concurrent chemoradiotherapy versus concurrent chemoradiotherapy for locally advanced squamous cell carcinoma of head and neck: a meta-analysis. *Sci Rep.* 2015;5:10798.
37. Williams M, Liu ZW, Hunter A, et al. An updated systematic review of lung chemo-radiotherapy using a new evidence aggregation method. *Lung Cancer.* 2015;87:290–295.
38. Spithoff K, Cummings B, Jonker D, et al., Gastrointestinal Cancer Disease Site Group. Chemoradiotherapy for squamous cell cancer of the anal canal: a systematic review. *Clin Oncol (R Coll Radiol).* 2014;26:473–487.
39. Tannock IF, Browman G. Lack of evidence for a role of chemotherapy in the routine management of locally advanced head and neck cancer. *J Clin Oncol.* 1986;4:1121–1126.

PART II

PRINCIPLES OF RADIATION THERAPY PLANNING AND DELIVERY

CHAPTER 4

Preparation for Radiation Treatment Planning

INTRODUCTION

Some of the most important steps in gynecologic radiation treatment planning occur well before the first radiation field or target volume has been designated. Adequate preparation prevents wasted time but, more importantly, reduces the likelihood of suboptimal, potentially ineffective treatment. Key steps in the preplanning preparatory period include the following:

- *Information gathering.* In every case, the quality of treatment depends critically on the quality of information about the nature and extent of the patient's tumor. The most detailed plan can fail if a region of gross or high-risk microscopic disease is overlooked and therefore treated to an inadequate dose.
- *Development of an overall radiation treatment strategy.* As discussed in Chapters 7, 8, and 10 to 15, some final decisions about the method of boosting gross disease may be delayed until the initial tumor response has been evaluated in the fourth or fifth treatment week. However, a decision tree mapping out potential strategies should always be developed before the initial plan is determined.
- *Patient set-up and preparation for external beam radiation therapy.* Features of the initial simulation, including the patient's position, placement of orienting radio-opaque markers, location of the central axis, and other factors, strongly influence the quality of the final treatment plan.

This chapter focuses on this initial stage of radiation therapy planning, with a focus on those aspects that are particularly relevant to the management of gynecologic cancers.

INFORMATION GATHERING—THE INITIAL PATIENT EVALUATION

What to Look for in the Clinical Record

Before processes of simulation, target definition, and treatment planning are begun, all potentially relevant clinical records (including pathology reports, operative reports, outside treatment records, and imaging studies) should be carefully reviewed to gain as much information as possible about the distribution of disease, recurrence risk, and any factors that could compromise treatment or contribute to the risk of treatment-related side effects.

Pathology Reports

Every treatment decision hinges on the findings described in a pathology report. Ambiguities can arise because of inexpert interpretation but also because of poorly articulated or erroneously transcribed findings. Modern synoptic reports reduce the potential for miscommunication. However, whenever there is doubt about the accuracy or clarity of the reported findings, the case should always be discussed directly with the examining pathologist or, if necessary, sent for review by an expert gynecologic pathologist.

Specific key features that guide decisions about treatment of various cancers are discussed in detail in the disease site chapters. However, in general, there should always be a clear description of the primary tumor, including:

- *Histology.* If unusual characteristics make the tumor difficult to classify, this should be clearly explained. For müllerian tumors, the histologic variant should always be described unambiguously (Chapters 1 and 13). For mixed tumors, the percentages of different variants within the tumor should be given. For adenocarcinomas, a histologic grade should always be specified (Chapter 1).

- *For biopsies, the adequacy of the biopsy specimen.* Would more tissue clarify the diagnosis?
- *The orientation of tumor within the specimen.* This should be part of the gross description. Orientation is particularly important if there are close or positive surgical margins following hysterectomy or wide local excision of a vulvar cancer.
- *The distance (in millimeters) between the surgical margin and the closest tumor within the specimen.* We have seen reports describing margins as "negative" when the tumor-free margin was <0.1 mm! The location of any close or positive margin should also be specified.
- *The depth of stromal invasion.* This should be described in millimeters and (for uterine and cervical cancers) as a percentage of the stromal thickness.
- *The size of the primary tumor.* For almost all gynecologic malignancies, tumor size is an important prognostic factor.
- *Lymph vascular space invasion (LVSI).* The presence or absence of LVSI should be noted. In some cases, this may be described as extensive or focal.

If a lymphadenectomy has been performed, the following details should always be specified:

- *The locations and numbers of recovered lymph nodes.* This description should include the nodal stations and laterality of recovered nodes. Reports that simply state "pelvic lymph nodes, no evidence of metastasis" are inadequate even if the number of nodes removed is described, because the adequacy of dissection within nodal stations cannot be ascertained. The original pathology report often contains more complete information about nodal counts than secondary reviews.
- *The number and location of positive nodes.*
- *The size of metastatic foci within nodes.*
- *The presence or absence of extranodal extension (ECE).* Although the importance of ECE has been particularly emphasized for vulvar cancers, it is undoubtedly an important prognostic factor for regional control of any carcinoma treated with adjuvant radiation therapy and is a key factor in determining the dose of radiation. If the location of ECE can be elicited from pathology, operative, or imaging reports, it can significantly reduce the size of the high-risk target volume.

Operative Reports

The reports of any potentially relevant operations should be obtained. Any ambiguities should be clarified through direct discussion with the surgeon. A thorough review of operative reports can provide key information about the following:

- *The location of tissues that may be at high risk for residual gross or microscopic disease.*
- *The extent of lymph node dissections.* In particular, the proximal extent of the dissection can often be determined from a careful review of the operative report.
- *The presence of adhesions or intraoperative events that could influence the likelihood of treatment-related side effects.* In particular, injury to bowel, bladder, ureters, or other critical structures should be considered when assessing the risk of late complications of combined modality treatment.

Outside Imaging Studies

Whenever possible, the original images from diagnostic studies should be obtained and reviewed, particularly if the results could have an influence on decisions about the treatment volume or radiation dose. Review of outside reports can be valuable but is often insufficient for the purposes of radiation oncology planning for a number of reasons.

- In many cases, the original studies are shown to be of poor quality or fail to include an area of interest.
- A second review can often pick up important findings that were missed in the initial interpretation.
- The initial extent and anatomic locations of tumors and lymph nodes are much more readily appreciated when the report is read while viewing the actual images.
- Digital imaging and communications in medicine (DICOM) images of contrast-enhanced CT scans, PET scans, and MRIs can be fused with treatment planning CTs, dramatically improving the speed and accuracy of target definition.

See the section, "Diagnostic Imaging Studies" for a discussion of indications for various imaging studies.

Outside Radiation Therapy Records

Detailed records should always be obtained before treating or denying treatment to a patient who has had radiation therapy in or close to the region of interest. Treatments described as, for example, "whole pelvic radiation" can vary widely. Detailed review of previous treatments often reveals that a lesion thought to represent an in-field recurrence is actually marginal to the prior radiation fields.

Written treatment summaries in the form of textual descriptions are insufficient unless previous treatment fields were far from the new area of interest. Color axial isodose distributions at intervals of 1 cm or less covering the entire treatment volume combined with central axis sagittal and coronal reconstructions may be sufficient to determine whether retreatment is possible. For patients who have had 3-D conformal treatment, digitally reconstructed radiographs showing the treatment fields are very helpful. In some cases, it is worthwhile to attempt to obtain original DICOM files; with some physics support and compatible treatment planning systems, these can be used to gain more detailed information about the doses of radiation delivered from previous treatments.

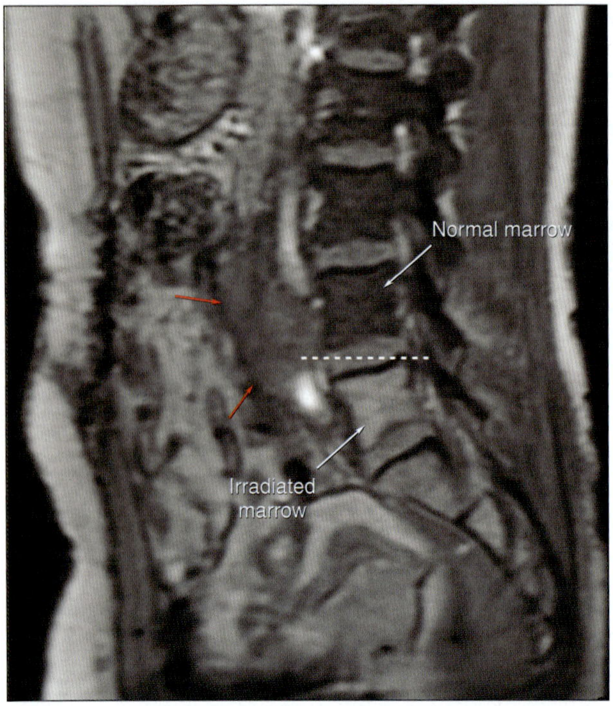

FIGURE 4.1 Use of MRI to evaluate the extent of previous radiation therapy. This patient was referred for possible treatment of a common iliac nodal recurrence of cervical cancer *(red arrows)*. She had a history of having received previous pelvic irradiation in another country, but her records proved to be unobtainable. However, T1-weighted MRI demonstrated bright signal in the marrow of the sacral and L5 vertebral bodies, indicating fatty replacement of irradiated marrow. The other lumbar vertebral bodies had normal dark signal intensity. This finding suggested that the proximal border of the previous pelvic field was at the L4–L5 interspace. The location of the tumor epicenter just above this level was consistent with a typical marginal recurrence just above the radiation fields.

If the radiation therapy records have been destroyed or are unobtainable for other reasons, an estimate of the proximal border of the treatment fields may be made using T1-weighted MRI (**Fig. 4.1**).

Clinical Examination of the Pelvis

A detailed pelvic examination is a critical part of the evaluation of every patient considered for radiation therapy of a gynecologic cancer. Because clinical descriptions cannot always impart the details required for treatment planning, the treating radiation oncologist should personally perform an examination before initiating treatment. Although high-quality MRI can provide remarkable anatomic detail, superficial vaginal disease and small vulvar lesions are poorly visualized on MRI. Clinical examination commonly complements the findings of diagnostic imaging, allowing evaluation of the mobility and tenderness of abnormal lesions and clarifying the relationship between tumor and critical structures. Pelvic examination also provides an excellent and inexpensive means of following tumor response and is used to assess a patient's suitability for brachytherapy.

The goal of pelvic examination is to define the extent of tumor involvement without causing the patient unnecessary discomfort or bleeding. The examination of a patient with probable or known cancer should include several steps:

- *Preparation and reassurance.* Ferric subsulfate (Monsel) solution, rectal swabs, and vaginal packing should be at hand in case they are required to achieve hemostasis after the examination. Several sizes of two-blade speculums should be available to accommodate narrow or spacious vaginas. A pediatric speculum may be needed to examine a very narrow or surgically reconstructed vagina, and extra-large Grave speculums may be required to visualize the cervix of obese patients. The patient should be placed in the lithotomy position with the perineum at the very edge of the table. She should be encouraged to relax her legs and perineal muscles. Before the examination, the patient should be reassured that she will be informed of each step of the examination and questioned about previous negative experiences or specific concerns about the examination. In every aspect, the examination should be approached at a careful pace with emphasis on obtaining high-quality information while causing the patient as little bleeding or discomfort as possible.
- *Inspection and palpation of the external genitalia and anus.* Describe the size, appearance, and location of any abnormal lesions and their distance (in millimeters) from critical structures (anus, urethra, or clitoris). Any evidence of infection should also be noted.
- *Initial evaluation of the vagina.* Before inserting a speculum, it is wise to gently place a finger in the distal vagina to evaluate the width of the vagina, determine the optimal speculum size, assess the presence of tumor near the introitus, and prepare the patient before inserting the speculum.
- *Speculum examination.* The purpose of speculum examination is to visualize the cervix and vaginal surfaces. The speculum should be gradually opened as it is inserted in the vagina until the cervix appears between the anterior and posterior blade, taking care to avoid inserting the speculum directly into an exophytic lesion or scraping the speculum blades against friable tumor (**Fig. 4.2**). The open speculum should then be gradually withdrawn while visualizing the vaginal walls. In some cases, the anterior and posterior walls can be better visualized if the speculum is rotated while it is withdrawn. Any vaginal lesions should be described in terms of their longitudinal location (proximal, middle, or distal third), distance from the apex or hymenal ring, and their circumferential (o'clock) location. In postoperative patients, the state of the healing vaginal incision should be noted.
- *Digital vaginal examination.* If there is a friable cervical or vaginal lesion, the vagina should be entered carefully with one or two fingers, avoiding direct contact with the tumor (**Fig. 4.3**); the examining finger(s) should be advanced to the fornix or apex of the vagina and then

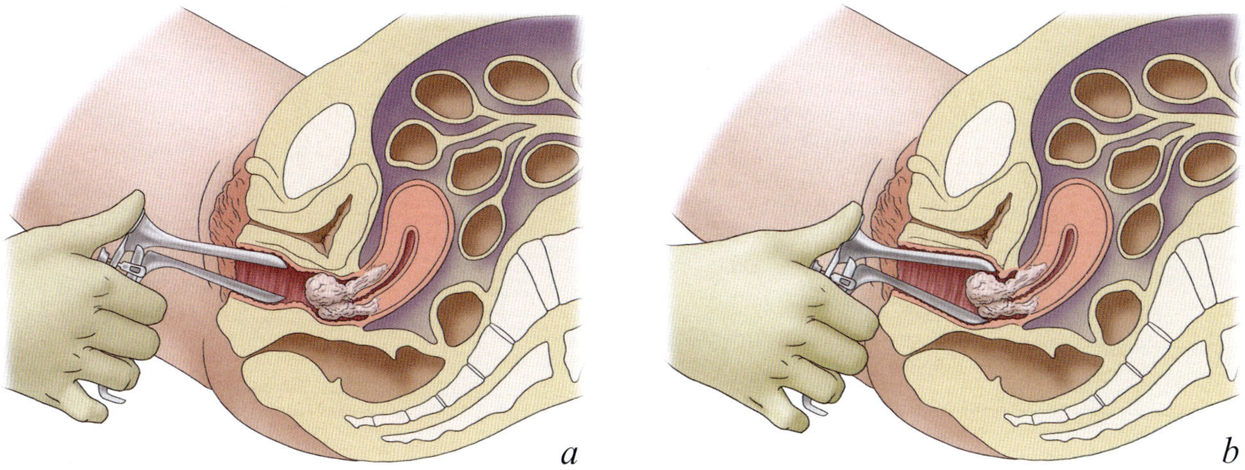

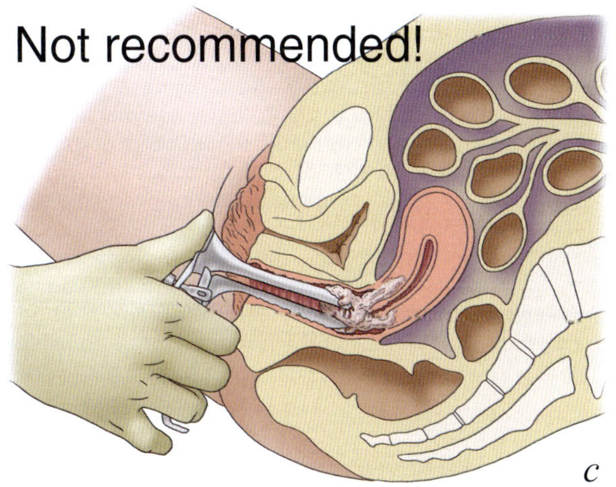

FIGURE 4.2 The speculum examination. During the speculum examination, the speculum blades should be separated immediately upon entry (*a*) and gently expanded as the speculum is advanced (*b*) to allow the cervix to come into view while minimizing trauma to friable cervical tumor. The open speculum should then be gradually withdrawn and, if necessary, rotated to provide a complete view of the vaginal walls. A closed speculum should not be inserted deep into the vagina of a patient who has cancer involving the cervix or upper vagina (*c*); insertion of the speculum blades directly into the midst of the tumor traumatizes friable tumor and can cause serious bleeding, particularly as the blades are separated. Also, a deeply inserted closed speculum blade frequently falls into the posterior fornix; when the speculum is opened, the cervix can be trapped above the anterior blade where it cannot be seen.

rotated with the palmar surface of the fingers in contact with the vaginal walls, assessing for any abnormal lesions. The relationship between the distal tumor extent and the introitus is important for determining the distal border of radiation therapy fields. However, palpation of tumor near the introitus does not necessarily mean that the distal vagina has been infiltrated by tumor (**Fig. 4.4**). The size of exophytic cervical tumors can be assessed between two intravaginal fingers (**Fig. 4.5**). However, the size of endocervical tumor can be assessed only by rectovaginal examination.

- *Rectovaginal examination.* The purpose of rectovaginal examination is to assess the diameter of the cervix, the mobility of pelvic tumor, the presence or absence of paracervical or paravaginal involvement, and the presence of disease in the rectovaginal septum. Rectovaginal examination is typically performed with an index finger in the vagina and middle finger in the rectum (**Fig. 4.6**). Right-handed examination tends to give better appreciation of the right parametrium and vice versa. The diameter of the cervix is estimated by comparing it with the diameter of the pelvis (usually about 12 cm). Tumor in the perineum can be effectively evaluated with one index finger in the distal vagina and the other in the anus.
- *Bimanual examination.* The size of the uterus and the size and mobility of the ovaries may be assessed by capturing these structures between one hand on the lower abdomen and two fingers in the vagina. This part of the examination is impossible in obese patients, and the status and size of uterus and ovaries are often better evaluated with ultrasound or tomographic imaging.

In some cases, pain, anxiety, obesity, or other factors make it difficult to obtain a satisfactory examination in clinic. In these cases, examination under anesthesia may be needed to determine the extent of disease and to define a treatment plan. We recommend examination under anesthesia for most patients with vaginal cancer and many patients with locally advanced vulvar cancers. Where appropriate, such examination can be accompanied by cystoscopy, proctoscopy, or placement of fiducial markers (discussed below).

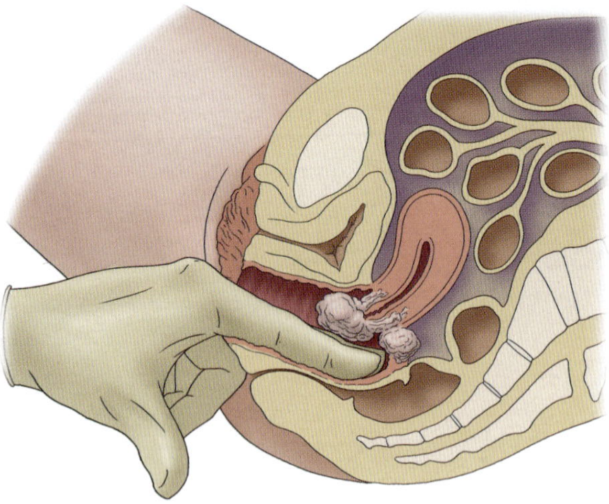

FIGURE 4.3 Digital vaginal examination. The digital examination should also be performed in a way that minimizes direct contact with the cervix. The primary goal of the digital vaginal examination is to evaluate for possible sites of vaginal involvement. After the distal extent of tumor has been assessed by gently inserting a single finger (palmar surface up) until it contacts tumor, the hand should then be turned palmar surface down and one or two fingers inserted into the posterior fornix while pushing posteriorly against the posterior wall as shown. The hand should then be rotated to the right and left to evaluate the right and left vaginal walls and fornices, all the while pushing toward the vaginal walls to minimize contact with the cervical tumor. A finger inserted directly into the face of the tumor provides no useful information and typically causes significant bleeding.

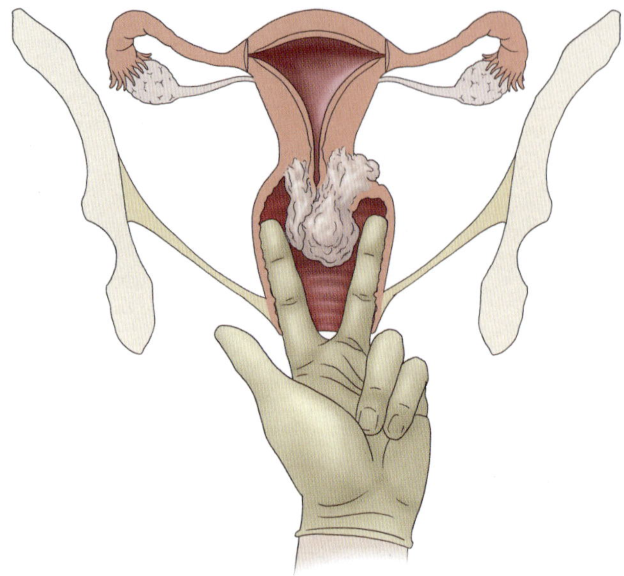

FIGURE 4.5 Estimating the diameter of intravaginal tumor. The diameter of exophytic disease can be estimated using two fingers in the vagina. However, the size of the cervix itself can be estimated only upon rectovaginal examination. Even massive endocervical tumors can easily be missed if rectovaginal examination is not performed.

Diagnostic Imaging Studies

This discussion focuses on some general principles and on some potential pitfalls associated with the use of diagnostic imaging studies, particularly for the assessment of possible regional metastases from gynecologic cancers. Disease site–specific diagnostic imaging strategies, particularly evaluation of the primary site, are discussed in detail in Chapters 10 to 15.

Evaluation of Regional Lymph Nodes

Gynecologic cancers commonly involve regional lymph nodes. However, even patients who have extensive regional metastases can frequently be cured if the treatment volume fully encompasses the region at risk for nodal metastasis and if the radiation dose is sufficient to control metastatic sites.

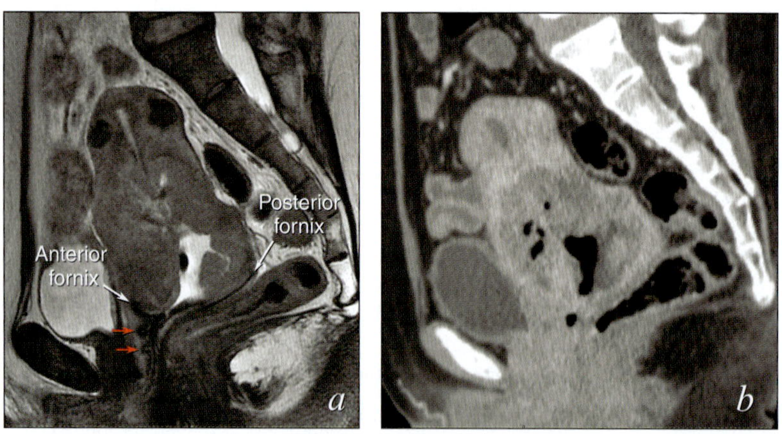

FIGURE 4.4 Estimating the distal extent of disease. Because the cervix inserts into the anterior wall of the vagina, expansile tumors typically compress the anterior vaginal wall and stretch the posterior wall. In this case, MRI shows that the anterior wall (*a, red arrows*) has been folded like an accordion; on examination, the tumor was encountered near the introitus at the level of the midpubis even though there was no mucosal vaginal involvement. The posterior vagina was stretched by the expanding tumor. This situation should always be differentiated from true infiltration of the distal vagina. In this, as in most cases, CT (*b*) provided no useful information regarding the presence or absence of vaginal involvement.

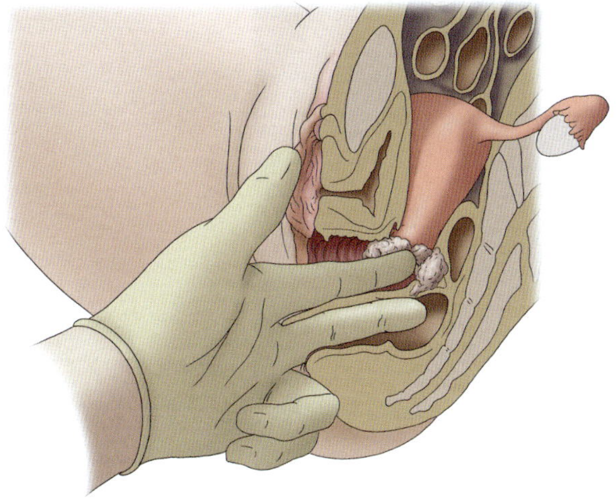

FIGURE 4.6 Rectovaginal examination. Rectovaginal examination permits evaluation of paracervical tissues, specifically the cardinal and uterosacral ligaments, which may be infiltrated by tumor. The index finger should be placed lateral to any exophytic cervical tumor in the vaginal fornix. The rectal finger is then used to palpate any nodularity that may be present superior to the fornix in the paracervical space. It is important to confirm that the rectal finger is high enough to palpate the paracervical tissues; nodular intravaginal tumor that is felt by the rectal finger should not be confused with parametrial tumor infiltration.

TABLE 4.1 Recommended CT and MRI Guidelines Regarding the Upper Limits of Normal Nodal Diameter

Site	Diameter, mm[a]
Upper paraaortic	9
Distal paraaortic	11
Common iliac	9
Internal iliac	7
Obturator	8
Presacral, paracervical, perirectal	Not seen
Inguinal	15

[a]The short-axis diameter as measured in the transverse plane.

From: Lai G, Rockall AG. Lymph node imaging in gynecologic malignancy. Semin Ultrasound CT MR. 2010;31:363–376.

The volume of regional treatment is based on an understanding of locoregional anatomy as discussed in Chapter 5.

The required dose of radiation depends heavily on the size of the metastatic deposit. Although a modest radiation dose of 45 to 50 Gy nearly always controls minimal microscopic nodal disease, lymph nodes that are enlarged by tumor typically require higher doses of 60 to 68 Gy. For the radiation oncologist, the goals of regional imaging are to identify lymph nodes that require these higher doses and sites of involvement that suggest the need to extend the volume of regional radiation. CT, MRI, PET, and ultrasound can all be helpful in making these determinations.

- *CT and MRI.* These noninvasive studies are generally widely available and remain the most frequent methods for nodal evaluation. Both depend heavily on nodal size (measured as the short-axis diameter in the axial plane) to distinguish benign from malignant. Using recommendations for the upper limits of normal size (Table 4.1), the specificity of readings can approach 90%.[1] However, infection or reactive hyperplasia can cause benign enlargement of lymph nodes, and "normal-" sized nodes can be heavily infested with tumor. For nodes of borderline size, an irregular nodal border, rounded shape (short-to-long axis ratio > 0.8), loss of the normal fatty hilum, or the presence of central necrosis may suggest tumor involvement. However, the diagnostic accuracy is poor in this size range, contributing to overall sensitivity rates of only 50% to 60% for most studies of CT or MRI.[1,2] Nodes that fall in the borderline size range pose some of the greatest challenges to the radiation oncologist because, if they are heavily infested with carcinoma, 45 Gy may be insufficient to prevent recurrence. In general, such nodes should be investigated further or, if they lie in a first echelon nodal site or adjacent to known sites of involvement, treated as if they were involved (CS 10.8, 10.9, 12.1, 13.7).
- *Positron emission tomography (PET).* PET uses ^{18}F-FDG as a tracer to detect the increased glucose metabolism that results from overexpression of glucose transporter-1 in most malignant tumors. The study is usually combined with a noncontrast CT, although in some cases, it can be combined with a contrast-enhanced CT, which is particularly helpful for image fusion and target definition. PET has consistently been found to be more accurate than CT or MRI for detection of lymph node metastases from cervical cancer, with reported sensitivities generally ranging between 75% and 85% and specificities of about 95%.[2,3] PET is particularly useful for radiation oncologists, because it helps to identify nodes of borderline size that contain metastases requiring a boost dose of radiation. It is also often the best study for the evaluation of possible nodal metastases in very obese patients, highlighting involved nodes that may be impossible to detect on CT, the quality of which is often severely degraded in very obese patients (CS 13.5 and 13.10). However, PET has several limitations. The accuracy is poor for the assessment of inguinal nodes, primarily because of a relatively low specificity (about 60% to 70% for patients with vulvar cancer).[2] Infection, commonly present in patients who have locally advanced cancers, can cause FDG-avid inflammatory responses in the draining lymph nodes (Fig. 4.7). Postoperative inflammation can also cause false positives, so PET is usually not recommended for the evaluation of the operative field for at least 6 to 8 weeks after surgery. Care must be taken not to misinterpret physiologic uptake in normal structures (e.g., ureters, ovaries, bowel) as

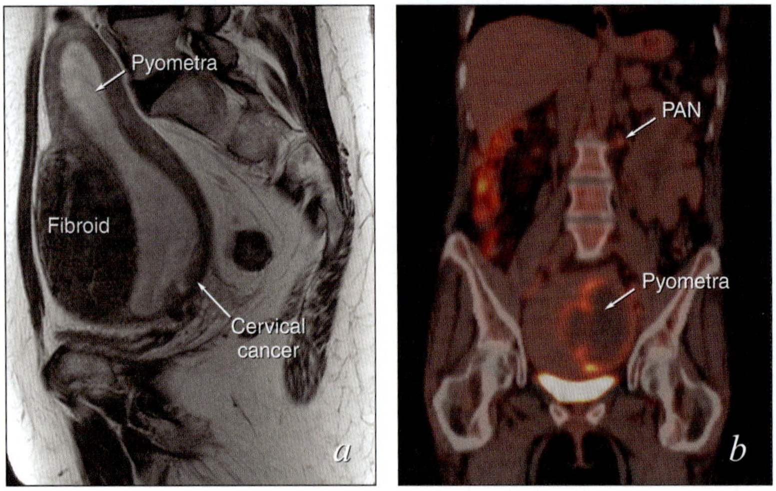

FIGURE 4.7 False-positive PET findings due to inflammation. PET has proven to be an extremely powerful tool, particularly for the assessment of lymph node involvement in patients with locally advanced gynecologic cancers. However, care must be taken not to overreact to potential false-positive findings. In this case, a patient with cervical cancer and a large uterine fibroid was found to have a massive pyometra with puss filling the uterine cavity (*a*). A PET–CT that was performed as part of her initial evaluation (*b*) demonstrated a single hypermetabolic lymph node in the infrarenal paraaortic region. This would be an extremely unlikely pattern of metastasis for a tumor confined to the cervix but is not a surprising finding for a patient who has active infection in the uterine fundus (Chapter 5). Biopsy of the node showed only inflammation, and the patient was treated to the pelvis only (PAN, paraaortic node).

indicating abnormal lymph nodes. However, we have also seen FDG-avid nodes misinterpreted as ovaries with normal physiologic uptake—this distinction can be very difficult to make on a noncontrast CT. One of the greatest disadvantages of PET is its cost; although U.S. insurers generally accept the value of PET for the initial staging of cervical and vaginal cancers, it is often not approved for initial staging of endometrial cancer or for follow-up of other gynecologic cancers unless there is already suspicion of recurrence. However, we generally recommend that PET be obtained for any patient who will be treated for gross disease involving lymph nodes.

- *Ultrasound.* Ultrasound can be extremely helpful, particularly for the evaluation of groin nodes that are interpreted as equivocal on other studies. The reported sensitivities of 80% to 85% and specificities of 80% to 90% are far better than for any other noninvasive study, including PET (**CS 12.10**).[4] In experienced hands, when coupled with fine needle aspiration, the accuracy of ultrasound can exceed 95%. Ultrasound is also helpful as a guide for biopsy of supraclavicular nodes. Unfortunately, it is useful only for the evaluation of superficial lymph nodes.

To summarize, PET is the study of choice to evaluate the lymph nodes of any patient who has locally advanced cervical cancer, vaginal cancer, or regionally recurrent carcinoma from any site that is being considered for definitive radiation therapy. CT with contrast is a reasonable second alternative if PET is unavailable and is probably the best initial study for regional evaluation of vulvar cancer, although ultrasound is the most sensitive method for the evaluation of equivocal inguinal lymph nodes. Ultrasound-guided biopsy (for superficial nodes; **CS 12.10**) or CT-guided biopsy (for deeper lesions) (**Fig. 4.8**) should be considered if the results would change treatment; however, the yield from these techniques is related to the skill of the interventional radiologist performing the study.

Evaluation of the Primary Lesion

The diagnostic imaging methods used to evaluate primary disease are detailed in Chapters 10 to 14. However, some general principles will be discussed here.

- *MRI.* The excellent soft tissue contrast achieved with MRI makes it the most useful study for evaluation of primary disease in the cervix, vagina, uterus, and other soft tissue sites. However, the preparation of the patient, coil selection, timing of contrast administration, and method of acquisition can dramatically influence the quality of the study.[5] Communication with the diagnostic imager with a clear description of the purpose of the study is critical. For example, the images from a pelvic MRI typically do not include the entire vulva unless this has specifically been requested. The insertion of aqueous gel in the vagina greatly improves the ability of MRI to define vaginal wall lesions and to differentiate vaginal involvement from exophytic cervical disease, but this may also need to be specifically requested (**CS 10.5, 10.7, 10.8, 11.2, 11.9, 11.10, 13.3**).[6] MRIs obtained in the treatment position can be fused accurately with the CT simulations to facilitate definition of the target volume. However, this may require some compromise in the set-up design to accommodate the bore size of the MRI unit, particularly

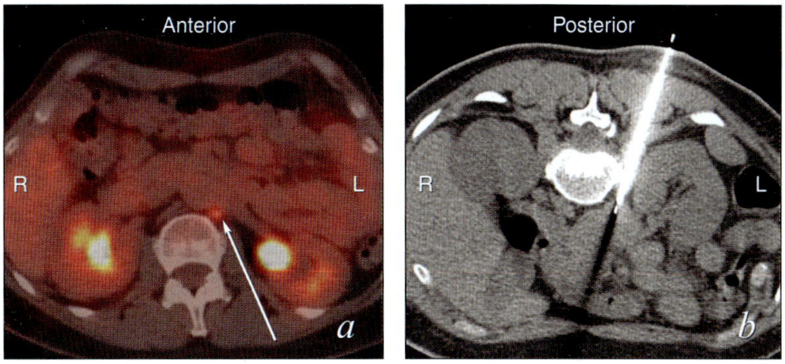

FIGURE 4.8 CT-guided fine needle aspiration biopsy. It is usually recommended that the first site of recurrence be documented histologically. In the hands of a skilled interventional radiologist, even small suspicious nodes often can be successfully biopsied. In this challenging case, a small FDG-avid lymph node was noted 4 months after the completion of radiation therapy for cervical cancer. This node was just above the margin of the previous radiation field. Under CT guidance, a biopsy needle had to be inserted through the narrow space between the left kidney and the adjacent vertebral body. Histologic examination revealed recurrent squamous carcinoma. The treatment and outcome of this patient are discussed in **CS 10.7**.

for patients who will be treated in a frog-leg position. A variety of new techniques can improve the utility of MRI in specific circumstances. Thin slice (1 to 2 mm) volumetric, T2-weighted sequences permit processing on different planes with a minimal slice thickness; this type of sequence can provide very satisfying, relatively artifact-free fusions with planning CTs and is particularly useful for image-guided brachytherapy but requires longer acquisition times. A variety of newer functional imaging techniques, including dynamic contrast-enhanced MRI and diffusion-weighted imaging, are currently being explored for their diagnostic and prognostic value.[7]

- *CT.* Contrast-enhanced CT can often be used to estimate the size of cervical and other pelvic tumor masses. Poor soft tissue contrast often limits the value of CT for precise definition of central pelvic target volumes (**Fig. 4.4**). However, modern high-resolution, contrast-enhanced CT with coronal and sagittal reconstructed views provides much clearer images than older units and can be helpful for planning of many cases.
- *PET.* Unassociated PET scans are of limited value for treatment planning because of the study's poor spatial resolution and the inability to coregister an unassociated PET scan with the radiation planning CT. Fortunately, most modern PET scans are acquired with a CT scan. Such studies, when accurately fused with the planning scan, can be extremely helpful for target volume definition, particularly for extrauterine soft tissue masses (**CS 11.8, 13.10, 14.1, 15.2**). However, because the CT and PET are acquired sequentially, internal organ motion and differing breathing protocols for the two studies can affect the accuracy of the attenuation corrections and of the registration between CT and PET. More recently, an increasing number of facilities are acquiring dual-modality PET–MRI units. PET–MRI has a number of at least theoretical benefits over PET–CT for imaging of pelvic malignancies. The most obvious is the ability to combine the superior soft tissue detail of MRI with the functional information of PET. Also, because the PET and MRI are acquired simultaneously, misregistration errors are eliminated. Early studies of the diagnostic value of these studies for patients with recurrent pelvic malignancies have given mixed reviews[8,9]; however, this technology holds considerable appeal for radiation oncology treatment planning and deserves additional study.

Preplanning Review of Imaging Studies

Before simulation and well before treatment planning is initiated, the radiation oncologist should personally review all of the relevant diagnostic materials, scrolling carefully through axial, coronal, and sagittal views to identify any positive or equivocal findings mentioned in the report and to identify potential areas of concern that may not have been mentioned in the radiology report.

Ideally, all studies needed to define the local and regional target volumes and to rule out distant metastases should be completed before the radiation therapy simulation is performed. If the patient's symptoms or scheduling limitations make it necessary to obtain a simulation before all the diagnostic information has been acquired, the radiation therapy simulation should be performed in a way that can accommodate the most likely findings; in particular, if unexpected nodal involvement could necessitate extended radiation fields, the patient's position and scanning range should be designed to allow for this possibility (see "Patient Set-up and Simulation for External Beam Radiation Therapy").

When to Seek Additional Consultation with a Diagnostic Radiologist

The simple answer to this question is, whenever there is any sense of uncertainty about the nature or location of the findings. In-field recurrences can rarely be salvaged; a misinterpretation or miscommunication between the radiologist and radiation oncologist can easily mean the difference between cure and uncontrollable disease progression. For very complex cases, an in-person consultation with an expert tomographic imager can be extremely helpful. In other cases, the radiologist can be asked to provide very specific information about the series, slice number, and anatomic locations of abnormal or equivocal findings. If the radiologist and radiation oncologist are in different locations without a shared picture archiving and communications system (PACS), e-mail communication through annotated screen grabs from the PACS or treatment planning system can often resolve ambiguities.

Fusion of the Planning CT with Diagnostic Imaging Studies

Each of the available imaging studies should be evaluated to determine whether fusion with the treatment planning CT would facilitate or improve the accuracy of target volume definition. Because positions of the pelvis relative to the spine and legs usually differ between studies, the dosimetrist should be given guidance regarding the areas of greatest interest (e.g., pelvis or paraaortic nodes). If necessary, more than one fusion can be performed focusing on different areas or the clinician can learn to use the fusion adjustment tools, which are straightforward for most planning systems. Alternatively, several vendors have developed fusion tools using deformable image registration to obtain optimized fusions throughout the region of interest.

Image fusion is most helpful for the designation of nodal or fixed central targets. However, variations in the positions of tumor and critical structures on various studies can be helpful in designing internal target volumes (ITVs).

DEVELOPMENT OF AN OVERALL RADIATION TREATMENT STRATEGY

Treatment Intent—Curative or Palliative?

The decision whether to treat with curative or palliative intent is a critical one that needs to be made before treatment has begun. For gynecologic oncology patients, this can be a very difficult choice. Once a palliative hypofractionated treatment course has been started, it is often impossible to convert to a curative treatment approach; even two or three fractions of 3 or 4 Gy delivered to the central pelvis significantly compromise the ability to deliver definitive treatment and potentially reduce the likelihood of complication-free cure. For this reason, *we do not recommend the use of small hypofractionated fields to control bleeding from locoregionally confined tumors*—a short course of hyperfractionated pelvic radiation therapy (1.8 to 2 Gy b.i.d. for 2 to 3 days) usually controls bleeding and is much easier to integrate into the patient's curative treatment (Chapters 10 and 16).

As a rule, most patients who have indications for radiation therapy and who have locoregionally confined disease should be treated with curative intent. Today, modern imaging techniques have improved our ability to define the extent of disease, and conformal radiation treatment methods, often combined with concurrent chemotherapy, have made it possible to control even extensive locoregional disease, curing many patients who would have been considered for only palliative treatment 15 or 20 years ago **(CS 10.10, 11.2, 12.8, 15.1, 15.2)**.

However, for some patients who have many major adverse risk factors, the chance of cure may be so small that it is insufficient to justify a curative treatment course. For example, cervical cancer patients who have supraclavicular metastases **CS 10.10**, massive nodal disease **(CS 15.1, 15.2)**, or stage IVA local disease **(10.11, 11.10)** can sometimes be cured of their disease. However, for a patient with all these findings, the chance of cure is extremely low (probably <1% or 2%) and may not justify a curative treatment approach, particularly if the patient also has a poor performance status. In such cases, a short course of palliative radiation may be considered for symptom relief (Chapter 16), or the patient may be treated with chemotherapy and perhaps reconsidered for consolidative radiation at a later date (Chapter 3).

Patients who have widespread hematogenous metastases are usually incurable with modern treatments. However, histologic confirmation of metastatic disease is recommended because the imaging findings caused by benign conditions and some curable or low-grade malignancies (e.g., lymphoma) can be indistinguishable from metastatic carcinoma.

Treatment that is begun with curative intent can be converted to a palliative schedule if distant disease is discovered. In particular, it is usually recommended that patients who have equivocal findings that are too small to biopsy be started on definitive treatment and periodically reevaluated for progression. However, large pelvic or extended fields and protracted treatment courses can alter the patient's quality of life and reduce bone marrow reserve that may be needed for future palliative chemotherapy. For these reasons, the decision to embark on "heroic" treatments should be considered very carefully.

External Technique

The intended external beam technique will influence choices about the patient's treatment position, method of immobilization, use of bolus, and other considerations. After all the relevant clinical information has been gathered, a tentative treatment volume and technical approach should be determined. Although choices about external beam technique may, in some cases, change during the treatment planning process, it is important to have a plan in mind before the simulation to avoid unnecessary repeat studies.

Brachytherapy

Brachytherapy plays a key role in the treatment of many gynecologic cancer patients. As will be discussed in later chapters, the decision whether or not to use brachytherapy may sometimes be made after there has been an opportunity to evaluate the patient's initial response to external beam therapy. The importance of advance scheduling and monitoring in advance of this decision is discussed in Chapters 7 and 8.

However, the initial external beam technique, dose, and fractionation influence the options for subsequent brachytherapy. This should be considered in advance of external beam treatment planning. If brachytherapy may be performed by a consulting radiation oncologist, decisions about external beam treatment parameters should be made in cooperation with the brachytherapist, after they have had an opportunity to evaluate the patient.

PATIENT SET-UP AND SIMULATION FOR EXTERNAL BEAM RADIATION THERAPY

Preparation for Simulation

The quality of a patient's final treatment plan often heavily depends on the quality of the initial simulation. Several key features of the patient's history and clinical evaluation should always be considered before the patient is brought into the simulator.

What is the proximal limit of the nodal target volume? The answer to this question influences the patient's arm position, the scope of the scan, and the location of the isocenter. Determination of the proximal limit requires detailed review of diagnostic imaging studies and surgical findings, if pertinent. Clinical parameters used to determine the upper field border are discussed in detail in Chapter 5 and in site-specific chapters.

What is the distal limit of the target volume? The answer to this question determines the distal margin of the simulation scan, the location of the isocenter, and often the optimal leg position. It requires careful review of imaging and detailed pelvic examination, with particular attention to the distal extent of the primary tumor. In most cases of vaginal involvement, fiducial markers should be placed to document the distal limit of disease (discussed below).

Will a large field-of-view be needed? Patients who are obese or who will require simulation in a frog-leg position usually require simulation in a wide-bore scanner. If available simulators cannot image the entire contour in a single scan, a complete contour can usually be obtained by rescanning after shifting the patient on the table and then fusing scans to achieve a complete contour[10] (**Fig. 4.9**).

Administration of Oral or Intravenous Contrast Agents

Although administration of intravenous or oral contrast agents during CT clearly improves identification of lymph node compartments, intrapelvic tumors, and critical structures, contrast administration is unpleasant for the patient, requires extra nursing support, and is probably unnecessary if the patient has already had high-quality diagnostic imaging

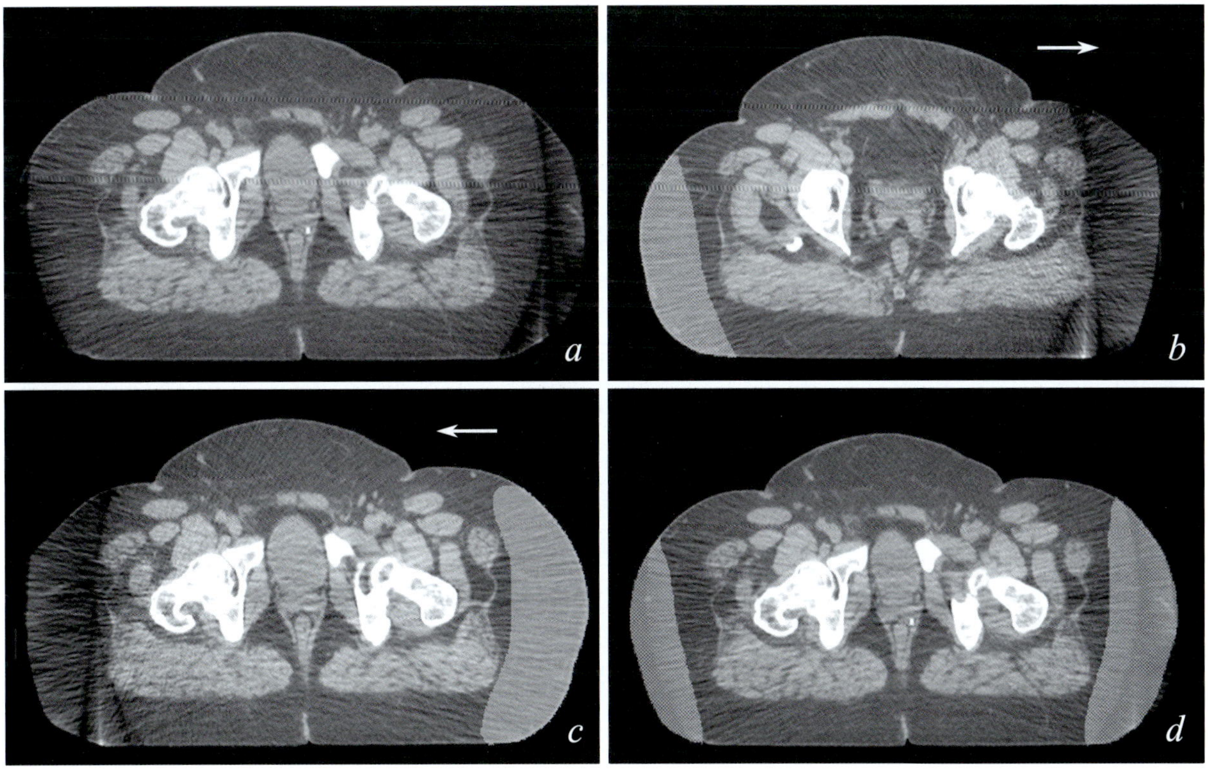

FIGURE 4.9 Technique for obtaining complete contours for patients whose diameter exceeds the CT simulator field of view. If portions of the lateral contour are missing on the initial planning CT scan (*a*), the patient can be shifted to the right (*b*) and left (*c*) and rescanned. The three scans can then be fused and used to create a complete external contour (*d*), which can then be filled in with a tissue-equivalent density.

studies. DICOM files from diagnostic CT, PET, or MRI scans can easily be fused with the patient's planning CT images. Although there may be slight degradation of the image quality during fusion, this approach has several advantages:

- The diagnostic scans have been reviewed by a qualified diagnostic imager and can easily be referenced in discussions about uncertain findings.
- The patient is not subjected to the additional time, discomfort, and risk associated with administration of contrast material.
- The scan that is used for treatment planning calculations does not contain high-Z materials that will cause aberrations in heterogeneity-corrected dose calculations; this is a particular problem after the administration of oral or rectal contrast and can be avoided only by obtaining a second, contrast-free scan or by laboriously subtracting the regions of contrast from the images.

Patient Positioning and Immobilization

When positioning and selecting an immobilization method for individual patients, several factors must be considered. No single setup is ideal for all clinical situations.

Supine versus Prone

For several reasons, supine positioning tends to be favored for the treatment of gynecologic patients. Many patients find it more comfortable, and it tends to be more reproducible, particularly for obese patients. Although prone belly board techniques may decrease the volume of bowel exposed to high dose in the central pelvis, the inclusion of anterior structures (external iliac nodes and uterus) and abdominal lymph nodes tends to decrease the advantage for many gynecology patients. When an open-leg position is desired to protect the perineum, the patient must be supine. That said, sometimes a prone position (with or without belly board) does provide better separation between bowel and target. In rare cases, a partial lateral decubitus position also may be useful.

Open- or Closed-Leg Position

The most reproducible leg position is with the legs apposed in a standardized cradle (**Fig. 4.10a**) or a customized vacuum cradle (**Fig. 4.10b, c**). Patients who have distal vaginal involvement can be placed in a frog-leg or open-leg position that decreases radiation exposure to the medial thighs and inguinal skin folds, significantly reducing local skin reactions (**Fig. 4.10d**); bolus may be needed to ensure that an adequate dose is delivered to any skin at risk for tumor involvement (Chapter 6). The frog-leg position is prone to small errors in leg position that can cause added uncertainty in the position of inguinal nodes. For this reason, a greater planning target volume margin may be required for these lateral targets, particularly in obese patients.

Upper Body Positioning

If paraaortic nodes are included in the target volume, the arms should be positioned above the head using a second customized cradle (**Fig. 4.10c**). It is key that the upper arm position be reproducible because even fairly minor alterations in arm position can change the arch of the spine and position of the paraspinous targets.

Radio-Opaque Markers

Whenever possible, radio-opaque markers should be used to delineate structures that are relevant to target volume or critical structure definition.

Vaginal Apex

The apex of the posthysterectomy vagina can be very difficult to appreciate on axial or even reconstructed CT slices unless the vaginal incision has been closed with radio-opaque material. For this reason, we typically insert two small gold or platinum marker seeds at 3 o'clock and 9 o'clock, ideally at the ends of the vaginal scar (**Fig. 4.11**). These markers add confidence to our delineation of the vaginal clinical target volume and ITV. They are also very helpful in determining accurate positioning of intracavitary applicators. We prefer this method over contrast-impregnated tampons, which distort the vagina, alter heterogeneity calculations, and may not remain in contact with the apex during simulation; however, the tampon method may be useful for the simulation of AP–PA or four-field techniques, which are less dependent on accurate localization of the apex. Intravaginal gel also distorts the vaginal contour. Rigid devices (e.g., cylinders) should never be used to localize the vagina during simulation unless the device will be used and precisely repositioned throughout treatment—these devices significantly distort the shape and position of the vagina and can lead to serious errors in target delineation (Fig. 6.2).

Vaginal Tumor Involvement

Although MRI usually provides excellent imaging of gross tumor involvement, it does not always visualize more superficial mucosal involvement by tumor. Fiducial markers inserted at the margins of vaginal tumor can be extremely helpful for the treatment planning and subsequent daily image guidance. For tumors that involve the mid- or distal vagina, we typically surround the lesion with radio-opaque markers, often placed during examination under anesthesia (**Fig. 4.11**; **CS 11.2–11.7**). These markers can be critically important to the planning of subsequent brachytherapy, which often must be designed and planned after the tumor has responded to radiation therapy, obscuring the location of the high-risk target volume.

Surface Landmarks

If accurately placed, anal and urethral markers can be helpful guides in target volume and field designation (**CS 12.4, 12.8**). Also, any target that involves the skin (e.g., vulvar lesions,

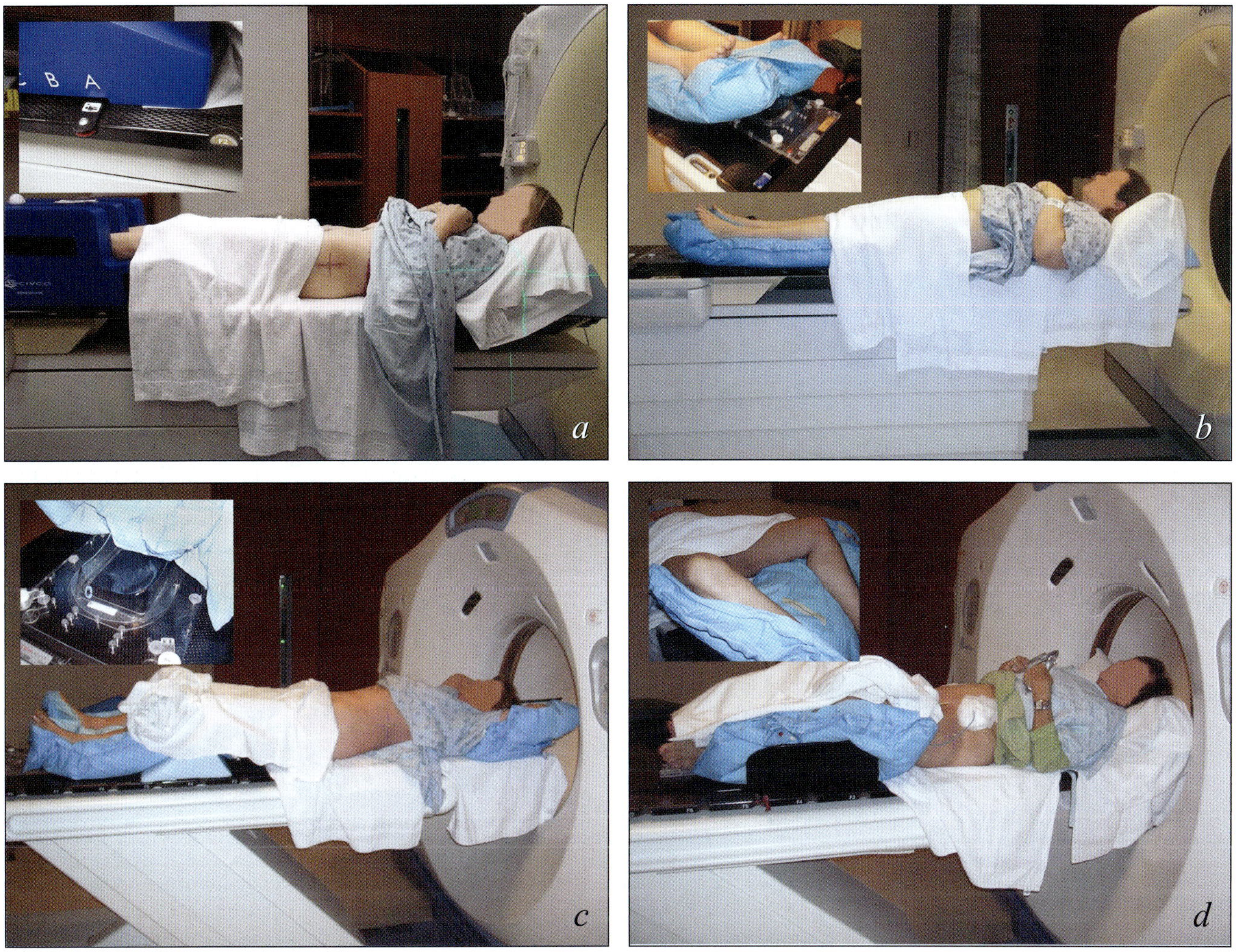

FIGURE 4.10 Samples of typical setups for patients with gynecologic tumors. For pelvic radiation, the legs can be immobilized in a fixed geometry device *(a)* indexed to the table or in a custom cradle *(b)*. In *(c)*, the arms are positioned above the head in a custom cradle for extended field irradiation. In *(d)*, the legs are placed in a frog-leg position in a custom cradle supported by a wing board. Both cradles are indexed to the table *(insets)* and marked to facilitate alignment with longitudinal lasers.

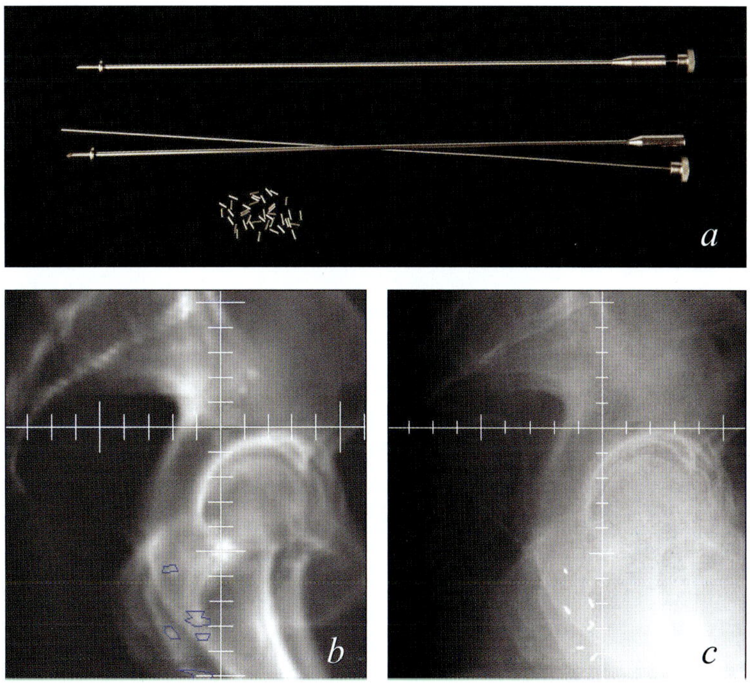

FIGURE 4.11 Insertion of vaginal fiducial markers. An elongated seed inserter *(a)* can be used to place fiducial markers in the cervix or vagina. Small seeds made of platinum *(a, bottom)* or gold can be readily seen on CT scans; although they may be difficult to see on digitally reconstructed radiographs (DRRs), they can be contoured on the treatment planning CT and displayed on DRRs as contours *(b, blue)* for comparison with on-treatment alignment images *(c)*. The contours in *(b)* include positions of the seeds on full and empty bladder scans. Comparison with *(c)* shows excellent alignment of bony structures, which are good indicators for the alignment of the nodal target. A small shift in positions of the vaginal fiducials was within the margins used for the ITV.

groin nodes with skin involvement, incisional recurrences) should be carefully marked with wires or multiple BBs surrounding the lesion. Any scar that may have been contaminated during removal of gross tumor should be marked with a wire and included in the target volume.

Other Landmarks

Any other surface landmarks that may help define the location of the target volume or avoidance structures should be marked with wire or BBs.

Bolus

Bolus is required to achieve full dose to any portion of the target volume that lies within the radiation build-up region. Commonly used bolus materials include SuperFlab and moistened gauze. However, the thickness, shape, and even the need for bolus frequently depend on the beam energy and incident angle of the treatment beams. For this reason, optimal bolus design may not be possible until a treatment plan has been developed. Nevertheless, it is often helpful to apply bolus prior to simulation to facilitate planning and to evaluate whether a selected bolus material can be closely apposed to the surface. If bolus is applied during simulation, we frequently obtain a second scan without bolus to permit visualization of surface details on skin renderings used during contouring (Fig. 6.10).

Selecting an Isocenter

The central axis of the radiation beam should not be selected arbitrarily but rather to optimize the relationship of the divergent beam to the target volume. Several characteristics of the radiation beam and isocentric setup should be carefully considered when selecting an isocenter:

- *Peripheral beam divergence.* In most cases, the ideal isocenter location is in the approximate center of the target volume. This placement minimizes divergence at the cephalad–caudad extremes of the radiation field and improves conformality at the periphery of the target volume.
- *Lack of divergence at the central axial plane.* The nondivergent center of the beam can be exploited in several special situations:
    - When two different techniques will be used to treat the cephalad and caudad portions of the target (**CS 10.2**).
    - When proximity to a particularly sensitive critical structure demands minimal divergence at one end of the target volume. In gynecologic treatment, the most common use of this "split-beam" technique is when the gross tumor volume is immediately adjacent to a previously treated region (**CS 10.6**).
- *Reproducibility of positioning.*
    - *Stability of initial setup.* Ideally, the isocenter should be placed in a location where the relationship between the skin surface and underlying boney structures is relatively constant. This can be a challenge in gynecologic patients whose primary targets may occur in a region underlying steeply sloping or unsteady body surface areas.
    - *Accuracy of image-guided setup.* Image-guided radiation therapy generally permits very accurate positioning of the isocenter of the radiation beam. However, in gynecologic applications, where large field sizes are frequently required, even slight tilts, rotations, or variations in the curvature of the spine can result in significantly greater positioning uncertainty at the periphery of the target volume (Fig. 6.5). In some cases, judicious placement of the isocenter may permit use of a relatively small planning target volume margin in a critical location (e.g., where gross disease is in very close proximity to a critical structure or previous radiation field edge) (**CS 10.7, 15.3**).

Assessing and Defining Internal Organ Motion—Imaging for ITV Designation

One of the greatest challenges to precision in gynecologic radiation therapy planning is the substantial, often unpredictable intertreatment and (to a lesser extent) intratreatment motion of the upper female genital organs. It is important to remember that the female reproductive organs are suspended in the central pelvis on elastic supporting ligaments; the ability of the uterus and vagina to make major positional adjustments during coitus, with pregnancy, and during filling and emptying of adjacent hollow viscera is essential to their design. The uterine fundus is subject to large translational and rotational changes in position that are influenced by filling of the bladder and small and large bowel, particularly rectosigmoid (**Fig. 5.14**). The cervix and upper vagina can also move by as much as 4 to 5 cm (**Fig. 5.15; CS 10.1**). *A single CT scan should never be assumed to be representative of the day-to-day position of central pelvic structures.*

The range of motion due to bladder filling, the extent of which varies considerably from patient to patient, can be estimated by performing sequential planning CT scans with full and empty bladder.[11] This information can be supplemented by fusing relevant diagnostic studies with the planning CT. For short vaginal boosts, a Foley catheter can be inserted and, after emptying the bladder, a fixed volume of saline (usually 200 to 250 cc) instilled for the simulation and daily treatment. Less precise control of bladder filling can be achieved by instructing the patient to empty her bladder and drink 16 oz of water 1 hour before simulation and treatment; however, bladder volumes need to be verified with ultrasound to obtain reproducible results (Chapter 7).

The influence of rectal filling is more difficult to estimate. Because daily enemas and rectal balloons tend, in our experience, to be poorly tolerated by patients receiving large field pelvic radiation, we account for the influence of changes in rectal volume by including a portion of the bladder or rectum

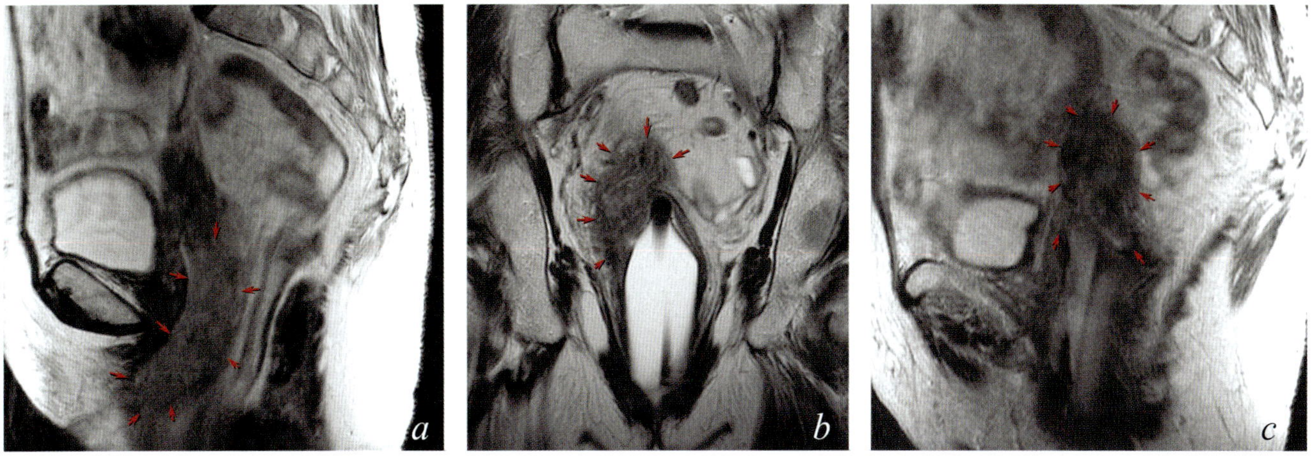

FIGURE 4.12 Correction for vaginal prolapse. In this case, a patient with severe vaginal prolapse developed an invasive squamous cancer, which was anatomically located at the apex of a posthysterectomy vagina. However, because of her prolapse, the vagina (and a portion of the tumor) varied markedly in position, often visibly protruding through the vulva, as seen here on MRI (*a, arrows*). During simulation and treatment, a rectal balloon was placed in the vagina, displacing the tumor higher in the pelvis (*b, c*).

in the vaginal or uterine ITV. This is discussed in greater detail in Chapter 5, "Vaginal Movement and Designation of a Vaginal ITV." However, if the patient is noted on initial scan to have a large bubble of gas in the ampulla, a rectal tube may be used to decompress the rectum. The rectal tube should not be left in place for the scan because it can cause the patient to tense the buttocks, potentially causing a pelvic tilt that cannot be easily reproduced.

Correction of Uterine or Vaginal Prolapse

Patients who have descensus (prolapse) of the uterus or vagina pose special problems for radiation therapy. Although the target may be the vaginal apex or cervix, severe prolapse can cause these structures to protrude through the introitus. Unless this is corrected, the entire vulva must be treated in order to encompass the target. However, a variety of methods can be used to return these structures to the pelvis during treatment. Some women with partial descensus use a pessary routinely and can be asked to continue this through treatment. Alternatively, a rectal balloon or vaginal dilator can be used (Fig. 4.12). Ideally, these should be indexed to the cradle to maintain consistent positioning. Fiducial markers in the cervix or vaginal apex can be monitored during the treatment to verify the reproducibility of the setup.

References

1. Lai G, Rockall AG. Lymph node imaging in gynecologic malignancy. *Semin Ultrasound CT MR.* 2010;31:363–376.
2. Selman TJ, Mann C, Zamora J, et al. Diagnostic accuracy of tests for lymph node status in primary cervical cancer: a systematic review and meta-analysis. *CMAJ.* 2008;178:855–862.
3. Grant P, Sakellis C, Jacene HA. Gynecologic oncologic imaging with PET/CT. *Semin Nucl Med.* 2014;44:461–478.
4. Selman TJ, Luesley DM, Acheson N, et al. A systematic review of the accuracy of diagnostic tests for inguinal lymph node status in vulvar cancer. *Gynecol Oncol.* 2005;99:206–214.
5. Sala E, Rockall AG, Freeman SJ, et al. The added role of MR imaging in treatment stratification of patients with gynecologic malignancies: what the radiologist needs to know. *Radiology.* 2013;266:717–740
6. Brown MA, Mattrey RF, Stamato S, et al. MRI of the female pelvis using vaginal gel. *AJR Am J Roentgenol.* 2005;185:1221–1227.
7. Wakefield JC, Downey K, Kyriazi S, et al. New MR techniques in gynecologic cancer. *AJR Am J Roentgenol.* 2013;200:249–260.
8. Grueneisen J, Schaarschmidt BM, Heubner M, et al. Implementation of FAST-PET/MRI for whole-body staging of female patients with recurrent pelvic malignancies: a comparison to PET/CT. *Eur J Radiol.* 2015;pii:S0720-048X(15)30083-8; doi: 10.1016/j.ejrad.2015.08.010.
9. Kitajima K, Suenaga Y, Ueno Y, et al. Value of fusion of PET and MRI in the detection of intra-pelvic recurrence of gynecological tumor: comparison with ^{18}F-FDG contrast-enhanced PET/CT and pelvic MRI. *Ann Nucl Med.* 2014;28:25–32.
10. Fisher CM, Fortenberry BR, Jhingran A, et al. Novel technique for simulation and external beam treatment planning for obese patients. *Pract Radiat Oncol.* 2011;1:152–155.
11. Jhingran A, Salehpour M, Sam M, et al. Vaginal motion and bladder and rectal volumes during pelvic intensity-modulated radiation therapy after hysterectomy. *Int J Radiat Oncol Biol Phys.* 2012;82:256–262.

CHAPTER 5

Applied Anatomy and Target Volume Definition

During most of the 20th century, radiation therapy treatment plans were based on external beam fields whose borders were drawn directly on x-ray films. For most gynecologic treatments, the borders of pelvic fields were drawn in relation to skeletal landmarks and fixed reference points on AP–PA and lateral x-ray films. Treatments designed in this way cured many gynecologic cancers, and the outcomes of treated patients confirmed that these conventional fields encompassed the central and regional targets that were most likely to harbor microscopic disease.

As demonstrated below, pelvic fields designed using these traditional methods are remarkably similar to fields that are shaped to conform to precise CT-guided target volumes. However, the traditional two-dimensional method of treatment planning can lead to underdosage of unappreciated regions of gross disease. Furthermore, early experiences with conformal treatment quickly revealed the dangers of implementing new technology without fully understanding the anatomy of the target region. For example, in the 1980s, a move to use electrons to treat the groins of patients with vulvar cancer rapidly revealed that the traditional prescription depth of 3 cm, used for many years to prescribe photon treatment of the groin, was not a good surrogate for the inguinofemoral target volume when the beam actually conformed to that depth. Unfortunately, the evidence came in the form of fatal groin recurrences.[1,2]

The 21st century has witnessed a sea change in gynecologic radiation therapy treatment planning. Intensity modulated radiation therapy (IMRT) is increasingly being used to generate plans that conform closely to physician-designated CT-based target volumes. Although IMRT can reduce the side effects of radiation therapy, its effectiveness is highly dependent on the accuracy of the designated target volumes and, therefore, on the radiation oncologist's understanding of regional anatomy and patterns of disease dissemination. Image-based planning also requires an appreciation for the value and limitations of diagnostic imaging modalities. Even when relatively simple three-dimensional plans are used for pelvic treatment, serious errors and unnecessary recurrences can occur if the field borders are based on inappropriate target volumes. For this reason, it is helpful to understand the relationship between target volumes and the traditional, long-tested fields that were based on bony landmarks.

In this chapter, relevant structures will be depicted in several ways to demonstrate not only their appearance on CT or MRI but also their relationships to bony, surface, and vascular anatomy. The influence of internal organ motion on target volume designation will also be discussed. The developmental origins of müllerian and lymphatic structures will be described to help explain adult anatomy and characteristic patterns of regional metastasis.

TARGET VOLUME DEFINITION

Accurate target volume definition requires a thorough understanding of:

- Locoregional anatomy, including normal variations,
- Gynecologic diagnostic imaging modalities,
- Operative findings and associated histologic findings,
- The natural history and patterns of spread of various disease processes,
- The nature of internal organ motion,

- The potential for tumor response and other anatomic changes during treatment, and
- Uncertainties in daily setup accuracy.

This information is used to determine an overall treatment strategy and to define various components of the final radiation therapy target volumes. In clinical practice, these components are not always defined consistently. This can lead to miscommunications in target volume definition. For this book and in our practice, components of the target volume are defined as follows:

Clinical target volume (CTV): A region with sufficient risk for containing disease to warrant targeted treatment. The CTV includes solely those tissues, as seen on the treatment planning CT scan, that are considered at risk for primary involvement, lymphatic spread, or direct extension to adjacent tissues. In most cases, for definitive treatment of gynecologic carcinomas, the CTV receives a minimum dose of 40 to 45 Gy of fractionated radiation therapy.

High-risk CTV: A region of potential microscopic disease for which doses of more than 45 Gy may be required to achieve high rates of disease control. Examples include positive or close resection margins, equivocal lymph nodes, and sites of extracapsular extension.

Internal target volume (ITV): An expanded target volume designated to account for intertreatment and intratreatment motion of a CTV or GTV. This often involves the integration of information from two or more imaging studies.

Gross tumor volume (GTV): An area of gross disease identified by imaging, physical examination, or intraoperative findings. Several GTVs may be designated to define regions requiring different radiation doses.

Planning target volume (PTV): A CTV, ITV, or GTV plus a margin added to account for variability in patient setup and table alignment. In our practice, the physician usually designates the targets described above and specifies a margin to be added by the dosimetrist prior to inverse planning (Chapter 6).

Nested interior GTV: This term will be used to describe internal target volumes that are sometimes specified to treat the interiors of very large tumor masses at a higher dose per fraction than the GTV–PTV; typically, this is a PTV that excludes all vulnerable critical structures (and therefore excludes a portion of the GTV–PTV). The goal is to accelerate the tumor response to facilitate boost planning although the ultimate impact on local tumor control is not known.

In general, bone, muscle, intraperitoneal contents, and other tissues not suspected of harboring disease are not included in the designated CTVs or GTVs. However, an ITV is designated where appropriate to account for internal organ motion, and *a PTV margin is always added to GTVs, CTVs, and ITVs to account for other uncertainties, particularly setup inaccuracies.*

Throughout this chapter, suggested target volumes should be viewed as examples that may vary with the clinical situation.

REGIONAL LYMPH NODES

Regional lymph nodes are included in the target of most definitive gynecologic radiation treatments. Radiation therapy is an effective tool in the treatment of many gynecologic malignancies in large part because regional spread frequently occurs well before the development of hematogenous metastasis, increasing the likelihood that effective regional treatment will be curative.

Overview of Vascular and Lymphatic Development

The lymphatic system develops in parallel with the embryonic venous (not the arterial) system in a fashion that explains many anatomic features of the adult (Fig. 5.1). At the end of the 5th week of fetal development, endothelium-lined lymphatic sacs appear in the jugular, retroperitoneal, and iliac regions; from these sacs, lymphatic vessels emerge and grow along the course of embryonic veins. Subsequently, clusters of lymph nodes develop in the regions of the lymph sacs and eventually along the course of major lymph vessels. Most of the lymphatic vessels supplying the central pelvic organs originate from paired posterior lymph sacs located at the junction of the primitive supracardinal and iliac veins. This region, at and just below the junction of the common iliac, internal iliac, and external iliac veins, is the most frequent site of pelvic node metastases from cervical cancer and other central pelvic malignancies (Fig. 5.2).[3]

Fetal venous development is also the best context in which to understand the asymmetric distribution of the paraaortic nodes and patterns of paraaortic lymphatic spread. The inferior vena cava is a compound structure formed by the fusion of right supracardinal vein and other portions of the early venous system (Fig. 5.1). Although the left supracardinal vein eventually disappears, it is present during the most active period of lymphatic development, and its associated lymphatic vessels and nodes persist, forming the left paraaortic lymphatic chain. Whereas the paracaval nodes are virtually always in direct contact with the vena cava, the left infrarenal paraaortic nodes can be found anywhere within the 1- to 2-cm space between the aorta and the left psoas muscle, reflecting their association with the supracardinal vein that once occupied this space.[4] The drainage of the left ovarian vein into the renal vein and the distribution of aortic nodes at the renal level are also evidence of this asymmetric development. These features have important implications for contouring of nodal CTVs in this region.

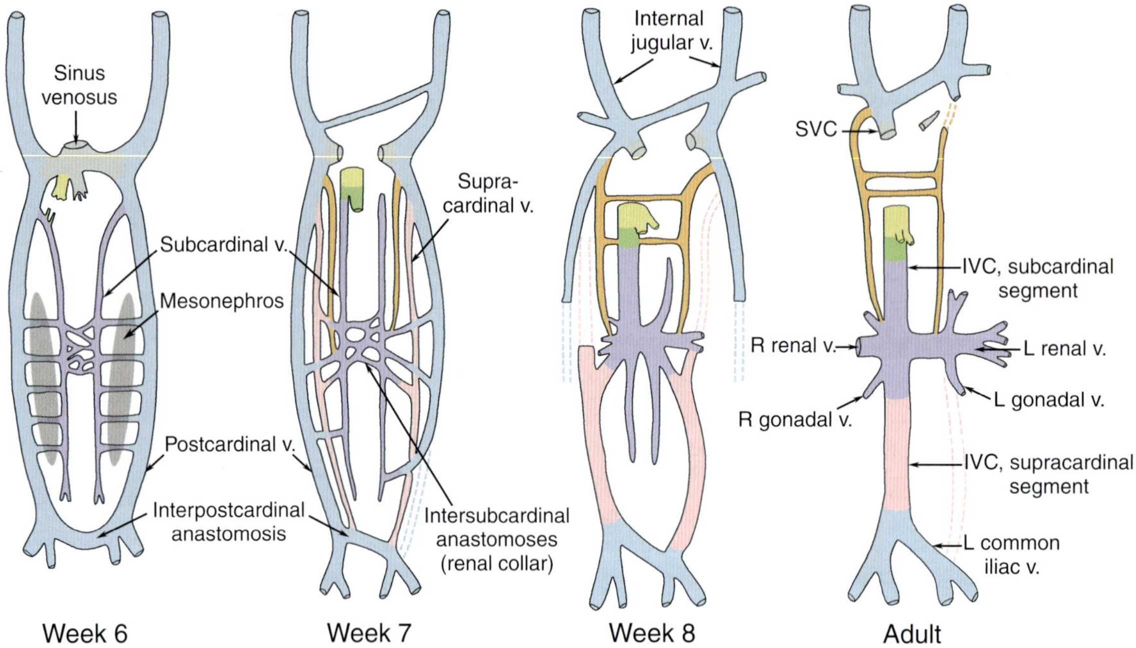

FIGURE 5.1 Venous development. Comparison of embryonic venous structures during weeks 6, 7, and 8 and venous structures in the adult. The abdominopelvic veins develop from longitudinal pairs and anastomoses of subcardinal *(purple)*, postcardinal *(blue)*, and supracardinal *(pink)* veins. Various segments expand, coalesce, diminish, and even disappear as the fetus matures. The lymphatic system begins to develop in the 5th week, when lymphatic vessels emerge from primitive fetal sacs and extend to follow the paths of the fetal veins. Lymphatics to the left of the aorta follow the course of the left supracardinal vein, which subsequently disappears. Note that the origin of the left common iliac vein from the interpostcardinal anastomosis differs from that of the right common iliac vein. This explains the greater length and near horizontal path of the left common iliac vein and possibly the asymmetric distribution of common iliac nodes described in Figure 5.2. (Adapted from Standrig S. *Gray's Anatomy: The Anatomical Basis of Clinical Practice*. 40th ed. Philadelphia, PA: Churchill Livingstone; 2008.) (IVC, inferior vena cava; L, left; R, right; SVC, superior vena cava; v., vein.)

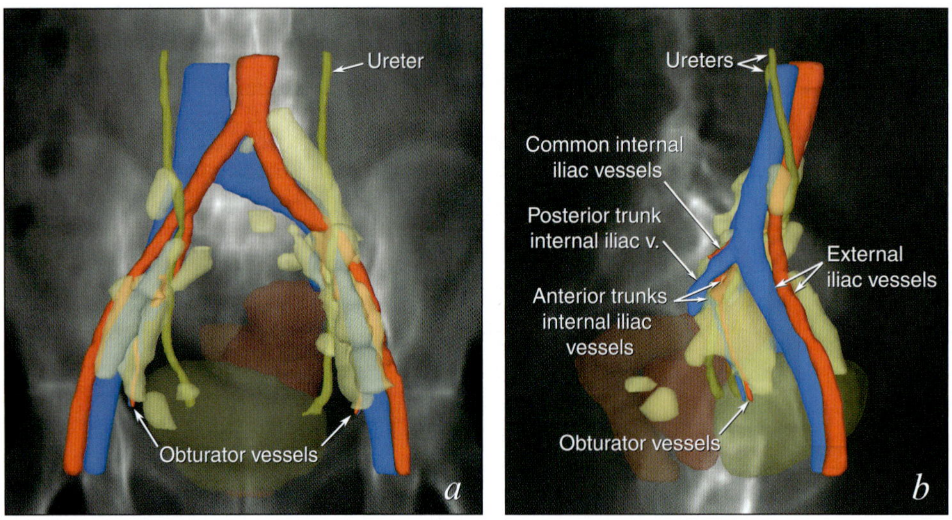

FIGURE 5.2 Relationship between pelvic structures and regional lymph nodes. Using data from a patient with stage IB2 cervical cancer, reconstructions of selected pelvic organs were superimposed on anterior–posterior *(a)* and lateral *(b)* digitally reconstructed radiographs.

The *khaki* structures represent the amalgamated contours of more than 150 PET-positive lymph nodes in 40 patients with cervical cancer. Nodal contours were applied to this single patient's CT scan using deformable image registration and then edited to refine their relationships to vascular structures.

Most primary echelon nodal metastases are found in the space between the internal iliac and external iliac vessels, anteromedial to the external iliac vessels, and surrounding the obturator vessels. Common iliac nodes can be involved secondarily and, at least in the distal (junctional) region, can be involved primarily by cancers of the cervix and other sites.

Note the path of the ureters as they cross over the iliac vessels into the pelvis. The ureters are particularly vulnerable to compromise from cancer-bearing lymph nodes in this region of frequent metastatic involvement.

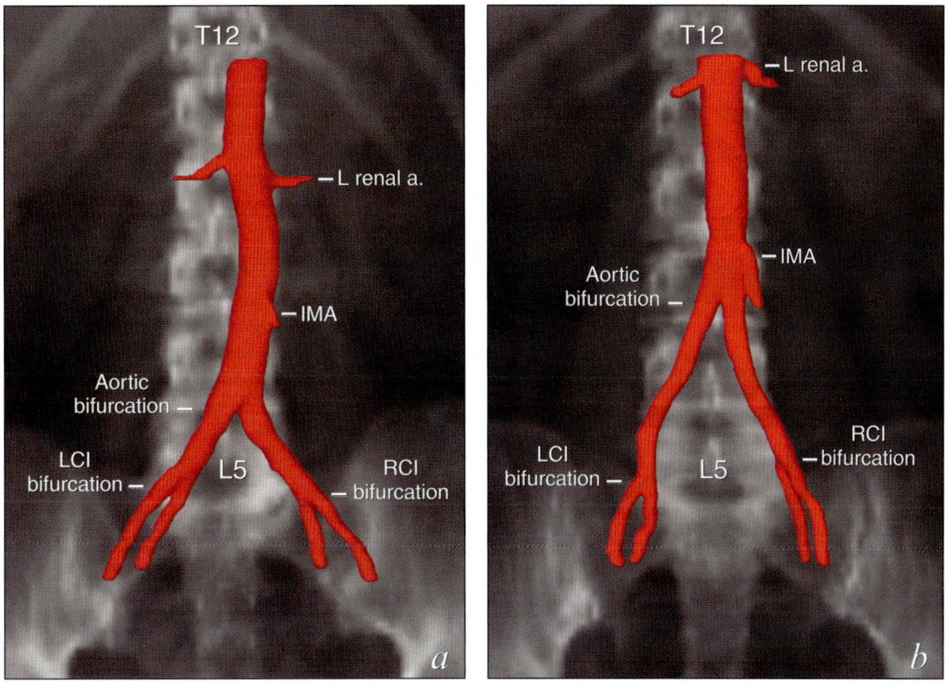

FIGURE 5.3 Variations in vascular anatomy. The levels of the renal arteries, inferior mesenteric artery, and aortic bifurcation vary widely, as shown in digitally reconstructed contours from 2 patients (*a, b*). Although the aortic bifurcation is most often located anterior to L4, it is frequently located above or below that level (though rarely distal to the L4/L5 interspace). The bifurcations of the common iliac arteries are somewhat less variable, usually occurring between the L4/L5 and L5/S1 interspaces. A review of CT scans from 80 patients showed that in 53 the common iliac bifurcations were at or above L5/S1, placing the common iliac nodes entirely outside the true pelvis. (IMA, inferior mesenteric artery; LCI, left common iliac; RCI, right common iliac.)

Although it is common to describe the locations of lymph nodes in terms of their relationships to arterial landmarks, this practice can lead to erroneous assumptions. During development, branches of the dorsal aorta migrate considerable distances as the corresponding organs develop. As a result, the final locations of the origins of the mesenteric and renal arteries and the lengths of intervening aortic segments vary significantly between patients (**Fig. 5.3**). The vertebral level of the aortic bifurcation is also highly variable, and the bifurcations of the common iliac arteries, though usually within 1 to 1.5 cm of the L5/S1 interspace, can also be found outside that range. For these reasons, the proximal vertebral level of radiation field borders does not always provide an accurate estimate of the adequacy of nodal coverage.

It is important to note that the common iliac vessels are not located in the true pelvis. Although clinicians frequently refer to sites of possible nodal involvement as "pelvic" or "aortic," the common iliac nodes do not fit into either of these designations. Studies of patients treated with pelvic radiation for cervical cancer demonstrate that the common iliac nodes immediately above the treatment field are common sites of nodal recurrence.[5] These "iliac" recurrences are frequently misidentified as pelvic and may be incorrectly assumed to be located within the previous pelvic radiation treatment field. To avoid confusion, nodal recurrences should be specified in terms of their precise anatomic location (external iliac, internal iliac, common iliac, or para-aortic) as well as their vertebral level and relationship to radiation treatment fields.

Definition of Nodal Clinical Target Volumes

Optimal nodal target volume definition requires an understanding of the patterns of lymphatic drainage and of the tissue compartments that house the pelvic, paraaortic, and inguinal lymph nodes.

Nodal target volumes cannot be defined accurately by simply surrounding the major vessels with a fixed margin. The distribution of lymph nodes around the major vessels is not symmetric, and although many relevant lymph nodes do lie immediately adjacent to large vessels, others do not. The hypogastric vessels, sacral vessels, and relevant branches of the femoral vessels are difficult to identify on axial CT slices but are associated with important sites of regional metastasis from gynecologic cancers.

Also, although contouring atlases can be helpful to clinicians who are developing their skills, the appearance of the nodal target volumes on an axial plane can vary dramatically according to the configuration of the pelvis (**Fig. 5.4**). *For this reason, axial contouring should be performed while the clinician references coronal and sagittal reconstructions to be certain that the target volumes are consistent and make sense in three dimensions.*

Finally, although the positions of the pelvic and abdominal lymph nodes tend to be fairly constant, lymph nodes can be displaced by large soft tissue masses. In addition, hyperexpansion of the bladder can compress the psoas muscles and displace iliac vessels and lymph nodes (**Fig. 5.5**); for this and other reasons (Chapter 4), patients should be discouraged from having an uncomfortably full bladder during treatment. Treatment

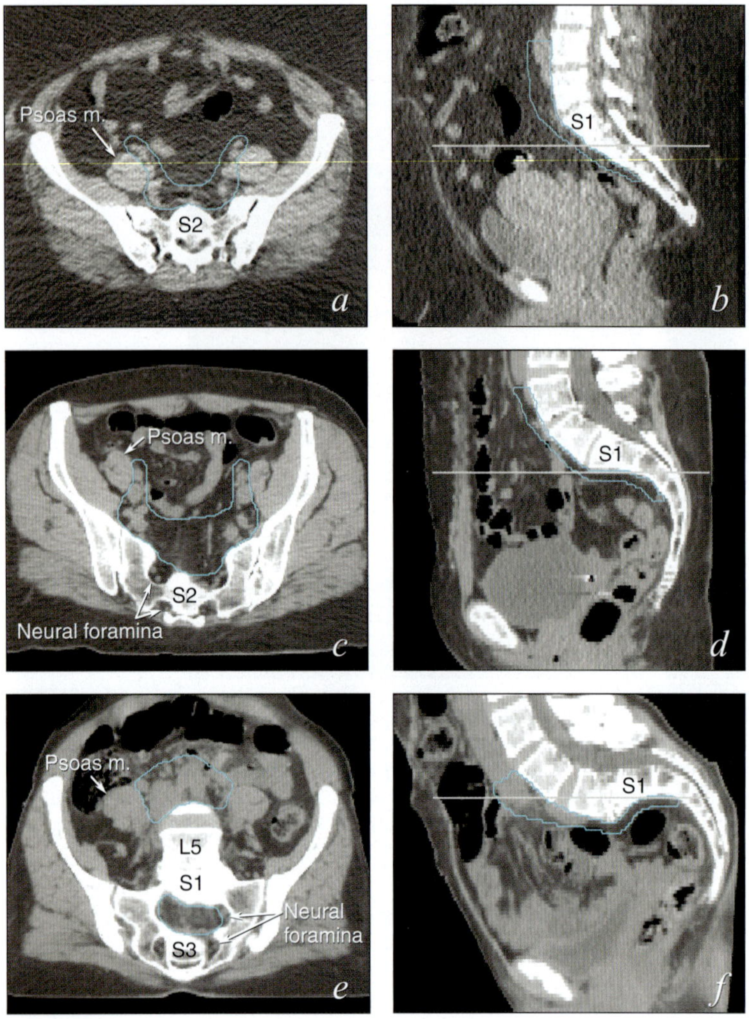

FIGURE 5.4 Influence of pelvic configuration on the axial appearance of regional target volumes. (*a, c, e*) Nodal CTV contours are displayed on an axial CT slice through the anterior S1/S2 interspace for each of three patients. (*b, d, f*) The plane of each axial slice is shown on a midline sagittal view. All the three patients were scanned in a supine position on a flat table.

Although the presacral nodes are always located within 1 cm of sacral bone, the amount of tissue that must be contoured to specify the presacral space *in the axial plane* varies widely according to the tilt of the pelvis and curvature of the sacrum. In the first patient (*a, b*), the sacrum is nearly straight, and the presacral space is adequately covered using a relatively constant 1- to 1.5-cm margin anterior to the bone. In the second patient (*c, d*), the anterior face of S1 is nearly parallel to the axial plane; the presacral space associated with S1 is located and must be contoured on the adjacent (caudad) slices, requiring that the contour extend several centimeters anterior to bone at this level. In the third patient (*e, f*), the extreme lumbar lordosis and pelvic tilt pose particular challenges; the nodal CTV can only be contoured correctly by careful attention to the axial and sagittal planes. Failure to recognize variations in the tilt and curvature of the sacrum will lead to contouring errors, with undertreatment of the nodal compartment or overtreatment of bowel.

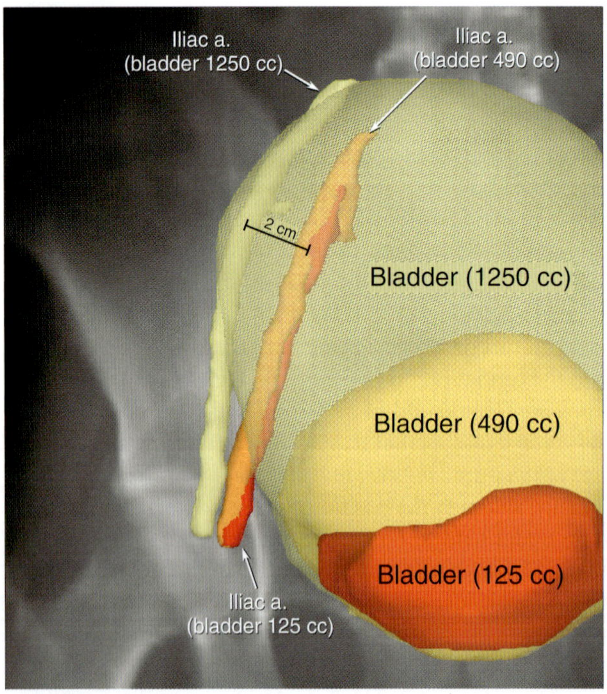

FIGURE 5.5 Relationship between bladder filling and the position of the iliac vessels. Shown are the locations of the iliac vessels reconstructed from three CT scans obtained with different degrees of bladder filling on the same day in the same patient. The locations of the iliac vessels with the bladder empty (*red*) or filled to a volume of 490 mL (*orange*) were very similar. However, hyperexpansion of the bladder (*khaki*) caused compression of the psoas muscles and lateral displacement of the iliac vessels and associated nodal compartments. Treatment plans that use contours based on CT scans obtained while the patient has a hyperexpanded bladder can lead to underdosage of associated nodal basins because this degree of bladder filling usually cannot be reproduced consistently over a 4- to 6-week treatment course.

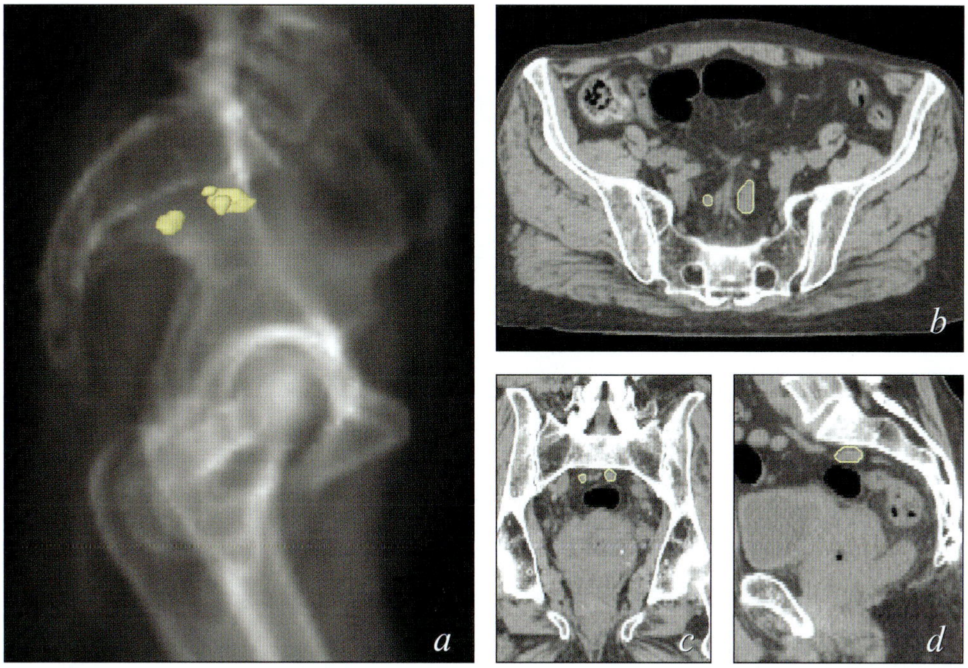

FIGURE 5.6 Presacral nodes in a patient with locally advanced vaginal cancer involving the rectovaginal septum. The nodes (outlined in *khaki*) lie within 1.5 cm of the anterior margin of the S1 and S2 vertebral bodies (*a, c, d*). However, on an axial view through mid-S2 (*b*), the nodes appear to be some distance from bone. When the presacral nodes are to be targeted, contours must cover a volume of tissue 1 to 1.5 cm from the anterior edge of the sacral vertebral bodies *as viewed in the sagittal plane* to avoid underdosage of the target volume. As viewed in the axial plane, the corresponding distance from bone to the anterior margin of the CTV may vary from 1 cm to more than 4 cm.

planning should not be based on a planning CT scan in which the bladder volume is more than about 500 to 600 mL (or extending above the base of the sacroiliac joints) without confirmation that vessel positions are similar when the bladder is less full. Large seromas can also displace adjacent vessels, and the displacement may change with seroma volume. Absent these special circumstances, intratreatment movement of the pelvic nodes tends to be <2 to 3 mm. Because day-to-day variations in lymph node positions are usually small, generalized, and difficult to quantitate for individual patients, this is one type of internal organ motion that may reasonably be accounted for with an adequate (6 to 7 mm) PTV margin (Chapter 6).

Pelvic and Common Iliac Lymph Nodes

The lymphatic drainage of the vulva, vagina, uterus, and ovaries is discussed in detail with the anatomy of these structures later in this chapter. The pelvic nodes most commonly affected by metastasis from the reproductive organs are those that lie between the internal and external iliac vessels near the bifurcations of the common iliac veins and those associated with the anterior branches of the internal iliac vessels (**Fig. 5.2**)[3]; however, other nodes, including sacral, gluteal, and pararectal nodes, can be involved under some circumstances (**Figs. 5.2 and 5.6; Table 5.1**). A detailed discussion of the CTV for postoperative regional treatment of uterine cancers is included in the annotations accompanying **Figure 5.7**. The three-dimensional appearance of this CTV and its relationship to typical AP and lateral pelvic fields is shown in **Figure 5.8**. However, the axial appearance of the pelvic node CTV can vary considerably according to the position of the pelvis (**Fig. 5.4**).

Paraaortic Lymph Nodes

The lymph nodes adjacent to the vena cava and aorta receive lymphatic drainage from the pelvis and also, as discussed below, can be sites of primary lymphatic drainage from the uterine fundus, tubes, and ovaries. A detailed discussion of paraaortic target volume definition is included in the annotations accompanying **Figure 5.9**. The three-dimensional relationships between lymph nodes and associated vascular structures and the appearance of typical AP and lateral fields designed to cover the paraaortic CTV are illustrated in **Figure 5.10**.

Inguinal Lymph Nodes

The inguinal lymph nodes receive lymphatic drainage from the vulva, distal vagina, mons pubis, and distal anterior abdominal wall (**Table 5.1**). Lymphatics of the external genitalia reach the groin via the superficial external pudendal and external epigastric lymphatic vessels. The more lateral (superficial circumflex) lymph nodes are rarely if ever the initial site of involvement but can be involved secondarily. A detailed discussion of inguinal target volume definition is included in the annotations accompanying **Figure 5.11**. The relationships between vascular structures, bony landmarks, and a three-dimensional view of a suggested CTV for comprehensive treatment of the relevant inguinal nodes are shown in **Figure 5.12**.

(*text continues on page 66*)

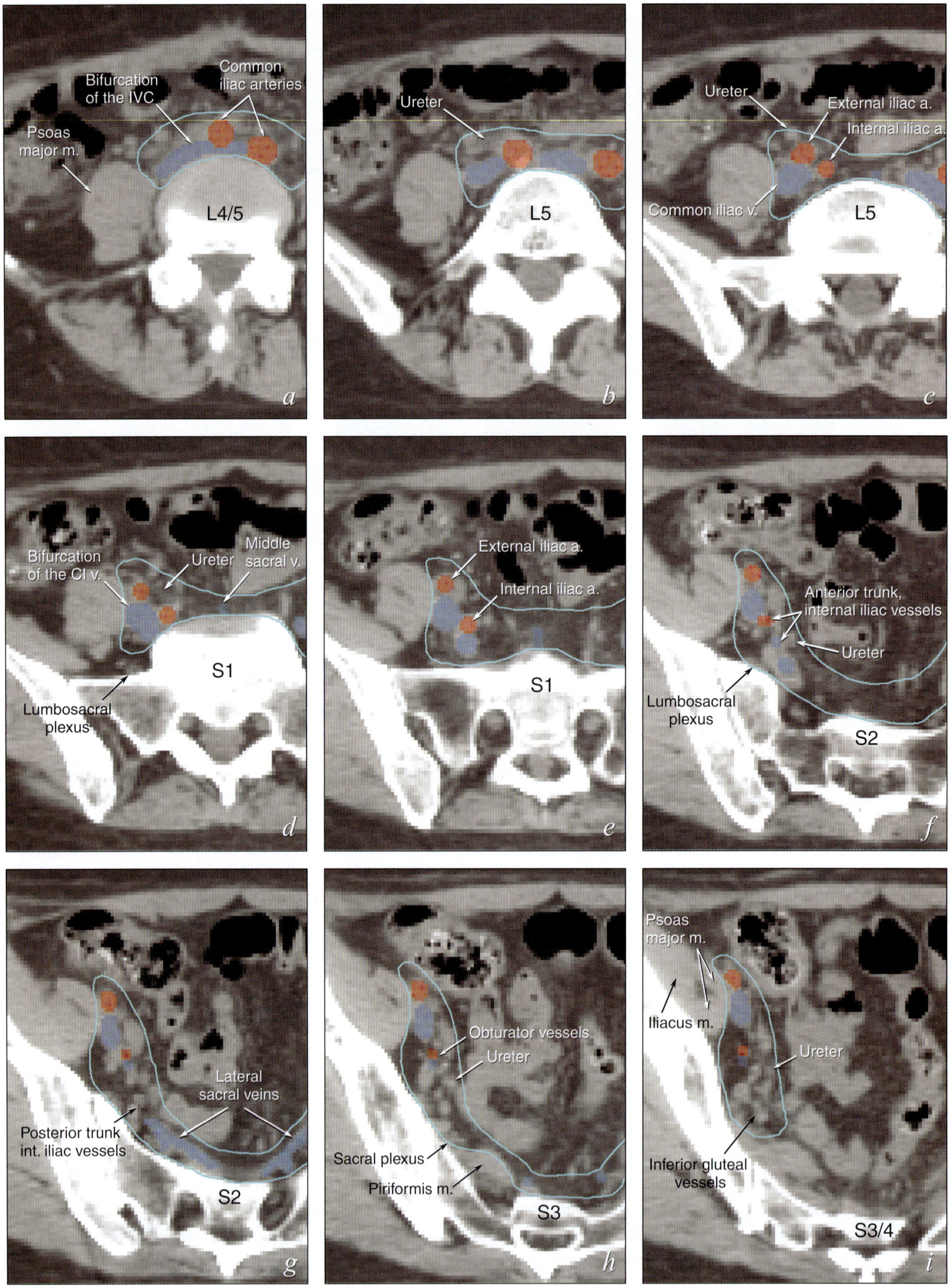
Bifurcation of the IVC
Common iliac arteries
Psoas major m.
L4/5
a
Ureter
L5
b
Ureter
External iliac a.
Internal iliac a.
Common iliac v.
L5
c
Bifurcation of the CI v.
Ureter
Middle sacral v.
S1
Lumbosacral plexus
d
External iliac a.
Internal iliac a.
S1
e
Anterior trunk, internal iliac vessels
Ureter
Lumbosacral plexus
S2
f
Lateral sacral veins
Posterior trunk int. iliac vessels
S2
g
Obturator vessels
Ureter
Sacral plexus
Piriformis m.
S3
h
Psoas major m.
Iliacus m.
Ureter
Inferior gluteal vessels
S3/4
i

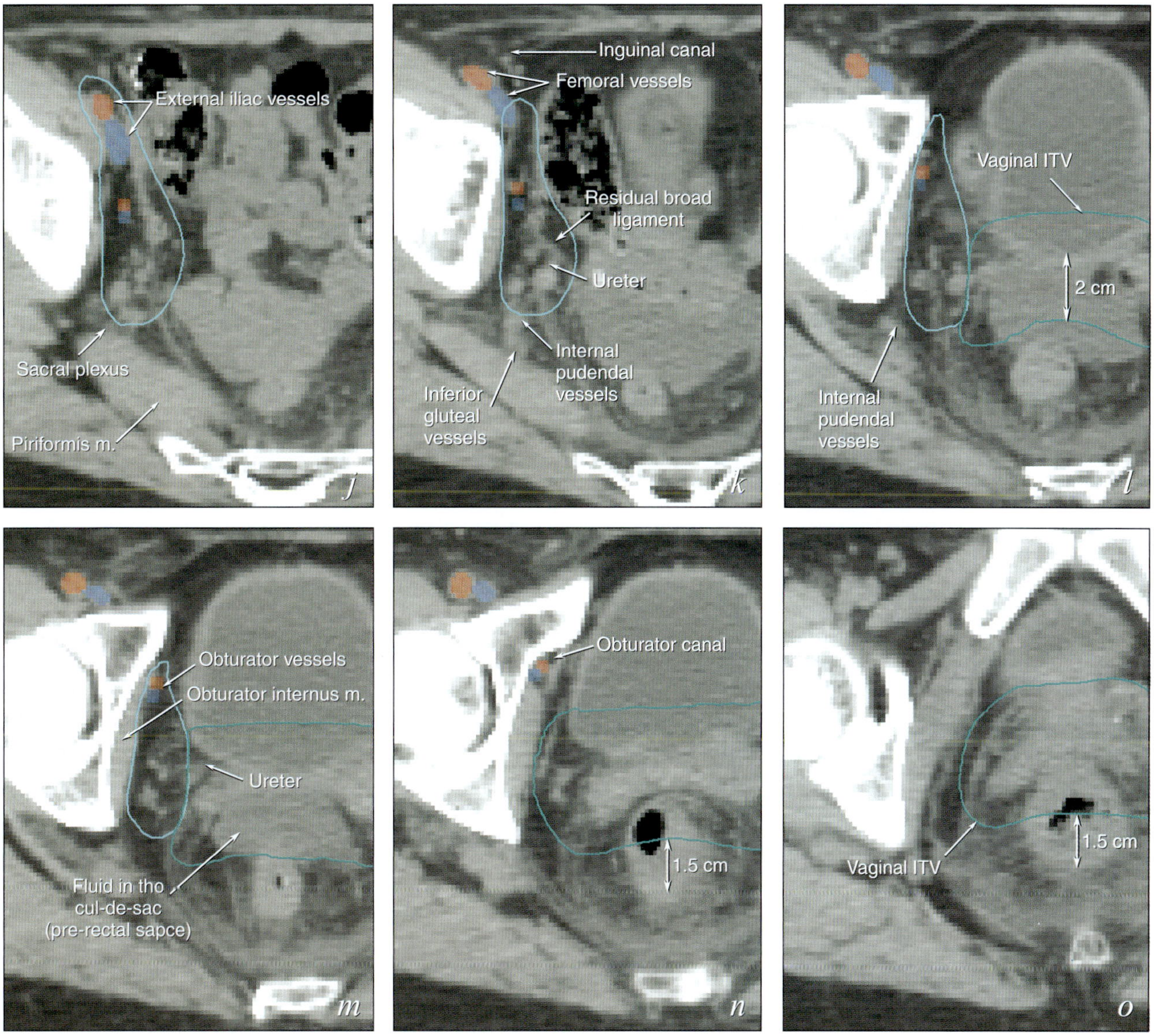

FIGURE 5.7 Pelvic anatomy and target volume definition after hysterectomy. Shown are axial CT sections from just below the aortic bifurcation *(a)* to the midpubis *(o)* and reconstructed coronal and sagittal views through the midpelvis *(p, q)*. CT simulation was performed 4 weeks after the patient underwent simple hysterectomy and pelvic lymph node dissection. Pelvic veins and arteries are highlighted in *blue* and *red*, respectively. *Cyan lines* indicate suggested limits of a nodal CTV for a patient who requires regional treatment after hysterectomy for cervical cancer or endometrial cancer involving the cervix. Except for the presacral region (discussed below), the nodal CTV would be similar for a cancer confined to the uterine body. (CI, common iliac; int., internal; IVC, inferior vena cava.)

Cervical and endometrial cancers often metastasize to nodes in the region at and just distal to the bifurcation of the common iliac vessels *(c–f)*; therefore, this region should always be included in the regional target volume. In this case, the right common iliac artery divided to form the external and internal iliac arteries just above L5/S1 *(c, d)*. The internal iliac vessels typically divide into anterior and posterior trunks 1 to 2 cm distal to the common iliac bifurcation *(f, g)*.

Iliac node CTV. Branches of the anterior trunk of the internal iliac artery *(f)* supply most of the central pelvic structures, including the uterus, cervix, and vagina. The pelvic lymph nodes that are most commonly involved with cancers originating in the uterus and cervix are the nodes lying near the origins of the anterior internal iliac vessels in the space between the external iliac, internal iliac, and internal pudendal vessels. Most of the branches of the anterior trunk (also termed hypogastric vessels) are difficult to identify on CT. However, the vessels are contained within the space between the external iliac vein and the piriformis muscle *(h–j)* and, more distally, between the external iliac and inferior gluteal vessels *(k, l)*, which can usually be identified on CT. The region anterior and posterior to the obturator vessels is frequently involved with metastasis; this region, which lies medial to the obturator internus muscle, should be covered distally to the point at which the vessels enter the obturator canal *(m, n)*.

Note the close proximity of the ureter to important node-bearing regions in the pelvis; from the point where the ureter crosses into the pelvis *(b, c)*, it is included in the CTV not because it is a target but because of its location within the nodal basin.

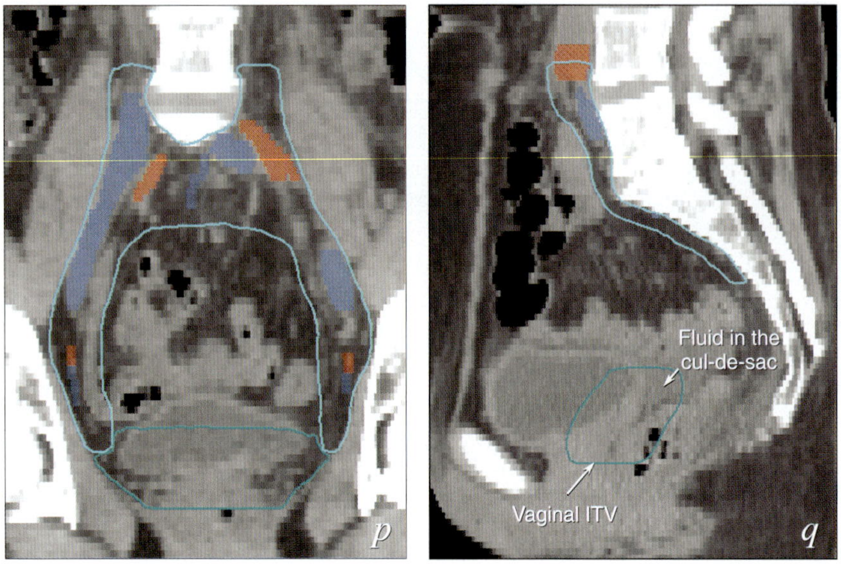

FIGURE 5.7 (*Continued*) The external iliac nodes typically lie posterior, medial, or occasionally anterior to the external iliac vessels but rarely if ever between the vessels and the psoas muscle. For this reason, the lateral border of the iliac CTV generally follows the medial border of the psoas muscle *(a–j)*. Particular care should be taken not to confuse the medial portion of the psoas muscle *(i)* with the external iliac vessels, whose location can sometimes be obscure on non-contrast-enhanced CT. Unless there are enlarged nodes, the CTV should be placed 3 to 4 mm from the external iliac vessels in the anterior and medial directions. Because the intra-iliac region (posterior to the external iliac vessels; *c–m*) is the most frequent site of pelvic node metastasis from gynecologic cancers, generous coverage of all the vessels in this space (typically at or near the interface with bowel and abutting adjacent muscle or bone) is necessary.

Just above the level of the acetabulum, the external iliac vessels begin to deviate laterally in their descent toward the inguinal canal where they become the femoral vessels (*k*); unless the distal vagina is involved with cancer, the CTV does not need to include the vessels distal to this level.

Presacral node CTV. Because the contours shown here are for a patient who has tumor in the cervix, the contours extend to cover the presacral nodes to mid-S3 *(d–h, q)*. For uterine body cancers, the distal presacral region may be reduced slightly, but the region anterior to S1 and S2 should still be treated. Coverage of the presacral nodes is also discussed in the legends for Figures 5.4 and 5.6.

Uterine ligaments. After simple hysterectomy, the residual broad ligament and associated parametrial tissues retract to a position medial to the obturator internus muscle and internal iliac vessels; for this reason, any soft tissue that remains between these structures and bladder or bowel should be included in the CTV *(j–m)*. Although the nodal CTV is usually discontinued distally at the level of the obturator canal, the paravaginal tissues must still be included in the CTV.

Vaginal ITV. Although the patient's bladder volume on the day of this simulation was only 100 mL, a diagnostic scan when the patient's bladder volume was 400 mL was used to estimate the influence of bladder volume on vaginal position. Teal lines *(l–p)* indicate a suggested vaginal ITV generated using the fused scans. The target included the vagina as well as paravaginal tissues at risk. Because the rectum was moderately full, the vaginal ITV was extended posteriorly to within 1.5 cm of the posterior rectal wall. At the apex of the vagina, the rectum reflects back toward the sacrum; the resulting prerectal space is typically filled with bowel or, as in this case, resolving postoperative fluid collections *(k–m)*. A 2-cm posterior margin was used in this region.

Scrutiny of reconstructed coronal views *(p, q)* provides an important check on the consistency and accuracy of axial contouring (see Figure 5.19). Reference to contrast-enhanced CT or MRI can be very helpful in identification of the vessels (discussed in Chapter 4).

Note: To account for setup uncertainties, the CTV and ITV must be expanded (usually by 6 to 7 mm) to account for setup variability; the resulting PTV should be used to generate the final plan.

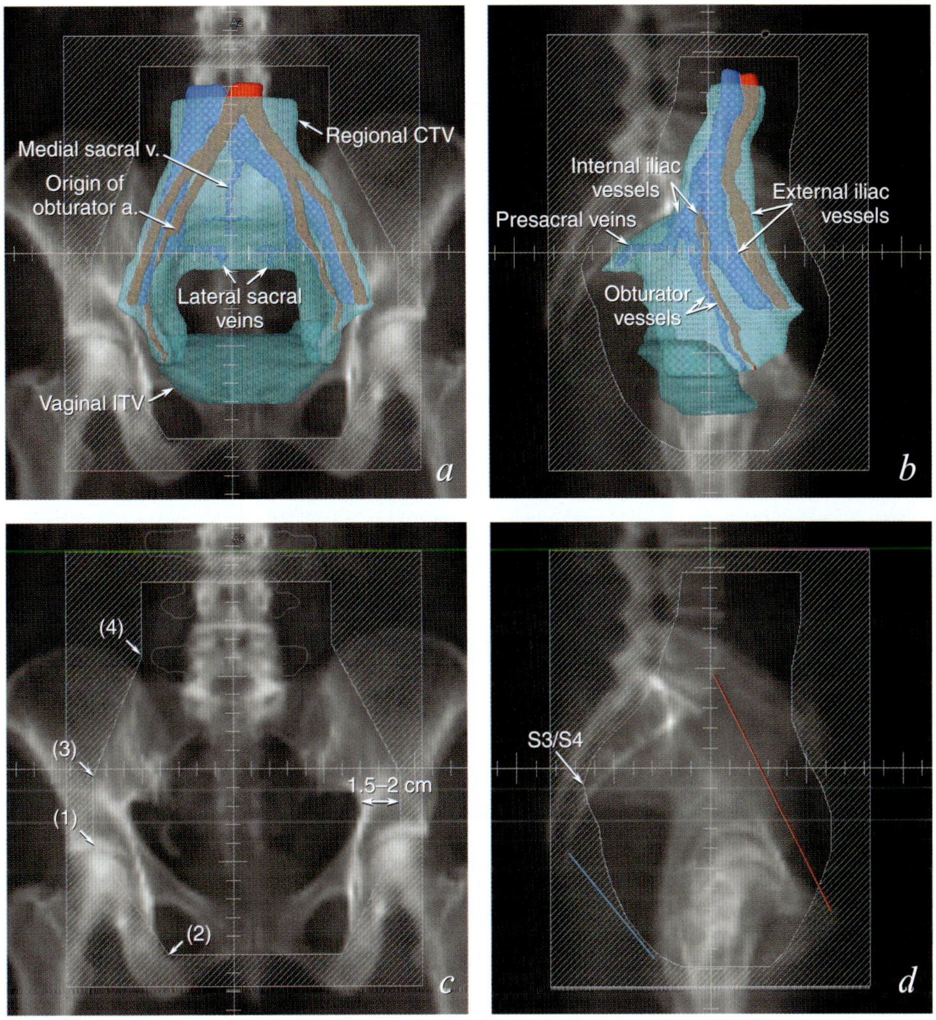

FIGURE 5.8 Relationship between regional target volumes and typical radiation therapy field arrangements for posthysterectomy pelvic treatment. (*a, b*) Three-dimensional reconstructions of the nodal CTV (*cyan*), vaginal ITV (*teal*), and selected vascular structures outlined in Figure 5.7 superimposed on a digitally reconstructed radiograph. Typical anterior and lateral fields that would be used for a four-field box arrangement have been added. Note how closely these fields conform to the designated target volumes, allowing margin for geometric penumbra and patient setup uncertainties.

In (*c*) and (*d*), fields are shown without superimposed structures to more clearly demonstrate the relationship between suggested field borders and bony landmarks.

Typical anterior fields (*c*) extend inferiorly to at least the mid-pubis or 4 cm beyond the vaginal apex; the lateral field border is usually 1.5 to 2 cm lateral to the pelvic brim. Each inferior corner block extends from a point at the intersection between the lateral field edge and the top of the acetabulum (*1*) passes along the outer margin of the obturator foramen and intersects with the inferior border of the field (*2*). Superior blocks extend proximally from the lateral edge of the field (*3*) to a point just outside the proximal SI joint (*4*), and then continue superiorly to intersect with the proximal border of the field.

The posterior border of the lateral fields is typically placed at the S3/S4 interspace; the anterior border is usually at the tip of the pubis but may need to be further anterior if the pelvis is severely lordotic. Corner blocks should be added to spare soft tissue: A block placed at the posterior margins of the sacral bodies usually provides adequate coverage of the sacral nodes. The anterior margin of the external iliac nodes typically lies along a line extending from mid-L4 to the tip of the pubis (shown in *red*); the anterior superior field margin should be placed at least 2 cm anterior to this line. The anterior inferior block can be placed at the posterior margin of the pubic ramus. The posterior inferior block is difficult to define without image-based planning but a small block extending from the tip of the coccyx to the inferior border (shown in *blue*) can be inserted for most posthysterectomy cases.

When image-based fields fail to meet these criteria, they should be carefully scrutinized for possible errors in target volume definition.

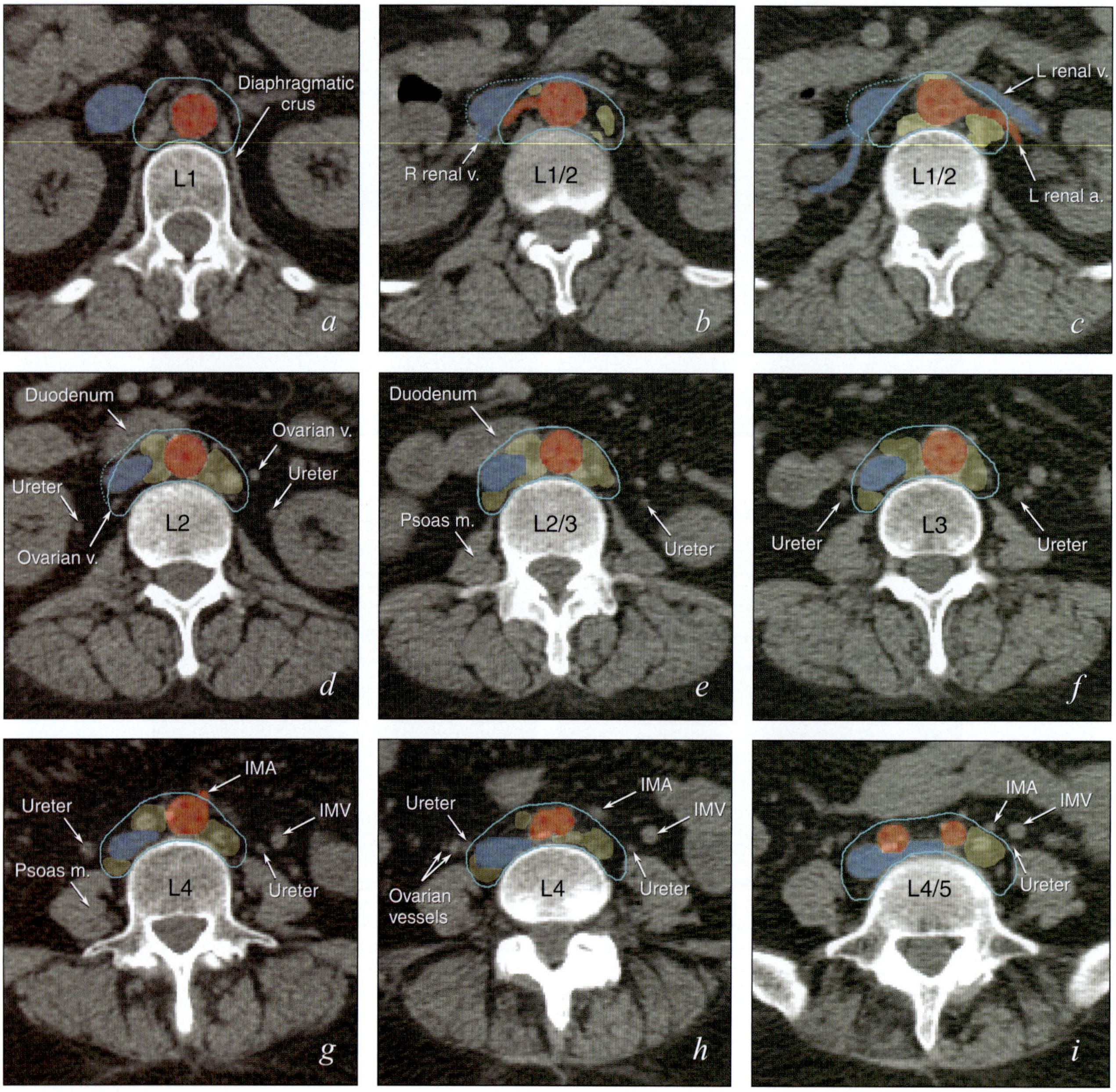

FIGURE 5.9 Paraaortic anatomy and target volume definition. Shown are axial CT slices from the diaphragmatic crus to the bifurcation of the aorta. Selected venous and arterial structures are highlighted in *blue* and *red*, respectively. The *khaki* structures represent the amalgamated contours of 35 PET-positive lymph nodes in 17 patients with cervical cancer. Nodes were mapped to a single patient's CT scan using deformable image registration; some node contours were edited to more accurately reflect their relationships to vascular structures and avoid overlap with adjacent bowel. Suggested CTV margins are indicated in *cyan*. (IMA, inferior mesenteric artery; IMV, inferior mesenteric vein.)

Most paraaortic nodal metastases are located to the left of the aorta or in the aortocaval spaces. However, metastases can also be found in the right retrocaval space, particularly distal to the right renal vessels. Nodes may be found well to the left of the aorta but are very rarely seen to the right of the vena cava, reflecting the asymmetric fetal development described in Figure 5.1. Therefore, because the aorta is typically at or slightly to the left of midline, the nodes are approximately centered over the vertebral bodies. Distal to approximately L2, the medial margins of the psoas muscles serve as useful guides for the lateral borders of the CTV (*d–i*). More proximally, the psoas muscle diminishes, but the CTV should still include at least a 1.5- to 2-cm lateral margin on the aorta (*a–c*).

The origin of the inferior mesenteric artery (*g*) is often used as a guide to describe the level of nodal metastases. However, the inferior mesenteric artery (*g, h*), inferior mesenteric vein (*f–i*), and ureters (*d–i*) are not associated with any lymph nodes per se; therefore, the CTV should not be expanded specifically to include these structures. Metastases directly anterior to the aorta (*c*) are rare.

FIGURE 5.9 (*Continued*) The ovarian vessels *(d, h)* follow the ureters during most of their intraabdominal course. Although the associated lymphatic vessels terminate in nodes adjacent to the renal vessels, there are no nodes along the distal course of the ovarian vessels and these vessels are not typically part of the regional target volume. The paths of the right and left ovarian veins differ. The left ovarian vein usually drains into the left renal vein 5 to 10 mm lateral to the aorta (between *c* and *d*); cancers from the ovary and uterine fundus can metastasize directly via this route to nodes in the space posterior and immediately distal to the left renal vessels *(c, d)*. From there, the lymphatic channels pass behind the renal vessels. Because nodes are rarely if ever seen anterior to the left renal vessels, we typically place our CTV border between the left renal artery and vein, minimizing the volume of bowel in the PTV in this region. In contrast, the right ovarian vein inserts directly into the vena cava distal to the renal veins *(d)*. On the right, metastases from ovarian cancer are usually posterior to the vena cava or in the aortocaval space. Nodal metastases are rarely seen to the right of the vena cava at this level; in patients with cervical cancer, it is reasonable to exclude the lateral vena cava in this region to spare kidney and duodenum *(dotted line, b–d)*. However, if there is extensive lymphadenopathy in the adjacent retrocaval or aortocaval space, it may be wise to use a more expansive target volume *(solid line, b–d)*, particularly for patients with adnexal primary tumors.

Note: To account for setup uncertainties, these nodal CTVs must be expanded (usually by 6 to 7 mm) to account for setup variability; the resulting PTV should be used to generate the final plan.

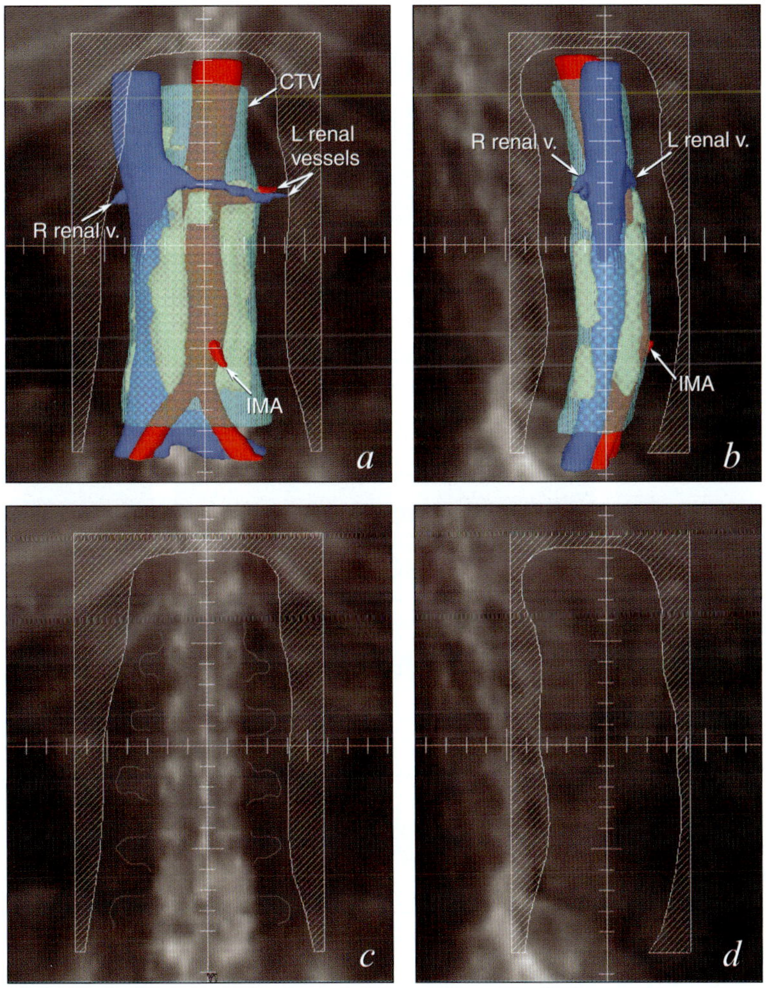

FIGURE 5.10 Relationship between regional target volumes and typical paraaortic field arrangements. AP *(a)* and right lateral *(b)* views of a three-dimensional reconstruction of CTV contours *(cyan overlay)*, selected vascular structures, and amalgamated nodal contours that were depicted as axial contours in Figure 5.9. Contours are superimposed on a digitally reconstructed radiograph with suggested AP and lateral fields. In *c* and *d*, fields are shown without superimposed structures to more clearly demonstrate the relationship between suggested field borders and bony landmarks. The transverse processes, which are difficult to appreciate on the reconstruction, are lightly outlined in *gray*. (IMA, inferior mesenteric artery.)

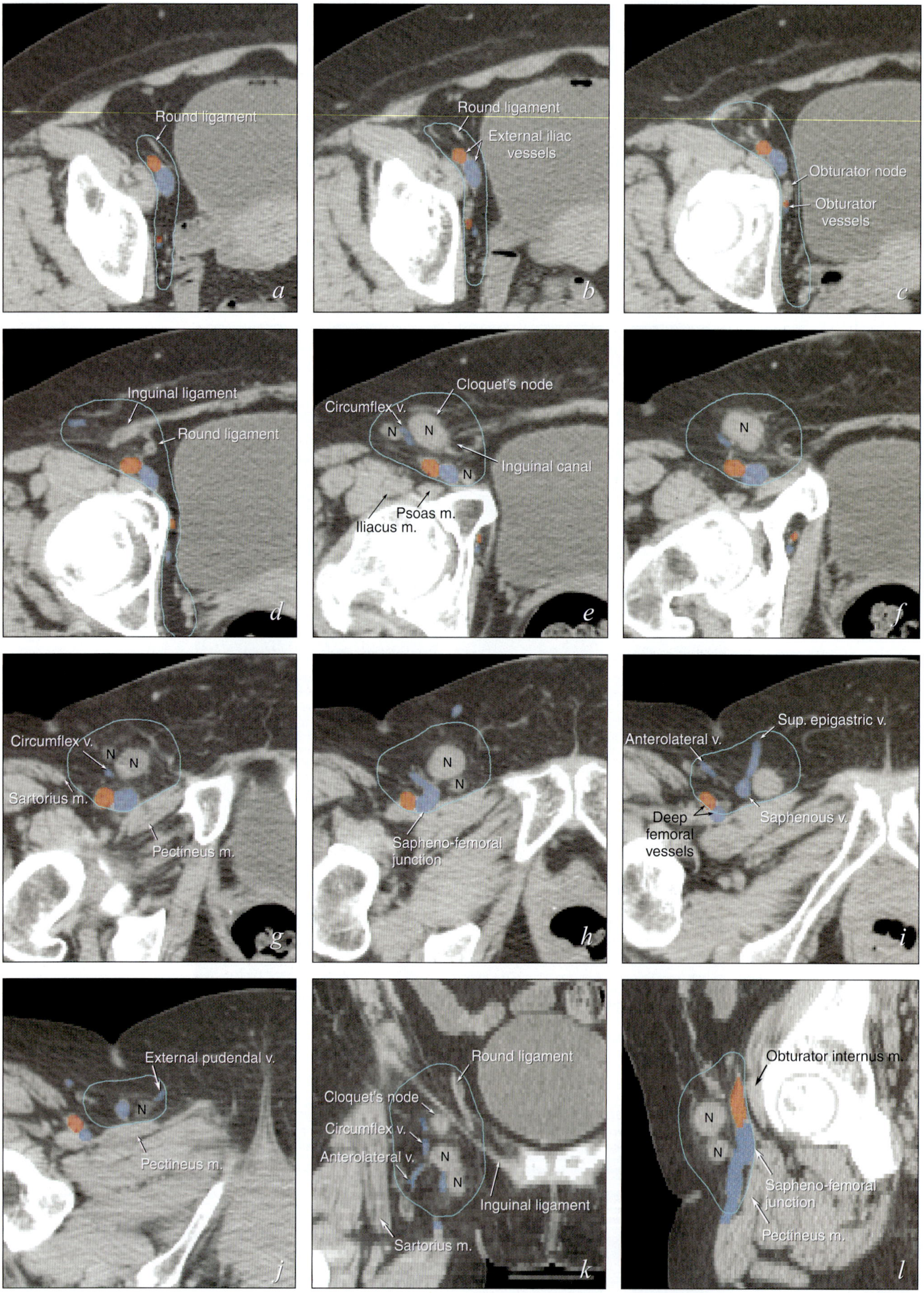
Round ligament
a
Round ligament
External iliac vessels
b
Obturator node
Obturator vessels
c
Inguinal ligament
Round ligament
d
Cloquet's node
Circumflex v.
N
N
Inguinal canal
N
Psoas m.
Iliacus m.
e
N
f
Circumflex v.
N
N
Sartorius m.
Pectineus m.
g
N
N
Sapheno-femoral junction
h
Sup. epigastric v.
Anterolateral v.
Deep femoral vessels
Saphenous v.
i
External pudendal v.
N
Pectineus m.
j
Round ligament
Cloquet's node
Circumflex v.
Anterolateral v.
N
N
Inguinal ligament
Sartorius m.
k
Obturator internus m.
N
N
Sapheno-femoral junction
Pectineus m.
l

FIGURE 5.11 (*Previous page*) **Anatomy of the inguinofemoral region.** Ten axial CT sections extending from the distal pelvis (*a*) to the level of the external pudendal vein (*j*) and digitally reconstructed coronal (*k*) and sagittal (*l*) views through the groin. This patient had abnormal nodes ("N") in many of the typical sites of vulvar nodal metastasis. The patient was scanned in a "frog-leg" position with legs abducted and externally rotated. *Cyan lines* indicate borders of the CTV suggested for patients who require comprehensive treatment of the inguinofemoral nodes for gynecologic cancer. To account for setup variability, this CTV would be expanded by 7 to 10 mm to create a PTV for treatment planning. (N, lymph node; Sup, superior.)

The inguinal nodal CTV cannot be adequately specified using a fixed margin around the femoral and saphenous vessels because important potential sites of nodal metastastasis lie along vascular tributaries that extend laterally and medially from the region of the sapheno-femoral junction.

The nodes most commonly involved in cases of vulvar cancer lie anteromedial to the femoral vessels and along the proximal portions of the saphenous, superior epigastric, and pudendal vessels. Cloquet's node (*e, f, k*) lies in the inguinal canal anterior to the femoral artery and is a frequent site of early groin involvement. The region anteromedial to the sapheno-femoral junction (*h, l*) is also a common site of involvement. Occasionally, nodes are seen immediately distal to the sapheno-femoral junction between the saphenous and deep femoral veins (*i*). In general, the medial border of the pectineus muscle is a useful guide for the medial limit of the inguinofemoral target volume unless there is massive lymph node involvement extending beyond this border.

The lateral nodes along the circumflex vessels (*e–g, k*) are not sentinel nodes for gynecologic cancers, but they are frequently secondarily involved in patients who have primary nodal metastases to the inguinofemoral region. The tissues adjacent to the circumflex vessels (up to the medial edge of the sartorius muscle) should always be included in the target volume for patients with vulvar cancer and for patients who have evidence of groin involvement from other gynecologic cancers. However, this region (lateral to the common femoral and saphenous vessels) may be excluded in most cases of distal vaginal cancer if gross disease does not extend distal to the hymenal ring and if the left and right inguinal regions are negative on imaging. Note that the suggested contours do not extend to include tissue posterior to the femoral vessels (*e–i*). Nodes are rarely if ever seen in this region, and expansion of contours behind the femoral vessels typically results in a higher dose to the femoral heads.

The first intrapelvic nodes that are typically involved in patients with vulvar cancer lie lateral to the round ligament and anterior and medial to the external iliac vessels as they enter the inguinal canal **(CS 12.8a)**. This nodal region is rarely involved in cases of localized cervical cancer but should be treated whenever the vulva or distal vagina is involved with cancer. The round ligament (*a–d, k*) provides a useful guide for designation of the medial border of the target volume as the external iliac vessels approach the inguinal canal from the pelvis.

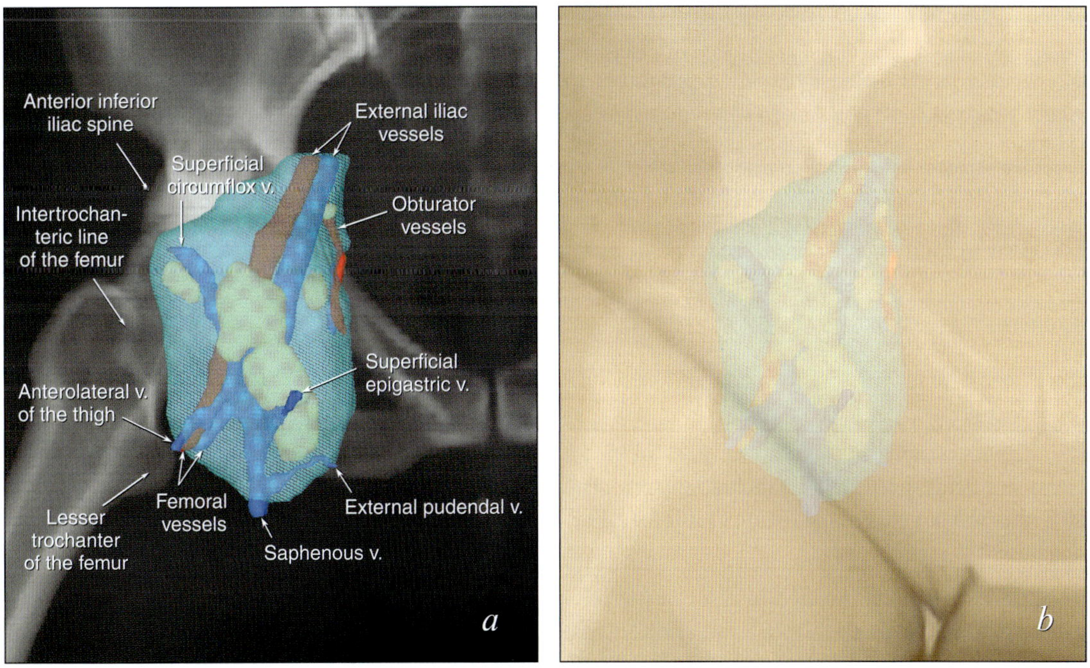

FIGURE 5.12 Three-dimensional anatomy of the inguinofemoral region. Three-dimensional view of the anatomy and contours depicted in Figure 5.11. (*a*) Volumes are superimposed on a digitally reconstructed radiograph to show the relationships between the vascular anatomy, CTV (*cyan cloud*), and underlying skeletal structures. Note the relationship between the inferolateral margin of the CTV and the intertrochanteric line; an inferolateral border through or just below this line on an AP field generally provides adequate margin around the target volume but also includes the entire femoral head and neck. For this reason, a various techniques have been developed to spare the femoral heads when this volume is treated. The anterior inferior iliac spine (not to be confused with the superior iliac spine) provides a landmark for the superolateral margin, and the lesser trochanter usually marks the distal limit of the target volume. The nodal GTVs for this patient were contoured in *khaki* and included to give a sense of the relationship between the nodes and vessels. Additional information about this patient's history and outcome are in Case Study 12.8. (*b*) A transparent skin rendering has been superimposed to demonstrate the relationship between surface landmarks and the target volume. Note that most of the target is superior to the inguinal skin fold. Skin landmarks are not a reliable guide for placement of inguinal radiation treatment fields.

TABLE 5.1 Direct Sites of Nodal Drainage According to Sites of Tumor Involvement[a]

Site of involvement	Lymph node regions						
	Aortic[b]	**Common iliac**	**Internal iliac**	**External iliac**	**Presacral**	**Pararectal**	**Inguinal**
Ovary	+++	+	++	?			+ (rare)
Fallopian tube	+++	+	++	?			+ (rare)
Uterus							
Fundus	++	+[c]	+++	+	+ (rare)		+ (rare)
Isthmus	?	+[c]	+++	++	+ (rare)		
Cervix		+[c]	+++	++	+	+ (rare)	
Uterosacral ligament			+++		++	++	
Vagina							
Apex		+[c]	+++	++			
Middle			+++	+			
Distal[d]			+++	+			++
Posterior wall			+++	++	+[e]	+[e]	
Vulva			+ (rare)[f]				+++
Anterior abdominal wall				+			++
Nodal regions							
Inguino-femoral			++	++			
Internal iliac		+++					
External iliac		+++					
Common iliac	+++						

[a]*If tumors involve multiple sites, all of the nodes that those sites drain to must be considered at risk. Plus signs indicate the relative frequency of metastases to each site, with +++ indicating the most frequent sites of nodal metastasis.*

[b]*Including the right paracaval, aortocaval, and left paraaortic nodes.*

[c]*Nodal metastases are very frequently found at the point where the common iliac vessels bifurcate into the external and internal iliac vessels. These "junctional" nodes are sometimes labeled as common iliac. Whether the more proximal common iliac nodes are ever direct sites of metastasis from the cervix is uncertain, but they are frequently involved at least secondarily.*

[d]*The vestibule of the vagina drains primarily to the inguinal nodes. Because there is an extensive plexus of anastomosing lymphatics bridging the vestibule and distal vagina, the inguinal nodes that lie medial to the femoral and saphenous veins should be treated if tumors involving the vagina are close to the hymenal ring. If the medial nodes are suspicious or involved, the lateral nodes should also be treated.*

[e]*Particularly frequent for tumors involving the rectovaginal septum.*

[f]*Theoretically, tumors involving the vestibule and clitoris can metastasize directly to internal iliac nodes, although this is vary rare.*

Definition of the Proximal and Distal Limits of the Nodal Target Volume

In general, treatment fields should at least include any *primary echelon nodes* within the targeted nodal region (Table 5.1). For example:

- When pelvic nodes are being targeted in cases of uterine, cervical, or proximal vaginal cancers, radiation fields should at least encompass all primary echelon nodes, including those found at the junction between the external iliac, internal iliac, and common iliac vessels (at the common iliac bifurcations). Pelvic treatments that are delivered using fields that extend proximally to the L4/L5 interspace typically include this region with a 1- to 2-cm margin. However, a more extended field is required to achieve full coverage of the common iliac nodes.
- When paraaortic nodes are included in the target volume for cancers involving the uterine fundus, tubes, or ovaries, the CTV should include primary echelon nodes at and just below the renal vessels (Figs. 5.9 and 5.10). Because the level of insertion of the renal vessels is inconsistent (Fig. 5.3), the vertebral level of the proximal field border may vary.

In many cases, the proximal field border (or CTV) is extended to encompass *secondary echelon nodes* that receive lymphatic drainage from the primary echelon region. In these cases, the upper limit of the CTV must be based on an estimate of the probability of microscopic nodal infiltration, which generally diminishes with increasing proximal distance from the region of primary echelon drainage. In most cases, the target should extend at least 4 cm proximal to known sites of involvement. However, many factors can influence decisions about placement of the proximal field border, including the following:

- The extent of distal lymph node involvement.
- The sensitivity of imaging studies used to evaluate lymph node involvement.

- The histologic subtype and grade of the cancer.
- After lymph node dissection, the quality of information about the location(s) of involved nodes and the several nodes examined proximal to involved nodes.
- The risk of short- and long-term side effects of extended-field treatment.

Because valves in the lymphatic vessels direct flow proximally from the pelvis (toward the thoracic duct), the distal limit of the nodal CTV is usually defined by the primary echelon drainage. However, under rare circumstances, massive lymphadenopathy can be associated with retrograde metastasis; in these cases, some distal extension of the nodal CTV may be justified. For example, if massive external iliac lymphadenopathy is present, the CTV may be extended to cover the proximal femoral nodes.

Targeting of Grossly Involved Lymph Nodes

Because there are rarely curative options for in-field nodal recurrences, the importance of correct identification of grossly involved nodes cannot be overstated. In recent years, new imaging modalities, including PET–CT, have improved our ability to identify involved lymph nodes and IMRT has improved our ability to deliver a sterilizing radiation dose without serious side effects. These tools have greatly facilitated the treatment of patients with gross lymph node involvement. Today, even patients with extensive pelvic and aortic metastases can often be cured (**CS 10.6, 10.10, 11.2, 13.7**). However, the contouring of target volumes for such cases is labor-intensive and requires attention to detail.

In general, the dose required to achieve local control of a lymph node involved with carcinoma increases with the size of the metastasis. Although 45 Gy is usually sufficient to control microscopic lymph node involvement, this dose is not adequate to control involved lymph nodes larger than about 1 to 1.5 cm in minimum diameter, even with administration of concurrent chemotherapy and may be insufficient to control smaller nodes if they are heavily involved. Whenever possible, lymph nodes that are believed to be grossly involved with tumor should be treated to a minimum dose of 60 Gy. For nodes larger than 3 to 4 cm in diameter, doses of 65 Gy or more are probably required to achieve high control rates, although the dose must often be tempered if there are concerns about normal tissue tolerance.

When tumor has invaded adjacent soft tissue or bone, a generous CTV margin (usually at least 1 cm beyond known gross disease) should be added to account for possible microscopic tumor infiltration.

Nodes that have apparently responded completely to chemotherapy probably still require more than 45 Gy. Although data on this subject are sparse, sites of initial gross lymph node involvement should receive a dose of 55 to 60 Gy, depending on the size of the resulting target volume and normal tissue constraints. However, unless they were directly infiltrated by tumor, critical structures that have fallen into the pretreatment location of responding lymph nodes should not be included in the CTV.

Before contouring is begun, all diagnostic imaging studies, including any performed before surgery or chemotherapy, should be reviewed and, if possible, fused with the planning CT scan (Chapter 4). PET is particularly helpful, but contrast-enhanced CT scans and MRI images can also facilitate identification of enlarged nodes. Lymph nodes at different risk levels (and potentially requiring different doses) should be contoured as separate targets for treatment planning.

When contouring is complete, coronal and sagittal reconstructed images should be carefully reviewed to check for accuracy and to confirm that grossly enlarged lymph nodes have been fully included in the contours. If there is any uncertainty about the interpretation of imaging findings, a diagnostic radiologist should be consulted.

Large nodes that are adjacent to critical structures should be monitored for their response to treatment. As large tumor masses regress, bowel or other uninvolved structures may shift into the region of high radiation dose (Chapter 6; **CS 10.6, 15.2**); in some cases, a mid-treatment adjustment of the plan can reduce the radiation dose of these structures.

For very large nodal masses, nested interior GTVs can be specified to treat the central portion of the node to a higher dose per fraction than the overall PTV-expanded GTV (**CS 12.8, 13.7, 14.8, 15.1–15.4**). Some practitioners use this approach in an effort to accelerate the response of very large tumor masses to facilitate boost planning. However the ultimate impact on local control is unknown; the periphery of the tumor (with PTV margin) must still be treated to a minimum dose of 60 Gy to achieve a reasonable probability of tumor control. Critical structures should be excluded from the hypofractionated volume and even modest hypofractionation of a portion of the target should be done only with close monitoring and adaptive planning as needed.

Special Considerations After Lymph Node Dissection

Factors influencing the decision whether to treat a patient with grossly involved lymph nodes using radiation alone or a combination of surgery and radiation are discussed in Chapter 3. However, if a patient is referred for treatment after resection or partial resection of involved nodes, several factors should be considered in the designation of targets for postoperative radiation therapy:

- *A thorough search should be performed for residual disease.* Even after lymph node dissection, enlarged lymph nodes are frequently left behind (**CS 12.1**). In particular, even the most experienced surgeon can have difficulty identifying or removing nodes in the distal obturator, posterior aortocaval, and left pararenal regions. Preoperative imaging should always be compared with postoperative imaging to confirm that all gross disease was removed.

- *Sites of residual disease or extracapsular extension (ECE) that require a boost dose should be identified.* Studies of radiation therapy for vulvar cancer and nongynecologic sites suggest that nodal ECE is a risk factor for recurrence after radiation therapy.[6–8] Although fewer data are available correlating ECE with disease control in the iliac or aortic nodes,[9] all regions of ECE should be considered to be at increased risk for recurrence; whenever possible, these areas should be boosted to a total dose of 55 to 60 Gy. Unfortunately, it is sometimes difficult to identify the precise site of ECE. Pathology reports, operative reports, and findings on preoperative imaging can yield important clues. If consulted preoperatively, the radiation oncologist should request placement of radio-opaque clips in sites of possible residual disease. However, surgeons also use metallic clips for hemostatic and other purposes; these should not be assumed to be markers of disease without confirmation by the surgeon.

- *Lymphocysts are common after extensive lymph node dissection.* The risk for involvement of the cyst itself is not well understood. If the lymph node dissection revealed no nodal metastases in the region of the lymphocyst, it should not be necessary to include the entire cyst in the target volume. If, however, there was extracapsular extension or extensive nodal disease in the bed of the lymphocyst, or if the relationship between the lymphocyst and site of nodal disease is uncertain, it may be wise to include the entire cyst at least in the CTV. Lymphocysts can enlarge or shrink during treatment; if fluctuation in the size of the lymphocyst would influence the validity of the treatment plan, lymphocysts should be monitored with CT every 1 to 2 weeks.

REPRODUCTIVE ORGANS

Ovaries

The ovaries first appear early during embryogenesis as indifferent gonads situated adjacent to the primitive kidneys on the dorsal abdominal wall. Peritoneal folds connecting the gonads to the labioscrotal swellings of the ventral abdominal wall form cords termed the *gubernacula*. In males, the gonads eventually descend via the gubernacula through the inguinal canal into the scrotal sacs. In females, each gubernaculum contacts and fuses with the lateral uterine fundus. This attachment restricts the descent of the ovary, which comes to rest near the uterine horn at the opening of the fallopian tube (**Fig. 5.13**). The proximal portion of the gubernaculum forms the *utero-ovarian ligament*; the distal portion forms the *round ligament*, which extends from the lateral uterine fundus and passes through the inguinal canal to terminate within the labium majus of the vulva (**Fig. 5.13**).

Lymphatic Drainage

The ovarian vessels follow the path of descent of the ovaries. For this reason, the lymphatic drainage of the left ovary is primarily to aortic nodes located at the insertion of the left ovarian vein in the renal vein, and the lymphatic drainage of the right ovary is primarily to aortocaval lymph nodes near the insertion of the right ovarian vein in the vena cava, usually just below the renal vessels. In the distal abdomen, the ovarian vessels run alongside the ureters lateral to the anterior psoas muscles until they turn medially to terminate in the aortic nodes. The ovarian lymphatic vessels themselves are not punctuated by nodes in their distal lumbar course, are rarely if ever sites of metastasis, and do not need to be included in radiation target volumes (**Fig. 5.7**).

Anastomoses between ovarian and uterine lymphatics within the mesovarium (the portion of the broad ligament that encloses and suspends the ovary) also provide a path for metastatic spread of disease from the ovaries to the iliac nodes.

Because the normal ovary usually rests in a slight depression on the pelvic wall near the obturator vessels, it is sometimes mistaken for an enlarged obturator lymph node (or vice versa). Also, in young women, the ovary is typically at least somewhat fluorodeoxyglucose avid on PET.

Fallopian Tubes

The fallopian tubes develop from the proximal unfused portions of the embryonic müllerian ducts and are situated in the upper margins of the broad ligaments.

Lymphatic Drainage

The fallopian tubes are supplied by anastomosing branches of the uterine and ovarian vessels. Branches of the ovarian vessels within the mesosalpinx (the portion of the broad ligament between the ovary and tube) create a route of lymphatic metastasis from the tube and lateral uterine fundus directly to the aortic nodes that receive lymphatic drainage from the ovary (**Table 5.1**). The lymphatic vessels that supply the round ligaments also emanate from this region and provide a rare but well-recognized route of primary lymphatic metastasis from the tube, ovary, and uterine fundus to the groin.

Uterus

The caudal portions of the müllerian ducts fuse to form the fetal uterovaginal primordium, which eventually gives rise to the epithelium and glands of the uterus, cervix, and apical vagina; the stroma and myometrium are derived from the surrounding mesenchyme.

The adult uterus is pear-shaped and has a muscular wall that is usually 1 to 2 cm thick. A slight constriction in the middle of the uterus marks the *internal os*; the portion of the uterus above the internal os is the *body*, and the portion of the uterus below the internal os is the *cervix* of the uterus. The dome of the uterus (above the openings of the tubes) is termed the *fundus* (**Fig. 5.13**).

The normal uterus is highly mobile (discussed later in this chapter). However, when the bladder is empty, the uterus typically rests on top of the bladder at an approximately right angle to the axis of the vagina. This position can make it difficult to visualize and contour the cervix accurately on axial CT slices. Because the cervix projects into the anterior vaginal wall, the anterior lip of the cervix is usually inferior to

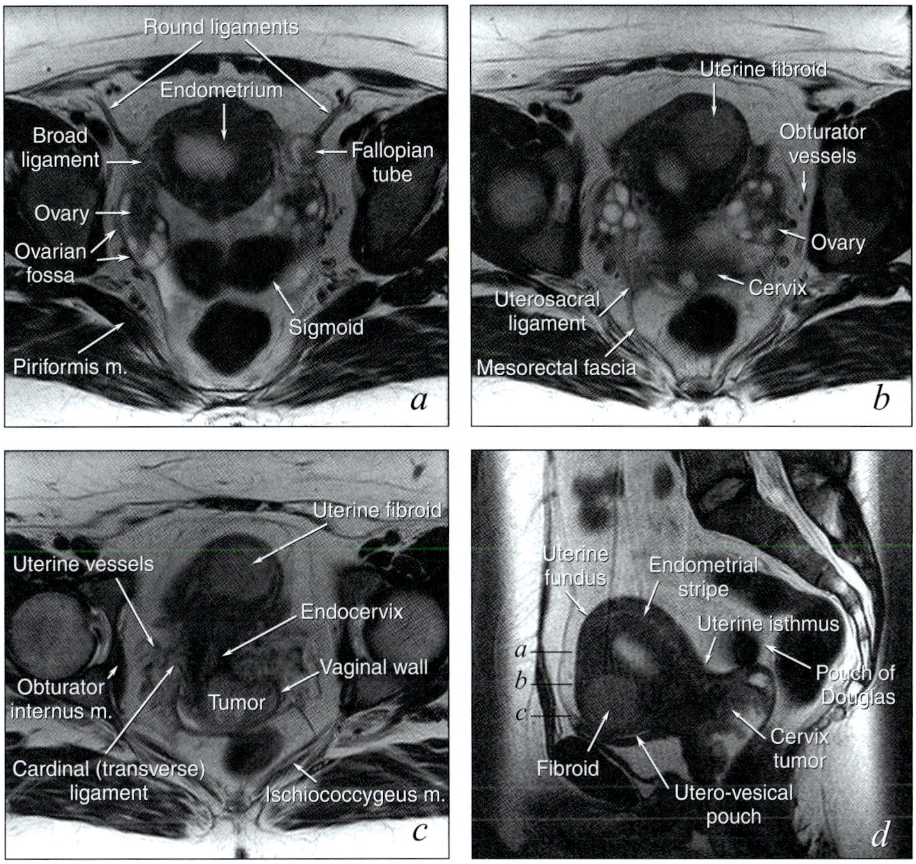

FIGURE 5.13 Anatomy of the uterus. Axial views (*a–c*) and a midline sagittal view (*d*) through the uterus of a 34-year-old woman with a stage IB2 carcinoma involving anterior and posterior lips of the cervix. The levels of the axial views are indicated on (*d*). The cardinal ligaments are located between the obturator internus muscle and the cervix (*c*), and the round ligaments extend from the horns of the uterus through the inguinal canal to their termination in the vulva (*a*). The uterosacral ligaments are continuous with the mesorectal fascia; advanced cervical cancers can extend directly to the cardinal and proximal uterosacral ligaments, which should be included in radiation fields.

The ovaries (*a, b*), of this young woman, included several corpus luteum cysts. Although they can be more medially located, the ovaries are often situated in a slight depression on the lateral pelvic wall where they can sometimes be confused with enlarged nodes. In this example, the bladder was nearly empty, and the uterus was in an anteverted position perpendicular to the axis of the vagina. The cervix usually protrudes into the anterior vaginal wall (*d*); in this typical position, the anterior lip of the cervix is located inferior to the posterior lip. The uterus, which in this case contains a small fibroid, is covered by peritoneum and is bounded anteriorly by the uterovesical pouch and posteriorly by the pouch of Douglas. The cervix is covered by peritoneum posteriorly but is separated from the bladder by only a thin layer of fascia anteriorly.

the posterior lip (**Fig. 5.13**). The uterus typically has a slight anterior curve; it can also in some cases have an anterior or, more rarely, posterior (retro) flexion at the level of the internal os. An awareness of the uterine position and degree of flexion is particularly important during sounding for intracavitary brachytherapy (Chapter 8).

The uterine body is covered with peritoneum. Posteriorly, the peritoneal surface extends downward from the body to cover the cervix and part of the apical vagina before reflecting onto the anterior rectal surface. The resulting *uterorectal pouch (pouch of Douglas)* typically contains portions of the sigmoid colon and terminal ileum. Anteriorly, the peritoneum reflects onto the bladder at the level of the internal os, forming the *uterovesical pouch*, which is typically empty but can also contain loops of bowel. The supravaginal portion of the anterior cervix is below this peritoneal reflection, separated from the bladder wall by a thin fascial layer that is continuous with the parametrium and cardinal ligament. This portion of the cervix is the most frequent site of a close or positive deep surgical margin after radical hysterectomy for cervical cancer. After hysterectomy, the space superior to the vaginal apex between the posterior bladder and anterior rectal serosal surfaces is sometimes termed the *cul-de-sac*.

The close anatomic relationships between the uterus, bladder, rectum, sigmoid, and terminal ileum have important implications for external beam radiation therapy and brachytherapy treatment planning.

Uterine Ligaments

As the müllerian ducts fuse, they bring together peritoneal folds that form the broad ligaments, cardinal ligaments, and uterosacral ligaments; these folds also form the boundaries of the uterorectal and uterovesical pouches (Fig. 5.13). The broad ligaments extend from the sides of the uterus to the lateral pelvic walls and contain a layer of connective tissue termed the parametrium. Bands of fibrous connective tissue at the base of the broad ligaments form the *cardinal ligaments* (also termed the Mackenrodt ligaments or transverse ligaments of the pelvis); the cardinal ligaments connect medially to the cervix and vaginal fornix and laterally to the connective tissues of the iliac vessels and fascia of the obturator internus muscles. When the cardinal ligament is involved by direct tumor extension, the clinical findings typically include both parametrial nodularity and infiltration of the ipsilateral vaginal fornix.

The *uterine artery* passes from its origin in the anterior branch of the internal iliac artery through the broad ligament at the superior margin of the cardinal ligament; the uterine artery crosses the ureter at approximately the level of the internal os of the uterus and then ascends along the lateral margin of the uterus, finally anastomosing with the ovarian artery at the uterine horn. Lymphatics from the uterus also pass through the broad ligament.

The uterorectal folds that form the lateral bounds of the pouch of Douglas contain fibrous tissue and nonstriated muscle fibers that pass from the uterus to the sacrum and piriformis muscles and constitute the *uterosacral ligaments.* Cancer can extend from the cervix through the uterorectal folds along the uterosacral ligament and, in advanced cases, can invade the piriformis muscle. This region must be included in the target volume for locally advanced cervical cancers.

Lymphatic Drainage

The lymphatics of the uterus are contained in three plexuses: one located beneath the basement membrane of the endometrium, one within the myometrium, and one beneath the serosal surface. There do not appear to be any lymphatic vessels within the endometrium itself; for this reason, nodal metastasis of cancers limited to the endometrium is extremely rare.

The lymphatic drainage patterns of the uterine body and cervix are similar except that the uterine fundus contains lymphatics that drain directly to the aortic nodes (via ovarian lymphatics) or, rarely, to the inguinal nodes (via round ligament lymphatics), whereas the cervix does not (discussed above, Table 5.1).

The primary lymphatic trunks from the uterine body and cervix pass into the broad ligament with the uterine vessels at the level of the internal os. Afferent lymphatics from the uterine body and cervix drain primarily to the internal and external iliac nodes (Fig. 5.2). Parametrial nodes, typically located where the uterine arteries cross the ureters, can be early sites of distant metastasis from cervical cancer.

After simple hysterectomy, the residual broad ligament and associated lymphatics retract and lie along the pelvic wall between the obturator internus muscle and adjacent bladder or bowel. This region should always be included in the postoperative target volume for uterine or cervical cancers (Fig. 5.7 k, l); if tumor is reported to be involving the posthysterectomy parametrial margin, this retracted tissue usually requires an increased dose of radiation (CS 10.2).

Cervical cancers can also metastasize to pararectal and sacral nodes (Figs. 5.2 and 5.6), although this is rare with tumors that are clinically confined to the cervix. Metastasis of cervical cancers to aortic lymph nodes is very rare in the absence of iliac node involvement.

Uterine Movement

The cardinal, uterosacral, and round ligaments, together with the muscles of the vagina and perineum, support the uterus and help to maintain its position in the pelvis. The uterine ligaments are also sufficiently elastic to accommodate large tilts and shifts in uterine position with coitus and pregnancy and with changes in bladder and rectal volume. Although the cervix is somewhat less mobile than the fundus of the uterus, shifts of 2 cm or more are not unusual (Fig. 5.14).[5]

Intratreatment uterine motion is difficult to predict but must always be considered when the uterus and cervix are included in a radiation therapy target volume. If inverse planning is being used to target the uterus and cervix, the following should be included in the ITV:

- A volume encompassing the positions of the uterus, cervix, and vagina (at least 3 cm beyond the most distal disease) as seen on full and empty bladder scans.
- At least the anterior rectum to within 1 to 1.5 cm of the posterior rectal wall (to account for variations in rectal volume; Fig. 5.14a, b).
- The uterosacral ligaments (Fig. 5.13); in cases of locally advanced disease, the entire pararectal space including the mesorectal fascia.
- The broad ligaments (i.e., all extraperitoneal tissue between the uterus and lateral pelvic wall).
- Regional lymph nodes as discussed above in the section "Regional Lymph Nodes."

In many cases, the large margins needed to account for uterine motion and possible sites of parauterine extension leave little or no room for IMRT to improve upon image-based four-field treatments of the pelvis (CS 10.6; Fig 6.7).

Vagina

The vagina extends from the vaginal fornices to the hymen. The *vestibule of the vagina* (sometimes called the *vaginal introitus*) extends from the hymen to the fimbrial edges of the labia minora and is generally considered to be part of the vulva; however, much of the vestibule is covered by epithelium identical to vaginal epithelium. The cervix projects into the anterior wall of the vagina, forming the vaginal fornices. Because of this, the posterior vaginal wall is usually considerably longer than the anterior vaginal wall. When the cervix is expanded by tumor, the distal, anterior aspect of the cervix can be mistaken for vaginal involvement leading to an overestimate of the tumor stage (Fig. 4.4).

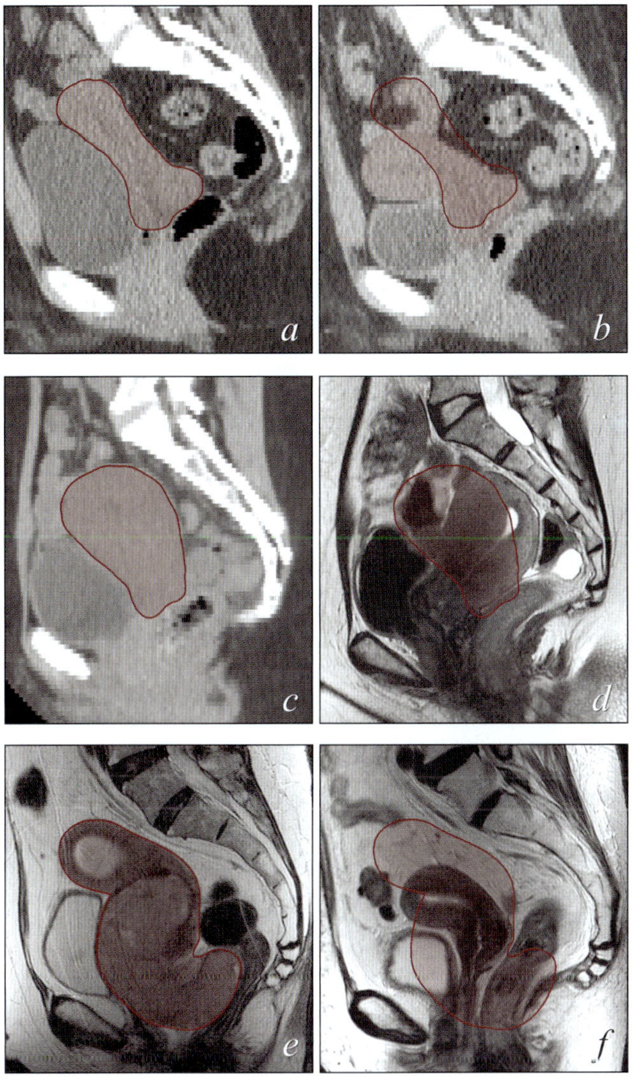

FIGURE 5.14 Variations in uterine position within the pelvis. Many factors can influence the position of the uterus within the pelvis. In each of the three cases illustrated in this figure, the position of the uterus outlined in the left panel (*a, c, e*) was superimposed on the right (*b, d, f*) to demonstrate the change in uterine position. Patient 1 (*a, b*). Simulation CT scans obtained before (*a*) and immediately after (*b*) the patient evacuated her bladder. The patient also appears to have passed some gas, contributing to an ~1-cm shift in the position of the cervix. In addition, the uterus, which initially appeared to have an axial configuration (*a*), has a marked anterior flexion in the second scan (*b*). Patient 2 (*c, d*). A planning CT scan and an MRI image obtained in the same week show a dramatic change in the position of the uterus from slightly anteverted to markedly retroverted and a shift in the position of the anterior and posterior cervical lips by more than 3 cm. In this case, a tightly conformal plan based on either position would have inadequately treated tumor that was grossly involving the cervix and distal two-thirds of the myometrium. Patient 3 (*e, f*). Images obtained before treatment (*e*) and after 4 weeks of chemoradiation (*f*). Some of the most dramatic shifts in uterine position occur as tumor responds to radiation therapy, as illustrated by this example. Potential variations in the position of the uterus must be considered whenever the uterus or cervix is a target for radiation therapy; to avoid underdosage of the target volume, a realistic uterine ITV must designated before a treatment plan is developed.

The posterior fornix of the vagina abuts the rectovaginal pouch and therefore has a serosal surface. Otherwise, the proximal portion of the vagina above the pelvic floor lies between the rectum and bladder, and the distal half of the vagina lies within the perineum between the urethra and anus. Because of these close relationships, the treatment of cancers involving the vagina can be particularly challenging.

Lymphatic Drainage

The vagina arises from müllerian tissue that comes into contact with the urogenital sinus at the site of the future vaginal hymen. Sinus cells proliferate to form the distal vagina and populate the vaginal epithelium. Distal to the hymen, the urogenital sinus shortens to form the vestibule of the vagina (considered part of the vulva). The vagina's complex pattern of lymphatic drainage reflects this embryological development and the close relationship between the vagina and adjacent structures.

Lymphatics of the apical vagina accompany the uterine vessels and drain to the external and internal iliac nodes; lymphatics of the middle vagina predominantly follow the vaginal branch of the anterior internal iliac artery and drain to internal iliac nodes; lymphatics of the vestibule drain via the internal pudendal vessels to the inguinal nodes; and lymphatics of the posterior vaginal wall, which receives part of its blood supply from the middle rectal branches of the internal iliac artery, drain to pararectal, presacral, and internal iliac nodes (Table 5.1).

These typical lymphatic drainage patterns are important, but treatment planning also must take into account the considerable anastomosis between lymphatics of these different segments of the vagina. If tumor involves the upper two-thirds of the vagina, the internal and external iliac nodes are generally treated in all cases. If tumor extends to involve the distal third of the vagina, it is customary to treat at least the medial inguinal nodes (CS 11.6, 13.9). If tumor involves the vestibule, the iliac and inguinal nodes are usually treated. If tumor involves the rectovaginal septum, the pararectal and presacral nodes should be treated in addition to the iliac nodes (Table 5.1).

Vaginal Movement and Designation of a Vaginal ITV

The vagina is mobile, and in some cases, can shift by as much as 3 cm with changes in rectal or bladder volume (Fig. 5.15).[10] For this reason, *it is never sufficient to use a simple contour of the vagina taken from a single planning CT scan for treatment planning*. However, methods that designate a vaginal ITV using a standard fixed margin tend either to underestimate vaginal motion or cover an unnecessarily large volume of bowel or bladder. For example, if the rectum is empty at the time of simulation, an anterior margin must be added to account for possible anterior displacement by rectal gas or stool; a posterior margin of similar magnitude is clearly unnecessary. Conversely, if the rectum is very full, a much greater margin will be needed posteriorly than anteriorly. Accurate assessment of the ITV requires an individualized approach that takes into account conditions at the time of simulation and potential day-to-day influences of bladder and rectal filling on the intrapelvic position of the vagina.

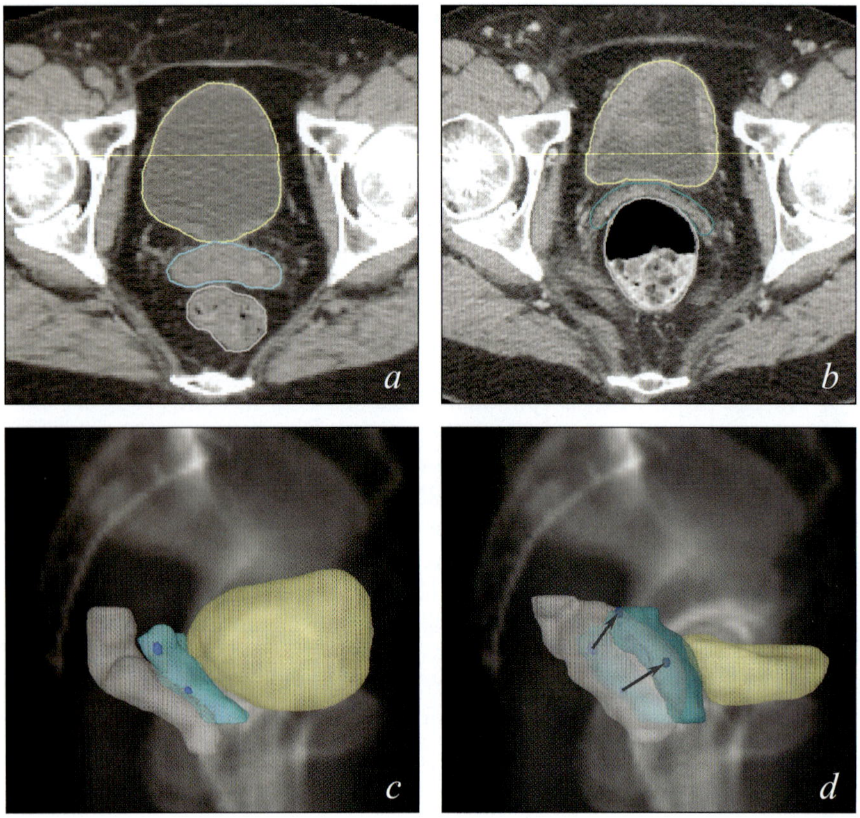

FIGURE 5.15 Influence of internal organ volume on vaginal position after hysterectomy. Images taken from treatment planning simulation (*a, c*) and from diagnostic CT performed the previous week (*b, d*) demonstrate a marked shift in the position of the vagina and changes in the volume of surrounding structures. Radio-opaque markers interstitially inserted in the vaginal wall (*dark blue* contours in *c* and *d*) shifted by 3 to 3.5 cm (*arrows, d*). The relatively full bladder in (*a*) and (*c*) contributed to the more posterior location of the bladder and rectum. Slight contraction of the perineal musculature in (*b*) and (*d*) also may have influenced the vaginal position.

Changes in rectal volume tend to move the vagina in an anterior–posterior direction. The following approaches should be used to account for changes in rectal volume:

- If the rectum is distended, the vaginal ITV should be extended posteriorly to within about 1.5 cm of the posterior rectal wall.
- If the rectum is empty, the ITV should be extended anteriorly into the bladder by at least 2 cm.
- Above the vaginal apex (at the level of the cul-de-sac), the rectum usually reflects backward toward the sacrum. Sigmoid, small bowel, or, immediately after surgery, peritoneal fluid (**Fig. 5.7**) may occupy the space between the vagina and rectum on axial view. In this region, the posterior ITV may be modified to parallel that of more distal apical slices.
- The distal third of the vagina, bounded anteriorly by the urethra and pubis (**Fig. 5.13**), is less mobile than the proximal two-thirds. However, contraction of the perineal musculature and expansion of the rectal ampulla can cause postero-inferior shifts that should be considered in target definition (**Fig. 5.15**).

Increases in bladder volume tend to extend the vagina cranially and, to a lesser extent, posteriorly although this effect varies greatly with the length of the vagina after hysterectomy and other factors.

- An excellent way to estimate the effect of bladder expansion on the vagina is to compare the location of the apex on full and empty bladder scans, ideally using fiducial markers inserted in the vaginal apex (Chapter 4, **CS 10.1**).
- Alternatively, simulation should be performed with a comfortably full bladder. A 1 to 2 cm apical (proximal) margin should be added to the ITV to account for motion and (if there are no vaginal markers) for uncertainty in the position of the apex. If the bladder is empty at the time of simulation, a much larger apical margin of 2.5 to 3 cm should be added.

Insertion of rigid vaginal obturators to identify the location of the vagina at the time of simulation is not recommended because this method can cause major deformations in the positions of the vagina, adjacent critical structures, and, if present, the uterus (**Fig. 6.2**).

Because the movement of the vagina is independent of the position of the regional lymph nodes, it is never appropriate to shift the isocenter to account for vaginal movement during treatment of the whole pelvis. However, platinum or gold interstitial fiducial markers can be used to confirm that the vaginal position remains between set boundaries (**Fig. 4.11**).

External Genitalia

In the absence of testosterone, the initially indifferent fetal genitalia develop female characteristics. The genital tubercle becomes the *glans of the clitoris*, the urogenital folds form the *labia minora*, and the labioscrotal folds form the *labia majora*, which fuse anteriorly and posteriorly to form the *labial commissures* of the mons and perineum, respectively.

The *vulva* consists of the clitoris, labia minora, labia majora, and the vestibule of the vagina (**Fig. 5.16**). The region between the posterior commissure of the labia and the anus is termed the gynecologic *perineum*. The *mons*

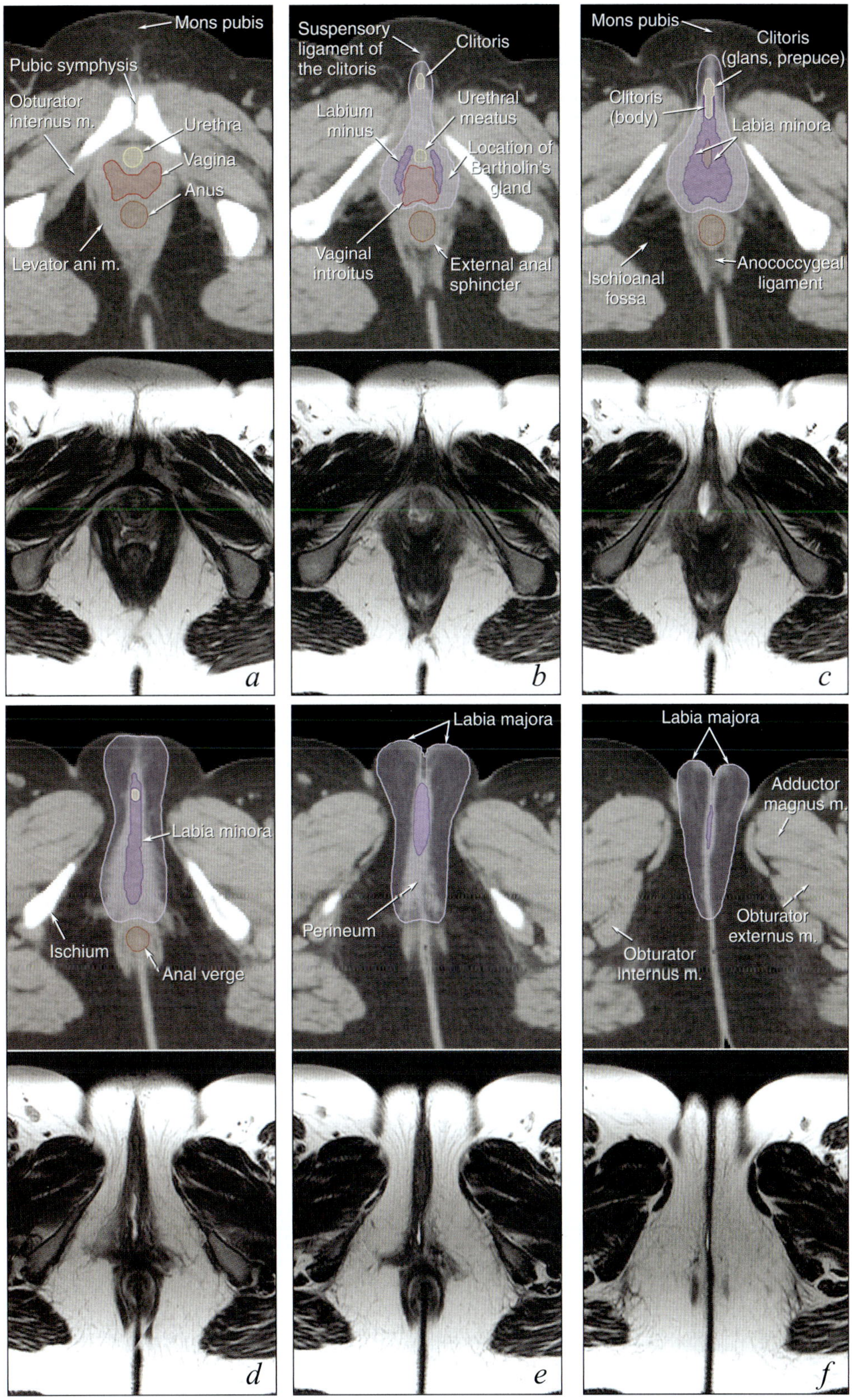

FIGURE 5.16 Anatomy of the normal vulva. Axial sections through the vulva in a 35-year-old woman with normal vulvar anatomy. A non-contrast-enhanced CT scan was digitally fused with a T2 MRI image; paired images represent comparable levels on the fused scans. On CT scans, most vulvar and perineal structures are of uniform density and therefore cannot be accurately discerned, although, the levator ani *(a)*, suspensory ligament of the clitoris *(b)*, and anus *(a–d)* can usually be identified and help to define the boundaries of the vulva. For this figure, the fused MRI images were used to locate and contour other labeled structures on the axial CT scans. Although reference to MRI can be very helpful in treatment planning, it is difficult to achieve a good fusion, particularly if a different leg position is used for the two scans. A critical part of the planning process is examination of the patient in the treatment position at the time of simulation with placement of orienting radio-opaque markers on key structures, tumor, and surgical scars. Whenever possible, this examination should be done by the same physician who will be using the simulation and reference markers to contour target volumes and critical structures.

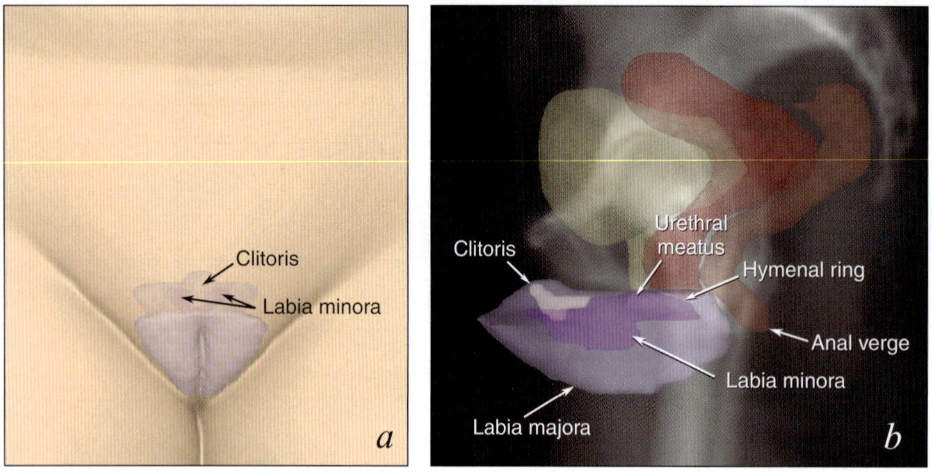

FIGURE 5.17 Three-dimensional anatomy of the normal vulva. For this figure, the contours shown in Figure 5.16 were reconstructed in three dimensions with a transparent surface rendering (*a*) and on a lateral digitally reconstructed radiograph (*b*). Note the relationships between vulvar structures, including the hymenal ring, urethral meatus, and anal verge, and the pubic ramus.

pubis is a mound of fatty tissue anterior to the anterior commissure, in front of the pubic symphysis. Although cancers involving the anterior vulva can secondarily involve the mons, it is very rare for cancers to have their origin anterior to the labial commissure.

Accurate target volume designation in the vulva is particularly challenging because the vulva lies approximately tangential to the axial plane. Also, because the individual structures of the perineum have very similar CT densities, it can be extremely difficult to identify landmarks on a planning CT scan. MRI can provide valuable information about tumor and normal structures but does not always visualize the full extent of vulvar involvement. Furthermore, if the patient is positioned differently for the two types of imaging, it can be difficult to translate the locations of tumor and other structures from a diagnostic MRI to CT scans obtained in the treatment position. In **Figure 5.16**, the locations of vulvar structures on CT scans and MRI images are compared. Careful study of the relationship between vulvar structures and landmarks that can be distinguished on CT—for example, the pubic symphysis, suspensory ligament of the clitoris, anal sphincter, and levator ani muscle—can also help to identify the boundaries

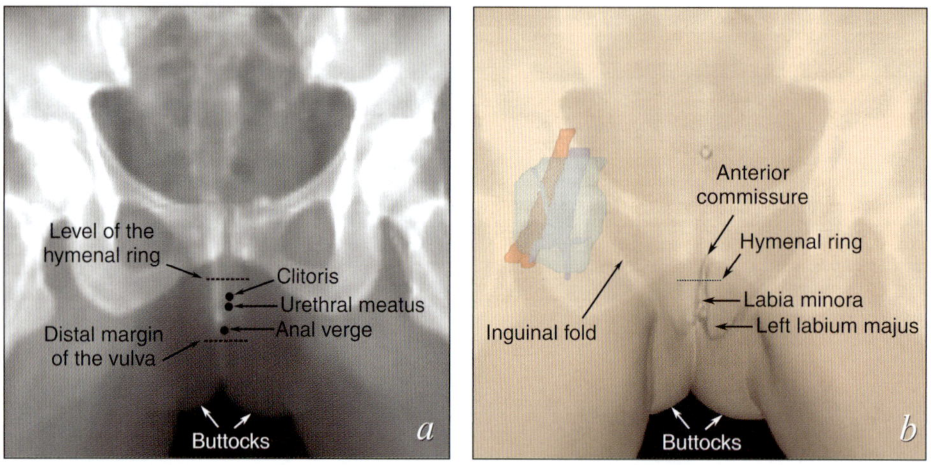

FIGURE 5.18 Location of vulvar structures with the patient in a "frog-leg" position. (*a*) *Dotted lines* and *dots* show the level of key landmarks on a digitally reconstructed radiograph. (*b*) A transparent skin rendering has been superimposed to show the relevant surface anatomy. The distances between these structures, particularly between the distal limit of the vulva and the pubic symphysis, vary according to the patient's body habitus; however in most cases, the distal median soft tissue shadow seen on AP x-rays represents the contour of the buttocks, not the vulva. Misinterpretation of this contour has frequently led clinicians to treat excessive skin and soft tissue in patients with distal vaginal or vulvar cancers. Perineal structures that will be used to define field borders should be localized using physical examination and careful placement of radio-opaque markers.

A rendering of the femoral arteries (*red*) and veins (*blue*) and an inguinal CTV (*cyan*) have been included on the right. Note how the relationships between the inguinal folds, femoral vessels, and femoral heads differ from those relationships in the patient depicted in Figure 5.12.

of the vulva. Fiducial markers should always be placed at the time of simulation to facilitate identification of tumor margins, surgical scars, and individual structures (e.g., the clitoris, urethral meatus, and anal verge). Reconstructed skin renderings also make it easier to relate axial contours to superficial landmarks (Figs. 5.17 and 5.18).

Lymphatic Drainage

A rich network of anastomosing lymphatics drain the vulva. The superficial external pudendal lymphatic vessels provide the primary route from the vulva to nodes medial to the femoral and saphenous veins, although the superior superficial epigastric lymphatic vessels also play a role (Figs. 5.11 and 5.12). Although anatomic studies suggest that there may be a direct path for lymphatic spread from the clitoris to the internal iliac nodes, in practice it is rare to see pelvic metastasis in the absence of inguinal node involvement (Table 5.1).

TARGET VOLUME DEFINITION: FINAL REVIEW

Target volume definition requires time and attention to detail. Although contouring is usually performed on axial slices, the axial plane is frequently not the best for visualization of anatomic structures and landmarks. Targets may be complex, and target volume definition often requires information gathered from several sources. In addition, it is not uncommon for the total length of gynecologic targets to exceed 25 cm, which means that the clinician must identify targets and critical structures on dozens of CT slices. Competing clinical demands are likely to interrupt or distract from this process.

For these reasons, it is useful to develop an organized approach to contouring and a systematic method of checking the final contours for consistency and accuracy (Table 5.2). It is always worthwhile to double-check that all high-risk targets suggested by imaging and other sources have been identified and correctly delineated. Also, during this process, the proximal and distal limits of the CTVs should be reviewed to confirm that the desired target volume lies within them.

Before contours are approved, it is important that the clinician scroll several times through axial, coronal, and sagittal views to verify that the contours are consistent; any abrupt change in the reconstructed sagittal or coronal contours should prompt a check for possible errors (Fig. 5.19).

Although modern techniques improve our ability to protect critical structures, it is important to remember that the primary goal of curative radiation therapy is to sterilize gross and microscopic disease in involved sites. With modern imaging studies, estimates of the extent of gross disease are undoubtedly improved but these studies do not reveal the limits of cancer infiltration. Once the primary GTVs (and associated ITVs) have been designated, generous CTV margins should be defined to account for possible infiltration of contiguous structures. Guidelines for specifying primary target volumes will be discussed further in disease site-specific chapters.

Finally, critical structures in the region of the target volumes must be contoured and reviewed, the margin determined for designation of the final PTV, and the dose and fractionation must be specified in a clearly articulated prescription. These final processes are further discussed in Chapter 6.

TABLE 5.2 Contouring Checklist

Contouring step	Materials to be reviewed
Initial contouring	
☐ Determine regions at risk	Pathology, operative reports, imaging, clinical findings
☐ List targets and desired doses	—
☐ Import and fuse relevant image sets	Diagnostic imaging; fusion accuracy
☐ Contour targets	—
☐ Contour critical structures	—
Final review	
☐ Proximal limit of nodal target volumes	Sagittal reconstructions
☐ Accuracy of nodal contours	Axial, coronal views
☐ Completeness of sacral coverage	Midline sagittal view
☐ CTV contouring consistency	Sagittal and coronal reconstructions
☐ Distal and proximal limits of vaginal/uterine target	Sagittal reconstructions
☐ Accuracy of GTV contours	Axial, coronal, sagittal reconstructions
☐ Adequacy of ITV	Full, empty bladder scans; rectal volume, etc.
☐ Assign margins to create PTV/draw fields	—
☐ Prescribe target doses; select number of fractions	Pathology, operative reports, imaging, clinical findings

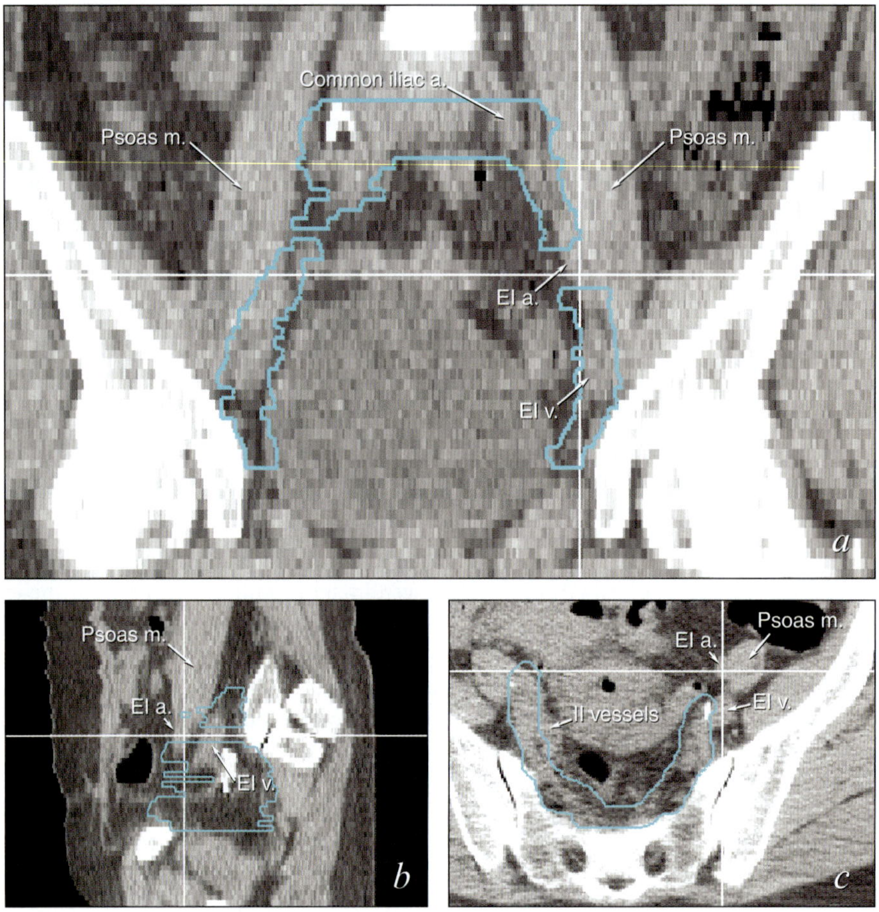

FIGURE 5.19 Monitoring coronal and sagittal views for contouring inconsistencies. Reconstructed views can highlight contouring errors that are difficult to appreciate on sequential axial CT slices. In particular, a sudden change or gap in reconstructed coronal or sagittal contours often indicates an inconsistency in interpretation of CT findings. In this example, a large gap can be seen in the left pelvic contour on coronal reconstruction *(a)*. Placement of the cross-hair in this region directs scrutiny to the left iliac region *(c)*, where a serious error has been made: the external iliac (EI) vessels and surrounding tissue were excluded from the contour at a level immediately distal to the left common iliac bifurcation. This area can be particularly confusing on axial view because of the extensive branching and crossing of vascular structures (Fig. 5.6). In this case, review of more posterior coronal views also detected inadequate medial coverage of the right internal iliac (II) vessels *(c)*. Even after addition of a 7-mm margin, these gaps were sufficient to cause underdosage of nodes in these regions; the errors were noted during quality assurance review of the contours and a final plan was designed using corrected CTVs.

The coronal plane is extremely helpful for review of iliac nodal contours. The sagittal view, which in this case also clearly demonstrates a contouring inconsistency *(b)*, is particularly valuable for review of presacral and aortic node contours and central targets. Note that even minor inconsistencies in the contoured vascular compartments adjacent to the psoas muscles are readily appreciated on the coronal reconstruction.

References

1. Koh WJ, Chiu M, Stelzer KJ, et al. Femoral vessel depth and the implications for groin node radiation. *Int J Radiat Oncol Biol Phys.* 1993;*27*:969–974, doi:10.1016/0360-3016(93)90476-C.
2. Stehman FB, Bundy BN, Thomas G, et al. Groin dissection versus groin radiation in carcinoma of the vulva: a Gynecologic Oncology Group study. *Int J Radiat Oncol Biol Phys.* 1992;*24*:389–396, doi:10.1016/0360-3016(92)90699-I.
3. Fontanilla HP, Klopp AH, Lindberg ME, et al. Anatomic distribution of [(18)F] fluorodeoxyglucose-avid lymph nodes in patients with cervical cancer. *Pract Radiat Oncol.* 2013;*3*: 45–53, doi:10.1016/j.prro.2012.02.003.
4. Takiar V, Fontanilla HP, Eifel PJ, et al. Anatomic distribution of fluorodeoxyglucose-avid para-aortic lymph nodes in patients with cervical cancer. *Int J Radiat Oncol Biol Phys.* 2013;*85*:1045–1050, doi:10.1016/j.ijrobp.2012.11.032.
5. Beadle BM, Jhingran A, Salehpour M, et al. Cervix regression and motion during the course of external beam chemoradiation for cervical cancer. *Int J Radiat Oncol Biol Phys.* 2009;*73*:235–241, doi:10.1016/j.ijrobp.2008.03.064.
6. Peters LJ, Goepfert H, Ang KK, et al. Evaluation of the dose for postoperative radiation therapy of head and neck cancer: First report of a prospective randomized trial. *Int J Radiat Oncol Biol Phys.* 1993;*26*:3–11, doi:10.1016/0360-3016(93)90167-T.

7. Raspagliesi F, Hanozet F, Ditto A, et al. Clinical and pathological prognostic factors in squamous cell carcinoma of the vulva. *Gynecol Oncol.* 2006;*102*:333–337, doi:10.1016/j.ygyno.2005.12.027.
8. van der Velden J, Lindert ACM, Lammes FB, et al. Extracapsular growth of lymph node metastases in squamous cell carcinoma of the vulva. The impact on recurrence and survival. *Cancer.* 1995;*75*:2885–2890, doi:10.1002/(ISSN)1097-0142.
9. Horn LC, Hentschel B, Galle D, et al. Extracapsular extension of pelvic lymph node metastases is of prognostic value in carcinoma of the cervix uteri. *Gynecol Oncol.* 2008;*108*:63–67, doi:10.1016/j.ygyno.2007.08.086.
10. Jhingran A, Salehpour M, Sam M, et al. Vaginal motion and bladder and rectal volumes during pelvic intensity-modulated radiation therapy after hysterectomy. *Int J Radiat Oncol Biol Phys.* 2012;*82*:256–262, doi:10.1016/j.ijrobp.2010.08.024.

Suggested Reading

Anatomy and embryology, general references:

Moore K, Persaud TVN, Torchia MG. *The Developing Human. Clinically Oriented Embryology*. 9th ed. Philadelphia, PA: Elsevier Saunders; 2013.

Plentl, AA, FriedmanEA. *Lymphatic System of Female Genitalia.* Philadelphia, PA: W.B. Saunders: 1971.

Smith RP, Turek PJ. *The Netter Collection of Medical Illustrations. Reproductive System*. 2nd ed. Philadelphia, PA: Elsevier Saunders; 2011.

Standrig S. *Gray's Anatomy: The Anatomical Basis of Clinical Practice.* 40th ed. Philadelphia, PA: Churchill Livingstone; 2008.

Torigian DA, Hammell MK. *Netter's Correlative Imaging. Abdominal & Pelvic Anatomy*. Philadelphia, PA: Elsevier Saunders; 2013.

CHAPTER 6

External Beam Radiation Treatment Planning

INTRODUCTION

The overarching goal of curative external beam radiation therapy planning is to create a plan that will comprehensively and consistently treat cancerous tissues without damaging uninvolved critical structures.

The steps involved in preparation for the planning process, including identification of gross target volumes (GTVs), clinical target volumes (CTVs), and internal target volumes (ITVs), were addressed in Chapters 4 and 5. In Chapter 7, we have discussed how to assure that the treatment is being delivered according to plan throughout its course. Chapter 6 focuses, in part, on the collaborative process that produces an optimized external beam treatment plan. The entire process of treatment plan creation and implementation requires a highly functioning team with all the characteristics discussed in Chapter 3. This team consists of a radiation oncologist, radiation therapy dosimetrist, radiation therapists, and a radiation physicist. Each member brings specialized expertise to the process and each helps to assure that high-quality treatment is administered safely. As with any multidisciplinary team, the quality of the end result depends on the quality of communication between team members. **Figure 6.1** summarizes the steps involved in the development of a high-quality treatment plan.

THE TREATMENT PLANNING DIRECTIVE

Before target volumes are finalized, the radiation oncologist should carefully double check each aspect of the patient's contours (Table 5.2). For complex IMRT plans, peer review of the proposed planning directive and target volumes is recommended before the case is transmitted to a dosimetrist (**Fig. 6.1**). This evaluation can reduce the chance for error and can markedly improve the efficiency of the planning process by decreasing the need for subsequent revisions to the treatment plan.

Many factors influence the choice of planning target volumes (PTVs) and external beam technique. As the planning process progresses, some of these factors may be adjusted to meet technical and anatomic constraints. However, every plan should begin with a clearly articulated, precise *treatment planning directive* that is transmitted in writing from the radiation oncologist to the radiation dosimetrist. In this directive, the radiation oncologist should specify:

- A list of CTVs and GTVs with designations that are matched precisely to the labels on the respective contours in the treatment planning system.
- The margin(s) to be added to each GTV or CTV to generate a final PTV.
- The desired dose and dose per fraction for each PTV.
- Normal tissue constraints with emphasis on areas of particular concern.
- A suggested field arrangement (e.g., four-field, AP–PA, or appositional electrons) or inverse planning approach (e.g., IMRT).
- Information about previous treatments or areas that may receive additional exposure from sequential boosts or future brachytherapy.
- If the skin is to be included in the target volume, this should be specified and the need for bolus discussed.

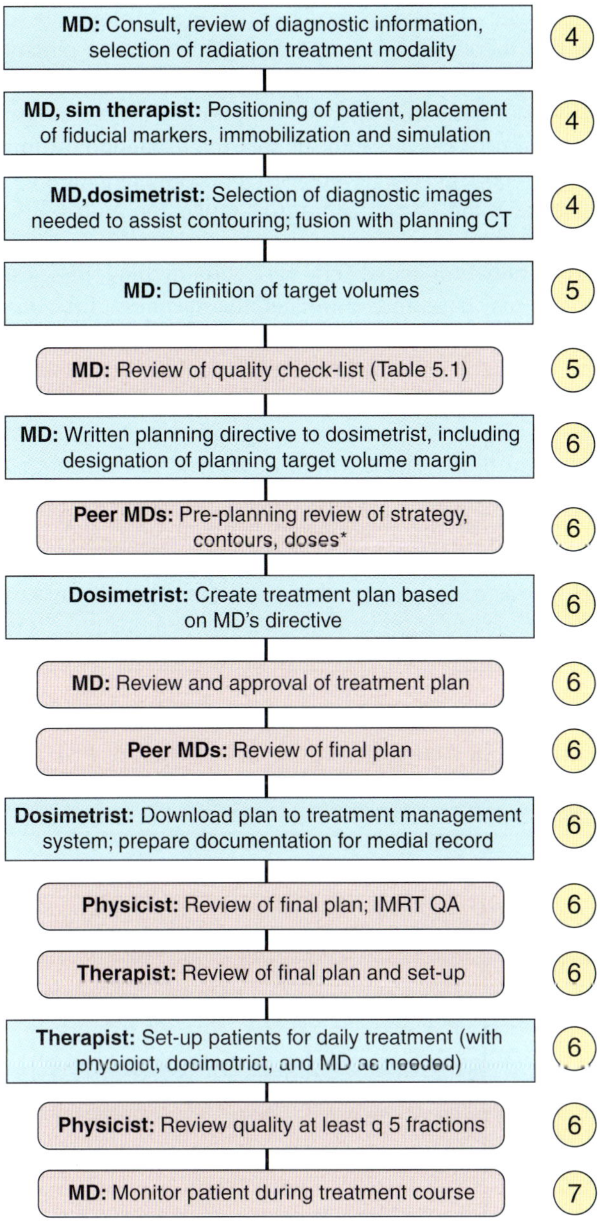

FIGURE 6.1 A diagrammatic representation of some of the process (*blue*) and review (*rose*) steps involved in treatment planning for gynecologic radiation therapy. Numbers to the right indicate the chapters that address each phase of the process. *We recommend this extra preplanning peer-review step for IMRT and other complex cases. (Adapted from Moran JM, Dempsey M, Eisbruch A, et al. Safety considerations for IMRT: executive summary. *Pract Radiat Oncol.* 2011;1:190–195.)

ACCOUNTING FOR UNCERTAINTIES—DESIGNATION OF THE PTV

Safe external beam radiation therapy requires a thorough understanding of the uncertainties underlying the treatment planning process and a recognition of the impact that even small errors can have on the ratio between the probabilities of tumor control and normal tissue complications. A failure to respect these uncertainties results in plans that look impressive but that fail to address the realities of neoplastic behavior and treatment delivery and that can easily lead to recurrence of disease inside or at the margins of the radiation treatment field (Figs. 6.2 and 6.3). Uncertainties that must be considered in the planning process include the following:

- Uncertain boundaries of gross disease due to ambiguous diagnostic findings or distortion and degradation of reconstructed images. In general, these uncertainties are addressed in designation of the GTV.
- Uncertainties about the extent of microscopic spread to lymph nodes or other tissues at risk for tumor involvement; these are addressed in the CTV.
- Uncertainties caused by internal motion of target structures. These are usually incorporated in an ITV based on diagnostic findings and an understanding of the nature of internal organ motion (Chapter 5).
- Uncertainties caused by inconsistent positioning of the patient (setup error). A PTV margin is typically added to the GTV, CTV, or ITV to account for these uncertainties.

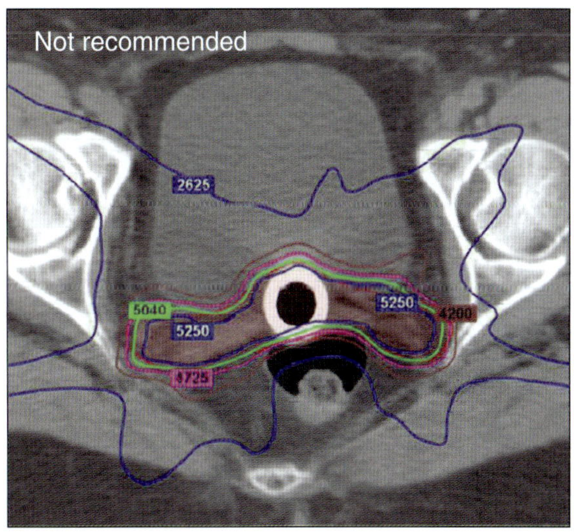

FIGURE 6.2 With IMRT, it is possible to achieve radiation dose distributions that conform tightly to unrealistic target volumes. This patient was referred for an infrarenal paraaortic node recurrence of endometrial cancer 2 years after completing adjuvant pelvic IMRT for a stage IAG2 endometrioid cancer. Only three central axis views of the doses from her previous treatment were available. However, this axial view suggests that her treatment was planned without sufficiently considering possible positioning uncertainties. The vaginal target was designated with no margin for internal organ motion or patient setup error. The patient also was simulated with a rigid obturator in the vagina; this is not recommended because such devices cause substantial vaginal distortion (Chapter 4). The distal obturator nodes also appear to have been excluded from the nodal target volume. Fortunately, the patient did not have a pelvic recurrence and has no evidence of disease 4 years after definitive treatment for her paraaortic node recurrence.

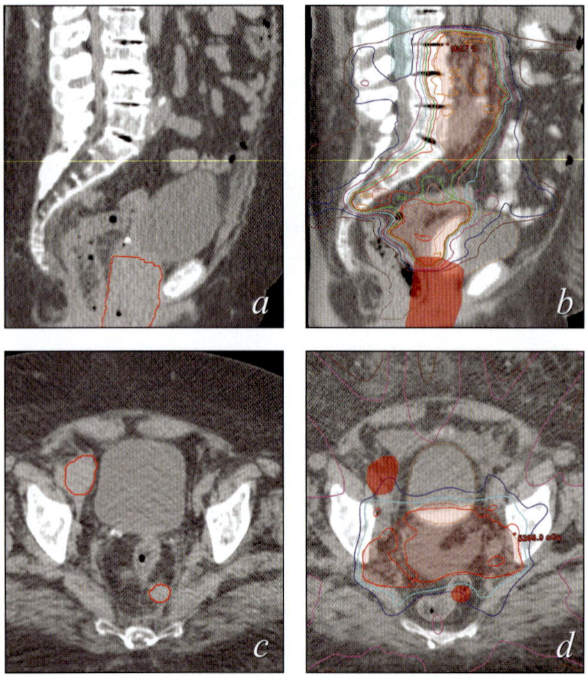

FIGURE 6.3 A woman who had a hysterectomy and adjuvant pelvic RT for stage IA, grade 3 endometrial cancer was subsequently referred for evaluation and treatment of pelvic recurrence. She had three sites of disease involving the vagina (*a*), a pararectal nodule (*c*), and a distal external iliac node (*c*). Outside records contained only one axial and one sagittal view of the dose distributions from her IMRT (*b*, *d*). However, these demonstrated that all three recurrence sites were on the margins of her previous treatment (red overlay, *b* and *d*). To minimize the risk of such recurrences, it is important to completely cover primary echelon nodes and to treat central structures with sufficient margin to account for motion and setup uncertainties.

Many of these issues are discussed in Chapter 5. The first section of this chapter focuses primarily on the last group of uncertainties, external factors that can cause the distribution of radiation dose within the patient to differ from that depicted in the radiation therapy treatment plan. The size of the PTV margin depends on the magnitude of these uncertainties, their impact on the delivered radiation dose, and on the probability of an adverse outcome if the actual dose that is delivered to the tumor is less than the prescribed dose. In the following section, factors that are used to determine a safe PTV margin are discussed with recommendations regarding the size of the PTV margin to be used under various conditions.

The Relationship between Radiation Dose and the Probability of Tumor Control

The range of doses that can achieve complication-free cure of gynecologic cancers is narrow, particularly if gross disease is present. Although high-quality dose response analyses are not available for external beam radiotherapy of gynecologic carcinomas, analyses of other tumor sites suggest that there is a very steep relationship between radiation dose and the probability of controlling macroscopic disease. Analyses of patients with gross lymph node metastases from head and neck cancers indicate that the likelihood of tumor control increases very steeply with increasing radiation doses between 55 and 65 Gy; within this range, the probability of tumor control appears to increase by at least 4% to 6% per 1 Gy of radiation added (**Fig. 6.4**).[1–3] If anything, these early analyses may have underestimated the steepness of the dose–response relationship because radiation treatment plans that were generated without image guidance may have overestimated the dose delivered to gross nodal disease in some cases.

For the past 20 years, the range of doses used at MD Anderson to treat gross lymph node metastases from gynecologic cancers has been too narrow to permit a meaningful analysis of the relationship between dose and tumor response. However, in the 1980s, patients with gross paraaortic node metastases from cervical cancer usually received only 55 Gy because previous studies had demonstrated unacceptable complication rates when extended fields were treated to a dose of 60 Gy. A retrospective review of patients treated during this period demonstrated a high rate of paraaortic recurrence. In contrast, after the introduction of PET imaging, IMRT (using policies described in this book), and image guidance, nodal metastases were routinely boosted to at least

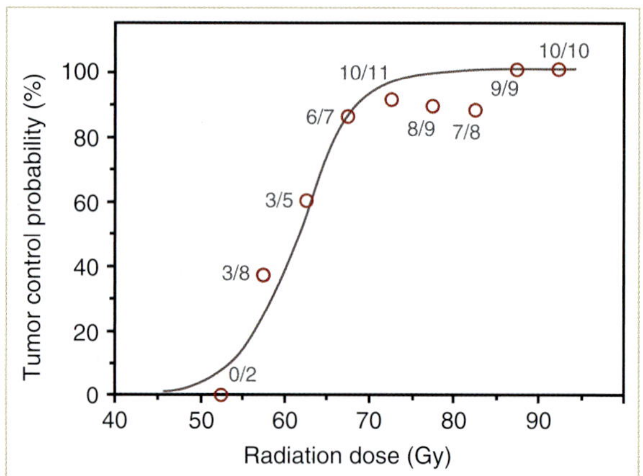

FIGURE 6.4 This figure was drawn using single institution data from patients who were treated with radiation for carcinomas of the pyriform sinus metastatic to lymph nodes that measured <3 cm in diameter. Although the number of patients is small, these data suggest that in the range between 55 and 65 Gy, the relationship between radiation dose and tumor response was very steep. Similar patterns have been reported for other types of carcinoma, although few data are available for gynecologic cancers. (Adapted from Van Dyk J, Battista JJ, Bauman GS. Accuracy and uncertainty considerations in modern radiation oncology. In: Van Dyk J, ed. *The Modern Technology of Radiation Oncology*. Madison, WI: Medical Physics Publishing; 2013:61–416. Using data from Bataini P, Brugere J, Bernier J, et al. Results of radical radiotherapeutic treatment of carcinoma of the pyriform sinus: experience of the Institut Curie. *Int J Radiat Oncol Biol Phys.* 1982;8:1277–1286.)

60 Gy; with these changes, the rate of infield paraaortic nodal recurrence dropped dramatically to <5%.[4] These results also suggest that there is a very steep relationship between radiation dose and the likelihood of tumor control.

The probability of bowel complications also tends to be strongly correlated with the dose of radiation, with a steep dose–effect relationship between 40 and 55 Gy, when large volumes of bowel are irradiated, and between 60 and 70 Gy, when small volumes (e.g., single loops of bowel) are treated. Because the doses required for tumor control can also cause significant side effects in normal tissues, highly conformal treatment plans that minimize the volume of incidentally irradiated normal tissue are likely to be of value.

However, although IMRT, image guidance, and other modern advances have increased the precision of radiation therapy delivery, they have not eliminated positional uncertainties. The steep relationship between the dose of radiation and the probability of recurrence means that even a few treatments that fail to encompass a site of active tumor could increase the probability of recurrence. Because even the best immobilization and localization systems cannot eliminate uncertainty, it is critical to understand the limitations of our techniques and to build in safety margins that minimize the chance that a target will receive less than the prescribed dose. *Incremental sparing of normal tissues at the expense of tumor recurrence is generally not an acceptable trade-off.*

Factors that Influence the Reproducibility of Daily Treatment Setup

Although modern radiation therapy techniques have improved the reproducibility of treatment setup and delivery, residual uncertainties continue to demand a margin for error.

One of the most important sources of uncertainty is day-to-day variation in the position of the patient. Kim et al.[5] evaluated the daily accuracy of clinical laser setups in 52 women treated with RT for gynecologic cancers; patients in their study were positioned with their feet together and a sponge under their knees. Accuracy of the initial setup was assessed using onboard KV imaging or cone beam CT to determined the shifts required to bring the patient's isocenter into correct alignment with adjacent boney landmarks. In general, right-to-left directional errors were greater than anterior–posterior (AP) or superior–inferior errors, probably reflecting the fact that only one skin mark is available for right–left alignment, while two lateral points of reference are used to align the patient in other directions.[5] Based on their determination of the frequency of random and systematic errors, the authors used the method of van Herk[6] to estimate required CTV-to-PTV margins of between 7 and 10.5 mm. In a similar study, Santanam et al.[7] concluded that a CTV-to-PTV margin of 7 mm was needed. However, it should be noted that both of these calculations were based strictly on the translational table shifts required to bring the isocenter into to the correct position. Possible rotational and tilt errors were not considered in these analyses.

Several factors can influence the magnitude of positional errors:

- *Body habitus.* In their analysis, Kim et al.[5] reported a significant correlation between a patient's body habitus and the magnitude of positional errors.
- *Field size.* Studies of pelvic setup reproducibility have focused on the translational shifts that are required to bring the isocenter into the correct position. However, as demonstrated in Figures 7.5 and 7.6, tilt errors and rotational errors can be equally important sources of errors in the setup of patients who have large fields. A mere 2-degree right-to-left tilt error will cause a shift of 5 mm at 15 cm from the isocenter and a shift of 7 mm at 20 cm (**Fig. 6.5**). Right-to-left rotational errors (Fig. 7.6) can also result in underdosage, particularly of presacral or inguinal targets. Because these errors are much more difficult to detect and correct than translational errors, they remain a significant problem even when treatments are set up using daily image guidance.
- *Immobilization method.* In a comparison of several different pelvic immobilization methods, Malone et al.[8] reported very little difference between the mean isocenter shifts required to achieve pubic alignment of prostate cancer patients treated in generic leg support devices (similar to that shown in Fig. 4.10a) or molded devices (similar to that shown in Fig. 4.10c). However, patients who were immobilized in HipFix thermoplastic devices were less likely to require large error shifts than patients immobilized in the other two types of devices. The ability to mark the isocenter directly on this type of device is a relative advantage of the thermoplastic device. The authors of this Canadian study did not report whether the device was equally effective for obese or thin patients.
- *Image guidance.* The practical application of image guidance is addressed in Chapter 7. Daily image guidance is an important tool that significantly reduces the magnitude of alignment errors. However, *image guidance does not eliminate all setup errors* for several reasons:
  - Even the most acute observer cannot always detect 1- to 2-mm errors in isocenter alignment and will occasionally miss even 3- to 4-mm errors, particularly if the isocenter is not close to a clearly visualized boney landmark.
  - The relatively poor image quality and low resolution of reconstructed pelvic images and cone beam CTs often makes it difficult to accurately identify the borders of key landmarks.
  - As discussed above, rotations and tilts are important sources of potential errors in gynecologic treatments; these are easily missed during review of onboard images that have a limited field of view (**Fig. 6.5**). These complex positioning errors can also be difficult and time consuming to correct, particularly if the entire spine and pelvis must be brought into alignment; this process can easily exceed the patient's tolerance.

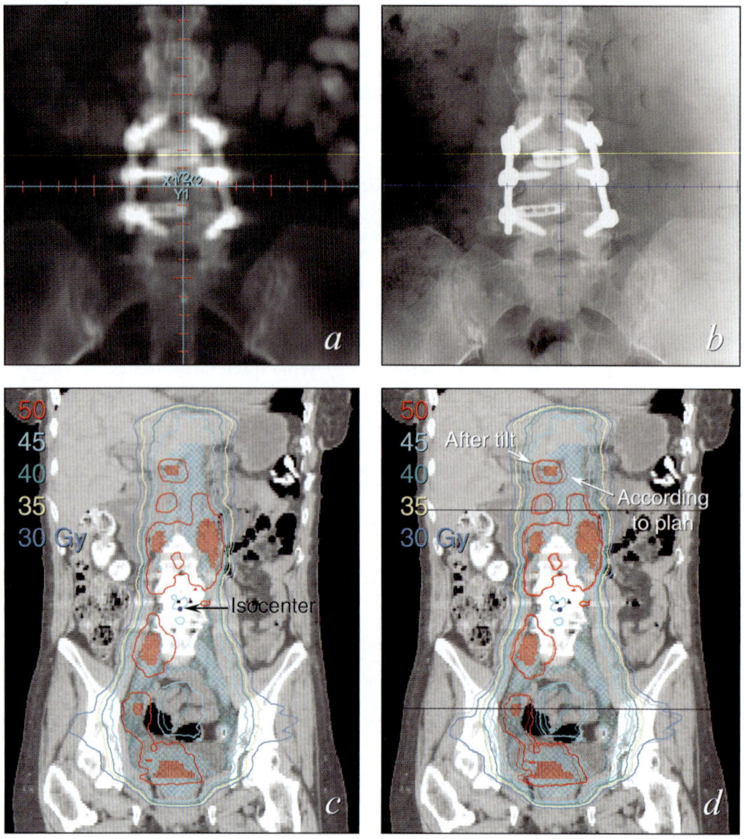

FIGURE 6.5 Even very small rotational errors can cause significant misalignments at the periphery of large radiation fields. This illustration shows a digitally reconstructed radiograph *(a)* and a coronal view of the isodose distribution *(c)* from a patient treated for extensive gross nodal metastases from vaginal cancer. In *b*, an onboard KV image demonstrates a counterclockwise tilt error that was measured to be 2 degrees. From the 20 × 20 cm field of view, this error appears to be very subtle; it is probably best appreciated by noting the distances between the iliac crests and the horizontal axis. In *d*, the isodose distribution has been tilted by 2 degrees and superimposed on the original plan. The horizontal black lines indicate the limits of the 20-cm field-of-view for on board KV imaging. Note that the shift appears very subtle within this range; however, at the periphery of the target volume, even this small error caused a 5 to 6 mm displacement. If the plan did not incorporate an adequate PTV margin, an error of this magnitude could cause involved nodes to receive an inadequate dose.

Sources of Inaccuracy in the Treatment Machine

The Science Council of the American Association of Physicist in Medicine (AAPM) has published quality assurance guidelines for medical linear accelerators.[9] Their recommendations included tolerance standards for the accuracy of localization lasers on the simulator and treatment machines (±1 mm for IMRT; ±2 mm for non-IMRT), accuracy of the port film graticule tray (±2 mm), coordinance of the onboard imaging and treatment coordinates (≤1 mm for stereotactic body RT [SBRT]; ≤2 mm for non-SBRT), and other features.[9] With recommended daily and monthly monitoring routines, systematic errors should not occur because of these uncertainties. However, they do make a finite contribution to the overall uncertainties that must be considered in the determination of a PTV margin.

Other Sources of Uncertainty

Other factors can introduce small variations in the target position. Breathing is not a major cause of target motion for most gynecologic cancer treatments; however, the breathing cycle can cause small changes in the position of the upper abdominal spine and nodes. Patients may clench their gluteal or perineal muscles during treatment; these actions can displace distal target structures by several millimeters.

Changes in hydration and blood pressure cause small changes in the diameter of the inferior vena cava and other major veins, potentially displacing adjacent lymph nodes. Some accounting for these variations is considered in the designation of the nodal CTV, but the PTV margin adds an additional margin of safety. It is important to note that injection of intravenous contrast can cause much more dramatic expansion of venous structures than normal hemodynamic variations; as discussed in Chapter 4, we do not recommend contrast administration during simulation to avoid this potential source of systematic error.

Recommended CTV-to-PTV Margins

Recommended target-to-PTV margins for 3-D conformal and IMRT treatments are summarized in **Table 6.1**.

Note that a somewhat smaller GTV-to-PTV margin is recommended when the GTV boost is integrated within a larger CTV. This is because the steepness of the dose gradient

TABLE 6.1 Recommended CTV/GTV/ITV to PTV Margins for Radiation Therapy Planning[a]

Target diameter (greatest dimension)	Weekly port films[b]	Daily image guidance
CTV >15 cm	10–12 mm	7 mm
CTV or ITV 10–15 cm	9–10 mm	6–7 mm
CTV or ITV <10 cm	8–10 mm	5–7 mm
GTV or HRCTV, integrated boost[c]	7–8 mm	4–5 mm
GTV or HRCTV, sequential boost	Same as CTV margins	Same as CTV margins

[a]*Assuming that the clinical target volume (CTV), gross target volume (GTV), and internal target volume (ITV) are defined and delineated as shown in Chapter 5.*

[b]*For patients who are obese (BMI greater than about 30), at least 5 mm should be added to these recommended margins.*

[c]*Assuming that the integrated GTV is contained within a CTV that is treated using a wider margin (see text for additional discussion).*

surrounding the GTV is less if the GTV is surrounded by a larger CTV–PTV that receives only a slightly lower dose than the GTV. This is also the rationale for occasional use of nested GTVs to treat large tumors that are close to critical structures (Chapter 5; CS 10.11, 14.1, 14.8, 15.1, 15.2).

NORMAL TISSUE CONSTRAINTS FOR EXTERNAL BEAM PLANNING

Although the primary objective of definitive radiation therapy is to cure the patient's cancer, the goal is always to accomplish this with as few side effects as possible. Because most gynecologic cancers involve or are in direct contact with critical structures, because even the best immobilization and image guidance techniques do not obviate the need for a PTV margin, and because every radiation beam passes through some normal tissues on its way to the target, a high probability of cure cannot be achieved without at least some risk of causing acute or late side effects. However, a well-designed treatment plan that minimizes the dose of radiation to structures outside the PTV can undoubtedly reduce the probability of life-altering side effects.

Although many investigators have attempted to correlate radiation dose, radiation volume, and radiation-related side effects, it is very difficult to generate practical guidelines from the results. Some of the factors that contribute to this include the following:

- For most studies, a single CT was used to calculate organ doses and volumes. These calculations do not accurately represent the doses delivered to mobile critical structures during a protracted course of radiation treatment.
- Inconsistent methods have been used to designate normal tissue volumes.
- Results that were based on site-specific multimodality treatments for nongynecologic cancers may not be broadly applicable to gynecologic cancer patients.
- Many factors other than dose and volume contribute to the risks of side effects (Chapter 9).
- The level of risk that is considered acceptable may vary according to the clinical situation (i.e., the potential benefit of a treatment).

Some general guidelines are discussed in the following sections. Where data are available to suggest very specific radiation dose or volume constraints (e.g., for kidney or duodenum), these will be emphasized. *However, the goal should always be to conform the radiation dose as tightly as possible to the PTV in order to minimize the dose to uninvolved critical structures.*

Bladder

In the course of four-field pelvic RT, most of the bladder usually receives the prescribed dose of 45 to 50 Gy. Although this appears to be tolerated fairly well, even 45 Gy has been associated with short- and long-term side effects (Chapters 7 and 9). Boothe et al.[10] demonstrated markedly decreased rates of urinary tract infection in patients treated to the whole pelvis with IMRT versus four-field conformal treatment. The lack of data and the variable volume of the bladder make it difficult to make strict recommendations regarding the volume that should receive <45 Gy. However, with IMRT, it is often possible to reduce the volume of bladder receiving 30 Gy or more to <50%, particularly if the bladder is full during treatment (Figs. 6.6 and 6.8).

Patients who require a high dose of radiation dose to treat gross vaginal disease usually receive a similarly high dose to at least a portion of the bladder. Most of the data concerning the tolerance of the bladder to external beam doses of more than 65 Gy are based on studies of prostate cancer treatment[11]; based on these results, it has been recommended that no more than 50% of the bladder receive more than 65 Gy and no more than 35% receive more than 70 Gy.[11] Patients who receive these relatively high doses should be treated with a full bladder (at least 200 cc, if possible).

Dose recommendations for patients receiving brachytherapy are summarized in Chapter 8.

Rectum

The rectal contour should extend from the anal verge superiorly to the point where it looses its round shape in the axial plane and turns toward the sigmoid.[12]

Because the rectum is intimately associated with common cervical and vaginal targets, it is rarely possible to prevent at least 50% to 70% from receiving at least 45 Gy. Fortunately, this dose is not often associated with major side effects. When pararectal targets require higher doses, an effort should be made not to treat more than 25% of the rectum to >65 Gy. It may be necessary to treat a larger volume to high dose in some cases (e.g., CS 15.2); however, the patient should be warned that the risk of radiation proctitis or stricture may be greater than usual.

Bowel

Contouring Methods

Although some clinicians contour individual loops to create a bowel avoidance structure, this method is unrealistic because bowel is constantly moving within the peritoneal cavity. A more efficient and, probably, equally valid method is to contour small and large intraperitoneal bowel as a single organ or "bowel bag." In obese patients, fat at the root of the mesentery and in the retroperitoneal space may displace bowel away from the iliac or paraaortic nodes; it is reasonable to exclude this region from the contour if it contains no bowel. The rectosigmoid is usually contoured separately from the bowel bag. To allow closer scrutiny, in some cases, a separate contour may be designated for a loop of bowel that appears to be fixed in a critical location (e.g., adjacent to a site of gross disease).

Dose Constraints

Because intraperitoneal bowel is usually moving in and out of any specific location, small portions of the bowel bag can usually be treated to 60 to 66 Gy without causing major complications; however, if a portion of the bowel is fixed by scarring or adhesions, the risk of obstruction is greater; if possible, an effort should be made not to treat the entire circumference of a fixed bowel loop to more than 60 Gy.

If a bowel obstruction does occur, surgical resection is easier and less likely to have long-term consequences if the rest of the bowel is healthy. For patients who require 60 Gy or more to a portion of bowel, it is particularly important to minimize the volume of adjacent bowel that receives intermediate doses of 35 to 50 Gy. Whenever possible, IMRT is recommended for such cases.

Although there are very few data available, it is likely that the side effects of large volume RT on bowel increase fairly steeply between 45 and 55 Gy.[13] In most cases, we do not recommend treating the whole pelvis to more than 45 Gy with AP–PA or four-field techniques because our data suggest that higher doses may be associated with a higher incidence of serious late effects.[13] If available, IMRT is recommended if a large pelvic volume requires more than 45 Gy **(CS 10.1)**.

Duodenum

At least the second and third portions of the duodenum should be contoured if paraaortic nodes are included in the target volume. The second (descending) portion of the duodenum is located to the right of the L1 to L3 vertebral bodies and the inferior vena cava; it then turns medially at about L3 (where it becomes the third part of the duodenum) and then passes anterior to the vena cava and aorta until it travels superiorly to the left of L3. Coronal views are typically very helpful for contouring the duodenum.[14]

It is recommended that no more than 15 cc of the duodenum receive more than 55 Gy and that no more than 2 cc receive more than 60 Gy.[15]

Femurs

The femoral heads and necks are vulnerable to radiation injury, particularly if the patient is osteoporotic. Whenever possible, no more than 25% of the femoral head should receive 45 Gy and no more than 50% should receive 30 Gy. Patients who receive more than 50 to 60 Gy to a significant portion of the femoral head, have a high risk of hip fracture.

EXTERNAL BEAM RADIATION TECHNIQUE

A review of the 54 case studies that are appended to Chapters 10 to 15 provides a sense of the wide variety of external beam treatment volumes, doses, and techniques that can be used to treat patients with gynecologic cancers. In each of the cases described in these studies, the final approach was chosen from among several options after weighing the advantages and disadvantages of each. Some of the more common uses of external beam radiotherapy for treatment of gynecologic cancer and the factors that influence the technical approaches to these treatments are discussed in the following sections.

Posthysterectomy Treatment of the Pelvis

The tissues that are typically at risk for recurrence after hysterectomy for cervical or uterine cancer include the vagina, paravaginal tissues, residual paracervical supporting ligaments, and the pelvic lymph nodes (Figs. 5.7 and 5.8). When these targets are combined, and consideration is given to internal organ motion, the final PTV takes the form of a bowl, the center of which is filled with bladder and bowel.

3-D Conformal Treatment

The traditional radiation field arrangement for treatment of the pelvis after hysterectomy is a four-field "box" technique, consisting of opposing AP, posterior–anterior (PA), and lateral fields (Figs. 5.8 and **6.6**).

Four-field arrangements are generally superior to AP–PA, two-field techniques, because the lateral fields of a four-field box can be shaped to spare posterior soft tissue and, in most cases, anterior small bowel. However, this comes at the price of a greater dose to the femoral heads and other lateral pelvic bones (and bone marrow). Also, for thin women with a scaphoid anterior abdominal wall, the amount of bowel spared by lateral fields is typically slight because of the relatively anterior location of the external iliac nodes. In such cases, if care is not taken, lateral fields can easily flash the anterior abdominal wall, causing significant skin reaction. Although four-field arrangements usually treat the entire bladder to the prescribed dose, some sparing of the anterior bladder and, often, considerable sparing of small bowel can sometimes be achieved if the patient is treated with a comfortably full bladder (**Fig. 6.6a,d**).

High-energy beams (10 to 18 MV) are usually preferred for pelvic treatment although, for very thin women, the dose distributions achieved with 6-MV or 10- to 15-MV beams are only slightly different, with the main advantage from high-energy beams being a somewhat reduced dose to subcutaneous tissues. In most cases, equalization of the monitor units from the four fields provides the most homogeneous dose distribution. This typically results in delivery of somewhat less radiation to target through the lateral fields than through the AP and PA

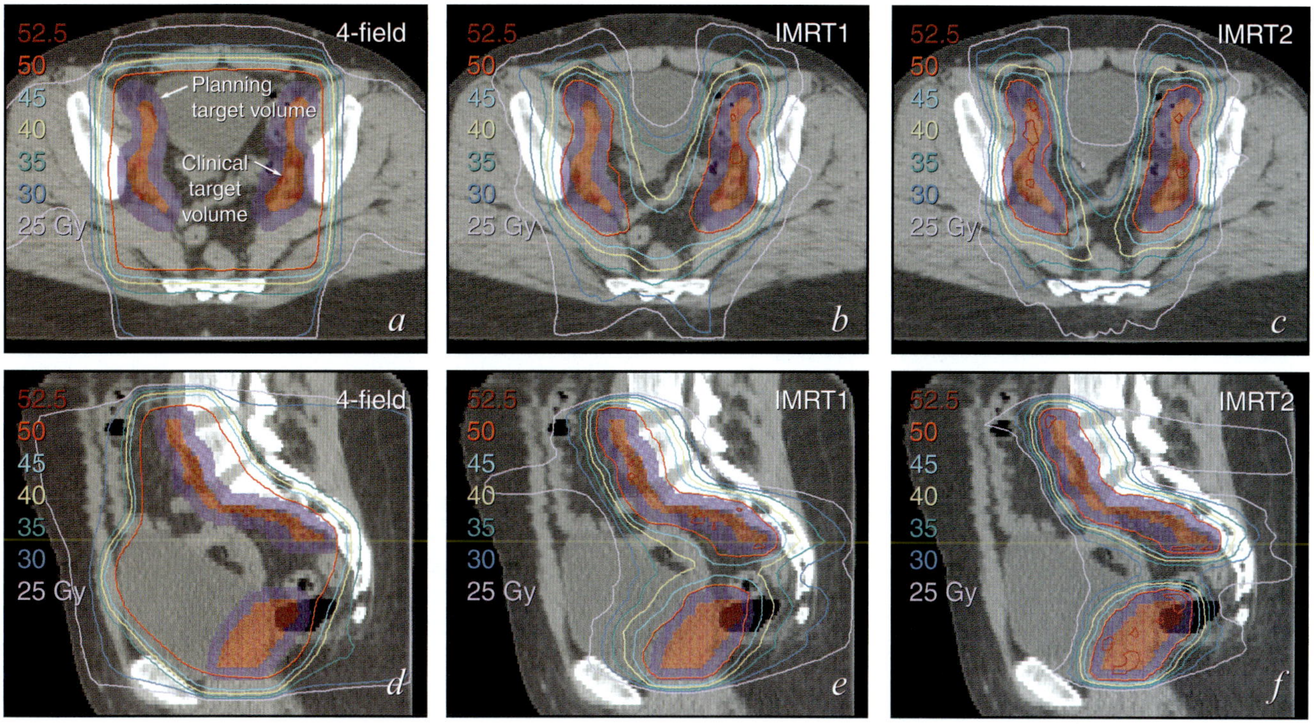

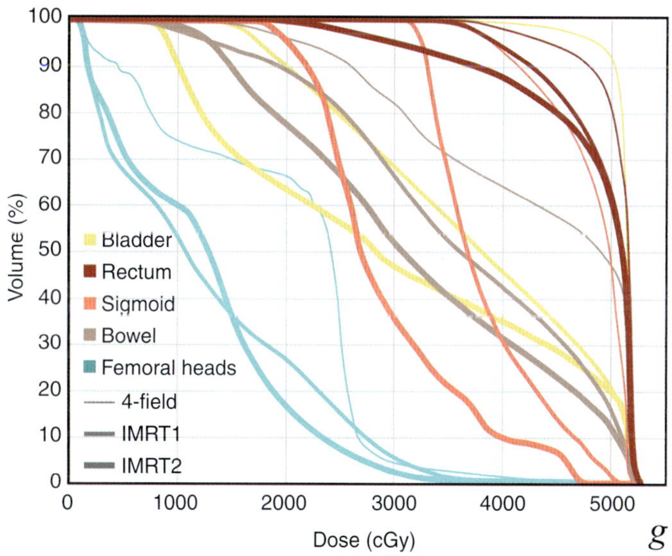

FIGURE 6.6 A four-field (*a, d*), and two volumetric modulated arc (VMAT) IMRT plans, that could be used to treat a patient after hysterectomy for high-risk cervical cancer (CS 10.1). Target coverage was similar for the three plans. However, a comparison of the three sets of DVHs (*g*) demonstrates that the IMRT plans provided greater sparing of normal tissues than the four field plan. IMRT1 (*b, e*), which was planned using a fairly simple VMAT optimization technique, met commonly accepted normal tissue dose constraints. However, additional effort aimed at maximizing conformality yielded a plan (IMRT2; *c, f*) that markedly reduced the doses to sigmoid, bladder and bowel when compared with IMRT1.

fields. If the lateral contour of the patient is sloped, wedges, or a step-and-shoot, field-in-field technique may be needed to achieve an acceptably homogeneous dose distribution.

IMRT

The main disadvantage of four-field, fixed beam arrangements for postoperative pelvic irradiation is that the walls of the bowl-shaped target volume cannot be treated without irradiating uninvolved central pelvic contents. Sparing of these intrapelvic tissues is the primary goal of modern IMRT treatments of the posthysterectomy pelvis.

In almost all cases, a well-designed IMRT plan can provide substantially greater sparing of normal tissues than can be achieved using a four-field approach. However, the amount of normal tissue sparing from IMRT is highly dependent on the techniques used by the radiation dosimetrist (Fig. 6.6). We have seen IMRT plans that exposed more bowel to moderately high radiation doses of 25 to 40 Gy than would be expected with a typical four-field plan. When reviewing a posthysterectomy IMRT plan, it is helpful to look at the degree to which the 50% and 70% isodose lines (e.g., the 25- and 35-Gy isodose lines in Fig. 6.6) dip between the external iliac node contours.

We currently prefer to use IMRT for most patients who require pelvic RT after hysterectomy. However, IMRT is particularly helpful in cases where the risk of treatment-related side effects is greater than usual, such as:

- Patients who have had major abdominopelvic surgery (including transperitoneal lymph node dissection).
- Patients who have a history of pelvic infection, autoimmune disease, heavy smoking, very low BMI, or other characteristics that increase the risk of bowel complications.
- Patients who require more than 45 Gy because of extracapsular node extension, positive surgical margins, gross disease, or other features (e.g., CS 10.1, 10.2, 11.4, 13.8).

Pelvic Treatment in Patients Who Have an Intact Uterus

When the uterus is still in situ, a number of factors can influence the choice of external beam technique including:

- The size and position of the uterus and cervix.
- The extent of central disease.
- The mobility of the central targets.
- The body habitus of the patient and the abdominal contour (e.g., scaphoid, rounded, or protuberant).
- The presence and extent of nodal metastases and the proximal extent of the nodal CTV (discussed in Chapters 5 and 10).
- Risk factors for major complications of radiation (e.g., infection, heavy smoking, or a history of major transabdominal surgery including lymphadenectomy).
- Institutional resources, including the energy of available treatment machines.

The balance of these considerations tends to be very different than it is for posthysterectomy pelvic treatments, in part because the uterus and cervix typically fill much of the central pelvis. Factors that influence designation of the CTV, GTV, and ITV contours are discussed in detail in Chapters 5 and 10. The following sections address the pros and cons of various external beam techniques.

AP–PA and Four-Field Techniques

For patients with intact cervical cancer, pelvic RT is usually given using AP and PA fields or with a four-field combination of AP, PA, and laterals fields. Most clinicians in the United States have adopted the four-field approach as standard and are convinced that it is in all cases far superior to two-field treatment. It has become almost heretical to suggest that AP–PA treatment arrangements be used for any patient with cervical cancer. However, actual review of comparative dose distributions suggests that there are some patients for whom AP–PA treatment is comparable or may even be superior to a four-field approach if treatment is delivered using high-energy (i.e., ≥15 MV) beams (Fig. 6.7).

For most cases of intact cervical cancer, very little intrapelvic tissue can be spared once the nodal CTVs, uterine and vaginal ITVs, and paracervical CTVs have been encompassed with an appropriate PTV margin. For this reason, the primary goal of four-field treatment is to reduce the amount of anterior small bowel that receives high-dose radiation. If the abdomen is rounded or protuberant, a substantial amount of bowel can usually be shielded with lateral fields; in these cases, four-field plans also tend to produce a more homogeneous dose distribution than AP–PA plans, although the magnitude of this improvement depends on the energy of the radiation beam and the AP diameter of the patient.

On the other hand, if the abdomen is flat or scaphoid, the amount of bowel that can be shielded by lateral fields is usually very small (Fig. 6.7b, e; CS 10.4, 10.5, 10.6). In such cases, the main advantage of four-field over 15 to 18 MV AP–PA treatment is elimination of the transient intergluteal skin reaction that usually occurs toward the end of a course AP–PA external beam pelvic treatment. If thin patients require inguinal node treatment because of distal vaginal involvement, AP–PA treatment is almost always preferred, to avoid flashing the skin of the mons pubis and groins.

Although four-field pelvic RT usually treats a smaller volume of bowel to high dose than AP–PA treatment, the volume of bowel, bone, soft tissue, and bone marrow treated to intermediate doses of 10 to 25 Gy is always substantially greater when four fields are used (Fig. 6.7j). Several studies have suggested that the likelihood of severe hematologic toxicity from chemoradiation is correlated with the volume of bone marrow treated to doses of radiation within this range.[16,17]

IMRT of the Pelvis for Intact Cervical Cancer

In recent years, there has been increasing interest in the use of IMRT for the regional treatment of patients with intact cervical cancer. Before prescribing inverse-planned treatment of cervical cancer, it is absolutely necessary to have a thorough understanding of the patterns of local and regional spread and, above all, a keen appreciation for the magnitude of internal organ motion (Chapters 5 and 10). We have seen many examples of inverse-planned treatments that severely underestimated the volume of tissue that was at risk for tumor involvement; the result has often been marginal recurrence and disease progression.

Even with aggressive treatment plan optimization performed by a highly skilled dosimetrist, the advantage of IMRT over 3-D conformal treatments is usually modest. The IMRT plan shown in Figure 6.7 demonstrated modest improvement over 3-D plans in terms of the volumes of bowel and bone receiving more than 30 Gy but still treated lateral structures to a much higher dose than the AP–PA plan.

There are several circumstances in which pelvic IMRT may have a substantial advantage over simpler techniques.

- Patients who have a very small or retroverted uterus and a greater than usual amount of bowel in the central pelvis.
- Patients who have stage IVA disease with a fistula (Chapter 10, CS 10.11).
- Patients who have extensive pelvic and paraaortic lymph node involvement who may benefit from an integrated boost to regions of gross disease (see "Nodal Boost Techniques" section below).

One way to determine whether IMRT is likely to have a major advantage over four-field pelvic RT is to view

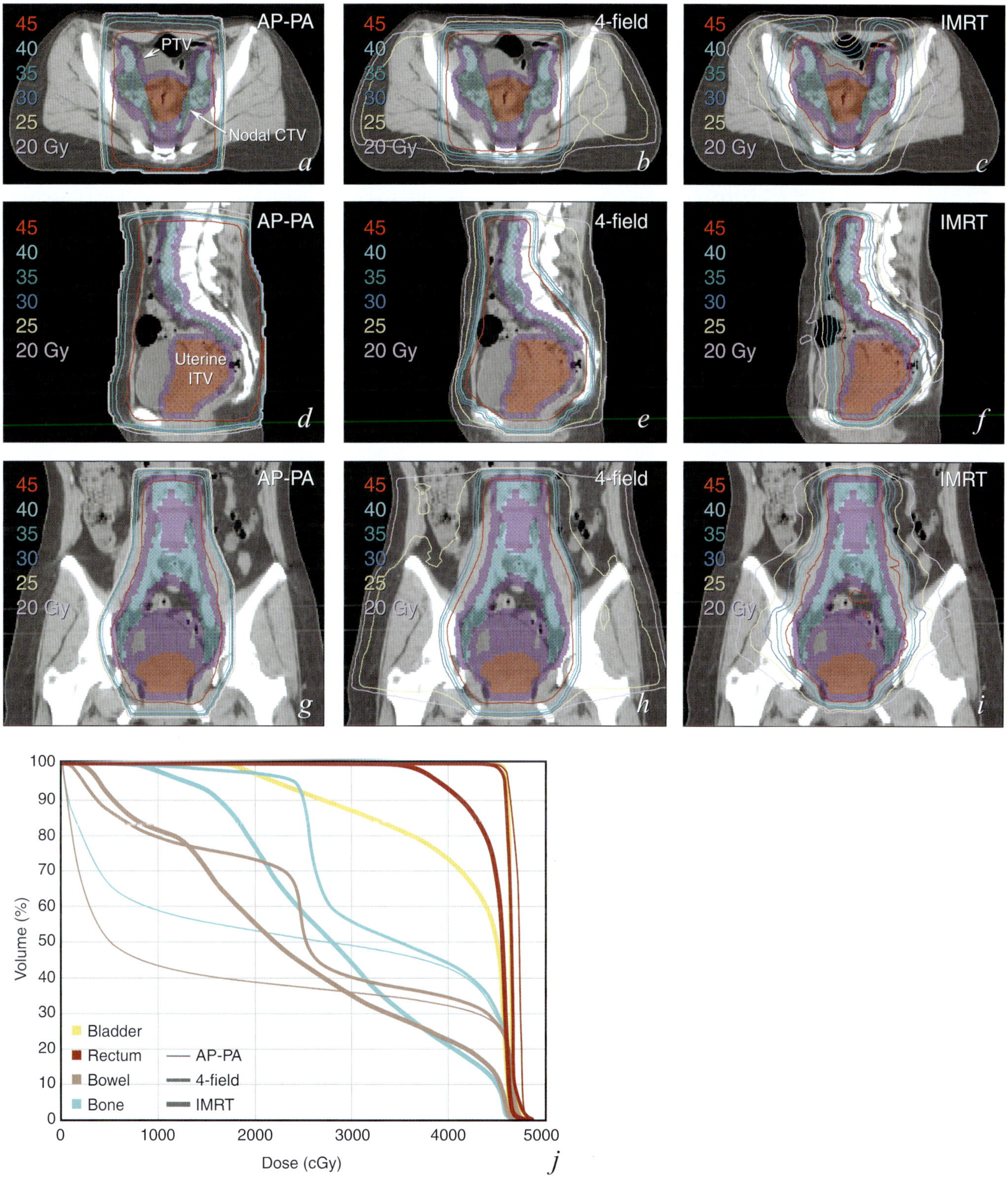

FIGURE 6.7 Three possible treatment planning approaches to pelvic RT for a patient with a 6-cm diameter, node-positive, stage IIB carcinoma of the cervix—the first (*a, d, g*) used two AP and PA 18-MV beams; the second (*b, e, h*) used four 18-MV beams; the third (*c, f, i*) is a 6-MV IMRT plan. In this case, the PTV extended anteriorly nearly to the abdominal wall (*a*). Because this anatomy permitted very little anterior shielding of lateral fields (*e*), the AP-PA plan was actually superior to the four-field plan, particularly in terms of the dose to bowel and bone marrow (*j*). IMRT was able to provide some reduction in the volumes of bone, bowel, bladder, rectum, and soft tissue receiving >30 Gy. However, had the uterus been larger, more anteverted, or more mobile, IMRT would have yielded very little advantage over the 3-D plans.

wireframe or transparent contours of the uterine and nodal CTVs or PTVs on a lateral 3-D reconstruction. If the uterine target volume extends to or nearly to the anterior limit of the nodal target volume, the distribution achieved with pelvic IMRT is unlikely to be superior and may actually be inferior to an optimized four-field plan.

Treatment of the Paraaortic Lymph Nodes

At least a portion of the paraaortic lymph node chain is frequently included as a target in gynecologic radiation therapy treatment plans. In many cases, the region is treated prophylactically to control suspected microscopic disease. However, even patients who have gross paraaortic metastases have a good chance of cure if grossly involved nodes can be treated to at least 60 Gy **(e.g., CS 10.6, 10.10, 11.2, 13.7, 14.5, and 15.1)**. The treatment of gynecologic cancers is the only setting in which radiation oncologists are routinely required to deliver more than 40 Gy to the paraaortic nodes of patients who have a high probability of cure.

The boundaries of the typical paraaortic CTV are discussed in Chapter 5 (Figs. 5.9 and 5.10). Because this region is surrounded by dose-limiting structures (kidneys, spinal cord, small bowel, and duodenum), it can be challenging to design plans that can deliver the necessary radiation dose without exceeding normal tissue tolerance limits; in our experience, this is one of the settings in which IMRT has been most helpful, making it possible to deliver definitive treatment to patients who would, in the past, have often been considered incurable.

If the paraaortic region is treated solely to eradicate possible microscopic disease, the recommended dose of 45 Gy can usually be delivered using a four-field technique without exceeding maximum normal tissue dose constraints **(CS 10.7, 13.4)**. However, it is often necessary to place greater weighting on the AP and PA fields than on the lateral fields to avoid exceeding the maximum tolerated dose to the kidneys. Two-field (e.g., AP–PA) treatment is not recommended for paraaortic RT because the volume of bowel irradiated to a high dose is excessive and because the prescribed dose usually exceeds accepted limits on the maximum dose to the spinal cord. When the paraaortic nodes are treated in conjunction with the pelvis, it may be necessary to use a step-and-shoot (field-in-field) technique to obtain a homogeneous distribution of dose throughout the entire target volume.

IMRT can usually improve on the distribution achievable with four-fields even when the prescribed dose is only 45 to 50 Gy; in these cases, IMRT is particularly helpful if the kidneys are in a relatively anterior position (i.e., lateral to the PTV). IMRT is indispensable for most cases that require treatment of gross paraaortic lymphadenopathy, particularly if the disease is extensive or if enlarged nodes are situated between the kidneys and posterior to the duodenum. In such cases, the duodenum, which typically crosses the vena cava and aorta just below the renal vessels, tends to be a critical dose-limiting structure. Although, with IMRT, it is usually possible to treat nodes in this region to 60 Gy without exceeding duodenal tolerance, several measures can help to achieve a favorable result.

- Referral to a contrast-enhanced CT, fused to the planning CT, can facilitate accurate definition of the duodenum and nodal target volumes.
- IV contrast should not be administered *during* simulation, because its high-osmolar load causes unnatural expansion of the vena cava, displacing nodes and duodenum anteriorly by as much as 5 to 6 mm. These structures can be expected to return to their more usual locations during treatment, resulting in a systematic error that can cause the duodenum to receive a higher than expected dose.
- As discussed earlier in this chapter, a slightly smaller than usual PTV margin may be used for integrated boosts if they are incorporated within a somewhat larger CTV–PTV. However, fractional doses of more than 2 Gy are not recommended in the region of the duodenum.
- Daily KV imaging that visualizes the proximal (paraaortic) portion of the target volume can be used to minimize misalignments that could prevent the prescribed dose from being delivered to the entire target.
- Adaptive planning of large nodes that regress during external beam treatment can reduce the total dose delivered to the duodenum **(CS 10.6)**.

Treatment of Paraaortic Node Recurrences after Pelvic RT

Paraaortic or common iliac recurrences that occur at the superior border of a previous pelvic RT field pose special treatment planning challenges **(CS 10.7, 13.5, 15.3)**. IMRT can help to minimize the volume of normal tissue treated in the region of overlap between the radiation treatment fields. However, special steps must be taken to optimize inverse planning in the region of potential overlap.

Marginal recurrences often occur near the lower poles of the kidneys just above the border of a previous pelvic radiation field. If the planning for paraaortic RT is performed using usual parameters, the typically strict constraints placed on the radiation dose delivered to the kidneys will drive an undesirably high dose of RT to anterior and posterior structures in the overlap region. This can be overcome by creating strict avoidance structures (usually in the form of a ring) that surround the target volume(s) in and for about 1 cm above the overlap region. In some cases, it may also be helpful to leave out a small portion of the distal kidney when setting renal avoidance criteria for inverse planning; the entire renal volume should, however, be used to create the final dose–volume histogram (DVH).

When planning for treatment of a marginal recurrence, it is also helpful to place the isocenter of the new treatment as close to the distal margin as possible. This decreases divergence into the previous field and places the isocenter in the most reproducible location, permitting use of a somewhat smaller than usual PTV margin (Chapter 4).

Treatment of the Vulva, Distal Vagina, and Inguinal Lymph Nodes

The locoregional treatment of vulvar cancer poses some unique technical challenges and deserves special attention for several reasons.

- The irregular butterfly-shaped target volume is wrapped around the dose-limiting femoral heads, requiring special techniques to achieve adequate groin coverage without exceeding normal tissue dose constraints.
- A key portion of the target volume is tangential to the axial plane. This unique relationship requires special techniques to assure that an adequate but not excessive dose is delivered to the target.
- Superficial tissues that are at risk for tumor recurrence must receive an adequate dose of radiation. However, treatment is better tolerated if the dose of radiation to skin that lies beyond the PTV is minimized. An open leg position facilitates this but creates its own set of challenges, particularly in terms of setup reproducibility and control of skin sparing within the target volume.

Clinicians have struggled for years to find an ideal solution to this treatment planning challenge. In the following sections, the advantages, disadvantages, and technical aspects of 3-D and IMRT approaches are discussed. Target volume delineation and indications for regional and local treatment are discussed in Chapters 5, 11, and 12.

3-D Fixed Beam Treatments

The introduction of electron beam treatments in the mid-1980s led to improved 3-D fixed beam solutions; these addressed some but not all of the issues discussed above. The classic approach (Fig. 6.8; CS 12.6) has three components:

- A wide anterior field that encompasses the entire local and regional target volume. In most cases, a relatively low-energy beam is selected (usually 6 MV) to limit the dose to the femoral heads and to place the superficial portions of the groin target beyond the buildup region of the radiation beam.
- A narrower posterior field that includes the vulva, pelvic lymph nodes, and medial groins, with lateral borders that are usually placed 1 to 1.5 cm lateral to the pelvic brim. A 10- to 18-MV beam is usually used for this posterior field.
- Anterior appositional electron fields that supplement the dose to the lateral portions of the groins. The medial borders of these fields are approximately matched with the exiting lateral edges of the posterior photon fields. Usually, about 30% of the dose to the lateral groins is supplied by these supplementary electron fields. The electron energy is chosen to cover the posterior margin of the inguinal target.

Although this technique provides fairly good sparing of the femoral heads, the full prescribed dose of radiation is delivered to the entire bladder, rectum, and distal small bowel (Fig. 6.8). The dose distribution produced with this technique is also relatively heterogeneous. The dose to anterior structures may be up to 10% higher than the dose at the central axis (Fig. 6.8); also, the sloping anterior contour usually causes a hot spot in the vulva, unless some form of compensation is used.

If the proximal pelvic nodes require treatment, a split-beam technique can be used to decrease the bowel dose; with this approach, the isocenter is placed at approximately the S2–S3 interspace and a four-field technique is used for the upper half of the field. Although an open-leg position can be used to achieve some sparing of the skin of the medial thigh, AP–PA fields always treat the intergluteal skin to full dose.

A major disadvantage of this approach is that it cannot be used to treat obese patients whose lateral inguinal nodes are too deep to be treated with electrons. If IMRT is not available, obese patients can be treated with high-energy beams using AP–PA or four-field techniques, but these solutions are suboptimal because they tend to expose a great deal of skin to full dose, particularly on the medial thighs and in the infrapannicular folds and usually deliver a higher than recommended dose to the femoral heads.

IMRT

Today, IMRT is increasingly been used to optimize the distribution of radiation in these complex cases. If it is skillfully planned, IMRT produces a dose distribution that is far superior to most 3-D conformal plans, with substantial sparing of the bowel, bladder, and femoral heads (Fig. 6.8). It also permits much greater control of the dose to uninvolved skin, particularly for obese patients. In our experience, both acute and late side effects can be significantly reduced with IMRT.

However, vulvar cancers pose some of the most difficult inverse planning problems in gynecologic radiation oncology. Overall, the amount of time required for contouring, planning, and quality assurance of these cases is probably greater than for any other type of gynecologic IMRT. As discussed in Chapters 5 and 12, accurate identification of the vulvar target volume can be very challenging. Once the targets have been defined, creation of an optimized treatment plan that is homogeneous, spares critical structures, and delivers an adequate dose to the targets also requires skill and patience; for this reason, these cases are usually planned by our most experienced dosimetrists. Once a plan has been devised, care must be taken to assure that superficial tissues in the vulvar target volume are receiving the desired dose.

The Use of Bolus and False Structures to Obtain an Adequate Dose to Superficial Structures

Treatment of superficial tissues of the vulva and, in some cases, inguinal target volumes pose special challenges for treatment planning for two reasons:

- Treatment planning algorithms tend to be inaccurate in the radiation buildup region, potentially underestimating or overestimating the delivered dose by up to 20%.[18] During inverse planning, this can result in plans that administer a significantly higher or lower dose than intended to superficial tissues.

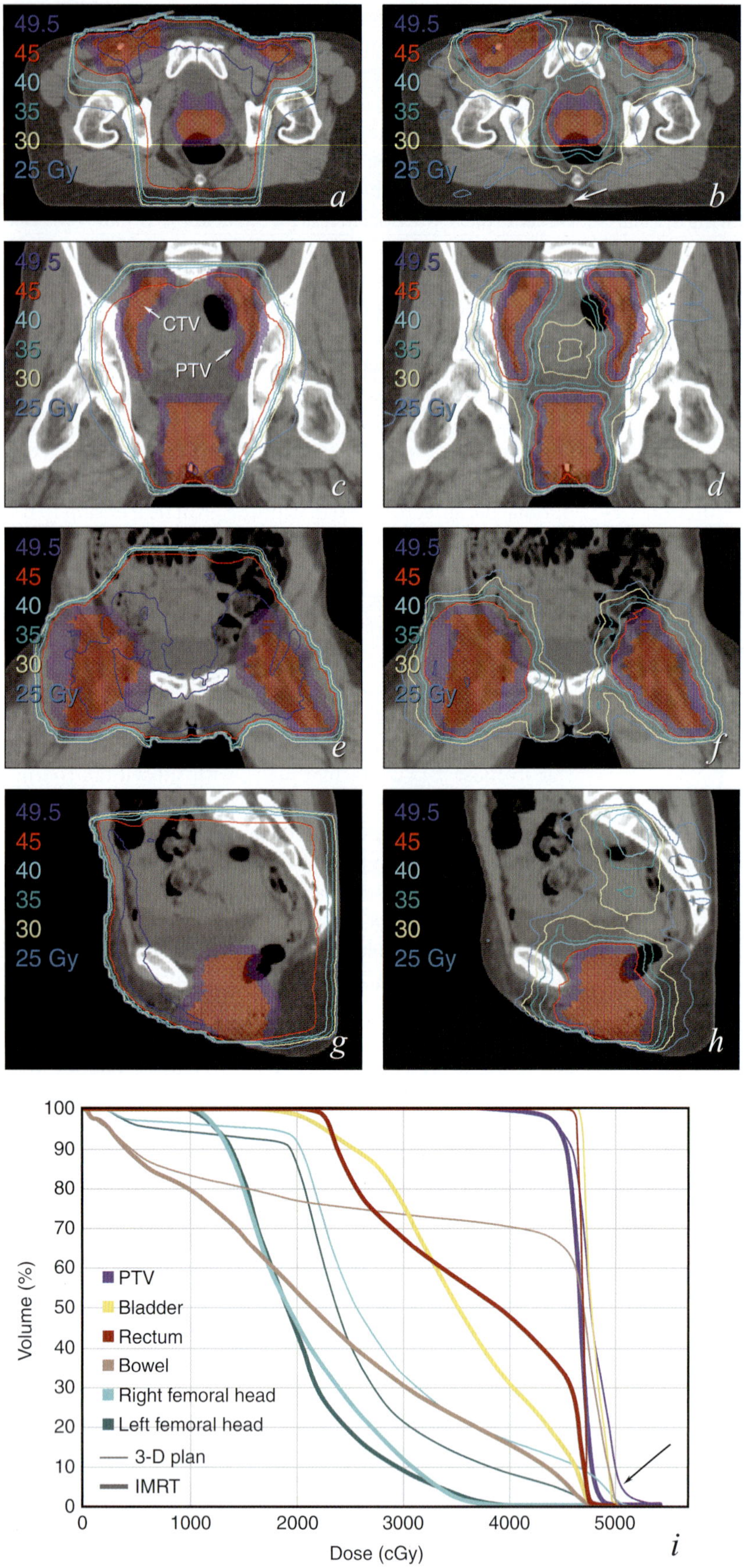

FIGURE 6.8 This figure shows axial (*a, b*), midpelvic coronal (*c, d*), anterior coronal (*e, f*), and midline sagittal views from two different treatment plans that could be used to treat the vulva, bilateral groins, and pelvic nodes. Because this patient's primary tumor was limited to the posterior vulva, the anterior mons was not included in the target volume. Before RT, a large left inguinal node metastasis was excised from the left groin; because there was evidence of extracapsular extension, the right inguinal CTV was expanded to include the entire operative bed. The treatment plan on the left is an example of a common 3-D conformal approach to this target volume. A wide 6-MV anterior field incorporated the entire target volume. To reduce the dose delivered to the femoral heads, a narrower 18-MV PA field included the vulva, pelvic nodes, and medial inguinal nodes but excluded lateral portions of the inguinal target volume. Because the AP field delivered only about 65% of the dose required to treat the lateral groins, small 16-MeV electrons were added to make up the dose to these regions. With this technique, anterior structures typically receive about 8% to 10% more than the prescribed dose (*g; arrow, i*). This heterogeneity can be factored into the prescribed inguinal dose, but it also results in a relatively high dose to anterior small bowel. The plan on the right was created using IMRT. Note that the IMRT plan delivered much lower radiation doses to the bladder, rectum, bowel, and femoral heads that the 3-D plan (*i*). By sparing uninvolved portions of the intergluteal fold (*arrow, b*) and other soft tissues, acute and late skin changes can be reduced. This patient's actual IMRT plan is shown in **CS 12.4**.

- If the plan does not provide an adequate margin or "air gap" beyond the skin surface, minor errors in the setup or alterations in the external contour caused by vulvar inflammation and edema can cause the target to fall outside the radiation field.

If 1 to 1.5 cm of bolus is added to the vulva at the time of simulation, a PTV can be added that will fall within the bolus. However, this thick bolus material tends to conform poorly to the skin surface; also, in some cases, elimination of all skin sparing may not be desirable.

An alternative solution is to digitally apply a virtual bolus or "false structure" that can accommodate an adequate PTV margin during the inverse planning process (**Fig. 6.9**). After an optimized plan has been calculated with the false structure in place, the plan should then be reapplied with the structure removed to confirm that its elimination has not caused unacceptable heterogeneities in the final dose distribution (**Fig. 6.9d**).

Because with this method the patient is simulated without bolus in place, the surface anatomy can be viewed on digital renderings of the vulvar surface (**Fig. 6.10a**); this can be a very helpful aid during contouring (Chapter 5). A digital skin rendering with the false structure in place (**Fig. 6.10**) can then be used to shape bolus for the actual treatment.

During the first week of treatment, thermoluminescent dosimeters (TLDs) should be used to measure the dose to various portions of the vulvar skin with and without the bolus applied **(CS 12.2)**. Because of the tangential incidence of the beams, 3 mm of bolus is almost always sufficient to eliminate skin sparing in the vulva; 3-mm bolus is also easier to conform to the surface contour than thicker bolus. If the surface radiation doses are inadequate with 3-mm bolus, the plan and light fields should be re-checked to confirm that there is an adequate air gap distal to the vulva (i.e., that the collimator is not shielding a portion of the target); once this has been confirmed, 5-mm bolus should be applied and TLD measurements repeated.

Large, cavitating cancers may have irregular surfaces that are inadequately bolused with standard sheets of tissue equivalent material. To achieve a more homogeneous distribution in these cases, the cavity can be packed with wet gauze during simulation and daily treatments **(CS 12.7)**.

Treatment of Extremely Obese Patients

Extreme obesity poses special problems at almost every phase of radiation therapy planning and treatment. Poor-quality CT and x-ray images decrease confidence in the accuracy of target volumes and in the reproducibility of daily setup during treatment. Many treatment tables cannot accommodate patients who weigh more than 350 to 400 lb. Extreme obesity also limits the options available for treatment planning. The field of view of CT simulators is commonly too narrow to encompass the entire contour of very obese patients. Although this problem can sometimes be overcome (Fig. 4.9), a more serious impediment is posed by limits in treatment planning algorithms, which typically do not accommodate extremely large patient contours. In these cases, the available treatment beam angles may be severely limited because lateral soft tissue cannot be modeled in the treatment planning system.

Simple AP–PA techniques are usually technically feasible but are not desirable for several reasons:

- AP and PA fields that pass through the subpanicular and intergluteal folds are likely to case severe skin reactions. Although local care and management of yeast infections

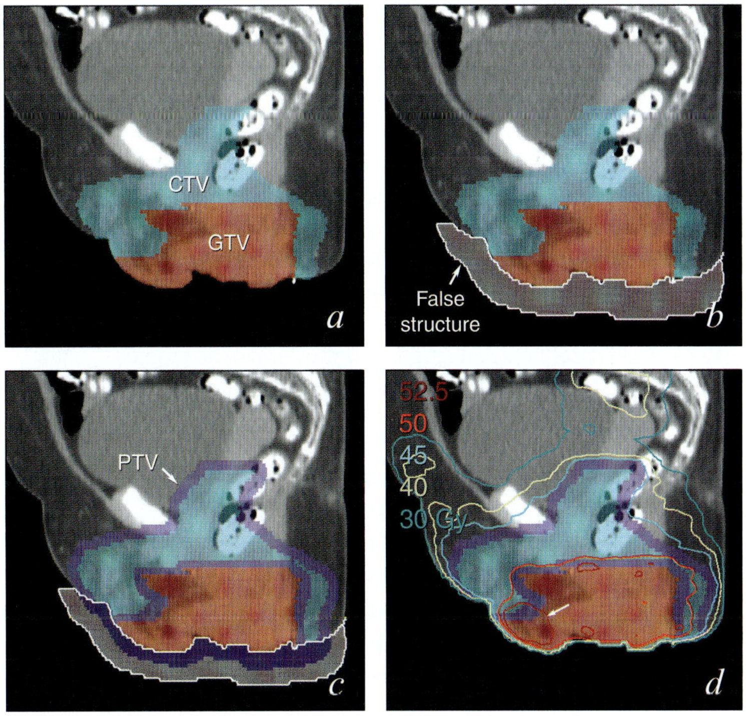

FIGURE 6.9 Addition of a false structure to facilitate inverse planning of vulvar IMRT. The patient depicted in this figure had a locally advanced vulvar cancer with extensive skin involvement that tracked into the left groin *(a)*. Before inverse planning was started, a false structure of tissue-equivalent density was added to the target surface *(b)*. When a 7-mm margin was added, the PTV extended into the false structure *(c)*. Before it was approved, the treatment plan was recalculated without the false structure to confirm adequate target coverage and homogeneity *(d)*; a localized 5% hot spot within tumor *(arrow)* was considered acceptable. Thermoluminescent dosimeters were subsequently used to measure the surface dose with and without 3 mm of bolus. Based on the results, bolus was applied daily during the first 2 weeks and then every other day until the end of treatment.

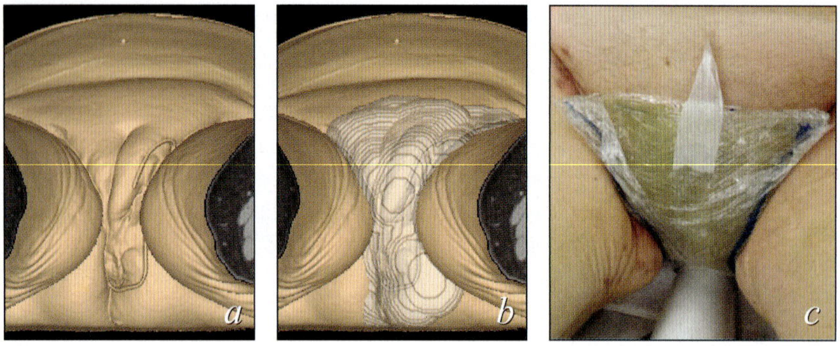

FIGURE 6.10 Digitally reconstructed surface renderings can be used to assist contouring and to design and accurately place bolus for treatment. From the patient discussed in Figure 6.9, a surface rendering of the vulva (*a*) shows tumor-related deformity and wires that were used to demarcate visible skin lesions. In *b*, the false structure has been added to the reconstructed image. The final 3-mm thick bolus was fashioned and positioned using the reconstructed images for guidance (*c*).

can provide some relief (Chapter 7), these reactions are best avoided whenever possible.

- The radiation dose tends to be very heterogeneous, with the dose to subcutaneous tissues sufficient to cause late fibrosis, even when high-energy (e.g., 15- to 18-MV) beams are used.
- AP–PA fields typically deliver the full prescribed dose of RT to a large volume of bowel and to the entire bladder and rectosigmoid.

For these reasons, multiple field techniques are always preferred. **Figure 6.11** demonstrates two different techniques that can be used to treat the whole pelvis.

3-D Conformal Treatment Using Four Oblique Fields

The recommended technique for pelvic treatments of very obese patients involves four oblique fields. Although the ideal angles of incidence are usually 45, 135, 225, and 315 degrees, it may be necessary to shift the beams slightly toward the midline to have a complete external contour within the full width of each beam. In almost all cases, unmodified beams produce significant areas of overdosage anteriorly and posteriorly; these hot spots, which usually fall in small bowel or rectum (**Fig. 6.11a, d**), can be eliminated with appropriate use of wedges or step-and-shoot, field-in-field techniques (**Fig. 6.11b, c**). Oblique fields work less well if more than 40 Gy needs to be delivered to extended fields, because the spinal cord cannot be easily protected without compromising coverage of the paraaortic target volume. In some cases, there is sufficient lateral contour visualized proximal to the pelvis to enable the use of a split field technique; with this approach, AP, PA, and lateral fields are applied to the paraaortic targets. Alternatively, IMRT may provide an acceptable solution.

IMRT

Because of the restricted beam angles and the need for relatively wide PTV margins, IMRT usually does not improve a great deal on a 3-D oblique treatment approach. Even when the lateral diameter of the patient can accommodate a standard four-field approach with AP–PA and lateral fields, the benefit of IMRT tends to be less for patients whose BMI is >30 than for thinner patients.[19] Also, because high-energy beams (>10 MV) are often required to achieve an acceptable IMRT plan in obese patients, collateral neutron exposure from IMRT may be greater than with a 3-D technique. However, for patients who require higher than usual doses to treat gross disease, IMRT may hold some advantage **(CS 13.10)**.

Because setups based on skin marks and lasers are poorly reproducible in very obese patients, daily KV image guidance is recommended in all cases. However, cone beam CT imaging is of little value because of the very poor quality of the images in obese patients.

Nodal Boost Techniques

Localized boosts are often required to supplement the radiation dose to involved or suspicious lymph nodes or, after lymphadenectomy, to sites of extracapsular nodal extension. A variety of techniques can be used according to the site and extent of the disease, the required dose, the proximity of critical structures, and the technique that is used for initial comprehensive nodal RT. For patients who also require brachytherapy to boost central disease, particular care must be taken to avoid critical structures that will be receiving a significant dose of radiation from the brachytherapy (**Fig. 6.12**).

Techniques Used for Patients Who Are Treated with External Beam RT Only

For patients who have only one or two relatively small nodes, 3-D conformal treatment approaches are often adequate. Small common iliac boosts of 15 to 20 Gy may be accomplished using four (AP, PA, and laterals) beams or three nonconvergent beams. Unilateral distal pelvic nodes can be boosted with three or more beams arranged in a variety of ways. In general, the use of nonconvergent beams decreases the volume of bowel and other critical structures treated to high dose. This is particularly true for bilateral pelvic node boosts because in this situation converging lateral fields tend to treat a large volume of central pelvic bowel to a higher than necessary dose (**Fig. 6.12**).

As the size and number of nodes increases, it becomes increasingly difficult to achieve an adequate dose to high-risk targets without exceeding normal tissue tolerance limits. This is particularly true in the paraaortic region, where renal, duodenal, and spinal cord constraints can rarely be met with 3-D techniques even when six or more fields are used.

For this reason, IMRT is strongly recommended for patients who have extensive nodal metastases. For these complex cases, experienced dosimetrists typically can produce a superior plan

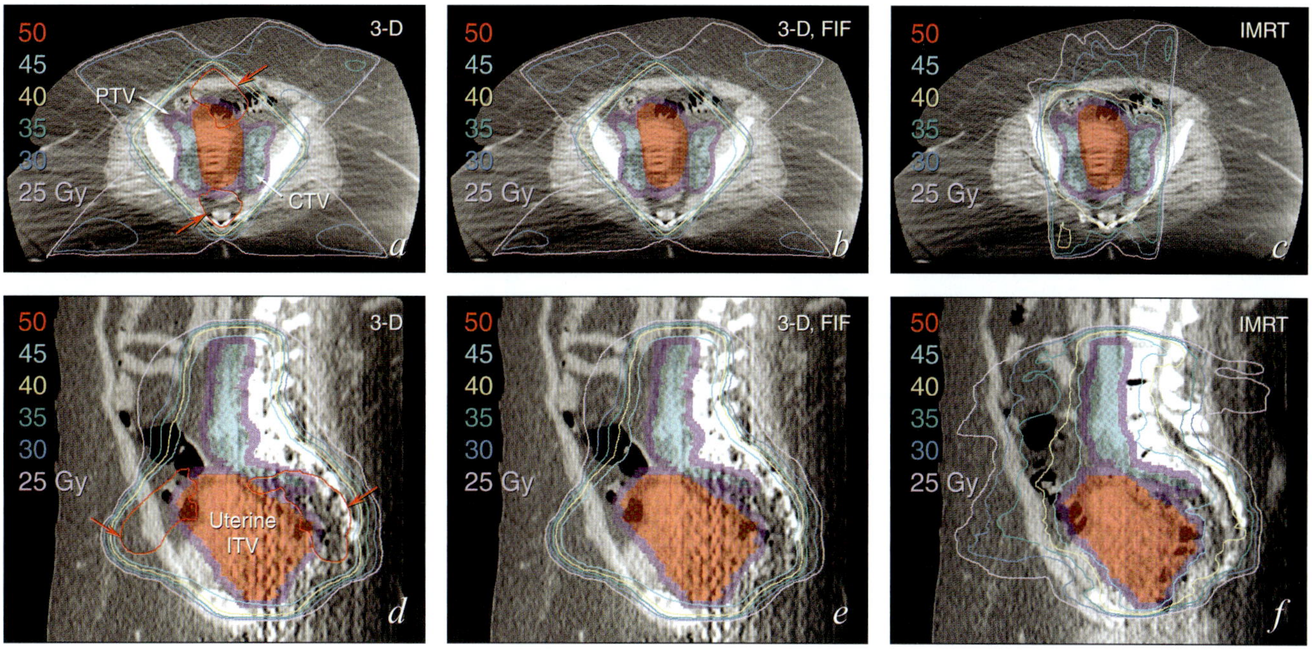

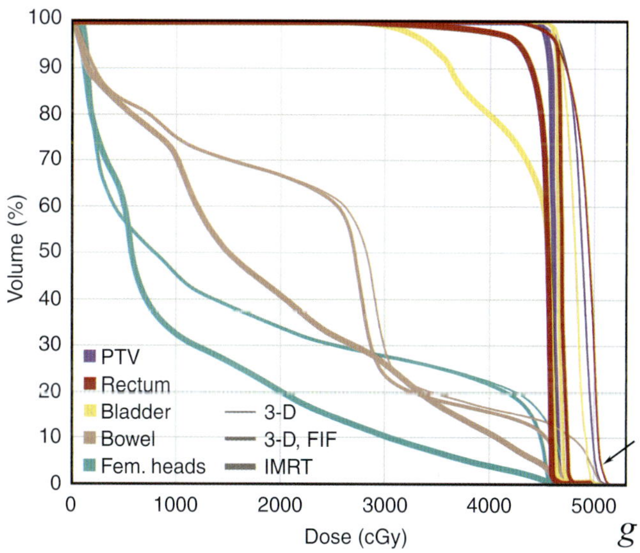

FIGURE 6.11 Three treatment plans designed to deliver 45 Gy of pelvic RT for a uterine cancer that was medically inoperable because of extreme obesity. In *a* and *b*, four oblique fields (45, 135, 225, and 315 degrees) of 18-MV photons were used without compensation; this plan produced unacceptable hot spots *(red arrows, a, d; arrow g)*. Field-in-field (FIF) compensation produced a more homogeneous dose distribution *(b, e)*. Because of the limited beam angles and intact uterus, IMRT *(c, f)* was only slightly better than the optimized 3-D plan *(g)*. However, this patient, who had grossly positive pelvic nodes, was treated with IMRT for reasons discussed in **CS 13.10**. PTV, planning target volume; CTV, clinical target volume; ITV; internal target volume.

with inverse planning and can do so in less time than would be required to produce an acceptable 3-D conformal plan.

If IMRT is used for the entire treatment course, it is often advantageous to integrate at least a portion of the boost dose with the initial locoregional treatment. This reduces the total treatment time and, as discussed earlier in this chapter, permits use of a slightly smaller PTV margin than is required for a sequential boost. Most commonly, we use an integrated boost to treat high-risk CTVs or GTVs to 50 Gy at a rate of 2 Gy per fraction while the larger CTV receives 45 Gy at 1.8 Gy per fraction; this is followed by five or more treatments of 2 Gy each that are given as a sequential boost. Many examples of this approach are illustrated in the case studies associated with Chapters 10 to 15.

It is probably not wise to treat integrated or sequential nodal boosts at rates of more than 2 Gy per fraction if the abnormal nodes are closely adjacent to hollow viscera. However, larger daily fractions of up to 2.2 Gy may be considered for targets that are surrounded by soft tissues (e.g., adipose and muscle) if nearby critical structures are not exposed to fractional doses of more than 2 Gy.

Pelvic Node Boosts for Patients Who Are Receiving Brachytherapy

The dose contributed from intrauterine brachytherapy should always be considered when prescribing boosts to pelvic node metastases. If brachytherapy is begun before boosts are completed, the total brachytherapy dose contribution can usually be estimated from the first procedure.

In the past, standard doses of low-dose rate (LDR) brachytherapy for cervical cancer usually delivered 10 to 12 Gy to

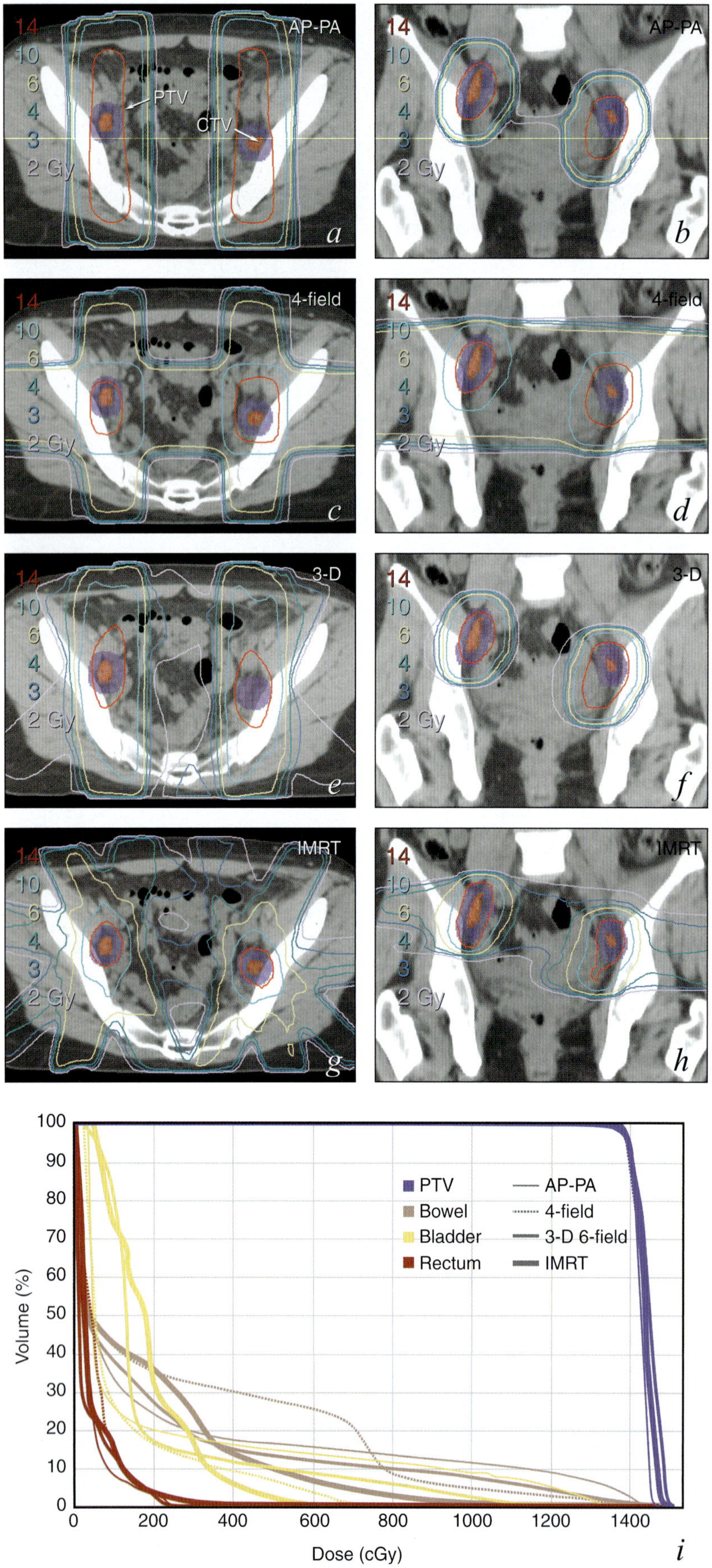

FIGURE 6.12 Four different techniques that can be used to boost bilateral pelvic node metastases after 45 Gy of pelvic RT. Unless the required dose is <10 Gy, AP–PA fields (*a, b*) usually result in an unacceptably high total dose to anterior small bowel. A four-field technique is often used to boost high common iliac or paraaortic nodes but is not ideal for treatment of midpelvic nodes because of the relatively high-dose delivered to central pelvic bowel (*c, d, i*). The eight-field 3-D technique shown in *e* and *f* is more complex but provided some sparing of the central pelvis with less anterior dose than was delivered with the AP–PA technique. Because brachytherapy also contributed a significant dose to midline bowel, the IMRT and eight-field conformal plans were the best solutions for this patient. Her final IMRT plan included several noncoplanar beams. Noncoplanar arrangements are sometimes particularly helpful when patients who are receiving brachytherapy require high-dose boosts to pelvic nodes. However, in this case **(CS 10.5)**, the noncoplanar arrangement was only slightly better than the coplanar plan shown in *g* and *h*.

the distal pelvic lymph nodes; this, combined with a typical course of pelvic RT, yielded a combined dose of 55 to 59 Gy to involved nodes. The additional 4 to 8 Gy required to treat distal pelvic nodes could usually be safely given with an AP–PA technique using 15- to 18-MV photons.

However, today, rapid responses to chemoradiation lead to smaller central targets, and brachytherapy is often given using high dose-rate techniques that deliver lower nominal doses of RT than LDR brachytherapy. These changes have resulted in brachytherapy treatments that, on average, deliver significantly lower doses to the pelvic sidewall than was the case in the past. As a result, patients who have pelvic node metastases from cervical cancer now routinely require boost doses of 12 Gy or more after 45 Gy of pelvic RT.

In general, if a boost dose of more than 10 Gy is required, AP–PA fields are not recommended, because they usually expose a significant volume of anterior small bowel or sigmoid to the full dose of radiation (**Fig. 6.12**). For this reason, multiple field techniques using oblique or noncoplanar fields are usually more satisfactory. IMRT can also be used, but in most cases, two isocenters are required to treat bilateral pelvic nodes.

Whenever distal pelvic nodes require boosts, care must be taken to minimize the dose delivered to central pelvic structures. Any dose that is delivered to midline must be considered during brachytherapy dose calculations; boost treatments that expose a portion of the bladder or rectosigmoid without fully encompassing the high-risk target volume can necessitate unwanted compromises in the dose delivered to the primary cancer. In general, boosts should be designed to deliver no more than 3 Gy to midline critical structures. *Dose distributions should always be reviewed with this in mind*; boost treatment plans should always display several isodose lines in the range between 2 and 6 Gy.

Other Factors that influence the Choice of Technique

Although the most important determinants of treatment technique relate to anatomic considerations, a number of other factors must be considered.

- *Resources.* In some settings, complex inverse-planned techniques such as IMRT are unavailable either because the facility lacks necessary equipment or sufficient personnel. In some cases, referral to another facility that has the necessary equipment and expertise may be worthwhile if IMRT is felt to be necessary to achieve complication-free locoregional control.
- *Expertise.* Although IMRT can be a valuable tool, particularly for the treatment of recurrent and regionally extensive gynecologic cancers, the methods and techniques are complex and require specialized training. In many cases, a well-designed 3-D plan is better than an ill-conceived IMRT plan that is performed by an inexperienced team.
- *Insurance coverage.* In the United States, most gynecologic applications require peer-to-peer discussion with insurers to obtain coverage for IMRT. IMRT is a costly resource that should always be used with discretion. However, the large volumes irradiated, the frequent need to administer high doses of radiation to areas of gross disease, and the significant probability of cure, even in the face of advanced disease, are all compelling arguments for the use of IMRT in selected cases. It is often helpful to remind insurers that the lack of level 1 data supporting use of IMRT reflects the rarity of many of these conditions, which are unlikely, because of the small number of patients, to ever be investigated in phase III trials.

Hypofractionation and Stereotactic Body RT

The hallmarks of SBRT include rigid patient immobilization, inverse treatment planning, attention to respiratory motion of thoracic and mobile upper abdominal targets, and onboard imaging. It should be noted that all of these are also characteristic elements of high-quality, standardly fractionated IMRT as it is used in the treatment of many gynecologic cancers.

The final element of SBRT is extreme hypofractionation, typically using radiation fractions of 10 Gy or more. Highly accurate, hypofractionated treatment has proven particularly useful as an ablative alternative to surgical resection of metastatic lesions in the lung parenchyma, liver, or noncritical portions of the brain. For patients who have small isolated metastatic lesions to these sites, SBRT may be a convenient and effective palliative treatment; in rare cases of oligometastatic disease, SBRT may even be curative.[20,21]

However, extreme hypofractionation is contraindicated for most potentially curative gynecologic radiation therapy applications, for several reasons:

- Most gynecologic cancers have already infiltrated adjacent tissues or regional nodes by the time a gross lesion is detected. Treatments that focus only on a primary or nodal GTV are rarely curative, and the large fields that are needed to encompass potential sites of microscopic disease cannot be safely treated with definitive hypofractionated schedules.
- Most central targets are extremely mobile. Movements of the vagina and uterus can be erratic, involving tilts as well as translational shifts (Figs. 5.14 and 5.15); significant shifts can occur even during the course of a single treatment. In an elegant MRI-based study of intrafraction motion of central structures, Kerkhof et al.[22] reported shifts in the positions of the uterus, cervix, and vagina of up to 1 cm during a 16-minute treatment.
- Most gynecologic targets lie within 0 to 5 mm of vulnerable hollow viscera. Ablation of even very small portions of these critical structures (e.g., rectum, sigmoid, small bowel, duodenum, or bladder) can cause potentially fatal perforations.

- Patients who are cured or who survive for many years after SBRT may begin to demonstrate late side effects that are rarely seen with standard treatment schedules (Fig. 9.9).

Hypofractionated Treatment of Isolated In-Field Recurrences

Hypofractionated schedules may be used to treat selected patients who have an isolated, potentially curable, in-field recurrence if the target is small and the nearest critical structure is at least 5 mm from the target (**CS 13.5**). In such cases, the following approach is recommended:

- Generate a "best plan" (e.g., a maximally conformal plan that covers the target *with a realistic margin for possible setup uncertainties*).
- Determine what percent of the prescribed dose is received by the nearest critical structure.
- Calculate the dose per fraction that will provide the greatest difference between the biologically effective dose (BED) to the target and the BED to the highest dose 2 cc of the nearest critical structure.
- Renormalize the plan to deliver a definitive dose to the target using the selected dose per fraction.
- Evaluate the safety of treatment after reviewing the DVHs for all critical structures in the context of previous treatment.

If the resulting treatment plan is deemed unsafe, alternative treatments should be reconsidered, such as resection followed by IORT, chemotherapy, or palliative RT using a less than definitive dose.

Proton Beam Therapy for Gynecologic Cancers

Although proton therapy is a conceptually appealing approach to the treatment of gynecologic cancers, there have as yet been very few reported cases of patients treated with protons for routine gynecologic problems. Theoretical comparisons between proton and photon distributions are encouraging, but these hypothetical plans have not always taken into account the uncertainties that can result from internal organ motion, changes in body contour, and potential variations in the density of material in pelvic bowel. Comparisons invariably conclude that the volume of tissue exposed to relatively low doses is smaller with protons than with IMRT; however, this is sometimes at the expense of a somewhat larger volume of bowel and bladder that is exposed to a relatively high dose.[23] Because many major complications of gynecologic radiation therapy are correlated with the volume of tissue receiving high-dose radiation, it is not entirely clear that these proton plans would be beneficial. However, much more study is needed to clarify the role of proton therapy in treatment of gynecologic cancers.

TREATMENT PLAN EVALUATION, DOCUMENTATION, AND QUALITY ASSURANCE

In most cases, there is only one chance to deliver curative radiation therapy for gynecologic cancers. The quality of the treatment delivered will be an important factor in determining whether the patient survives her cancer and maintains a high quality of life. Plan optimization, documentation, and quality assurance are key steps in the planning process of any radiation treatment (**Fig. 6.1**). This is particularly important for the complex plans used to treat gynecologic patients.

Evaluation of the Treatment Plan

Once the dosimetrist has created a treatment plan, it must be reviewed by the physician to determine whether the treatment objectives have been met. It is wise to develop a systematic approach to this review process. In most cases, thorough review involves scanning of the entire treatment volume by slowly scrolling through axial, sagittal, and coronal views. Critical features of the DVHs should then be reviewed; if the DVHs suggest that some tissues may be receiving an inadequate or excessive dose, the isodose contours should be reexamined to locate the areas of concern. Before reviewing the treatment plan, the display should be optimized to provide all the necessary information:

- Isodose distributions should include at least one line every 10 Gy and usually one line every 5 Gy in the high-dose region. For boosts that are treated to <20 Gy, one line every 2 to 4 Gy is needed to obtain a full sense of the plan quality.
- The point of maximum dose should be displayed.
- Target volume contours should be displayed in a way that makes it easy to differentiate them from isodose lines. We prefer to review plans with the CTVs and GTVs visible but with the PTV margins and most of the critical structure contours turned off. This enables a clearer view of the isodose contours and of the doses delivered to critical structures within the PTV margins.

The following features should always be considered in the physician's review:

- *Inclusiveness*: Have all the target volumes been incorporated in the treatment plan? Has the appropriate PTV margin been added to each? Although previous quality assurance measures should have eliminated errors in contouring (**Fig. 6.1, Table 5.2**), the time of treatment plan review provides another opportunity to verify the accuracy of target volume designations.
- *Coverage*: *Is the entire PTV receiving the prescribed dose?* There is often some trade-off between ideal PTV coverage and normal tissue protection. However, any compromises should be carefully considered in the context of the patient's clinical situation. If areas of inadequate coverage

are found at the margins of the treatment volume, it is usually better to increase the field size than to renormalize the plan to a different isodose line; when the entire plan is renormalized to address a localized problem, the result is usually increased dose heterogeneity and exposure of critical structures to a higher than necessary dose.

- *Conformality*: Conformality should be scrutinized throughout the treatment volume and throughout the range of doses delivered. It is not enough to have a prescription isodose line that conforms to the shape of the target—IMRT plans that only display the 90% to 100% isodose lines may look very conformal, but hide the fact that the rest of the plan is exposing critical structures to higher than necessary doses. Even plans that meet minimum standards for conformality can often be improved (**Fig. 6.5**). The goal should always be to seek the maximum degree of conformality that can be achieved *without compromising the dose delivered to the PTV*.
- *Homogeneity*: Whenever possible, the volume of tissue receiving more than 105% of the prescribed dose should be small. Technical limitations posed by some 3-D techniques can result in somewhat greater dose heterogeneity (**Figs. 6.8** and **6.11**), but this can often be improved by using a step-and-shoot, field-in-field compensation technique (**Fig. 6.11**). IMRT plans that are not adequately optimized can result in extremely heterogeneous dose distributions with scattered regions that receive 110% or more of the prescribed dose. These hot spots can almost always be eliminated through the creation of special avoidance structures in high-dose areas. With modern treatment planning algorithms and experienced dosimetry staff, more than 5% heterogeneity is rarely necessary and should be considered unacceptable in most settings.
- *Radiation doses to critical structures*: An initial scan of treatment isodose contours usually provides a sense of any problem areas. However, DVHs should always be scrutinized to confirm that normal tissue dose constraints have been met. For small, dose-limiting structures such as the duodenum or sigmoid, a tabular view of the DVHs provides more detailed information than the histogram curves.

IMRT requires specialized training for all members of the treatment planning team. Many of the methods and "tricks" used to optimize IMRT plans are difficult to find in textbooks. Recently, automated plan optimization algorithms have helped to streamline the planning of complex multitarget IMRT treatments. However, in our experience, plans generated in this way still do not always match the quality achieved by a very experienced dosimetrist. Whenever possible, dosimetrists who were trained more than 10 to 15 years ago should be afforded opportunities to obtain specialized training in IMRT and, specifically, in the optimization techniques used for gynecologic applications.

Treatment Summary Documentation

Clear, detailed written documentation of the radiation treatment plan is important for several reasons:

- Recurrences at the margins of external beam treatment fields may be curable. However, the risks of retreatment are impossible to estimate if the extent of previous treatment is unknown.
- Safe planning of palliative treatments also requires knowledge of previous treatment.
- The risks of surgical salvage treatments are better understood with knowledge of previous radiation doses and volumes.
- An understanding of the dose and volume of radiation can shed light on posttreatment diagnostic findings.
- Interpretation of possible late treatment-related symptoms is facilitated by accurate information about the doses received by critical structures.

Forward planned, 3-D conformal treatments can usually be reconstructed from films or digitally reconstructed radiographs of the radiation fields and a summary that documents the treatment dates, site(s) treated, patient position, beam modifiers and treatment aids, beam energy, doses delivered, and fractionation.

IMRT treatments require much more detailed documentation. Two or three central axis views of the isodose distribution never provide sufficient information to meet clinical requirements. The American Society for Radiation Oncology[24] has recommended that the IMRT treatment plan printout and treatment summary include all the information described above and:

- The doses prescribed to each target volume)
- Cumulative DVHs for targets and organs at risk
- Isodose distributions on CT images, including:
  - Axial planes at intervals of 1 cm or less, extending 1 cm beyond the superior and inferior limits of the treatment fields
  - Coronal and sagittal cuts through the center of the PTV and any dose-limiting normal tissue such as spinal cord
- Dose–volume statistics that include minimum and maximum doses to targets and organs at risk

Despite these recommendations, made in 2009, many treatment records lack this key information, complicating efforts to plan subsequent treatments (**Figs. 6.2** and **6.3**).

Peer Review and Quality Assurance

The importance of adequate peer review and quality assurance cannot be overestimated. In recent years, as part of its Target Safely Campaign, the American Society for Radiation

Oncology has published a series of white papers, stressing the importance of quality assurance and setting standards for high-quality radiation therapy delivery.[24–26]

Of particular importance, is the role of physician peer review. The many components of the complex treatments discussed in this book undoubtedly leave greater than usual room for error. The long period of focused concentration required to accurately contour the target volumes for cases of locoregionally extensive disease may not be easy to find in a busy clinical environment. For this reason, we strongly advocate the use of checklists such as that illustrated in Table 5.2—this first step of "self-review" can prevent many errors. Every case should also be reviewed by a physician peer. For complex IMRT cases, we recommend a two-step peer-review process—an initial review of proposed doses and contours and a second review of the completed treatment plan. These reviews should occur at a dedicated time, with minimal distractions and with resources that permit reference to diagnostic images, pathology reports, and other critical features of the medical record. Physician peer review should include the following:

- An evaluation of the overall treatment plan including the treatment intent (curative vs. palliative), the appropriateness of proposed adjuvant treatments, and the need for multidisciplinary treatments.
- An assessment of the completeness and accuracy of each target volume.
- A review of the prescribed doses and fractionation.
- A review of the quality of the treatment plan in terms of coverage, conformality, and homogeneity.
- A review of critical structure doses.
- Confirmation that key quality assurance measures have been completed (e.g., quality assurance checks of IMRT treatments).
- A description of future brachytherapy or external beam boost treatments and the measures that have been taken to plan for these future needs. A quality assurance conference is a good place to arrange for scheduling for diagnostic studies, operating room time, or resimulations that will be required to complete the entire course of treatment.

The peer-review process is not confined to physicians but involves every member of the radiation oncology team, including therapists, dosimetrists, and physicists. A full accounting of key quality assurance and peer-review measures is beyond the scope of this chapter. However, **Figure 6.1** summarizes some of the key steps in the process and quality assurance of gynecologic radiation therapy delivery.[26]

References

1. Bataini P, Brugere J, Bernier J, et al. Results of radical radiotherapeutic treatment of carcinoma of the pyriform sinus: experience of the Institut Curie. *Int J Radiat Oncol Biol Phys.* 1982;8:1277–1286.
2. Okunieff P, Morgan D, Niemierko A, et al. Radiation dose-response of human tumors. *Int J Radiat Oncol Biol Phys.* 1995;32:1227–1237.
3. Van Dyk J, Battista JJ, Bauman GS. Accuracy and uncertainty considerations in modern radiation oncology. In: Van Dyk J, ed. *The Modern Technology of Radiation Oncology*. Madison, WI: Medical Physics Publishing; 2013:61–416.
4. Osborne E, Klopp A, Jhingran A, et al. Definitive extended-field radiation therapy for cervical cancer pateints with para-aortic lymph node metastases. *Int J Radiat Oncol Biol Phys.* 2015;93: S202–S203.
5. Kim H, Beriwal S, Huq MS, et al. Evaluation of set-up uncertainties with daily kilovoltage image guidance in external beam radiation therapy for gynaecological cancers. *Clin Oncol (R Coll Radiol).* 2012;24:e39–e45.
6. van Herk M. Errors and margins in radiotherapy. *Semin Radiat Oncol.* 2004;14:52–64.
7. Santanam L, Esthappan J, Mutic S, et al. Estimation of setup uncertainty using planar and MVCT imaging for gynecologic malignancies. *Int J Radiat Oncol Biol Phys.* 2008;71:1511–1517.
8. Malone S, Szanto J, Perry G, et al. A prospective comparison of three systems of patient immobilization for prostate radiotherapy. *Int J Radiat Oncol Biol Phys.* 2000;48:657–665.
9. Klein EE, Hanley J, Bayouth J, et al. Task Group 142 report: quality assurance of medical accelerators. *Med Phys.* 2009;36:4197–4212.
10. Boothe D, Patel SH, Stessin A, et al. Comparing the rates of urinary tract infections among patients receiving adjuvant pelvic intensity modulated radiation therapy, 3-dimensional conformal radiation therapy, and brachytherapy for newly diagnosed endometrial cancer. *Pract Radiat Oncol.* 2013;3:269–274.
11. Marks LB, Yorke ED, Jackson A, et al. Use of normal tissue complication probability models in the clinic. *Int J Radiat Oncol Biol Phys.* 2010;76:S10–S19.
12. Gay HA, Barthold HJ, O'Meara E, et al. Pelvic normal tissue contouring guidelines for radiation therapy: a Radiation Therapy Oncology Group consensus panel atlas. *Int J Radiat Oncol Biol Phys.* 2012;83:e353–e362.
13. Logsdon MD, Eifel PJ. Figo IIIB squamous cell carcinoma of the cervix: an analysis of prognostic factors emphasizing the balance between external beam and intracavitary radiation therapy. *Int J Radiat Oncol Biol Phys.* 1999;43:763–775.
14. Jabbour SK, Hashem SA, Bosch W, et al. Upper abdominal normal organ contouring guidelines and atlas: a Radiation Therapy Oncology Group consensus. *Pract Radiat Oncol.* 2014;4:82–89.
15. Verma J, Sulman EP, Jhingran A, et al. Dosimetric predictors of duodenal toxicity after intensity modulated radiation therapy for treatment of the para-aortic nodes in gynecologic cancer. *Int J Radiat Oncol Biol Phys.* 2014;88:357–362.
16. Albuquerque K, Giangreco D, Morrison C, et al. Radiation-related predictors of hematologic toxicity after concurrent chemoradiation for cervical cancer and implications for bone marrow-sparing pelvic IMRT. *Int J Radiat Oncol Biol Phys.* 2011; 79:1043–1047.
17. Rose BS, Aydogan B, Liang Y, et al. Normal tissue complication probability modeling of acute hematologic toxicity in cervical cancer patients treated with chemoradiotherapy. *Int J Radiat Oncol Biol Phys.* 2011;79:800–807.
18. Price RA Jr, Koren S, Veltchev I, et al. Planning target volume-to-skin proximity for head-and-neck intensity modulated radiation therapy treatment planning. *Pract Radiat Oncol.* 2014;4: e21–e29.

19. Ahamad A, D'Souza W, Salehpour M, et al. Intensity-modulated radiation therapy after hysterectomy: comparison with conventional treatment and sensitivity of the normal-tissue-sparing effect to margin size. *Int J Radiat Oncol Biol Phys.* 2005;62: 1117–1124.
20. Mayr NA, Huang Z, Sohn JW, et al. Emerging application of stereotactic body radiation therapy for gynecologic malignancies. *Expert Rev Anticancer Ther.* 2011;11:1069-1075.
21. Kunos CA, Brindle J, Waggoner S, et al. Phase II clinical trial of robotic stereotactic body radiosurgery for metastatic gynecologic malignancies. *Front Oncol.* 2012;2:181.
22. Kerkhof EM, van der Put RW, Raaymakers BW, et al. Intrafraction motion in patients with cervical cancer: the benefit of soft tissue registration using MRI. *Radiother Oncol.* 2009;93:115–121.
23. Lin LL, Kirk M, Scholey J, et al. Initial report of pencil beam scanning proton therapy for posthysterectomy patients with gynecologic cancer. *Int J Radiat Oncol Biol Phys.* 2016;95:181–189.
24. Holmes T, Das R, Low D, et al. American Society of Radiation Oncology recommendations for documenting intensity-modulated radiation therapy treatments. *Int J Radiat Oncol Biol Phys.* 2009;74:1311–1318.
25. Marks LB, Adams RD, Pawlicki T, et al. Enhancing the role of case-oriented peer review to improve quality and safety in radiation oncology: executive summary. *Pract Radiat Oncol.* 2013;3:149–156.
26. Moran JM, Dempsey M, Eisbruch A, et al. Safety considerations for IMRT: executive summary. *Pract Radiat Oncol.* 2011;1: 190–195.

CHAPTER 7

Monitoring During Treatment

INTRODUCTION

The treatments administered to patients with gynecologic cancers are among the most complex in a radiation oncologist's practice. Treatment of gynecologic cancers requires multidisciplinary collaboration, integration of multiple treatment modalities, and complex specialized radiation therapy (RT) techniques. The use of highly conformal external beam techniques requires close monitoring of radiation setup accuracy, organ motion, and tumor response. Brachytherapy, a component of treatment for many gynecologic cancers, often requires detailed advance planning to assure that patients are ready for the treatment. In addition, in many cases, radiation is used for definitive treatment of tumors that cause pain, bleeding, urinary tract compromise, or other symptoms; the optimal management of tumor and treatment-related side effects is an important component of high-quality care.

Careful monitoring during RT is essential and includes several components:

- Consideration of social circumstances, nutrition issues, and coexisting medical conditions that could influence treatment of the cancer
- Monitoring progress toward completion of the treatment plan to avoid delays
- Evaluation and management of acute treatment-related adverse effects
- Evaluation of the accuracy of daily treatment setup
- Monitoring of changes in body habitus and tumor response and preparation for sequential treatments including external beam boosts or brachytherapy

SOCIAL CIRCUMSTANCES, NUTRITION, AND COEXISTING MEDICAL CONDITIONS

Social circumstances, nutrition issues, and preexisting medical conditions can have major influences on patients' ability to tolerate and complete treatment of gynecologic malignancies. Whether or not these conditions are directly related to the cancer, they must be addressed from the onset of treatment for patients to have the best possible outcome.

Social Circumstances

Social and financial stresses frequently make it difficult for patients to complete 6 to 8 weeks of RT in a timely manner. Young single mothers and elderly women with disabled spouses can have difficulty managing the demanding schedule of chemoradiation. Victims of sexual or spousal abuse can have particular difficulty dealing with pelvic examinations and other invasive procedures. In patients with social circumstances that could jeopardize the success of treatment, an early social services consultation can be critical to a good outcome.

Nutrition Issues

Poor nutrition can result from social circumstances, from the side effects of combined modality treatments, or from the cancer itself. Patients should always be closely monitored for weight loss, which is often the first sign of dehydration or poor nutritional intake. Most patients with nutrition issues benefit from consultation with a dietician who can counsel them on dietary adjustments to help control diarrhea, nausea, and weight loss.

Coexisting Medical Conditions

For patients receiving complex treatments involving concurrent chemoradiation and brachytherapy, coexisting medical conditions can be major barriers to optimal care. The radiation oncologist must be aware of any condition that could influence the course of treatment, including those listed in the following paragraphs.

Cardiopulmonary Disease

Cardiac, respiratory, and other conditions that could influence the patient's ability to undergo brachytherapy should be evaluated early in the patient's course of RT to optimize the patient's condition prior to invasive procedures and to avoid delays in treatment. Patients with pacemakers and cardiac defibrillators require assessment by a cardiologist and close monitoring during RT to confirm that treatment does not cause these devices to malfunction.

Diabetes Mellitus

Even well-managed diabetes can become uncontrolled when corticosteroids are administered with chemotherapy. Management of diabetes can be complicated by adverse effects of cancer treatment, including nausea, anorexia, and changes in diet. Patients should be reminded to monitor their blood glucose level closely during this time. Close collaboration with the patient and with her medical oncologist and internist can reduce the risk of serious diabetes-related complications. In some cases, a reduction in the corticosteroid dose or even suspension of corticosteroid use may be necessary to manage brittle diabetes.

Deep Venous Thrombosis

Patients with cancer have an increased risk of developing deep venous thrombosis and pulmonary embolus. Patients with gynecologic cancers are at particularly high risk because bulky pelvic wall disease (which can obstruct venous flow; **CS 11.8**), pelvic lymphadenectomy, and prolonged immobility are all risk factors for clot formation. A new finding of peripheral edema, particularly if it is unilateral, should be evaluated promptly. Because clots often originate in the pelvis, peripheral Doppler studies may not detect the source of obstruction; pelvic imaging may be required to make a diagnosis. Patients who have a pulmonary embolus may present with hypoxia but often have less specific symptoms such as sudden onset of profound fatigue or tachycardia; these symptoms should be evaluated immediately. A computed tomography (CT) scan of the chest according to a pulmonary embolus protocol is usually used to confirm or rule out pulmonary embolus. If an embolus is confirmed, anticoagulation, usually with enoxaparin sodium (Lovenox), is required.

Need for Anticoagulation

Patients who will require brachytherapy and are receiving anticoagulants should be evaluated early to determine whether their medications will need to be adjusted prior to brachytherapy. If necessary, intracavitary applicator placement can be performed carefully while patients are receiving therapeutic doses of anticoagulants. However, whenever possible, patients who are taking warfarin, aspirin, or antiplatelet agents such as clopidogrel should have the drug held for 5 days prior to invasive procedures; reversible anticoagulation therapy with enoxaparin sodium or heparin can be administered and then stopped 12 hours prior to the procedure. Interstitial implants should not be placed while patients are receiving warfarin, clopidogrel, or similar anticoagulants.

MONITORING PROGRESS TOWARD COMPLETION OF THE TREATMENT PLAN

Before treatment is started, the overall treatment plan should be clearly articulated, and there should be clear communication between the members of the multidisciplinary team to confirm the details of the treatment plan and the start date.

Once treatment begins, the plan should be reviewed weekly to determine the following:

- Is the patient receiving chemotherapy as planned? If not, why not? Are members of the multidisciplinary team aware of the RT schedule, particularly as it affects the delivery of concurrent chemotherapy?
- Is the patient receiving radiation treatments on schedule? If not, why not? How can the delay be addressed?
- What are the most recent laboratory results? How are any abnormalities being addressed?
- Is the patient losing weight? Is she receiving adequate nutrition?
- Have necessary arrangements been made to facilitate planned external beam or brachytherapy boosts?
- Have any tumors or treatment-related adverse effects been adequately addressed?

Delays in RT should be avoided whenever possible; an effort should always be made to assure that the average weekly dose is at least 850 cGy per week. Radiobiologic principles and extensive clinical data[1,2] indicate that treatment protraction allows proliferation of surviving cells, increasing the risk of local recurrence. Although some investigators have suggested that treatment protraction may be less harmful for patients treated with concurrent chemoradiation,[3] these suggestions have been based on studies that were far too small to rule out clinically significant increases in recurrence rates caused by treatment protraction. Although there have been no adequately powered studies in patients receiving chemoradiation, a 2008 review of Gynecologic Oncology Group chemoradiation trials suggested a deleterious effect of treatment protraction.[4] Concurrent chemotherapy has reduced but not eliminated in-field recurrences, and there is no reason to believe that concurrent chemotherapy eliminates proliferation of surviving clonogens, some of which may be resistant to chemotherapy. If concurrent chemotherapy were sufficiently effective to reduce the recurrence risk to negligible levels, it would actually be more beneficial to reduce the dose of radiation, thereby decreasing the risk of late adverse effects, than to unnecessarily protract treatment.

In our experience, nearly all treatment breaks and delays are medically unnecessary and should therefore be avoided. The following steps can eliminate most delays:

- At the beginning of treatment, discuss with the patient the importance of not missing treatments. Ask the patient about transportation, dependent care, and other challenges to adherence to the prescribed schedule and enlist social services to work with the patient if necessary.
- Plan each step of treatment in advance to avoid delays related to planning or scheduling of boosts.
- Manage treatment-related adverse effects proactively.
- If concurrent chemoradiation causes depression of blood cell counts, RT should be continued even if chemotherapy has to be interrupted.
- If the patient has missed more than 2 days of treatment because of holidays or other reasons, attempt to schedule b.i.d. treatments (usually separated by a 6-hour interval) to make up some or all of the missed treatments (**CS 10.1**).

The overall duration of treatment is emphasized in site-specific chapters and in each of the case studies appended to Chapters 10 to 15.

EVALUATION AND MANAGEMENT OF ACUTE TREATMENT-RELATED ADVERSE EFFECTS

Most patients receiving RT for gynecologic cancers experience tumor- or treatment-related adverse effects.

Adverse Effects of RT by Treatment Location

The acute adverse effects of RT are directly related to the region treated.

True Pelvis

The most common adverse effect of pelvic RT is diarrhea, which usually worsens gradually over the course of treatment. Dysuria, usually associated with urinary tract infection (UTI), is less common. Skin reactions are rare unless patients are treated with anteroposterior–posteroanterior fields or have skin folds or vulva included in the high-dose region. Patients who are treated for gross cervical, vaginal, or vulvar disease may experience a foul-smelling discharge as the tumor responds to RT. Nausea is rare if treatment is confined to the pelvis and is not accompanied by chemotherapy.

Paraaortic Region

The most common adverse effect of irradiation of the paraaortic region is nausea, sometimes accompanied by belching and heartburn. Radiation-related nausea can have an abrupt onset, typically 30 to 60 minutes after RT. Diarrhea is infrequent and usually mild if treatment is confined to the paraaortic region.

Distal Vagina and Vulva

The most common symptoms of irradiation of the distal vagina and vulva are erythema and desquamation associated with pruritus and pain. Vulvovaginitis may cause dysuria or pain on defecation. As discussed below, the severity of local symptoms can be significantly lessened with local care and infection control.

Adverse Effects of Chemotherapy

Today, RT for gynecologic cancers is frequently administered with concurrent chemotherapy, usually cisplatin-based chemotherapy. Although other members of the multidisciplinary team administer the chemotherapy, the radiation oncologist is typically on the front line when patients coming for daily treatment develop symptoms. Therefore, radiation oncologists must be aware of the drugs being administered with radiation, understand the adverse effects of these drugs, and be prepared to treat symptoms as they occur. Acute and long-term side effects of chemotherapy are also discussed in Chapter 3.

Diarrhea

Most patients receiving pelvic RT experience at least mild diarrhea, usually beginning in the 3rd or 4th week of treatment. In severe cases, patients may have eight or more watery bowel movements per day; these symptoms can contribute to electrolyte disturbances and even dehydration. Diarrhea is often accompanied by lower abdominal crampy pain. Hemorrhoid flare-ups can contribute to the patient's discomfort. Patients who are receiving concurrent chemotherapy tend to have more severe diarrhea than patients treated with radiation alone, and concurrent multiagent chemotherapy may cause more severe diarrhea than weekly cisplatin (**Fig. 7.1**).

Patients who have very severe diarrhea, particularly early in the treatment course, should be evaluated to rule out another contributing factor, particularly infection with *Clostridium difficile*. Patients who have recently received intravenous antibiotics in the hospital are at particularly high risk for *C. difficile* infection (**CS 12.1**). In some cases, presumptive treatment with metronidazole may be warranted while cultures are in process.

Treatment and positioning techniques that minimize the dose of radiation to bowel can reduce the severity of diarrhea (Chapter 6). For patients who still experience symptoms, dietary management, and carefully titrated administration of antidiarrheal medications can usually control symptoms. Pretreatment counseling and a staged approach to medical management, as outlined in the following paragraphs, are important components of symptom management.

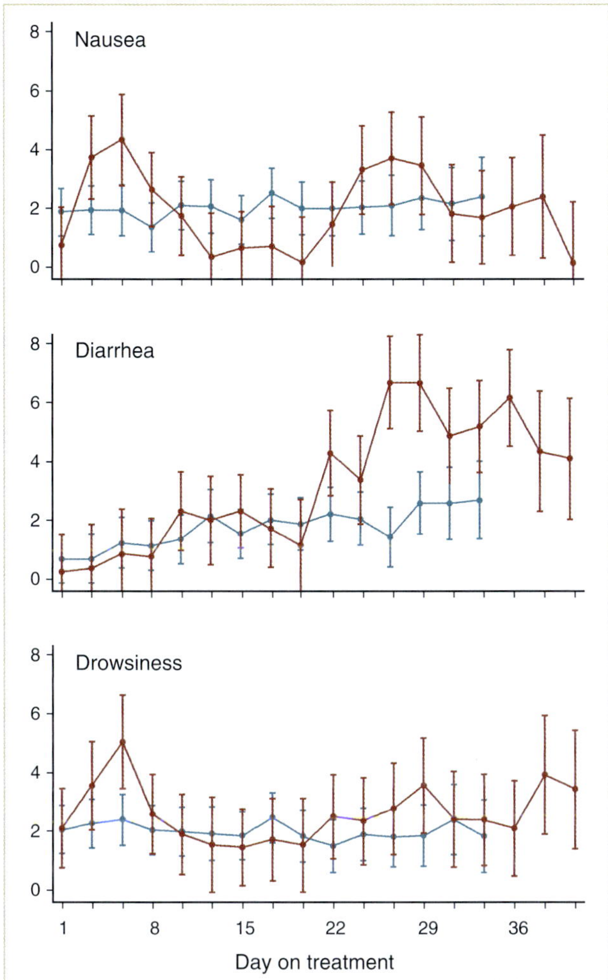

FIGURE 7.1 Patient-reported symptoms during chemoradiation for cervical cancer. In a prospective study, patients receiving chemoradiation were asked three times per week to estimate the severity of their symptoms on a scale of 0 to 10. Shown in *red* are the mean symptom scores for 37 patients who had pelvic RT with weekly cisplatin (40 mg/m^2); shown in *blue* are the mean symptom scores for 13 patients who had pelvic RT with a combination of cisplatin (75 mg/m^2) and 5-fluorouracil (in 2 cycles beginning on days 1 and 21). *Bars* represent the 95% confidence intervals for each time point. Patients treated with weekly cisplatin experienced relatively constant low levels of nausea and anorexia, while patients treated with cisplatin and 5-fluorouracil had peaks in their symptoms during the weeks after chemotherapy administration followed by a relatively symptom-free period. Both groups experienced a gradual increase in diarrhea despite the use of antidiarrheal medication, but diarrhea was significantly more severe for patients treated with two drugs. (Adapted from Likhacheva A, et al. Prospective study of symptom assessment among patients with cervical cancer during concurrent chemoradiotherapy with weekly cisplatin or every-3-week cisplatin and 5-fluorouracil. *Int J Gynecol Cancer.* 2013;23:1520–1527.)

Before Treatment

Before treatment, ask patients about their bowel habits and food sensitivities and advise patients to avoid any food that tends to cause diarrhea. Lactose intolerance tends to become more severe or may first become apparent during RT. Therefore, patients who have a history of lactose intolerance should be advised to avoid milk products during treatment.

Advise patients who are constipated to continue their laxative regimens as necessary, but counsel them that their medications will probably need to be modified as treatment progresses. Encourage patients to request guidance when their bowel habits begin to change. Advise patients to obtain loperamide to have on hand in case diarrhea develops suddenly.

Counsel patients to contact you immediately if symptoms are not well controlled. A visit with the radiation oncologist on Friday can avoid a weekend emergency room visit.

During Treatment

Ask patients about their bowel habits at each visit. A good way to estimate symptom severity is to ask, "How many bowel movements did you have, what was the consistency, and how many loperamide or diphenoxylate and atropine (Lomotil) pills did you take yesterday? the day before?"

Increase the use of antidiarrheals as needed. The following guidelines are recommended:

- Initially, 1 pill after each loose bowel movement up to 8 pills per day.
- If the patient requires more than 3 to 4 pills per day for 2 or more days, ask about the timing of diarrhea and suggest a schedule that anticipates the symptoms. The following regimen can be very effective:
  - One pill left on the bedside table at night taken as soon as the patient awakens in the morning
  - One pill 20 to 30 minutes before lunch
  - One pill 20 to 30 minutes before dinner
  - One pill at bedtime
- If diarrhea occurs between these intervals, an additional pill (loperamide or diphenoxylate and atropine) can be taken, or the dose can be increased to 2 pills at each time point.
- The total number of loperamide pills should not exceed 8 per day, but in rare cases of refractory diarrhea, up to 8 diphenoxylate and atropine pills can be added to this.
- In cases of very refractory diarrhea, other medications, such as tincture of opium or paregoric, can help, but such medications are very rarely necessary.

Manage the patient's diet. Patients should reduce intake of dietary fiber and any food that has caused diarrhea in the past. Foods that frequently exacerbate diarrhea are raw fruits (particularly pitted fruits and watermelon), salad greens, beans, onions, and spicy or greasy foods. In some cases, caffeinated beverages can stimulate diarrhea. A dietician should be consulted if one is available.

Monitor patients for weight loss. Sudden loss of more than 3% to 4% of the body weight usually is a sign of dehydration. Examine patients for orthostatic symptoms, decreased skin turgor, and dry mucous membranes. Check electrolyte levels. Give patients intravenous fluids if necessary. Management of late radiation enteropathy is discussed in Chapter 9.

At the End of Treatment

Counsel patients that in most cases, diarrhea resolves completely within 4 to 6 weeks of the end of treatment, although some patients may continue to have episodes of diarrhea beyond this period. Advise patients to proceed gradually when reintroducing previously avoided foods. Loperamide can be taken as needed.

Nausea, Vomiting, and Anorexia

Radiation-Induced Nausea

Patients who undergo only pelvic RT without chemotherapy rarely experience nausea. However, treatments that include the stomach or duodenum frequently do cause nausea. Typically nausea occurs during the 30 to 60 minutes after treatment, and it can usually be prevented by administration of an antiemetic 20 to 30 minutes before treatment. Patients rarely require round-the-clock antiemetic treatment for nausea unless they are also receiving chemotherapy.

Administration of proton pump inhibitors (PPIs) during and for several months after paraaortic RT may benefit patients by decreasing acid levels in the stomach and duodenum. Administration of PPIs is recommended particularly for patients who will receive more than 45 Gy to the duodenum. Although PPIs have not specifically been studied for such patients, they have been proven to assist in the healing of duodenitis stemming from other causes and likely aid in the healing of acute RT-induced duodenitis. Antacids may also help some patients who have nausea that is refractory to standard antiemetics, particularly if patients also have symptoms of heartburn.

Chemotherapy-Induced Nausea

The cisplatin that is often administered with RT is the cause of most treatment-related nausea. Although modern antiemetics usually prevent vomiting in patients receiving standard doses of weekly cisplatin, most patients have at least mild nausea and anorexia for several days after chemotherapy. When cisplatin is delivered at doses higher than 40 mg/m^2 or as part of a multiagent regimen, the symptoms may be more severe (Fig. 7.1). Patients who are refractory to front-line antiemetics may respond to other medications. The first week of treatment usually predicts how the patient will respond to future courses of cisplatin. However, failure to recognize refractory nausea during this first week frequently results in a weekend emergency room visit for dehydration.

Urinary Tract Symptoms

Patients who are receiving pelvic RT may experience bladder-related symptoms, including dysuria, frequency, urgency, hematuria, bladder spasm, suprapubic pain, incontinence, atony, or retention. Urinary tract symptoms can result from a number of different causes, as discussed in detail in the following paragraphs.

Symptoms Related to Tumor Invasion

Tumors that involve the cervix, vagina, or vesicouterine space can cause symptoms through infiltration of the bladder wall or obstruction of the ureters or urethra. Bladder invasion may cause pain, spasm, or, if the mucosa is involved, hematuria; secondary infection is common. Unilateral ureteral obstruction is often asymptomatic but may cause back pain or pyelonephritis causing flank pain and fever. Bilateral hydronephrosis can lead to acute renal failure. Ureteral obstruction necessitates placement of stents or a percutaneous nephrostomy to preserve renal function. Ureteral stents avoid the discomfort and inconvenience of percutaneous nephrostomy but can cause spasms and suprapubic pain and may increase the long-term risk of ureteral stricture. Urethral obstruction can cause severe bladder distension, hydronephrosis, and renal failure and constitutes an emergency necessitating placement of a urethral catheter or, if that is not possible, a suprapubic catheter. Pretreatment imaging usually reveals these conditions; however, ureteral obstruction can develop suddenly, especially in the first week of treatment, when inflammation in response to treatment precedes tumor regression.

Posthysterectomy Symptoms

After radical (type 3) hysterectomy, patients may experience bladder retention; in severe cases, long-term self-catheterization may be necessary (Chapter 3). Simple or modified radical (type 2) hysterectomy is rarely associated with prolonged atony, but patients may have mild bladder retention or develop bladder infections during the first few weeks after surgery. More commonly, patients describe a feeling of pressure in the retropubic area that can persist for weeks or even months.

Periurethral Irritation

Patients whose radiation fields include the vaginal introitus may experience dysuria because of local irritation of the urethral meatus. UTI and yeast infection should be ruled out. Phenazopyridine (Pyridium) may be helpful. Local treatments discussed below should be used to treat periurethral vulvar skin reactions.

Symptoms Related to UTI

A number of factors contribute to the increased risk of UTI during pelvic RT. Any disruption of the normal protective urothelial lining by instrumentation, tumor, or other factors described above can increase the risk of UTI; for this reason, infection should always be ruled out before another cause is assumed to be solely responsible for the patient's symptoms. Factors that decrease urine flow (e.g., postoperative hypotony, ureteral obstruction, or urinary diversion) can also facilitate infection. The degree to which direct effects of RT on the bladder mucosa or on local cell-mediated immunity play a role in UTI is uncertain. However, some evidence suggests that the risk of UTI is correlated with the volume of bladder irradiated.[5]

Typical symptoms of UTI include dysuria, urgency, or frequency; symptoms of UTI may also include suprapubic pain or hematuria. In some cases, the only symptom is the new onset of incontinence. Symptoms can progress rapidly and be intensely painful. Urinalysis usually shows pyuria and sometimes bacteria; nitrite is not always detected but, when present, is highly specific for UTI. If the patient has nausea, flank pain, fever, or white blood cell casts in the urine, acute pyelonephritis must be ruled out. If a patient complains of vaginal discharge or external rather than internal irritation, vaginitis should be considered as a possible cause of the patient's symptoms (discussed below).

Whenever possible, particularly in patients with recurrent UTIs, urine culture with evaluation of drug sensitivities should be performed to rule out drug resistance; a finding of more than 100,000 colony-forming units per milliliter in a properly collected specimen suggests the presence of infection.

Some immediate symptom relief can be obtained with phenazopyridine. However, patients who present with classic symptoms of UTI should be started on antibiotics immediately; if necessary, treatment can be discontinued or adjusted once culture results are available. In general, patients who have UTI in the setting of RT or tumor involvement should receive at least 7 to 10 days of antibiotics, usually at the doses recommended for complicated bladder infections.

Cranberry juice or pills, which contain proanthocyanidins that can prevent bacteria from adhering to the bladder mucosa, are frequently recommended to prevent UTI in high-risk patients, including those receiving RT. Although a 2012 Cochrane meta-analysis[6] failed to demonstrate clear benefit when cranberry was compared with placebo in high-risk patients, poor patient compliance and variations in the quantity of active substances in the administered pills may have limited the generalizability of the contributing studies. The studies reviewed also failed to demonstrate adverse effects, although cranberry may interact with warfarin to cause increased bleeding.

Sterile Dysuria

The acute development of sterile dysuria during pelvic RT is usually associated with vaginitis, vulvitis, or one of the other factors described above. Women who have a history of chronic interstitial cystitis may have worsening of their symptoms during pelvic RT. Avoidance of certain foods, including caffeine, hot peppers, and citrus, may be helpful.

Vaginitis

Candidal Vaginitis

Candidal vaginitis may occur in patients undergoing pelvic RT. Symptoms include dysuria, discharge, and intense pruritus. Patients usually describe the dysuria as superficial rather than the deep pain described by patients who have UTI, but the symptoms of candidal vaginitis can be confused with those of UTI. The discharge is typically odorless, thick, and white but may be clear. On speculum examination, there are usually white "cottage cheese–like" plaques with associated erythema or edema of the vaginal mucosa. Vaginal examination is often painful for patients who have active infection. Patients who have diabetes mellitus, have a compromised immune system, are receiving corticosteroid therapy (which is often administered with chemotherapy), or have been treated with antibiotics are at increased risk for developing a vaginal yeast infection.

Because short-course topical antifungal treatments are often incompletely effective in patients undergoing RT, a 7-day course of treatment is usually recommended. If symptoms are unresponsive to topical treatment or if the patient cannot tolerate intravaginal treatment, a 7-day course of oral fluconazole is usually effective if there are no medical contraindications to its use.

Bacterial Vaginosis

Bacterial vaginosis may occur in patients with gynecologic cancers. Patients who have infiltrative tumor involving the cervix or vagina often have superimposed infection causing a foul-smelling discharge that may increase during treatment. The usual treatment is oral metronidazole.

Radiation Dermatitis

Most patients who receive therapeutic doses of radiation to the vulva, groin, or skin folds experience inflammatory skin changes within the treated region. The skin's response to radiation is complex, and underlying mechanisms have not been precisely defined. However, the following factors probably contribute to the development of acute radiation dermatitis:

- Direct interference of RT with skin renewal via killing of epidermal germ cells
- Direct effects of RT on cutaneous vasculature
- Disruption of the mechanical keratinocyte protective barrier by tumor, surgery, and RT-mediated interference with normal skin renewal
- Disruption of local immune protective mechanisms that are mediated in large part by resident T cells
- Secondary infection with *Candida albicans*, *Staphylococcus aureus*, or other organisms that proliferate when normal skin defense mechanisms are compromised

Secondary infection contributes importantly to the skin inflammation associated with external beam RT for vulvar or distal vaginal cancer. The severity of symptoms can be dramatically reduced with intensive local care and prompt recognition and treatment of local infection. For this reason, the importance of infection control for any patient receiving more than 20 to 30 Gy to the skin surfaces cannot be overemphasized.

Patients who have locally advanced vulvar cancer or skin involvement from groin metastases usually have concurrent bacterial and yeast infections at the time of initial diagnosis; these infections are often the primary source of the patient's pain and can obscure the extent of cancer in the region (**Fig. 7.2**). If possible, cultures should be obtained, and the patient should be treated intensively with appropriate local care, antibiotics, and

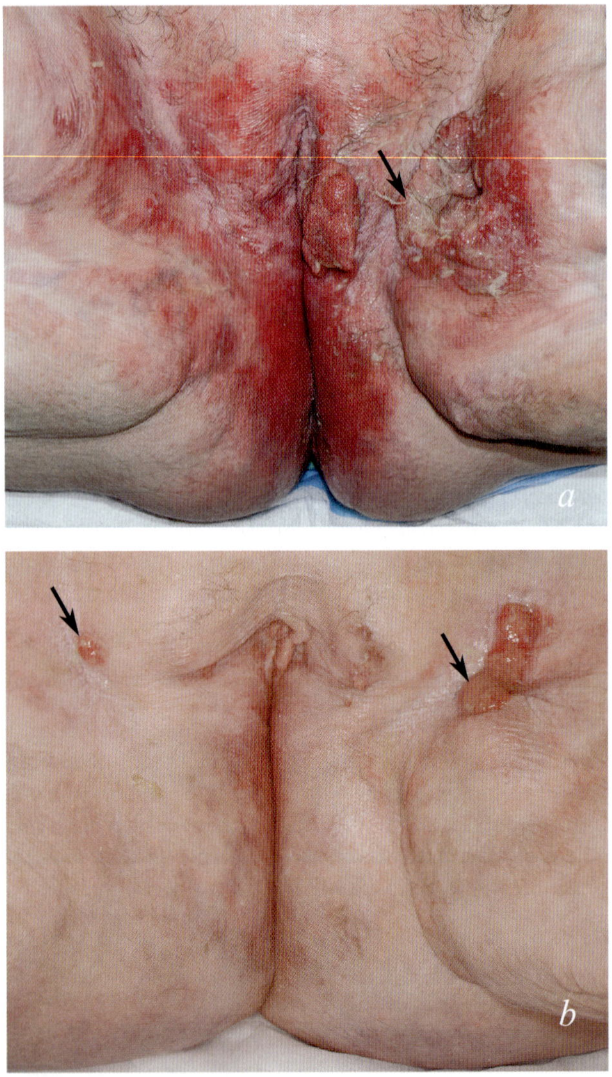

FIGURE 7.2 Severe infection in a patient with newly diagnosed vulvar cancer. This patient was referred for possible RT for a presumed locally advanced vulvar cancer. The patient was in severe pain from an extensive lesion *(a)* that included intense vulvar and perianal erythema and exophytic vulvar lesions, including a large one on the left labium majus and a 6 × 7 cm ulcerating lesion in the left genitocrural fold. Multiple biopsies of the vulva showed inflammation or dysplasia; only the biopsy from the left genitocrural fold *(arrow)* was positive for invasive squamous carcinoma. Because the patient appeared to have severe concurrent infection, she was started on intravenous antibiotic and antifungal therapy combined with intensive local care and pain management. After 10 days of inpatient care, she was discharged to receive outpatient treatment of her infection with involvement of a home health nurse.

During the following 8 weeks, the patient continued to show gradual improvement with marked diminution in the extent of her visible lesions. After 10 weeks of infection management but no cancer treatment *(b)*, repeat biopsies were taken of the left genitocrural lesion and of a small right-sided lesion that had been obscured by the initial infection *(b, arrows)*. Both biopsies showed invasive squamous carcinoma. Other random biopsies were negative for cancer.

antifungals to control infections before treatment of the cancer is initiated.

Once treatment is started, it is critical to avoid bacterial and yeast infections to minimize symptoms. For this reason, local care should be stressed from the first day of treatment. Sitz baths with a warm solution of baking soda (1 tablespoon per quart) or dilute Domeboro solution (1 packet per quart) should be initiated in the 1st or 2nd week of treatment and used two to three times per day, particularly after bowel movements. The vulva and skin folds should be kept as dry as possible, but cornstarch or similar powders are not recommended because they can encourage yeast proliferation.

Even with these precautions, most patients begin to develop mild erythema in the 3rd week of vulvar RT. These early reactions usually reflect overgrowth of *C. albicans*; they are usually limited to the treated region, although satellite lesions are sometimes seen outside the treatment field. Prompt treatment with a 7- to 10-day course of fluconazole usually results in improvement or resolution of symptoms despite continued RT. However, if this initial erythematous reaction is not treated promptly, moist desquamation follows rapidly, particularly in skin folds, which provide a favorable environment for fungal infection (**Fig. 7.3**). Once the skin surface has been breached by tumor or by the development of patchy moist desquamation, it is particularly susceptible to bacterial infection. Hill et al.[7] emphasized the important role of *S. aureus* in severe radiation dermatitis, but other organisms can be involved. Antibiotics, such as ciprofloxacin, can be effective at reducing dermatitis associated with bacterial overgrowth.

Hydrogel dressings can be applied to areas of moist desquamation to alleviate pain and to protect affected skin from further injury. The patient should be guided by a nurse or physician to ensure that she understands how to properly apply these dressings. For sites of moist desquamation adjacent to critical structures, such as the urethra and rectum, lidocaine cream compounded with Aquaphor can be applied to tender skin for symptom relief.

Hematologic Effects of Treatment

Anemia

In patients with gynecologic cancers, anemia is a frequent problem and is often due to one of the following causes:

- Spontaneous bleeding from friable uterine or lower genital tract cancers.
- Blood loss from operative procedures and clinical examinations.
- Chronic iron deficiency anemia unrelated to cancer. This is likely a major contributor in young, menstruating, often socially disadvantaged women.
- Bone marrow suppression from cancer treatments.

The well-documented correlation between anemia during RT and poor outcome of patients treated for cervical cancer has led clinicians to investigate a variety of methods designed

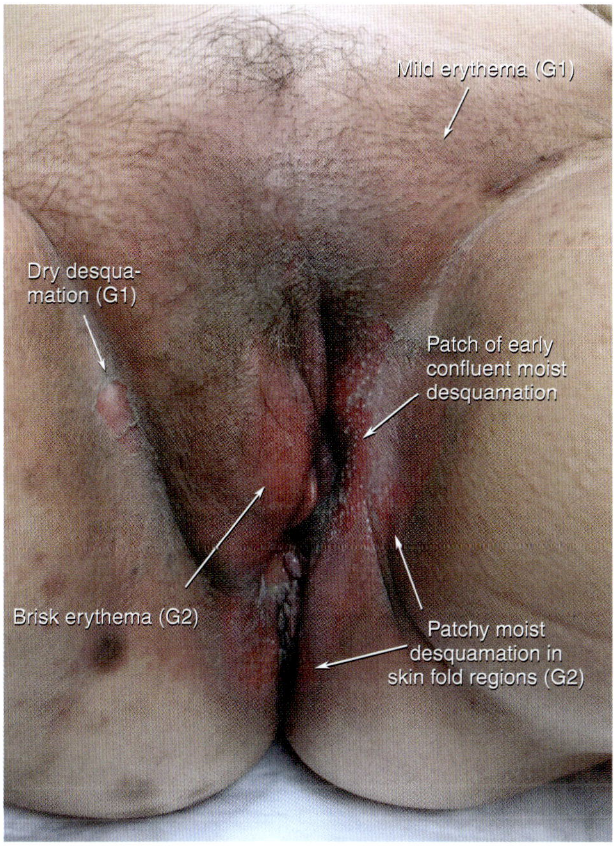

FIGURE 7.3 Acute dermatitis during postoperative RT for vulvar cancer. This image was taken on the 29th day before the 21st fraction of postoperative RT in a patient who had close vulvar margins and microscopic nodal metastasis from invasive squamous carcinoma of the vulva. At that point in the treatment course, the patient had received 42 Gy of a planned 50 Gy to the vulvar operative bed and 37.8 of a planned 45 Gy to the nodal and vulvar clinical target volumes; she had also completed four courses of weekly cisplatin. Significantly, before RT was begun, the patient had been hospitalized for perioperative cellulitis that responded to antibiotic treatment. At the start of RT, she was counseled to inform us immediately of any local change that could represent recurrent cellulitis. In fact, mild erythema and pruritus noted after the third treatment were correctly diagnosed as recurrent cellulitis and responded promptly to antibiotics. At the time of this photograph, the patient had been restarted on antibiotics and fluconazole for a second bout of infection, was using local cortisone-containing treatment for painful hemorrhoids, was taking opioid medication as needed for pain, and was taking frequent sitz baths containing baking soda. Note areas of brisk erythema and patchy moist desquamation in vulvar skin fold regions that had received 42 Gy. Milder erythema with a few patches of dry desquamation is visible in surrounding areas. The patient's symptoms improved after she was restarted on antibiotics, and she completed her last 4 days of treatment. However, she continued to have local pain. This pain had improved significantly by the 2nd week after completion of RT. At 3 months, the area was well healed, and the patient had no local symptoms.

to overcome the putative effects of hypoxia on local tumor control, including hypoxic cell sensitizers, tirapazamine, hyperbaric oxygen, neutron therapy, stimulators of erythropoiesis, and red blood cell transfusion. None of these interventions have been found to improve local disease control or survival. Retrospective studies suggested that anemia had an independent influence on outcome, but these studies generally did not have adequate correction for the large number of potential confounding factors, particularly tumor size. Nevertheless, because it was assumed that radiobiologically significant hypoxia contributed to the increased rate of local failures in anemic patients, for many years, it was considered standard practice to transfuse patients to maintain hemoglobin levels at least 10 g/dL during RT.

In 2015, Bishop et al.[8] published an analysis of 2,359 patients treated with radiation alone for intact cervical cancer at MD Anderson Cancer Center. In this very large study of well-characterized patients, no independent correlation was found between the minimum hemoglobin level during RT and freedom from central recurrence for the overall group or for the 678 patients who were treated with concurrent chemoradiation. When patients were grouped according to the estimated tumor diameter, no difference in tumor control rates was seen between patients with minimum hemoglobin levels 10 g/dL or greater or less than 10 g/dL, even within subgroups of patients who had large tumors (Fig. 7.4).

For this reason, we no longer recommend red blood cell transfusion to maintain hemoglobin levels above 10 g/dL. However, we do transfuse red blood cells if the hemoglobin level falls below 9 g/dL or if the patient has dyspnea on exertion. Also, because hemoglobin levels tend to fall during evaluation and treatment, we tend to transfuse red blood cells if the patient is actively bleeding and the hemoglobin level is less than about 9.5 g/dL at the start of the treatment.

That said, anemia is at least a contributor to fatigue during treatment. The following simple steps can be taken to minimize anemia in gynecologic oncology patients:

- Practice techniques that minimize trauma to bleeding tumors during physical examinations (Chapter 4).
- For patients who have evidence of iron deficiency, initiate iron supplementation. Significant recovery may be seen even during the week or so that it takes to initiate treatment. However, $FeSO_4$ can contribute to nausea during treatment and probably has less impact once chemotherapy has been started; $FeSO_4$ should probably be discontinued if it appears to contribute to the patient's symptoms.
- Discourage the patient from engaging in activities such as intercourse and douching that could traumatize friable tumor.

Thrombocytopenia

Thrombocytopenia is rarely a major problem for patients receiving RT for gynecologic cancers unless patients have previously received chemotherapy or are receiving concurrent

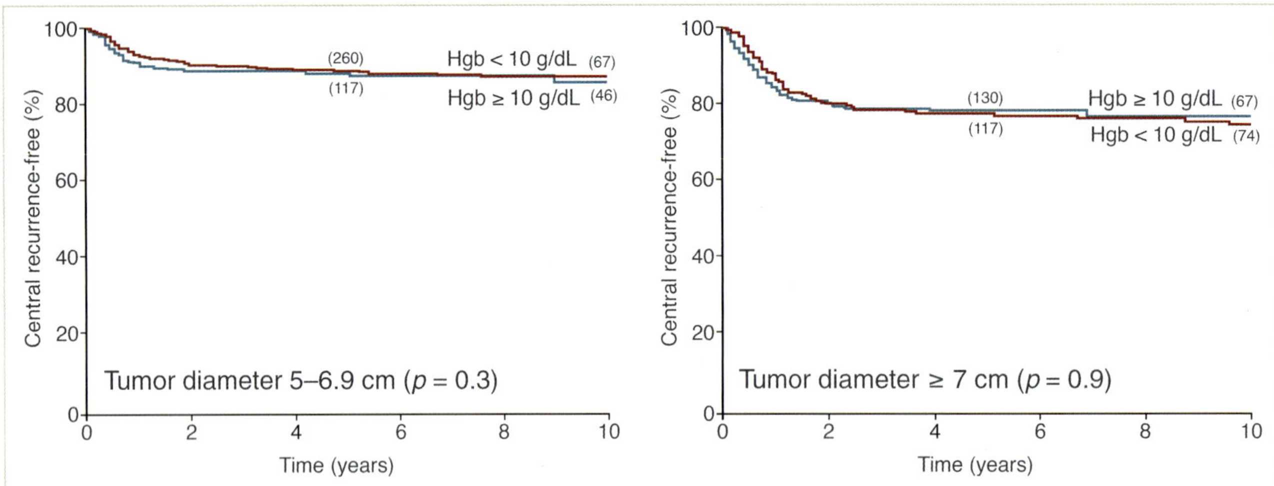

FIGURE 7.4 Hemoglobin level and recurrence risk. Shown is the influence of the minimum hemoglobin level during RT on freedom from central recurrence (FFCR) in a retrospective study of 2,454 patients treated with definitive RT or chemoradiation for cancer of the cervix. Although hemoglobin was strongly correlated with all outcome measures in univariate analysis, there was no significant correlation between FFCR and hemoglobin level after correction for other major prognostic factors. The Kaplan-Meier curves shown here depicting FFCR for subgroups of patients with bulky tumors. (From Bishop AJ, Allen PK, Klopp AH, et al. Relationship between low hemoglobin levels and outcomes after treatment with radiation or chemoradiation in patients with cervical cancer: has the impact of anemia been overstated? *Int J Radiat Oncol Biol Phys.* 2015;91:196–205.)

chemotherapy with extended radiation fields. Patients who develop profound thrombocytopenia during pelvic RT should be evaluated for other causes, for example, drug interactions, heparin-induced thrombocytopenia, or idiopathic thrombocytopenic purpura.

Patients with platelet counts of <40,000 to 50,000 platelets/μL may be at risk for bleeding with brachytherapy. A short delay in brachytherapy may be considered if there has been an acute decline in the platelet count; however, because platelet recovery can be slow, the risk of bleeding must be weighed against the risk of recurrence associated with protracted treatment. Consultation with a hematologist is recommended in these cases, with consideration of platelet transfusion in rare cases of profound thrombocytopenia.

Neutropenia

Even extended radiation fields rarely cause severe neutropenia unless the patient has previously received chemotherapy or is receiving concurrent chemotherapy. Concurrent chemoradiation with weekly cisplatin has a cumulative effect that usually results in some degree of neutropenia by the 4th or 5th week. Because the white blood cell count nadir occurs 10 to 14 days after cisplatin administration, the count usually continues to fall even after a weekly cycle is postponed because of neutropenia. This is an important consideration in the scheduling and preparation for brachytherapy (Chapter 8). Filgrastim administration usually returns the neutrophil count to a level acceptable for brachytherapy within 24 to 48 hours. For patients who are receiving concurrent chemoradiation, chemotherapy may need to be delayed until the absolute neutrophil count returns to an acceptable level. However, we generally continue with RT to avoid treatment protraction.

Dehydration and Electrolyte Depletion

Uncontrolled nausea, vomiting, and diarrhea can rapidly lead to dehydration and electrolyte depletion. Therefore, patients should be encouraged to seek immediate help from the radiation oncologist if such symptoms are not well controlled. A nursing visit several days after the first dose of chemotherapy (before the first weekend) can provide an opportunity to confirm adequate symptom control and potentially avoid a weekend emergency room visit. Any patient who has rapid weight loss associated with gastrointestinal symptoms should be considered for intravenous hydration; repletion frequently produces an immediate improvement in the patient's appetite and sense of well-being.

Even without dehydration, patients receiving chemotherapy can develop significant electrolyte disorders. Impaired renal resorption of magnesium is a common adverse effect of cisplatin chemotherapy[9]; although usually mild, it can in some cases be severe. The symptoms of hypomagnesemia, which include fatigue, anorexia, and depression, can easily be misinterpreted as general treatment-related malaise; hypomagnesemia should always be considered as a possible cause of worsening postchemotherapy symptoms in patients receiving weekly cisplatin. Prophylactic administration of intravenous magnesium with chemotherapy has been shown to significantly reduce the incidence and severity of hypomagnesemia and is generally recommended to avoid the need for oral supplementation, which can significantly increase symptoms of diarrhea and nausea during pelvic RT. However, in a small percentage of patients, magnesium wasting can be severe and resistant to supplementation. If oral magnesium must be given, magnesium lactate is preferred because it is a less potent laxative than magnesium citrate and has a high level of bioavailability. Because any form of oral magnesium can cause or exacerbate diarrhea, intravenous administration is preferred for most patients receiving pelvic RT.

Hypokalemia can also be a problem for patients undergoing cisplatin therapy, and potassium levels should be monitored throughout treatment.

MONITORING THE ACCURACY OF DAILY TREATMENT

An important component of monitoring during treatment is continuous monitoring of treatment accuracy. This includes monitoring of:

- The accuracy of daily treatment setup
- Changes in body habitus that could influence the dose delivered to targets
- Tumor responses necessitating adjustment of target volumes for boosts or adaptive planning

Maximizing the Accuracy of Daily Setup

The first step in assuring the accuracy of treatment setup is to have in place excellent quality assurance measures and communication between the physician, dosimetrist, and therapists. Alignment is particularly important in patients with gynecologic cancers, who frequently have very long fields that are subject to major tilt and rotational errors.

To assure accuracy throughout treatment, some form of imaging must be used to assure continued treatment accuracy.

In addition, thermoluminescent dosimeters can be used to directly measure the dose delivered to the skin. Because treatment planning systems cannot accurately calculate the dose to the surface of the skin, it is important to confirm that the skin surface is receiving the desired dose if it is included in the gross tumor volume or clinical tumor volume (Chapters 6 and 12, **CS 12.2, 12.5, and 12.6**).

Imaging options for maximizing setup accuracy are discussed in the following paragraphs.

Portal Imaging

At a minimum, patients must have weekly portal imaging or some other form of imaging to confirm that no major error has caused a discrepancy between the patient's external marks and internal landmarks. The dose delivered with portal images makes this a poor method for daily verification, so when portal imaging is used to verify treatment setup, a somewhat larger planning target volume margin must be allotted to account for possible errors on days when no imaging is performed. Also, even with enhancement, portal images can be very difficult to interpret in obese patients.

Daily Kilovoltage Imaging

Daily kilovoltage (kV) imaging is recommended for patients treated with intensity-modulated RT or proton plans, which typically use smaller planning target volume margins than standard conformal plans. Daily kV imaging is also recommended for obese patients because megavoltage image quality is usually poor and skin marks tend to correspond poorly with boney landmarks.[10] The large fields typically used in gynecologic applications require very careful review to detect errors. Although simple translational errors are usually easily detected and corrected by the therapists, tilt errors and rotational errors are more likely to be missed and can lead to errors of 1 cm or greater even when the isocenter is correctly positioned (**Figs. 7.5 and 7.6**).

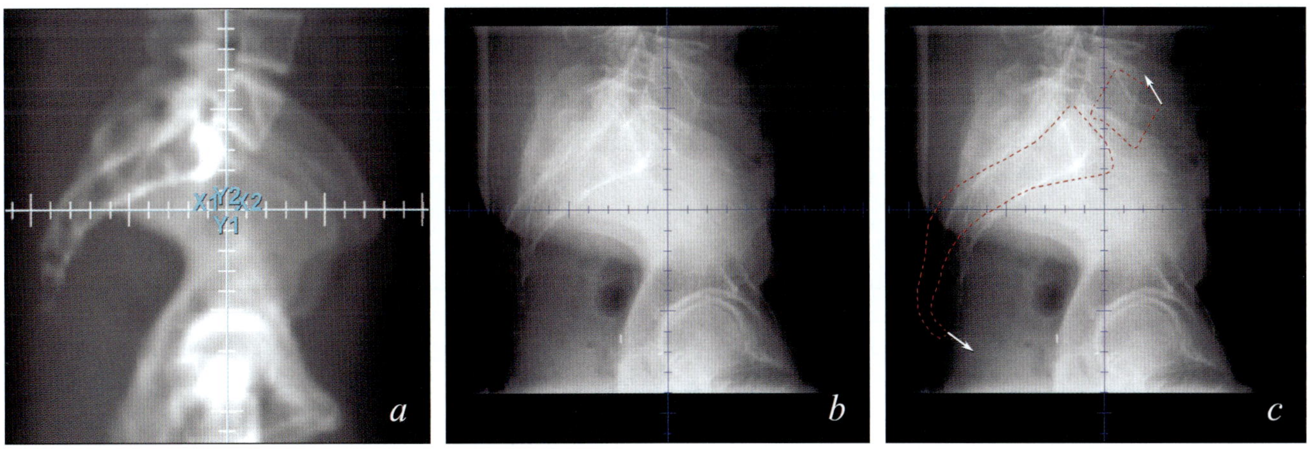

FIGURE 7.5 Positioning error—pelvic tilt. Digitally reconstructed radiograph (DRR) from the treatment plan of a patient receiving pelvic RT *(a)* and an online kV image taken in the 4th week of treatment *(b)*. If one only compares the intersections of the *x* and *y* axes with the sacrum, the error may appear to be subtle. However, closer examination of the shape of the presacral space and, more particularly, of the relative positions of the field axes versus L5 and the distal sacrum demonstrates a serious tilt error. In *(c)*, the correct position of the sacrum and L5 from *(a)* is superimposed *(red dotted line)* on the kV image; the tilt error measured ~11 degrees and resulted in an error of close to 2 cm at the proximal and distal margins of the treatment field. Prior to this, the patient had been setting up very well. However, in week 4, the patient was shifted to a new treatment machine after a hospital admission for pneumonia. The therapists were unaware that the patient tended to clench her buttocks when she was first placed on the treatment table. When she was reminded to relax, the tilt error disappeared.

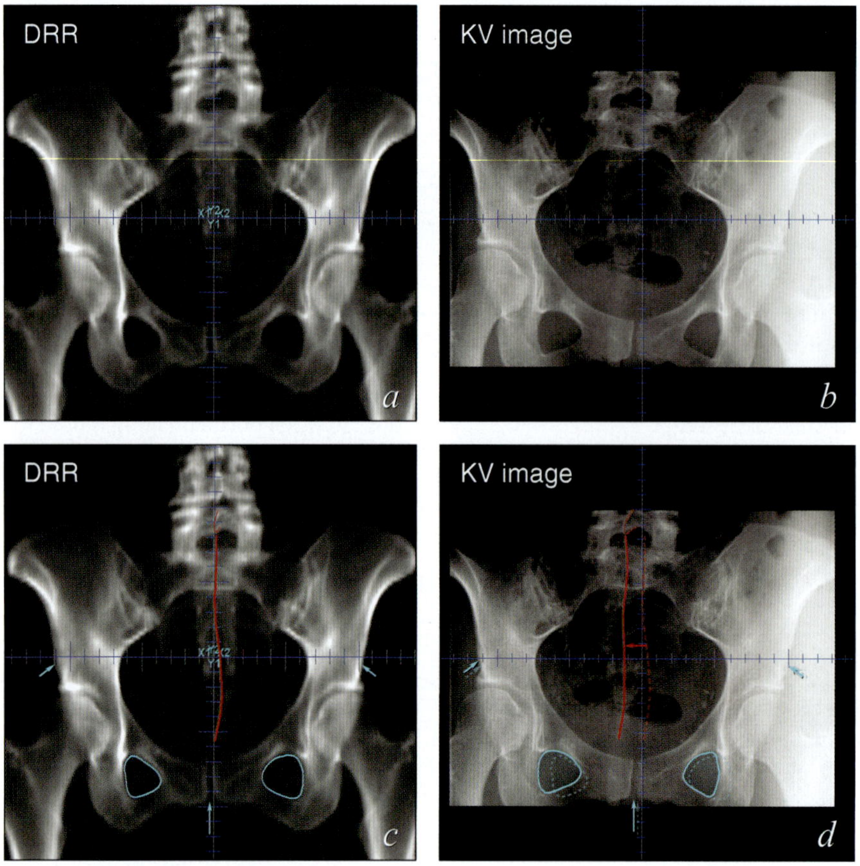

FIGURE 7.6 Rotational errors in patient positioning. Rotational errors can be some of the most difficult to detect. In *(a)* and *(b)*, the digitally reconstructed radiograph (DRR) from a patient's treatment plan is shown adjacent to an on-treatment kV image. The relationship between the central axis and the pubic symphysis appears to be off by about 1 mm; the position at L5 appears to be off by a slightly greater distance in the same direction. It would be easy to conclude that the error is only a slight shift and tilt to the right. However, in this case, there was also a serious counterclockwise rotational error, causing posterior structures to be displaced to the left by as much as 1.8 cm. To highlight this, in *(c)* and *(d)*, the same DRR *(c)* and kV images *(d)* are shown, but now with lines demarcating boney landmarks. The *solid lines* in *(c)* represent the midsacrum and L5 spinous process *(red)* and the obturator foramina *(cyan)*. The positions of these landmarks are transposed to the kV image *(dotted lines)* in *(d)*, allowing direct comparison with the position of the same structures on the on-treatment image. Note the change in shape of the spinous process and obturator foramina caused by the rotational shift, which displaced posterior portions of these structures more than anterior portions of these structures. In this case, the *cyan arrows* demonstrate that there were also very slight tilt and shift errors. The patient was repositioned in the cradle, and subsequent films lined up well. Examination of on-treatment images should always include an evaluation of the positions of posterior structures (e.g., coccyx, sacrum, and spinous processes) as well as anterior structures (e.g., pubic symphysis) to rule out rotational errors.

One disadvantage of daily kV imaging for gynecologic RT is the relatively narrow field of view (usually 20 cm). For patients treated with extended fields, it may be necessary to obtain a second set of films after displacing the intensifier to verify proper alignment along the entire length of the field.

Cone Beam CT

Cone beam CT can be very helpful in selected patients. For patients who have large tumors or potentially fluctuating body habitus, weekly cone beam CT can be used to determine when repeat simulation and adaptive planning are needed. When the target volume is small, particularly in the case of soft tissue boosts to mobile structures, cone beam CT can be very helpful. However, the image quality is so poor for obese patients that kV imaging is almost always preferred. Also, before routine cone beam CT is prescribed, the relatively small field of view, additional image acquisition time, and added radiation dose should be considered.

Ultrasound Imaging

Ultrasound imaging can be useful for monitoring bladder volumes in patients who have mobile uterine or vaginal targets. If possible, bladder volumes should be measured before the patient is on the treatment table. Because the suprapubic pressure caused by the ultrasound probe can cause patients to tense their buttocks, causing severe tilt errors, it is important to assure that the patient is relaxed before treatment and to check carefully for tilt errors (**Fig. 7.5**).

Fiducial Markers

Radioopaque markers placed in the cervix or vagina can be monitored on daily kV images or cone beam CT scans to assure that the structure is within the planning target volume (Chapter 4, CS 10.1, 11.1, 11.3).[11,12] *However, real-time adjustments should not be made to follow the position of the markers unless their positions are representative of the entire target volume.* For patients who have only a small central target that is well demarcated by fiducial markers, it may be appropriate to adjust isocenter position to follow the markers. For patients who are receiving comprehensive central and nodal treatment, alignment should be based on boney landmarks; in such cases, if imaging shows sufficient displacement of the markers to place the target outside the internal target volume (ITV), the patient should be taken off the table and the radiation oncologist should be called to determine the cause (e.g., change in bladder or rectal volume) so corrective action can be taken.

Monitoring Changes in Body Habitus and Tumor Response

Body Habitus

Changes in external contour can sometimes have a significant impact on the radiation dose distribution. Conditions that should be monitored for changes include the following:

- Weight changes. The patient's anterior–posterior and lateral separations should be monitored; a change of more than 2 cm should be evaluated to determine whether the change may have influenced the dose distribution sufficiently to warrant adjustment of the plan. This is particularly true for patients who are receiving intensity-modulated RT because of the relatively low beam energy.
- Lymphocysts. Fluctuating lymphocysts, particularly in the groin, can alter the external contour or, if enlarging, can displace the target outside the treatment field. Depending on the clinical situation, we recommend monitoring with clinical examination or cone beam CT to determine whether a plan adjustment is needed.
- Edema. Patient who are treated for vulvar cancer sometimes develop edema of the vulva, which can displace the vulvar surface outside the treatment field if the distal air gap is not adequate to cover the edematous vulva with a margin. Patients should be monitored clinically for this. In rare cases, the plan may need to be adjusted.

Tumor Response

Any patient who has a large tumor mass adjacent to critical structures, particularly bowel, should be monitored periodically for tumor response. If uninvolved critical structures have moved into the treatment volume because of a major tumor response, an adjustment in the plan is often warranted (Fig. 7.7; CS 10.6, 11.10, 12.7, 14.5, 15.1, 15.2, 15.3). For patients who have extensive vaginal or cervical disease, midtreatment examinations are used to choose the most appropriate modality and technique for delivery of a central boost.

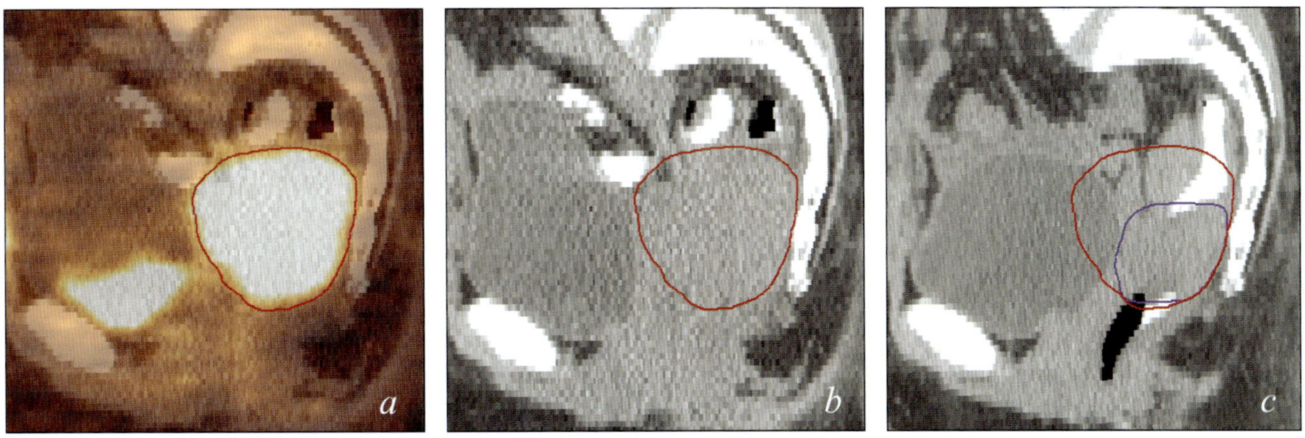

FIGURE 7.7 Intratreatment response of a large pelvic mass. Critical structures that are displaced but not infiltrated by expanding pelvic wall masses may fall within the region of high radiation dose as tumor responds to RT. Close monitoring with adaptive planning can significantly reduce the dose to bowel and other normal tissues. For this large precoccygeal squamous carcinoma, the initial gross tumor volume (GTV; *red line*) was defined using positron emission tomography (*a*) and planning CT (*b*). As part of the definitive treatment, the GTV plus a 7-mm margin was treated at 2 Gy per fraction, with a nested internal target treated at 2.2 Gy per fraction. On the 10th treatment day (after delivery of 20 to 22 Gy), the patient's pain and findings on clinical examination were noted to have markedly improved. A repeat CT scan with contrast was obtained the same day and demonstrated dramatic tumor regression with rectosigmoid now filling portions of the original GTV (*c*). The treatment plan was reoptimized using the new GTV, and the treatment was resumed after a 1-day break. A second adjustment was made 2 weeks later. See CS 15.2 for treatment details and outcome of this patient.

References

1. Chatani M, Matayoshi Y, Masaki N, et al. High-dose rate intracavitary irradiation for carcinoma of the uterine cervix. The adverse effect of treatment prolongation. *Strahlenther Onkol.* 1997;173:379–384.
2. Fyles A, Keane TJ, Barton M, et al. The effect of treatment duration in the local control of cervix cancer. *Radiother Oncol.* 1992;25:273–279.
3. Shaverdian N, Gondi V, Sklenar KL, et al. Effects of treatment duration during concomitant chemoradiation therapy for cervical cancer. *Int J Radiat Oncol Biol Phys.* 2013;86:562–568.
4. Monk BJ, Tian C, Rose PG, et al. Which clinical/pathologic factors matter in the era of chemoradiation as treatment for locally advanced cervical carcinoma? Analysis of two Gynecologic Oncology Group (GOG) trials. *Gynecol Oncol.* 2007;105:427–433.
5. Boothe D, Patel SH, Stessin A, et al. Comparing the rates of urinary tract infections among patients receiving adjuvant pelvic intensity modulated radiation therapy, 3-dimensional conformal radiation therapy, and brachytherapy for newly diagnosed endometrial cancer. *Pract Radiat Oncol.* 2013;3:269–274.
6. Jepson RG, Williams G, Craig JC. Cranberries for preventing urinary tract infections. *Cochrane Database Syst Rev.* 2012;10:CD001321.
7. Hill A, Hanson M, Bogle MA, et al. Severe radiation dermatitis is related to *Staphylococcus aureus. Am J Clin Oncol.* 2004;27:361–363.
8. Bishop AJ, Allen PK, Klopp AH, et al. Relationship between low hemoglobin levels and outcomes after treatment with radiation or chemoradiation in patients with cervical cancer: has the impact of anemia been overstated? *Int J Radiat Oncol Biol Phys.* 2015;91:196–205.
9. Lajer H, Daugaard G. Cisplatin and hypomagnesemia. *Cancer Treat Rev.* 1999;25:47–58.
10. Kim H, Beriwal S, Huq MS, et al. Evaluation of set-up uncertainties with daily kilovoltage image guidance in external beam radiation therapy for gynaecological cancers. *Clin Oncol (R Coll Radiol).* 2012;24:e39–e45.
11. Rash D, Hagar Y, Cui J, et al. Interfraction motion of the vaginal apex during postoperative intensity modulated radiation therapy: are we missing the target? *Int J Gynecol Cancer.* 2013;23:385–392.
12. Jhingran A, Salehpour M, Sam M, et al. Vaginal motion and bladder and rectal volumes during pelvic intensity-modulated radiation therapy after hysterectomy. *Int J Radiat Oncol Biol Phys.* 2012;82:256–262.

CHAPTER 8

Brachytherapy

INTRODUCTION

Brachytherapy plays a critical role in the definitive management of primary and recurrent tumors within the uterus and vagina. As a general principle, to deliver a boost dose to gross disease, brachytherapy is preferred over external beam radiation therapy (RT) whenever brachytherapy sources can be positioned closer to the tumor than to adjacent critical structures. With brachytherapy, the physical proximity of the source to the tumor makes it possible to take advantage of the inverse square law to create a steep dose gradient and thereby deliver much high doses to tumor than to adjacent critical structures. The advantages of brachytherapy over external beam RT include the following:

- *Delivery of a higher mean dose.* The steep dose gradient with brachytherapy means that it is often possible to deliver a higher dose to the tumor with brachytherapy than with external beam RT with the same normal tissue doses.
- *Reduced impact of internal organ motion.* In external beam treatment planning, an additional margin is added beyond the target to account for variation in setup accuracy and internal organ motion. Because the relationship between the brachytherapy applicator and the tumor is fixed, there is no need for this additional margin in brachytherapy treatment planning.
- *Acceleration of treatment.* Brachytherapy dose is typically given more rapidly than external beam treatment dose, reducing the opportunity for tumor cell repopulation.
- *Increased dose heterogeneity within the tumor.* Within the target volume, brachytherapy produces significant dose heterogeneity. The potential benefits of delivering a very high dose to a portion of the tumor have not been proven; however, this heterogeneity may offer biologic advantages through immunologic mechanisms, such as enhanced tumor antigen presentation.

In addition to these general advantages over external beam RT, brachytherapy for gynecologic cancers may offer several additional advantages. First, applicator placement for treatment of most gynecologic cancers does not require a major surgical intervention. Second, the presence of a central canal from the vagina through the uterus provides a natural cavity into which applicators can be placed. Finally, although functioning of the gynecologic organs is critical for childbearing, it is not critical for patient survival; thus, it is possible to deliver ablative doses of radiation to gynecologic organs. For all of these reasons, brachytherapy has a central role in the management of gynecologic cancers.

Brachytherapy also has a number of disadvantages or challenges. These include the following:

- *Need for technical expertise.* Brachytherapy requires a unique set of skills on the part of the physician, the dosimetrist, and the physicist. In particular, the placement of applicators in relationship to the tumor is critical and can be challenging in many cases. This is particularly true for interstitial brachytherapy.
- *Anesthesia and procedure risks.* There are risks of anesthesia and injury from applicator placement. However, these risks are generally very small and should rarely be a reason not to perform brachytherapy.
- *Capital costs.* Building a facility to perform brachytherapy and maintaining sources and applicators requires significant resources, necessitating a sufficient volume of patients to support a brachytherapy program.

- *Patient discomfort.* Discomfort from applicators can be a part of the patient's experience and requires a plan for management.

Specific indications for brachytherapy are discussed in detail in Chapters 10, 11, and 13. This chapter focuses on some general principles of gynecologic brachytherapy.

ESSENTIAL ELEMENTS OF A BRACHYTHERAPY TREATMENT PLAN

If brachytherapy is being considered as a possible treatment, it is critically important to begin preparations for brachytherapy as soon as the patient's initial evaluation is complete. Factors that need to be considered at initial presentation include the timing of brachytherapy, applicator types that may be needed, brachytherapy placement approach, delivery method, dose rate, and fractionation.

Many aspects of the brachytherapy treatment plan are governed by the initial extent of disease. Thus, the physician who will be performing brachytherapy should always be given an opportunity to assess the patient before any treatment (including chemotherapy or external beam irradiation) has been started. Ensuring up front that all the necessary expertise and supplies are available to perform appropriate brachytherapy prevents last-minute referral to a brachytherapist. Urgent referrals can leave the brachytherapist in the difficult position of having to glean information about the initial extent of disease from review of the patient record. Furthermore, urgent referrals often result in an undesirable protraction of treatment due to delays in establishing care with a new physician at a new facility.

High-quality brachytherapy requires a coordinated team approach. The necessary steps and resources are detailed in the *American Brachytherapy Society Consensus Guidelines for Locally Advanced Carcinoma of the Cervix. Part I: General Principles.*[1] Physicians who regularly perform brachytherapy usually work with a dedicated team of physicians, dosimetrists, and physicists using a set of established guidelines and procedures for gynecologic brachytherapy. For physicians who perform brachytherapy only occasionally, it is particularly important to explicitly verify the plan and procedures with all members of the team during each step of the procedure. Essential elements of a brachytherapy treatment plan include the following:

- *Anesthesia.* Although some practitioners give patients only oral anxiolytics and narcotics before intrauterine applicator placement, patient discomfort with this approach can be significant and may result in suboptimal applicator placement. Anesthesia can be obtained using conscious sedation, spinal or epidural block, or general anesthesia. In our practice, we use general anesthesia for most patients who do not have a high risk for complications from anesthesia due to medical comorbidities.
- *Timing.* It is recommended that all radiation treatment, including brachytherapy, be completed within 56 days. Brachytherapy should be started no later than 6 weeks after the start of pelvic RT. For patients with cervical cancer, the first implant can be performed after completion of external beam RT or earlier if the disease is small or has responded sufficiently to allow for good tumor coverage (e.g., if a central tumor has shrunk to <4 cm). Any nodal or parametrial boosts should be interdigitated between brachytherapy treatments. Prolonged treatment results in lower rates of local control and survival (Chapter 7).[2]
- *Applicator selection.* It is critical to select the best applicators for each patient's anatomy. The features of various gynecologic brachytherapy applicators are discussed in more detail below.
- *Physician expertise.* Optimal placement of intrauterine intracavitary applicators requires familiarity with the processes of sounding the uterus, often in the setting of extensive disease, and placing applicators within the vagina. Initial clinical and radiographic findings can help to identify cases that are likely to be particularly challenging. Challenging cases can often be identified prospectively through tumor factors, such as disease obstructing the cervical canal, and patient-specific factors, such as obesity, retroverted uterus, or narrow vagina (**Fig. 8.1**). For cases like these, it may be useful to arrange for a gynecologic oncologist to be present during applicator placement. Placement of interstitial needles is particularly complex and requires specialized expertise.
- *Intraoperative imaging.* Intraoperative imaging is critical to ensure that the tandem is well placed in the uterus, the vaginal applicators are flush with the cervix, and adequate vaginal packing is present to reduce the dose to the bladder and rectum. The combination of transabdominal sonograms and orthogonal films can provide a great deal of information about the applicator position (**Fig. 8.2**). Transabdominal ultrasonography is particularly helpful to allow visualization of tandem placement in real time during the procedure. Orthogonal radiographs can be used to identify the proximity of the vaginal applicators to the cervix as marked with radiopaque markers. An alternative approach is to use intraoperative axial imaging with magnetic resonance imaging (MRI) or computed tomography (CT). The relative advantages of these imaging techniques are discussed below.
- *Physics expertise.* Brachytherapy treatment planning is a unique discipline that requires dedicated physics support. It is important to ensure that a physicist with necessary expertise will be available for the procedure.

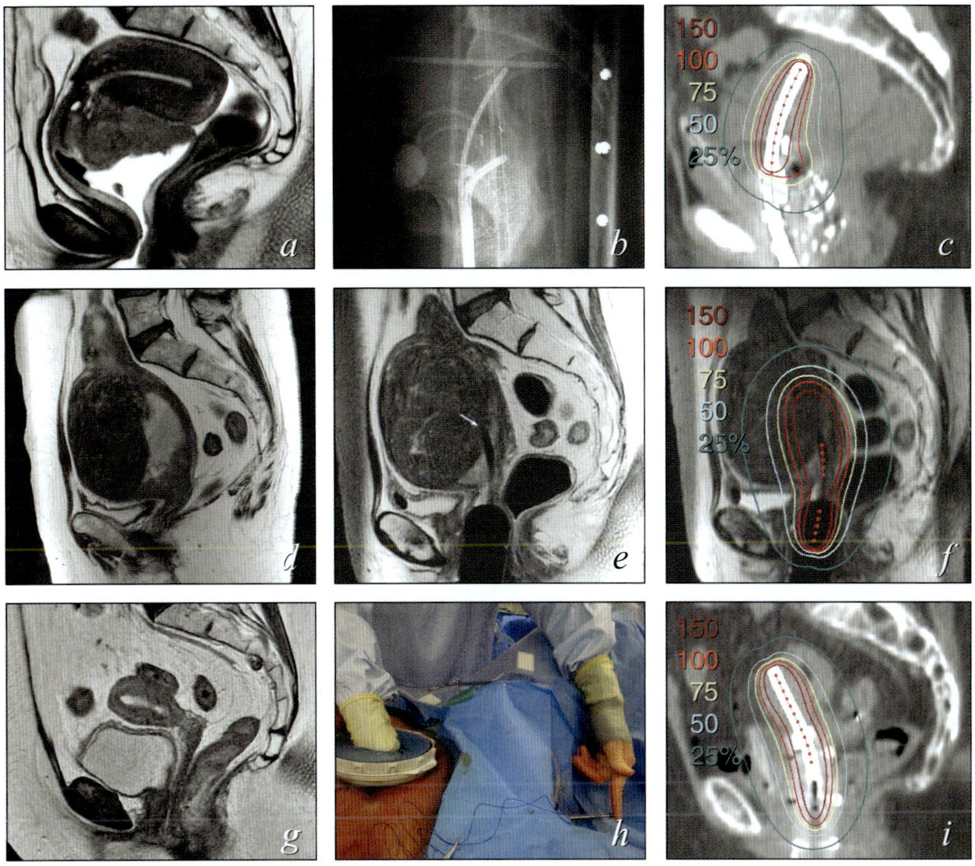

FIGURE 8.1 Initial imaging features may suggest cases that require special preparation for brachytherapy. The three patients illustrated here had rare anatomical features that were predicted to pose unusual challenges for brachytherapy. The first patient *(a–c)* had bulky disease involving the posterior lip of the cervix and a sharply retroflexed uterus that was essentially trapped in the sacral hollow *(a)*. MRI performed before brachytherapy showed an excellent response, but the uterine position was unchanged and, at brachytherapy, could not be moved to a neutral position. However, an unusual brachytherapy arrangement *(c)* provided excellent coverage of the posterior lip of the cervix. At this writing, the patient had no evidence of disease (NED) at 3 years. The second patient *(d–f)* had a large uterine fibroid, with pyometra above an obstructing cervical cancer and parametrial involvement (*d* and Fig. 4.7). It was anticipated that the fibroid would impede optimal brachytherapy applicator placement. Arrangements were made for pelvic RT followed by MRI-guided brachytherapy; the patient was counseled that she might receive either definitive brachytherapy or a reduced dose followed by hysterectomy. At 5 weeks, MRI and examination under anesthesia showed a near complete tumor response. PDR brachytherapy was performed, but the tandem could not be passed beyond the fibroid *(arrow, e)*. Minimal dwell times were allocated to positions close to the rectum; total HRCTV D90 and D_{2cc} rectal doses were 73 and 68 Gy, respectively. Four weeks later *(f)*, hysterectomy was performed. The third patient *(g–i)* had a narrow vagina and a tiny uterus with a small tumor that replaced the cervix and invaded the parametrium and vaginal fornix *(g)*. After external beam RT, no cervical os was visible, and initial efforts to sound the uterus failed. Because the surgeon felt the patient was still a poor candidate for hysterectomy, a second attempt was made to sound the uterus. Using a 4 cm incision made by the gynecologic oncologist, the radiation oncologist inserted a hand into the pelvis, grasped the cervix between the thumb and forefinger, and, using the opposite (left) hand, successfully threaded the tandem through the obstructed canal *(h)*. The patient received a single 66-hour treatment, bringing the total HRCTV D90 dose to 85 Gy, although Point A received only 63 Gy *(i)*; the D_{2cc} doses to bladder and rectum were 63 and 60 Gy, respectively.

GYNECOLOGIC BRACHYTHERAPY APPLICATORS

Intravaginal Applicators

Single-Channel Vaginal Cylinders

Single-channel vaginal cylinders are useful if the surface of the entire circumference of the vagina requires treatment to a similar dose. Because of the rapid falloff in dose with increasing distance from the surface, intracavitary cylinders are not appropriate to treat tumors that are more than 4 to 5 mm thick.

Vaginal cylinders that are placed in the vagina after hysterectomy typically have a domed apical surface. These dome cylinders can be purchased as a single unit that extends along the

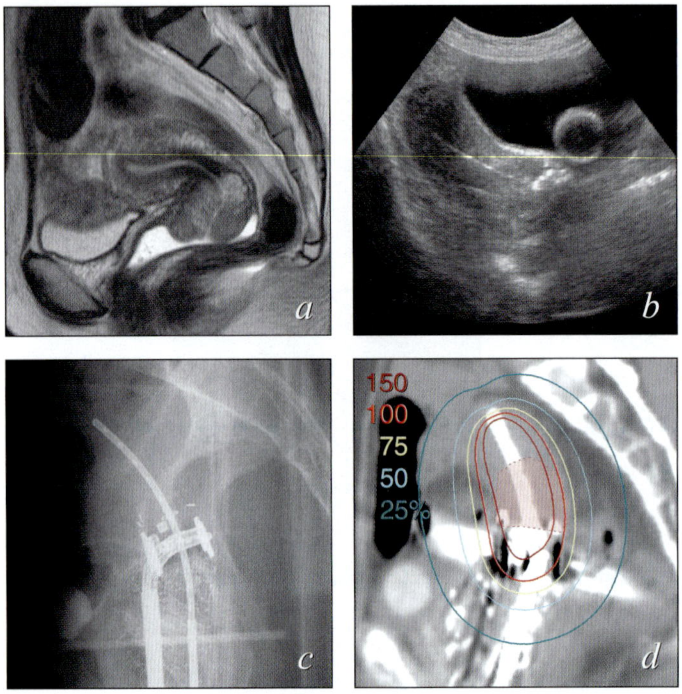

FIGURE 8.2 A variety of imaging tools can be used to inform brachytherapy. Pre-brachytherapy reexamination of initial diagnostic MR images can provide valuable information about the configuration of the uterus and uterine canal *(a)*. Intraoperative ultrasound guidance facilitates sounding of the uterus and helps to confirm accurate placement of the tandem in the uterus *(b)*. During applicator placement, some form of imaging should always be performed to rule out obvious problems. Plain films *(c)*, yield a wealth of information about the position of the applicator in the pelvis, the relationship of the applicator to the cervix (which contains three platinum fiducial markers), and the relationship between the tandem and ovoids; in this case, the position appears to be excellent. Image-based treatment planning with CT or MRI yields more precise information about the relationship between the applicator and surrounding structures *(d)*.

length of the vagina or as a dome that can be assembled with vaginal cylinders to create an applicator of the desired length.

Single-channel domed vaginal cylinders are ideal for prophylactic treatment of the apical vagina in patients who are at risk for vaginal recurrence after hysterectomy for endometrial cancer (Chapter 13). In selected cases, a domed cylinder may be used to deliver a boost dose to the vaginal surface after postoperative external beam RT for cervical or endometrial cancer (e.g., **CS 10.1, 13.1**).

Vaginal intracavitary brachytherapy may also be used in the definitive treatment of primary or recurrent cancers that involve the upper vagina if the disease is no more than 5 mm thick at the time of brachytherapy **(CS 11.1)**. If there is any uncertainty about the thickness of the lesion, it should be evaluated using MRI or ultrasonography before brachytherapy is performed. To accurately determine the lesion thickness, MRI should always be performed with an MR-compatible cylinder or gel in the vagina (Chapter 4).

For patients who have an intact uterus, vaginal cylinders may be placed in the vagina in conjunction with an intrauterine tandem. Cylinders are typically used in this way to treat patients with cervical cancer who have a narrow vagina or to treat areas of superficial vaginal involvement. Again, disease that is more than 5 mm thick should be treated using another method, usually interstitial brachytherapy.

Domed vaginal cylinders come in widths ranging from 1.5 to 4.5 cm to accommodate variations in vaginal capacity. For most patients with endometrial cancer, a cylinder with a diameter of 2.5 to 3.5 cm provides the best fit for posthysterectomy vaginal cuff treatment. Because of the rapid falloff of radiation dose from the surface of vaginal cylinders, the effectiveness of treatment depends on achievement of an accurate fit. Poor selection of an intracavitary applicator can lead to underdosage of the vagina in several ways:

- If a very small cylinder is placed in a capacious vagina, folds in the lateral vaginal mucosa will not be in contact with the cylinder and will, therefore, receive less than the prescribed dose of radiation. Failure to fully advance the dome can also cause a portion of the vagina to receive an inadequate dose (**Fig. 8.3**).
- A domed shape is optimal for most posthysterectomy vaginal cuff treatments; however, in some cases, the surgeon sutures the vagina in a way that leaves pockets or "rabbit-ears" at the lateral aspects of the apical vaginal incision site. The bases of these pockets may be displaced a sufficient distance from the dome surface to cause significant underdosage. In some of these cases, vaginal ovoids provide a better distribution of radiation dose than can be achieved with a domed cylinder; image guidance is particularly helpful in such cases.
- An overly large dome may not reach the vaginal apex. If the vagina is tapered at the apex, it is sometimes necessary to use different widths for the domed and distal cylinders, particularly if more than the apical vagina requires treatment.

Most cylindrical vaginal applicators can be purchased as stackable segments. Additional cylinders are added to the dome or are stacked distal to the stopper on an intrauterine tandem to tailor the applicator length to the length of the vagina. At a minimum, the applicator should extend at least 2 cm beyond the most distal source or active dwell position to ensure that the vagina does not collapse around active sources in the stem of the applicator, resulting in a high dose to the vaginal mucosa. Ideally, for prophylactic vaginal cuff treatment, the distal limit of the applicator

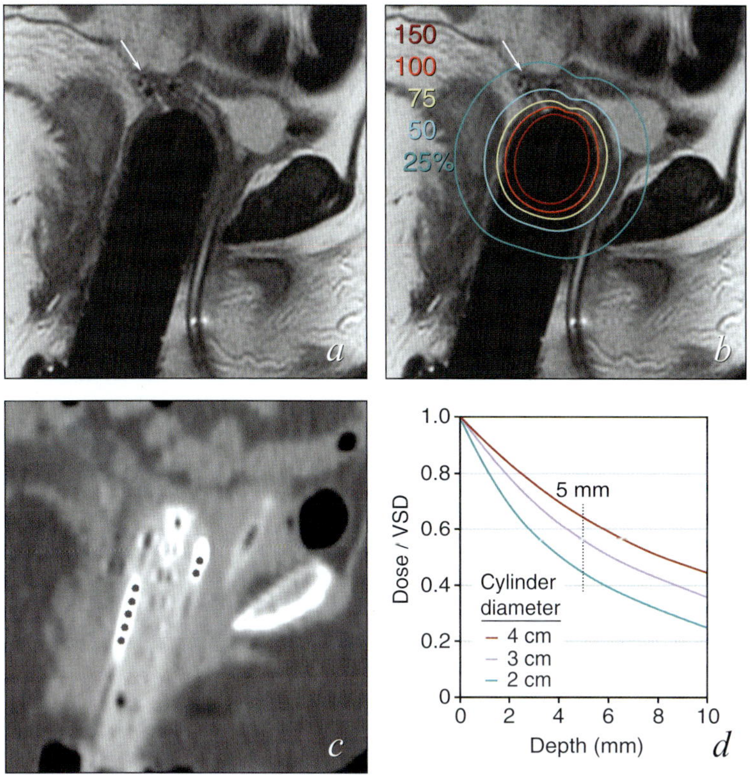

FIGURE 8.3 The dose of radiation declines rapidly with increasing distance from the surface of an intracavitary domed cylinder. For this reason, intracavitary therapy alone (without interstitial needles) is inadequate to treat tumors that are more than 4 to 5 mm thick at the time of brachytherapy. Care must always be taken to assure that the domed cylinder fits well and is flush against the vaginal mucosa. In this case, the 3-cm-diameter cylinder was not fully advanced, and a small portion of vagina remained folded above the dome *(arrow, a)*. This patient was actually being treated for a distal vaginal lesion; however, had the vaginal apex been included in the target, this placement would have been unacceptable. The isodose distribution from a typical apical vaginal treatment is shown in *b*; note that the dose to the vaginal fold is only 25% to 30% of the vaginal surface dose. The mucosal fold and the relationship between the bladder and the dome were poorly visualized on CT *(c)*. Panel *d* shows the relationship between dose (expressed as a fraction of the vaginal surface dose) and distance from the surface of a 2-, 3-, or 4-cm-diameter domed cylinder; the falloff in dose is particularly steep when the diameter of the cylinder is small.

should lie just inside the introitus. For treatment of gross disease, the dome and cylinders should fill the entire vagina and extend at least 2 cm distal to the distal limit of the target volume.

Fixation devices can be used to assure that the dome remains in the correct position throughout high-dose rate (HDR) treatment (Fig. 8.4). For patients receiving low-dose rate (LDR) or pulsed-dose rate (PDR) treatment, the applicator should be secured with a suture passed through the labia. Vaginal cylinders that protrude beyond the perineal ring must be secured during treatment. The position of a vaginal dome or tandem, and cylinders can shift slightly when the legs are brought down from the lithotomy position. For this reason, verification films or CT scans should always be obtained with the patient in the treatment position.

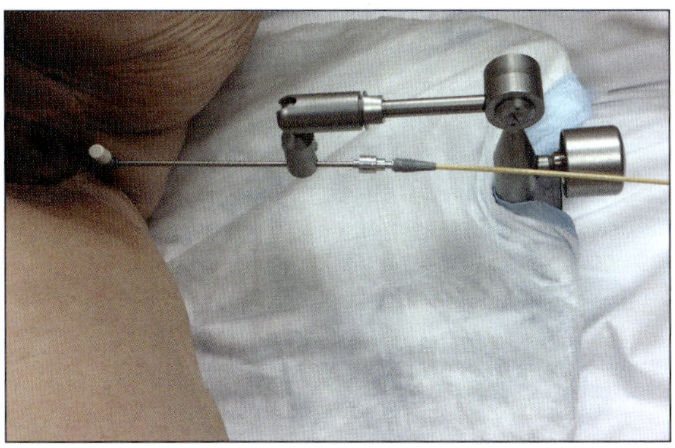

FIGURE 8.4 A fixation device used to ensure that the domed vaginal cylinder remained flush against the vaginal mucosa throughout treatment.

Fiducial markers inserted at the lateral edges of the apical vaginal incision (Chapter 4) can help to assess applicator position. The relationships between the dome and the mucosa can be appreciated on MRI but only roughly appreciated on CT (Fig. 8.3).

Multichannel Vaginal Cylinders

Vaginal cylinders with circumferential peripheral channels allow eccentric distribution of the surface radiation dose. In most cases, these channels do not reach into the dome itself.

Multichannel cylinders typically contain 5 to 6 channels that are evenly spaced 3 to 5 mm deep to the surface of the cylinder; however, cylindrical vaginal applicators have been manufactured that contain up to 13 channels.

For prophylactic vaginal cuff irradiation, multichannel cylinders offer few clinical advantages over single-channel cylinders because the goal of treatment, that is, to achieve a homogeneous dose to at-risk apical vaginal mucosa (Chapter 13), is achieved nicely with a single-channel domed cylinder.

Multichannel vaginal cylinders can be helpful for treatment of primary or recurrent cancers that superficially involve the midvagina. Because the peripheral channels are usually <5 mm deep to the cylinder surface, the falloff in dose beyond the vaginal mucosa is very steep: *typically the dose contributed from peripheral channels to tissues 5 mm deep to the applicator surface is <25% of the surface dose.* Depending on the depth and separation of the channels, the surface dose may also be quite heterogeneous, with hot spots overlying the activated channels. For these reasons, it is recommended that the peripheral channels be used only as a supplement to the dose delivered from the central channel, usually for lesions that are <3 mm thick (CS 11.2, 11.6, 13.3) or in combination with interstitial needles (CS 11.3, 11.5, 11.7).

Multichannel vaginal cylinders must always be secured during treatment to prevent rotation of the applicator.

Vaginal Colpostats or "Ovoids"

First developed in Paris in the early 20th century, colpostats, also known as "ovoids," are paired vaginal applicators that distance intravaginal sources from the mucosa and ideally fit adjacent to the cervix in the vaginal fornices. The goal of this arrangement is to maximize the dose to lateral parametrial tissues with relatively less exposure of anterior and posterior critical structures. Subsequent innovations led to adjustments in the shape of the ovoids and in the angle and position of the source channels; the addition of internal shielding; and the development of manual and remote methods of afterloading (Fig. 8.5).[3] Today, these applicators come in a wide variety of configurations. Although many are labeled "Manchester" or "Fletcher" ovoids, these frequently bear little resemblance

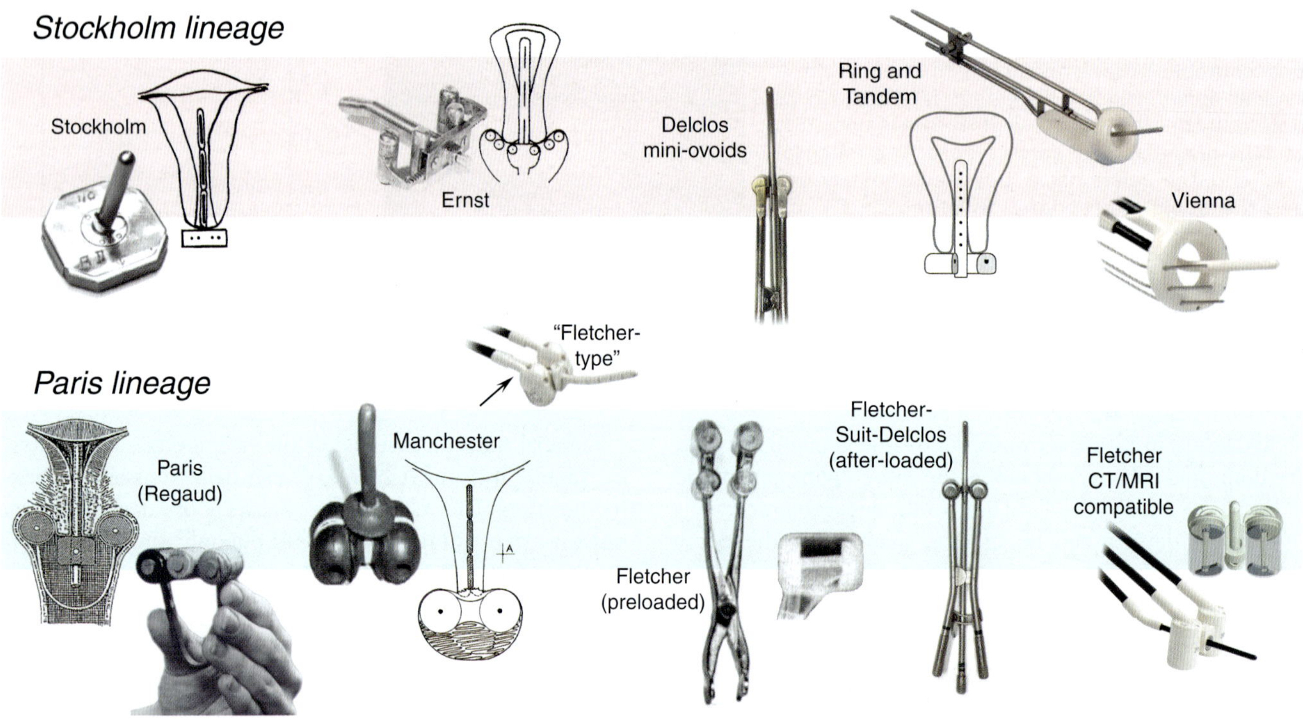

FIGURE 8.5 In the early days of radium treatment, groups in Paris and Stockholm championed two different approaches to design of intracavitary applicators for treatment of cervical cancer. These designs formed the beginnings of two lineages that extend to the present day. In the 1930s, Stockholm clinicians developed an applicator that positioned vaginal sources within a few millimeters of the surface of a rectangular vaginal packet; this applicator could be inserted quickly, but it required delivery of very high vaginal mucosal doses to treat parametrial disease. The Ernst applicator, which was popular in the 1960s and 1970s, and the modern ring applicator are descendants of this Stockholm lineage. However, with a fixed tandem length and vaginal sources that are near the mucosal surface, these compact systems tend to provide only a modest dose of radiation to deep paracervical tissues. Because of this, clinicians sometimes add interstitial needles to achieve better parametrial coverage when treating bulky tumors with ring applicators.

Also in the 1930s, at the Radium Institute in Paris, Regaud developed a system that placed vaginal sources at a greater distance (~10 mm) from the vaginal surface, leveraging the inverse square law to improve the dose to lateral tissues. At Manchester, investigators modified this arrangement with a system that allowed greater individualization of the tandem length and ovoid diameters. These innovations permitted delivery of higher parametrial doses than was possible with the Stockholm approach. The Manchester group also developed the concept of point A; however, this reference dose was meant to be an indicator of the risk of normal tissue complications—it was not considered to be a measure of tumor dose.

In the 1950s, Gilbert Fletcher developed an innovative applicator that paired an adjustable tandem with shielded cylindrical colpostats. These modifications of the Manchester system further improved the ability to treat large tumors and deep parametrial tissues without exceeding critical structure tolerance limits. The Fletcher applicator was subsequently modified for afterloading, remote-afterloading, and most recently, CT- or MRI-guided brachytherapy. It should be noted that some applicators that have been labeled as "Fletcher-type" are closer in shape to Manchester ovoids and lack internal shields, a key feature of all of the colpostats designed by Fletcher and his team. Also developed at MD Anderson were the Delclos mini-ovoids, which were made for use in patients whose vaginas could not accommodate Fletcher ovoids; mini-ovoids have a geometry similar to that of a ring applicator but with an adjustable tandem and slightly greater distance between the vaginal sources and the applicator surface.

to the applicators that were designed in Manchester or by Dr. Fletcher, respectively. For this reason, it is always preferable to look at the individual features to determine which type of applicator is best suited to a specific clinical setting.

Key features that influence the distribution of radiation surrounding vaginal colpostats include the following:

- *The angle of the source channels vis à vis the intrauterine tandem.* Most colpostats have been designed to position a 2-cm tube source or a line of source positions approximately perpendicular to the axis of the vagina and uterus (**Fig. 8.5**). This orientation takes advantage of the anisotropy of the sources and decreases the dose to rectum and bladder relative to lateral structures. In contrast, colpostats that have the source channel positioned in parallel with the vaginal axis tend to provide less sparing of critical structures. One example of such a colpostat is the Henschke applicator, an early afterloaded applicator that was originally developed at Memorial Sloan Kettering but is still available in several forms today.
- *The shape of the colpostat.* Early colpostats, such as those designed in Manchester in the 1930s, were truly ovoid. In the 1950s, Fletcher developed a cylindrical ovoid designed to provide greater distance between the rectovaginal septum and the radiation sources and to accommodate vaginal shields; this applicator was the most popular in the United States for several decades. The Fletcher-Williamson applicator, which has all the key features of earlier shielded applicators, was developed in the 2000s for use with remote afterloading units. In recent years, there has been increased use of unshielded ovoids similar in shape to Manchester ovoids; these are somewhat easier to insert in the vagina but generally accommodate less activity than true Fletcher ovoids because of the shape, lack of shielding, and other features (**Fig. 8.5**).
- *The size of the colpostat.* Most colpostats come in a variety of sizes, with a diameter ranging from 15 to 30 mm. Historically, it was recommended that clinicians use the largest ovoids that could be accommodated by the vagina because large ovoids could be loaded more heavily and achieve greater lateral penetration of dose than was possible with 2-cm ovoids. However, 25- to 30-mm ovoids also tend to expose a large vaginal surface area to a high dose of radiation. With the advent of chemoradiation, the cervix is usually small at the time of brachytherapy, and 2-cm ovoids are usually sufficient. Mini-ovoids were originally designed to be used in patients whose narrow vaginas did not accommodate 2-cm Fletcher-Suit-Delclos ovoids (**Fig. 8.5**). With similar source loadings, the dose at the surface of a mini-ovoid is two to three times the dose at the surface of a 2-cm Fletcher-Suit-Delclos ovoid. For this reason, and because mini-ovoids lack internal shields, mini-ovoids can safely accommodate only about half as much activity as a 2-cm Fletcher-Suit-Delclos ovoid or Fletcher-Williamson ovoid.
- *Internal shields.* Internal shields have been a hallmark of all variations of the 2-cm Fletcher, Fletcher-Suit, and Fletcher-Suit-Delclos colpostats. Internal shields have been demonstrated to reduce the dose to the rectum and bladder by as much as 25%.[4] Many of the applicators that are currently marketed as "Fletcher" or "Fletcher-type" ovoids lack internal shields and other signature features of true Fletcher colpostats.
- *Position of the source channel.* In order to accommodate limitations on the curvature of remote-afterloading applicators, some modern ovoids have source channels that are not perfectly centered in the ovoid, with the source closer to the surface posteriorly than at the center of the ovoid. This can cause higher than expected doses to be delivered to some portions of the vaginal mucosa and rectum, particularly if image guidance is not used.
- *Separation of the ovoids.* For any given source loading, the dose to the bladder and rectum increases markedly as the distance between the sources decreases. However, excessive separation of the ovoids creates a cold spot in the distribution of dose to the distal cervix.
- *MRI and CT compatibility.* Fletcher-Suit-Delclos ovoids (and Fletcher-Williamson ovoids, which were designed for remote afterloading) are not MRI compatible and cause substantial artifact on CT. At MD Anderson, we utilize a novel applicator with movable shields made of nonferrous metal.[5] These shields make it possible to obtain high-quality CT and MR images without sacrificing the dosimetric benefits of ovoid shields (**Fig. 8.6**). Most recently, unshielded ovoids have been developed that contain a passageway through which interstitial needles can be passed through the ovoid into the cervix.[6]

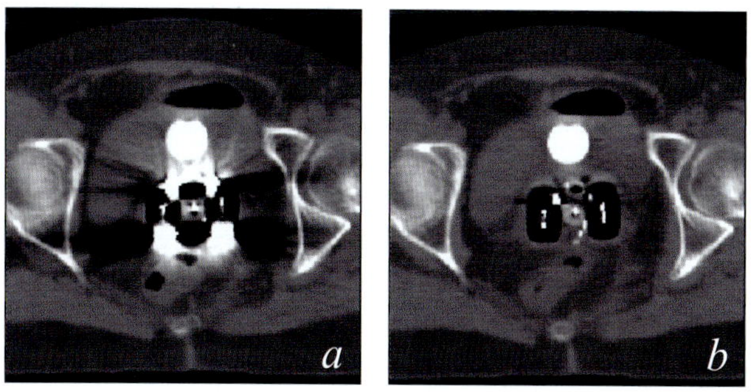

FIGURE 8.6 One disadvantage of shielded Fletcher ovoids is the CT artifact caused by the shields (Fig. 8.2d). To overcome this problem, ovoids have been developed with movable shields that can be shifted out of the image acquisition plane during CT. On the left *(a)* is an axial image with the shields in the treatment position throughout CT acquisition. On the right is an image taken with the shields shifted first anteriorly and then posteriorly to keep them out of the CT plane *(b)*. The ovoids are also MRI compatible.

Ring Applicators

Ring vaginal applicators were developed as an alternative type of vaginal applicator used to treat the cervix. Like mini-ovoids, ring applicators have geometry similar to that of early Stockholm applicators (**Fig. 8.5**). Ring applicators are some what easier to insert than tandem and ovoid implants because they have only two pieces and a fixed geometry. A disadvantage of ring applicators is that they are combined with fixed-length tandems (usually available in 2-cm increments). The tandems are also relatively straight, which can encourage perforation, particularly when the tandem is inserted in a sharply flexed uterus. The distance from the source channel to vaginal mucosa is very short, resulting in a higher vaginal surface dose to achieve the same dose at depth. Finally, the caudad side of the ring has an exposed source train, which could be a particular concern if the vagina is not adequately retracted, allowing it to come in contact with the source channel. For these reasons, we prefer ovoids over rings in most cases.

Intrauterine Tandem

The tandem is a hollow tube that accommodates a single line of sources within the endocervical and endometrial canals. Tandems are typically 3 to 6 mm in diameter. The thicker tandems usually require cervical dilatation to be inserted in the uterine cavity but are less likely to perforate the uterus. For this reason, they are sometimes preferred for patients who have a very thin uterine wall or a sharply flexed uterus.

Tandems are available in fixed or adjustable lengths, depending on the applicator type. The distal portion of most fixed-length tandems is perfectly straight, which in our experience often results in less optimal applicator placement. The fixed length may also compromise coverage of intrauterine tumor. As an example, because a patient with a 5.5-cm endometrial canal cannot accommodate a 6-cm fixed-length tandem, a 4-cm fixed-length tandem must be utilized; while a 4 cm tandem should provide sufficient dosimetric coverage for a very small cervical cancer, it might not allow adequate treatment of a barrel-shaped tumor that extends into the uterine body.

A short tandem, particularly when combined with a ring applicator or mini-ovoid, results in a compact system that accommodates relatively little activity; this in turn tends to limit the dose deliverable to paracervical tissues without exceeding normal tissue tolerance limits. In our experience, an adjustable-length tandem with a continuous curvature is easier to position and typically conforms better to the natural curvature of the uterine body. Adjustable tandems require a flange that can be moved to secure the tandem at the desired length.

For patients with inoperable endometrial cancer, it is critical that the tandem extends to the end of the endometrial canal. Patients with inoperable endometrial cancer often have an expanded endometrial canal that may be difficult to treat to full dose with a single tandem. In these cases, two slightly diverging tandems can be utilized. The Rotte "Y" applicator includes two tandems secured with a vaginal cylinder. These applicators may be useful for selected patients who have a relatively low body mass index and a very expanded uterus. However, for obese women with inoperable endometrial cancer, the connectors to the applicators tend to fall within the proximal vulva, where they can easily be contaminated by vaginal fluids.

Interstitial Needles

When intracavitary treatment methods cannot provide an adequate dose to deep tissues without exceeding the tolerance of proximate normal tissues, interstitial needles may be used, most often as a means of supplementing intracavitary treatments. Interstitial needles are typically 1 to 2 mm in diameter with a pointed closed end that can be inserted directly into soft tissues. A central obturator protects the center of the needle from body fluids but is removed when iridium sources are inserted or the needles are connected to a remote-afterloading device.

Interstitial needles may be supplied with an adjustable hub that is secured to the needle using a set screw; as will be discussed later in this chapter, the hub can also be used as a means of securing the needle to the perineum after transperineal insertion.

A variety of templates have been designed to guide and regularize interstitial needle placement. There are two main types of interstitial templates:

- *Perineal templates.* These templates consist of a plastic plate that has a central hole (to accommodate a vaginal obturator) and a series of smaller holes arranged in concentric circles. The template is sutured to the perineum and the central obturator is placed in the vagina. To prevent the target (usually the cervix or apical vagina) from being displaced as the needles are inserted or as the legs are brought down from the lithotomy position, a suture should also be placed in the cervix or apical vagina and secured to the template. Current commercially available templates include the Martinez Universal Perineal Interstitial Template (**Fig. 8.7**) and the Syed-Neblett template. One disadvantage of perineal templates is that the template itself interferes with examination of the tumor during needle placement. It is recommended that this type of implant be inserted under direct image guidance or laparoscopic guidance.
- *Vaginal applicators with needle guides.* More recently, applicators have been developed that allow interstitial needles to be placed into the cervix through a ring (**Fig. 8.5**) or ovoids.[6] These applicators may help to supplement the dose to paracervical tissues, particularly when compact intracavitary applicators (i.e., tandem and ring) are used to treat locally advanced cancers.

In most cases requiring interstitial vaginal brachytherapy, we use needles placed using freehand technique in combination with intracavitary applicators. The pros and cons of freehand versus template-guided vaginal implants are discussed further in Chapter 11. The process for placement of interstitial needles is described in detail below.

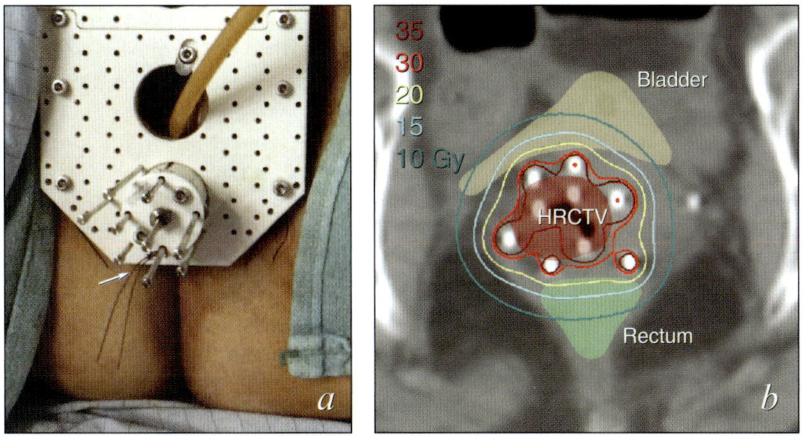

FIGURE 8.7 In this case, an interstitial template was used to treat a primary vaginal adenocarcinoma originating in the vaginal fornix adjacent to a cervical stump. Although there was a 50% response to 50 Gy of external RT and concurrent chemotherapy, the tumor was still 7 to 8 mm thick. A stitch *(arrow, a)* was placed in the cervical stump, held with a clamp during needle insertion, and tied around one of the template needles to keep the tumor in close apposition to the central cylinder during treatment. Under laparoscopic guidance, nine needles were inserted through the tumor until there was tenting of the peritoneum. The D90 for the high-risk clinical target volume (HRCTV) was 32 Gy (total tumor dose, 82 Gy). The total D_{2cc} doses for the bladder and rectum were 65.4 and 66.4 Gy, respectively.

APPLICATOR PLACEMENT

Anesthesia

The type of sedation that is recommended during applicator placement depends on the level of pain likely to be caused by the procedure, the need for relaxation to optimize the positioning of the applicator, and the need for a high-quality examination under anesthesia.

The insertion of a domed cylinder for vaginal cuff treatment generally does not require any sedation because the discomfort caused by the insertion rarely exceeds that of a normal pelvic examination. However, we often perform an examination under anesthesia prior to brachytherapy if we are treating tumors that grossly involve the vagina; if the patient is to be treated with PDR or LDR brachytherapy, the cylinder can be sutured in place at the same time.

Anesthesia of some form is usually required for placement of intrauterine applicators and is always required for insertion of interstitial needles.

Options for anesthesia include monitored anesthesia care, epidural or spinal anesthesia, and general anesthesia. In some cases, when medical comorbidities prohibit any respiratory depressant or regional anesthesia, a paracervical block may aid intracavitary placement. For most cases, we find that general anesthesia provides maximum patient comfort and provides the best conditions for optimizing brachytherapy applicator placement.

In some practices, intrauterine brachytherapy applicators are placed using monitored anesthesia care only. Placement of an indwelling intrauterine tube (e.g., a Smit sleeve) may decrease the pain associated with uterine sounding and facilitate applicator placement under monitored anesthesia care. However, in some cases, anesthesia is required to fully relax the patient and achieve optimal displacement of the rectum and bladder during the procedure. Spinal or epidural anesthesia may be used for pain management during placement of the applicator, but the induction and recovery times are longer than for monitored anesthesia care or general anesthesia. For some patients, such as those with pulmonary disease contraindicating general anesthesia, spinal anesthesia is a good alternative to general anesthesia.

Fiducial Marker Placement

Fiducial markers can be placed during examination under anesthesia to facilitate identification of soft tissue landmarks on postprocedure imaging. For patients with cervical cancer, platinum or gold markers can be inserted at 12 o'clock and 6 o'clock to mark the anterior and posterior lips of the cervix.[7] These markers are used to assure that the vaginal applicator is flush against the cervix (**Fig. 8.2**). For patients with cancer involving the vagina, fiducial markers are inserted at the peripheral limits of disease to ensure that the target volume is clearly defined at the time of treatment planning. Ideally, vaginal disease should be demarcated with fiducial markers prior to external beam therapy in order to maintain a record of the initial extent of mucosal involvement (Chapters 4 and 11).

Placement of the Intrauterine Tandem

Before an intrauterine tandem is inserted, the uterus must be sounded. This can be a difficult procedure, even for gynecologic oncologists, particularly in patients who have extensive tumor involvement obscuring the os or causing obstruction of the endocervical canal. However, in our experience, the uterus can be successfully sounded in more than 99% of cases.

Transabdominal ultrasound guidance is strongly recommended in all cases (**Fig. 8.2**, **CS 10.3**). For optimal visualization, the bladder should be filled with 200 to 300 mL of saline using a Foley catheter. Ultrasound guidance is not only useful for real-time guidance during insertion of the probe and tandem but also helps to assure that the tip of the tandem is in the correct position in the cavity. We usually set the tandem to be a few millimeters short of the fundus, but it must be long enough to permit adequate coverage of intrauterine disease.

The following additional steps can assist with successful probing of the uterus:

- If MRI has been performed, the MR image should be reviewed before the uterus is sounded, and special attention should be paid to the position and length of the uterine canal.
- Digital examination with careful attention to the location of the os can be very helpful. The cervical os is often easier to feel than to see, particularly when the cervix is involved with necrotic tumor.
- One of the most common causes of uterine perforation is the use of a very straight probe in a severely flexed uterus. In most cases, it is recommended that the distal inch of the probe be bent about 20 to 30 degrees; this facilitates passage of the probe through the flexure at the endocervical canal.
- Once the tip of the probe or tandem is in the cervical canal, it is typically much easier to navigate the canal if all the hardware (speculum, retractors) has been removed from the vagina. Further progress is guided by feel and ultrasonography, not direct visualization of the cervix. Retractors tend to limit maneuverability, particularly if the vagina is narrow.
- In patients with a very narrow vagina, it may be easier to insert the probe into the cervical os by feel with the retractors removed. With an index finger at the os, it is usually possible to slide the probe along the finger and guide it into the os. Ultrasonography is then used to guide the rest of the procedure.
- In some cases, if the uterus is extremely mobile, it may be helpful to place a tenaculum on the cervix to straighten the uterus and permit application of counter traction when the probe is being inserted.
- Unless the endocervical canal is truly obstructed, in which case there is usually fluid in the uterine cavity, relatively little force should be needed to probe the uterus. Typically, the canal can be found by maneuvering and adjusting the angle of passage using very gentle pressure under ultrasound guidance.
- Even the presence of a Smit sleeve does not guarantee accurate placement. We have seen several cases of unexpected perforation through the lower uterine segment immediately above a Smit sleeve.

If a 5- or 6-mm-diameter tandem is used, the cervix must be dilated after the canal has been located. Each dilator should be left in place for a minute to allow the cervix to relax; the next should be inserted as soon as the last has been removed. The correct length of tandem is selected on the basis of the uterine sounding. The tandem is then placed in the uterine canal, and it is ensured that the flange, if one is used, is flush against the cervix.

Correct placement of the intrauterine tandem should always be confirmed by CT or MRI after the procedure has been completed, particularly if the quality of ultrasound imaging was poor.

Placement of Intravaginal Applicators and Packing

After the tandem is in place, the vaginal applicators are inserted. Ovoids should be positioned flush against the cervix and centered on the cervix. In most cases, this means that the ovoids should be bisected by the tandem; however, if the tumor primarily involves the anterior or posterior lip, the ovoids may deviate from the bisected position by a few millimeters. Rings are advanced until they are in the apical vagina and are then secured to the tandem. Vaginal packing, balloons, or retractors are then placed in the vagina to push the rectum and/or bladder away from intravaginal sources. Treatment should not be delivered without some form of vaginal packing or retraction; if the rectum or bladder is allowed to prolapse around vaginal applicators, the applicators cannot be loaded without risking injury to critical structures.

We find that vaginal packing provides the most flexibility and is the most effective method for minimizing bladder and rectal doses. Gauze with a radiopaque central marker, impregnated with sulfa or Premarin (conjugated estrogen) cream, is placed anterior and posterior to the tandem between the ovoids and, as space permits, surrounding the ovoids. Additional packing should then be placed distal to the ovoids or ring until the vagina is filled to the perineal ring. As packing is added, the retractors should be gradually removed, with care taken not to dislodge the packing and to fill the space that was occupied by the retractors. For patients who have a very capacious vagina, a suture slipped through the cervix and secured with a clamp can be used to prevent the cervix from being displaced and to apply counter traction during packing (**Fig. 8.8**).

When MRI-based planning is performed, vagina packing is soaked in ultrasound gel to maximize contrast with the cervix (**Fig. 8.9**).[8] If cylinders will be used in the vagina, they should be added to the tandem after it has been inserted in the uterus. The tandem should never be inserted with cylinders in place because doing so is associated with a very high risk of uterine perforation. A distal flange is placed to keep the cylinders in place.

After the applicator has been positioned, it should be secured to prevent it from being displaced away from the cervix before treatment is complete. If PDR or LDR therapy will be used or if the patient will receive more than one HDR treatment using the same applicator placement, the system should be secured with a suture that approximates the labia and is secured around the arms of the applicator.

Placement of Interstitial Needles

A number of methods have been used to place interstitial needles. Brachytherapy technique, particularly interstitial brachytherapy technique, cannot be learned from a book. Only one-on-one experience with a brachytherapist who has specific experience with gynecologic implants can provide the training necessary for this specialized area of practice.

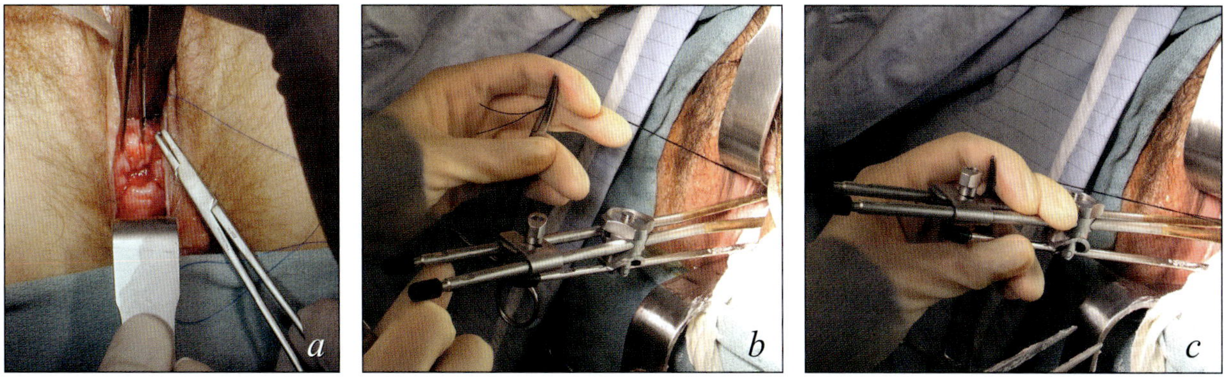

FIGURE 8.8 For patients who have a very capacious or relaxed vagina, a stitch can be placed in the cervix to provide counter traction and to prevent the cervix from being displaced away from the vaginal applicator during packing. Using a tenaculum, the cervix is pulled toward the introitus to facilitate insertion of the stitch *(a)*. Once the needle is removed, the stitch (which should not be knotted) is grasped with a clamp *(b)* and held during packing *(c)*. After treatment is complete and the packing has been removed, the stitch is slipped out of the cervix.

However, we offer the following specific guidelines and tips for successful gynecologic interstitial brachytherapy:

- In most cases, needles are inserted transperineally, parallel to the axis of the vagina. We never position needles parallel to the vulva because it is extremely difficult to control dose heterogeneities that can lead to ulceration and necrosis of the skin (Chapter 12).
- Ideally, needles should be parallel to each other and about 9 to 11 mm apart. Stepping-source remote-afterloading methods permit a great deal of optimization. During the planning process, dwell times can usually be adjusted to correct for needles that are closer than 9 mm to each other; however, needles that are more than 12 to 15 mm apart invariably result in very heterogeneous dose distributions and should therefore be avoided.
- Needles should be inserted distally several centimeters beyond the target for several reasons:
    - Most needles have a blind end that does not accommodate a source in the distal 7 to 10 mm.
    - When the patient's legs are brought down from the lithotomy position, the perineum is compressed between the legs, forcing the needles downward and potentially pulling them out of the target area. This is a major issue for perineal templates; for this reason, the apical vagina or cervix should always be secured to the template with a suture (usually threaded through the central obturator and tied to a corner of the template) (**Fig. 8.7a**). With freehand implants, the needles should be inserted at least 2 cm beyond the target but may still need to be advanced after the legs are down.
    - The final implant should allow the proximal source to be at least 0.5 to 1 cm beyond the portion of the target that requires deep coverage; additional superficial margin can be provided from intracavitary sources in the cylinder.
- Ideally, needles should also be placed at least 0.5 cm beyond the target radially. However, in some cases, additional coverage of superficial tumor can be achieved using channels in a central cylinder or obturator. This is often necessary if the tumor margin is close to the rectum.
- Needles should not be allowed to perforate hollow viscera, even if they will not be loaded.
- Needles that are in direct contact with hollow viscera and needles that are in the peritoneal cavity and could, therefore, come in contact with mobile hollow viscera should *never* be loaded with a radiation source. The dose at the surface of the needles is typically severalfold greater than the prescribed dose and will cause a perforation if there is contact with bowel.

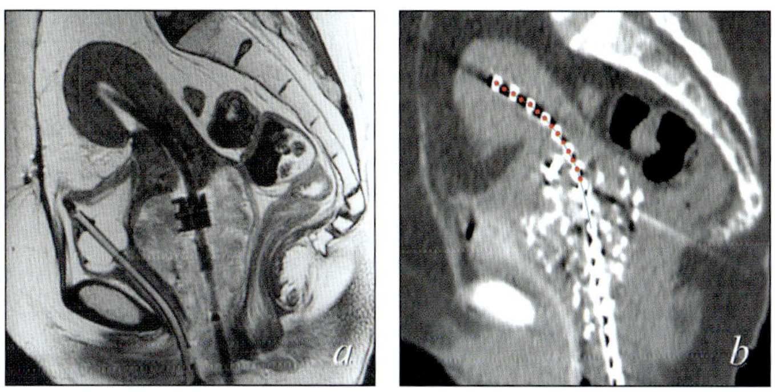

FIGURE 8.9 Vaginal packing impregnated with ultrasound gel provides excellent contrast between the packing and surrounding structures, as shown on a T2-weighted sagittal MR image *(a)*. For patients who will have prolonged treatment using LDR or PDR brachytherapy, a 50:50 mixture of ultrasound gel with antibiotic cream or estrogen cream also provides excellent contrast. For patients who will have treatment planning based on CT or plain radiographs, vaginal packing that contains a radiopaque thread facilitates identification of the vaginal walls *(b)*.

- Interstitial needles should never be inserted without some form of direct guidance. Depending on the type and location of the implant, this guidance can be provided by palpation (for freehand implants), ultrasonography, MRI, or laparoscopy.

For the reasons discussed in Chapter 11, we prefer to use a freehand method of needle insertion for most vaginal implants. This approach is described in **Figure 8.10**, Chapter 11, and **CS 11.3–11.5, 11.7, and 13.9**.

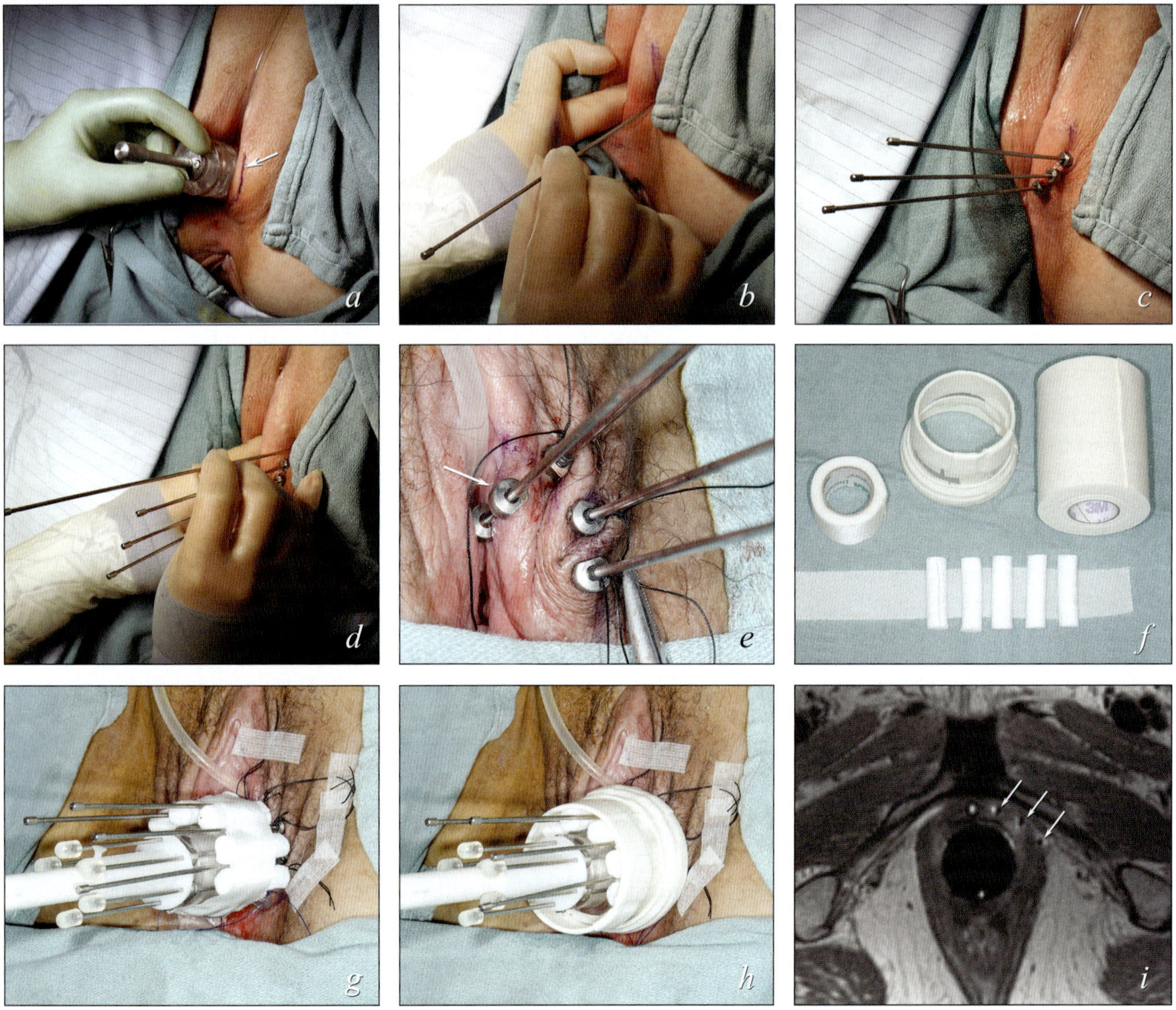

FIGURE 8.10 This figure illustrates some of the steps involved in the freehand insertion of interstitial needles for vaginal brachytherapy. An intracavitary cylinder fit to the diameter of the vagina is used to protect tissues outside the implant volume, as a vehicle for placing intracavitary sources, and as a means of stabilizing the needle positions. A dummy cylinder of the same diameter is usually substituted during the initial steps of needle insertion. To determine the points of needle insertion at the skin, a line is drawn 5 to 6 mm from the surface of the cylinder *(a)*. The first needle is inserted, usually through the center of the tumor, under direct palpation *(b)*. As the needle is advanced, the depth of the needle from the mucosa, the position of the tip, and the relationship of the needle to the tumor are monitored by the intravaginal finger. The angle of insertion should be approximately parallel to the axis of the cylinder. Additional needles are inserted 10 to 12 mm apart, at appropriate depth, with periodic checks with the cylinder in place to verify that the needles are parallel to each other and to the axis of the cylinder *(c, d)*. The individual needles are secured to the skin *(e)*: first, a suture is looped around the needle and tied distal to the needle hub; then, a small stitch is taken through the skin at the margin of the hub; and then, the two ends are tied to secure the needle without putting too much tension on the skin. If a needle is placed medially along the urethra, two hubs are used; one is placed at the surface of the urethra, and the other is placed near the surface of the vulva and used to secure the needle *(arrow)* (the stitch had not yet been placed in this example). When the needles have been inserted, the final cylinder is placed in the vagina and secured, usually with a collar that is sutured to the skin and fixed to the cylinder with set screws (shown in CS 11.4e). Using silk tape and dental spacers *(f)*, the needles are secured in position around the cylinder *(g)*. Added protection is provided by a specimen cup that is modified and cushioned with padded tape *(f, h)*. The patient is then imaged with the implant in place *(i)* for treatment planning.

BRACHYTHERAPY TREATMENT PLANNING

In 2005, the gynecologic working group of the European Society for Therapeutic Radiology and Oncology (ESTRO) proposed a set of guidelines for the use of tomographic imaging (specifically MRI) in brachytherapy treatment planning.[9] Since then, there has been a rapid expansion in the use of three-dimensional image-guided treatment planning for gynecologic brachytherapy.[10] This evolution is still under way but promises to yield significant improvements in the rate of complication-free local control for patients treated with brachytherapy. However, while data are being gathered to confirm the value of these new approaches, some grounding in the successful treatments of the past remains useful.

Traditional Two-Dimensional Treatment Planning Approaches

For decades, brachytherapy treatment planning was based on orthogonal radiographs that were used to document the geometry of the brachytherapy system. For patients receiving intracavitary treatment of cervical cancer, this approach depended on optimization of applicator placement (which remains important regardless of the treatment planning method) and on standardized loadings of brachytherapy sources within the intracavitary applicators. These standard loadings had been determined empirically from decades of experience and were designed to control the following:

- *The linear intensity of activity in the tandem (and therefore the dose rate or dose per fraction at the uterine serosa).* With LDR brachytherapy, a loading of 5 mgRaEq per cm generally achieved a dose rate <40 cGy per hour at the uterine serosa. Slightly higher activity (6–7.5 cGy per hour per cm) was usually used in the proximal tandem to improve lateral penetration of dose to treat bulky endocervical or parametrial disease. The sources were never allowed to protrude between the vaginal ovoids.
- *The vaginal surface dose.* This was usually limited to 100 cGy per hour or a total of 130 Gy. This value was determined from the geometry of the applicator because the dose gradient is too steep to obtain an accurate estimate from digitized images.
- *The integral dose to the pelvis (as measured by mg-hr or reference air kerma rate).* The purpose of this limit was to control the dose delivered to large pelvic volumes from brachytherapy applicators that accommodated a large amount of activity. This is rarely an issue unless a very long tandem (>8 cm) or large (>2 cm) ovoids are used.

With these methods, high cure rates could be obtained with relatively low complication rates, as evidenced by long-term outcome data from MD Anderson and elsewhere (Chapter 10).[11–13] With the emergence of image guidance, it now seems remarkable that relatively low complication rates were also achievable using only the information from physical examination and orthogonal films to adjust radiation source loadings (**Fig. 9.3**).

Point A

Point A is a reference point used to assess dose that is classically described as located in the parametrium at the approximate crossing of the ureter with the uterine artery. As developed in Manchester, point A was intended to be used merely as a reference point (**Fig. 8.11a**) and was considered useful only in the setting of strict rules about implant geometry, source loadings, and dose rate. However, clinicians who found it difficult to follow the plethora of rules devised to guide loadings under different conditions[14] increasingly began to use point A as a prescription point. As remote-afterloading HDR brachytherapy became increasingly popular, point A began to be used to prescribe intracavitary treatments under conditions that deviated substantially from long-established guidelines for the distribution of activity in intracavitary systems. The monitoring of doses to critical structures was typically limited to estimates of the doses delivered to bladder and rectal reference points (**Fig. 8.11b**).

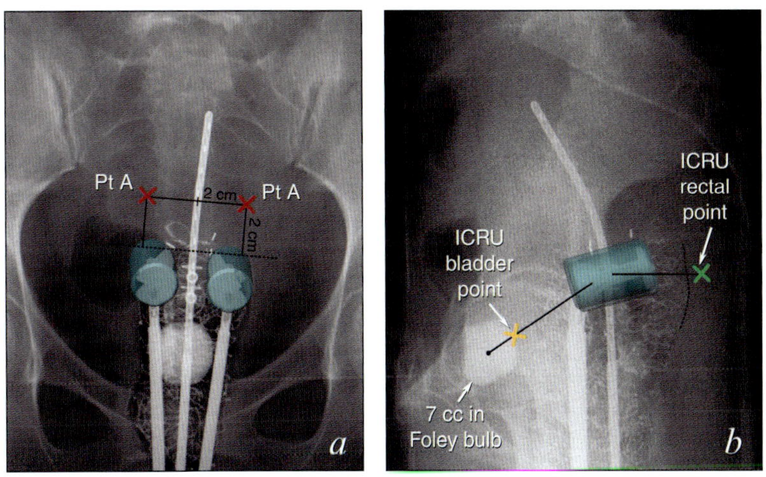

FIGURE 8.11 Common reference points used for two-dimensional intracavitary brachytherapy treatment planning. Point A (Pt A) is located 2 cm superior to the vaginal fornix (in this case at the surface of the ovoids) and 2 cm lateral to the tandem *(a)*. As defined by the International Commission on Radiation Units (ICRU), the bladder reference point is located on the surface of a Foley bulb filled with 7 mL of saline mixed with radiopaque contrast on a line drawn from the center of the Foley bulb to the closest source position in the vaginal applicator *(b)*. The rectal point is located 5 mm behind the vagina applicator or packing at the level of the center of the vaginal applicator sources.

Because point A bears little connection to the actual target volume, because bladder and rectal reference points can be wildly inaccurate, and because exposure of normal tissues to large doses per fraction can be particularly hazardous, traditional methods of treatment planning became increasingly unsatisfactory.

Two-Dimensional Imaging in Modern Practice

Although it is increasingly being replaced by MRI- or CT-guided three-dimensional treatment planning, two-dimensional planning based on kilovoltage images can be used successfully. Two-dimensional imaging may be most appropriate in very low resource settings. Orthogonal anteroposterior and lateral images are obtained in the operating suite or subsequently in the radiation oncology department. If the films are obtained in the operating room, a reference structure of known diameter can be used to determine the magnification factors of the films. Sources and reference points are then digitized into brachytherapy treatment planning software to perform dose calculations.

Source activities or dwell times are initially selected using standard loadings and can then be adjusted to achieve the desired distribution. Activity should usually be distributed fairly evenly along the length of the tandem. With cesium, the tandem is usually loaded with ~5 mg radium equivalents (mgRaEq) of activity per centimeter; increasing the activity of the apical source by 25% to 50% can improve coverage of deeply invasive lower uterine segment disease and increase the lateral parametrial dose. Small (2 cm) ovoids are usually loaded with 10 to 15 mgRaEq and mini-ovoids with 5 to 7 mgRaEq. With PDR therapy, we use a correction factor to select initial dwell times that mimic standard cesium loadings. For HDR therapy, it is reasonable to begin with dwell times that follow these same ratios. Although the times can be normalized to point A to achieve an initial tentative plan, the dose and dose per fraction must be adjusted for patients who have a small uterus or unacceptably high estimated bladder and rectal doses.

Point A, as defined in **Figure 8.11**, is classically described as located in the parametrium at the approximate crossing of the ureter with the uterine artery. However, uterine anatomy and the extent of cervical cancer are, of course, highly variable; for patients with small tumors, point A may lie well outside the tumor margins, but for patients with extensive disease, point A may be located in the middle of gross disease. For this reason, point A dose should never be considered a sufficient metric for assessing the adequacy of an implant. It should instead be regarded (as it was originally intended) merely as a reference point that should be evaluated in the context of the implant geometry, normal and tumor anatomy, distribution of radiation sources, and normal tissue doses. When the distribution of activity deviates a great deal from standard weightings, it is possible to undertreat the cervix and deliver very high doses to critical structures in the face of "acceptable" doses to point A and normal tissue reference points. To use an extreme example, a single source located in the tandem cephalad to the internal os could deliver the "desired" dose to point A and very low doses to the International Commission on Radiation Units and Measurements (ICRU) bladder and reference points but would deliver an extremely high dose to any sigmoid or small bowel lying in the rectouterine pouch and a relatively low dose to the portio of the cervix. For patients with stage IB2 to III cervical cancer who have relatively normal anatomy and a well-positioned applicator with standard loadings, a biologically equivalent combined external beam and brachytherapy dose of ~85 Gy to point A is usual. However, this dose may not be achievable in cases in which the anatomy is very unfavorable, such as those illustrated in **Figure 8.1**.

A major disadvantage of two-dimensional methods is that the standard normal tissue reference points (**Fig. 8.11b**)[15] yield very poor estimate of the actual doses to critical structures.[16] In particular, the bladder doses are significantly underestimated by these reference points. Poor placement of vaginal ovoids or inadequate posterior retraction or packing of the vagina can cause the rectum to prolapse around the applicator, resulting in higher than expected doses to regions adjacent to the reference point.

However, when point A and normal tissue reference points are used in the setting of optimal applicator placement, good vaginal packing, and standardized loadings, a dose distribution is generated that provides excellent tumor coverage and minimizes normal tissue doses for many patients. In many cases, CT- or MRI-based planning serves only to confirm that the applicator is in the proper intrauterine location and that standard loadings provide an optimal solution. However, in other cases, tomographic imaging reveals anatomical anomalies that demand dramatic alterations in the plan in order to achieve an acceptable ratio between the doses to tumor and normal tissues; several such examples are shown in **Figure 8.1**.

Three-Dimensional Image-Based Treatment Planning

The three-dimensional images provided when CT or MRI is performed with brachytherapy applicators in situ provide a much more realistic sense of the relationships between the applicators, tumor, and critical structures than can be gleaned from orthogonal plain films of the pelvis. High-quality MRI, in particular, can provide exquisite soft tissue detail that allows ready identification of critical structures and often permits clear visualization of gross tumor involving the vagina or uterus; this detail can greatly facilitate optimization of selected interstitial and intracavitary brachytherapy treatments. Emerging evidence suggests that this approach can also lead to significantly reduced side effects and improved tumor control rates.[17,18] Because it has greater soft tissue resolution than CT, MRI is considered the gold standard for image-based brachytherapy planning, although CT is more widely used because of its lower cost and more widespread availability.

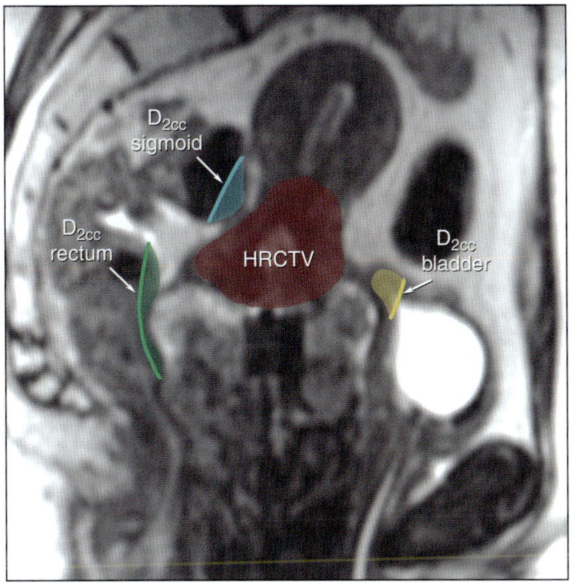

FIGURE 8.12 Sagittal MRI showing the high-risk clinical target volume (HRCTV) and normal tissue dose parameters as defined by GEC-ESTRO guidelines. Shaded areas represent the 2 mL high-dose volumes for the bladder, rectum, and sigmoid. The associated lines represent the isodose lines corresponding to the lowest doses within these 2 mL volumes.

MRI-Based Target Definition

The routine use of MRI-based planning of cervical cancer treatment has been standardized by the Groupe Européen de Curiethérapie (GEC)-ESTRO working group and tested in an international prospective trial, EMBRACE.[9] Results of these experiences are still emerging, but early results suggest that MRI-guided treatment planning is associated with high disease control rates and low complication rates.[17]

MRI-based treatment planning requires the delineation of target volumes and structures to be avoided ("avoidance structures") (Fig. 8.12). Volumetric dose constraints are then used to optimize the brachytherapy treatment plan. The following targets and avoidance structures are contoured according to the GEC-ESTRO approach.

- *High-risk clinical target volume (HR-CTV).* The HR-CTV is the primary prescription volume used for image-guided brachytherapy. The HR-CTV is defined to include the entire cervix plus any macroscopic residual tumor apparent at the time of brachytherapy. For a patient with central disease limited to the cervix (e.g., a patient with stage IB2 disease), this volume would consist of the cervix as visualized at the time of brachytherapy. For patients who had initial involvement of the parametrium, the HR-CTV would also include any residual parametrial disease seen on MRI at the time of brachytherapy.
- *Intermediate-risk CTV.* The GEC-ESTRO group defined a second target volume, the intermediate-risk CTV. This volume derived from the French practice of tracking the volume receiving 60 Gy. The volume is defined by GEC-ESTRO as the initial anatomical extent of disease including the HR-CTV with a 1-cm margin. This volume was felt to be a lower-risk volume and was thus recommended to receive an equivalent of 60 Gy. In the United States, the intermediate-risk CTV is used less frequently than the HR-CTV.

For patients with cervical cancer, a minimum dose delivered to 90% of the HR-CTV of 87 Gy has been associated with high rates of local control in patients treated with MRI-guided brachytherapy.[17] However, these doses are not always achievable within normal tissue constraints, and the relative risks of complications and tumor recurrence must be carefully considered.

Technically, the HR-CTV as defined by GEC-ESTRO does not include the vagina or endometrium that was initially involved if there is no visible residual disease. However, unlike paracervical tumor, areas of vaginal or myometrial infiltration cannot be expected to regress centripetally toward the cervix and may receive a negligible brachytherapy dose if source positions in the uterus or vagina are not loaded to cover these original sites of infiltration. For this reason, we recommend inclusion of initial sites of uterine or vaginal disease in the HR-CTV, particularly if an intermediate-risk CTV has not been used in treatment planning (Fig. 8.13).

The concept of the HR-CTV can also be adapted to the treatment of inoperable endometrial cancer; in such cases, the high-risk volume is considered to be the endometrium and any gross disease seen on MRI at the time of brachytherapy, although the initial extent of disease must also be taken into account.

MRI guidance of vaginal interstitial implants is particularly appealing because of the close proximity of the vagina to adjacent critical structures. Ideally, MRI guidance is performed in real time to allow for adjustments in needle position based on MRI guidance.[19] However, this approach requires extensive resources and planning because of the need for MRI-compatible materials for anesthesia and applicator placement. When planning is based on CT, target volumes should be defined while referring to initial and follow-up MRI scans (Fig. 8.7).

Although MRI-based treatment planning has many advantages, it also has several limitations. For one, it requires use of special MR-compatible devices. MRI is also more expensive and often less accessible than CT, which is available in nearly all radiation oncology departments. As a result, many radiation oncologists who perform brachytherapy base their treatment plans on CT, extrapolating principles from the MRI experience.[20] Many other physicians, including ourselves, use CT for relatively routine cases and save MRI for difficult applications or for the first of several treatments.

CT-Based Target Definition

CT can be used to verify that the applicator is satisfactorily positioned within the uterine cavity. In addition, CT can be used to volumetrically evaluate the doses to the bladder, rectum, and sigmoid. CT-based treatment planning may offer

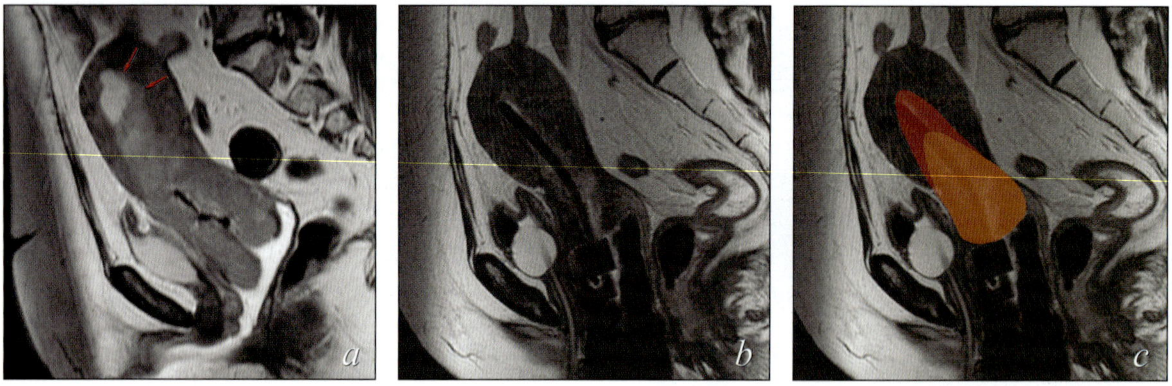

FIGURE 8.13 As defined by GEC-ESTRO, the high-risk clinical target volume (HRCTV) for treatment of intact cervical cancer includes the cervix and any residual disease seen on MRI at the time of brachytherapy. However, treatments prescribed solely on the basis of this definition may deliver inadequate doses to regions of initial involvement that are proximal or distal to the cervix, particularly if a relatively short tandem is used. In this case, initial MRI showed extensive involvement of the endometrium, extending to the fundus of the uterus *(a)*. MRI after the first brachytherapy applicator placement showed an excellent response with residual disease confined to the lower uterine segment and cervix *(b)*. Although a relatively short tandem could have been used to cover the GEC-ESTRO HRCTV (orange), it would have delivered a negligible dose to sites of probable residual microscopic disease in the fundus. For this reason, we recommend modification of the HRCTV in such cases, to include proximal and distal sites of initial involvement (*red color wash, c*).

many of the benefits seen with MRI-based treatment planning, but studies suggest that clinicians tend to overestimate the size of the target volume on CT.[20] In particular, care must be taken not to contour beyond the tumor into the vaginal fornix or into parametrium that is not grossly involved; the accuracy of CT-based contouring can be improved by referring to prior diagnostic MRI scans. The STIC trial was a prospective nonrandomized study in which outcomes following brachytherapy were compared between patients who had two-dimensional film-based treatment planning and patients who had three-dimensional, primarily CT-based treatment planning.[21] Higher rates of local control and lower toxicity were reported in the patients who had three-dimensional image-based planning. To date, no studies have directly compared outcomes of patients who had brachytherapy planned with CT versus MRI.

Critical Structure Definition

With MRI- or CT-based planning, the bladder, rectum, and sigmoid should be contoured after the applicators have been confirmed to be in an acceptable position. Available data suggest that the minimum dose to the maximally irradiated 2 mL of tissue (the D_{2cc}) is the best predictor of urinary and gastrointestinal toxic effects (**Fig. 8.12**). The entire bladder is contoured, including the full thickness of the bladder wall and the bladder contents. The rectum is contoured from the anal verge to the sigmoid flexure. Above the sigmoid flexure, the sigmoid contour extends to the region where the sigmoid is no longer in contact with the uterus. The position of the sigmoid is quite variable, and it is sometimes difficult to distinguish the sigmoid from the ascending colon. Also, the proximal sigmoid is usually mobile. In our experience, major sigmoid complications are rare. However, image-based brachytherapy has now demonstrated that portions of the sigmoid are commonly close to the brachytherapy system and calculated doses may be high.[22] For LDR and PDR implants, this means that the sigmoid dose may be significantly different than the treatment plan would suggest. For this reason, we place less emphasis on sigmoid than on rectal constraints. Whenever possible, we constrain the D_{2cc} to the sigmoid to <70 Gy. However, in some cases, it may be necessary to exceed this tolerance in order to deliver sufficient dose to tumor.

Because the portions of the rectum and bladder that receive the highest dose (i.e., the D_{2cc}) are close to the brachytherapy applicators in an area of the dose distribution where dose falls off rapidly, the accuracy of critical structure contours is critical. In some cases, artifacts caused by the applicators can make it very difficult to distinguish the interfaces between the applicator and normal tissues on CT, particularly if the applicator includes internal shields. The MD Anderson adaptive applicator was developed to circumvent this limitation by utilizing shields that can be shifted during CT image acquisition (**Fig. 8.6**). In cases in which the interface is difficult to visualize, it is useful to consider other parameters to evaluate the plan, such as point doses and source loadings.

Treatment Plan Optimization

Regardless of the treatment planning technique, the first step is to provide a planning directive for brachytherapy treatment. The planning directive should specify goals for the ratio of activity in each dwell position within the tandem and intravaginal applicators, the target doses, and dose constraints for organs at risk. For PDR and LDR treatment planning, the planning directive should specify goals for dose rate or total treatment time, and for HDR treatment planning, the planning directive should specify an overall goal for the final dose and fractionation. Once images are imported into the treatment planning system, points and volumes can be identified and optimization can be performed through one of the following approaches:

- *Iterative optimization techniques.* In many cases, a well-placed implant with standardized loading will deliver intended doses to target structures while meeting dose constraints for organs at risk, and few, if any, changes will be needed. When this is not the case, the treatment plan can be modified as needed to increase the dose to target tissues or reduce the dose to normal tissues. To accomplish this, dwell times can be iteratively increased or decreased by 10% to 50%, or weightings can be shifted anteriorly or posteriorly within the vaginal applicators until the dose constraints are met. In cases in which interstitial needles are placed, dwell times within the needles can be similarly adjusted.
- *Graphical optimization.* Treatment planning systems provide tools to facilitate image-guided brachytherapy treatment planning. Graphical optimization allows the planner to manually adjust the position of an isodose line; depending on the settings, the program may then renormalize the plan to achieve the desired dose to a given target, for example, point A. While graphical optimization may be an appealing option, it can cause dramatic shifts in the dwell times of sources, producing unusual loadings that can cause unexpected toxic effects. If this approach is used, it should only be used in the context of image-based planning with close attention to the effects of optimization on doses to the bladder, rectum, sigmoid, and targets. In general, adjustments should be subtle, and we recommend that renormalization features be turned off. In all cases, care should be taken to closely monitor the relative changes in source dwell times in response to use of graphical optimization tools.
- *Inverse planning simulated annealing dose optimization tools.* Inverse planning tools are also available in some brachytherapy treatment planning systems. As with graphical optimization techniques, if these tools are used, the source dwell times and all critical structure and target doses should be closely monitored to ensure that there are no unintended consequences.

Dose Fractionation

Options for brachytherapy dose delivery include LDR, PDR, and HDR. Each of these treatment delivery approaches can be effective, but each has distinct advantages and disadvantages in terms of complication risk, patient and physician convenience, radiation exposure, plan optimization potential, and radiobiology. LDR therapy usually delivers treatment at 40 to 60 cGy per hour, utilizing fixed-length cesium 137 sources that have to be manually placed into applicators. This process necessitates some exposure to personnel working with sources and during inpatient care. PDR brachytherapy was developed with the goal of mimicking the radiobiologic advantages of LDR while utilizing a 0.5 to 1 Curie iridium 192 stepping source similar to that used for HDR brachytherapy; PDR minimizes radiation exposure to personnel and has greater potential for dose optimization than LDR brachytherapy. HDR utilizes a high-activity (usually about 10 Curie) iridium 192 stepping source that delivers outpatient treatment over a few minutes. For these reasons and others, many practices have moved to HDR treatment.

The use of higher doses per fraction may be advantageous for situations where critical structures are far away from the sources. In these situations, the difference between the dose to the tumor and dose to normal tissue is maximized because of the higher relative biologic effectiveness of high-dose-per-fraction treatments. This opens up the potential to optimize the dose per fraction in addition to optimizing the relative dwell times in treatment planning.[22] Many radiation oncologists select one HDR fractionation regimen and use it for nearly all of their patients. In the United States, the most common fractionation scheme used for cervical cancer after 45 Gy of pelvic RT is five fractions of 5.5 to 6 Gy. However, the use of rigid fractionation schemes that are normalized to point A can be dangerous, because the effective dose to critical structures may be very high if unfavorable anatomy causes bowel or bladder to be close to the radiation sources.[22] For this reason, prescription to a carefully designated target volume with attention to the doses to critical structures is always preferred, particularly for HDR brachytherapy.

Calculating EQD2 Values

When HDR brachytherapy is performed, the nominal dose delivered needs to be converted into a biologically effective dose. The reference utilized is the equivalent dose per fraction when delivered at 2 Gy per fraction, or the EQD2. Doses delivered to the CTV and organs at risk should be converted into a radiobiologically weighted dose equivalent of 2 Gy per fraction (EQD2). This can be accomplished with the linear-quadratic model, using the following values: α/β of 10 Gy for target volumes and an α/β of 3 Gy for organs at risk. Worksheets for calculating equivalent doses are available through the American Brachytherapy Society (https://www.americanbrachytherapy.org/guidelines/). For intracavitary brachytherapy, five fractions can be utilized to keep the dose per fraction relatively low.[23] However, for cases that require invasive procedures, such as interstitial brachytherapy, it is impractical to reinsert the implants four or five times. In these cases, it is reasonable to admit the patient and deliver twice-daily treatments over 2 or 3 days. In our practice, we use PDR brachytherapy for all interstitial implants.

For intracavitary prophylactic vaginal cuff brachytherapy, a wide range of dose fractionation schemes is used with a wide range of effective doses. Sorbe et al. performed a randomized trial comparing the toxicity of vaginal cuff brachytherapy with five treatments of 5 Gy prescribed to 5 mm and five treatments of 2.5 Gy delivered to 5 mm depth (**Fig. 8.14a**). Five years after treatment, patients treated with 5 Gy to 5 mm had a significantly shorter mean vaginal

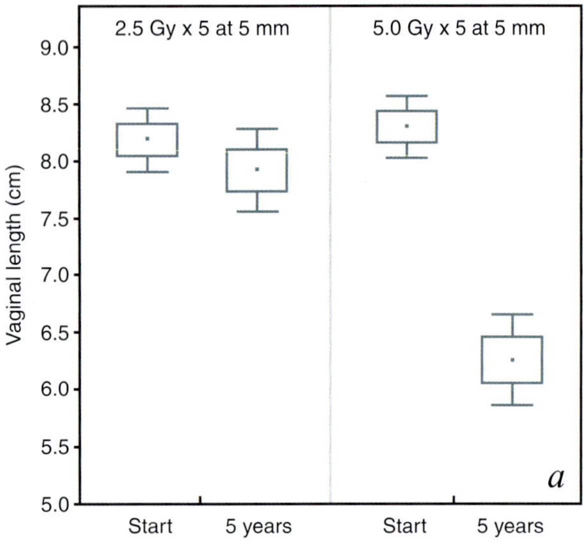

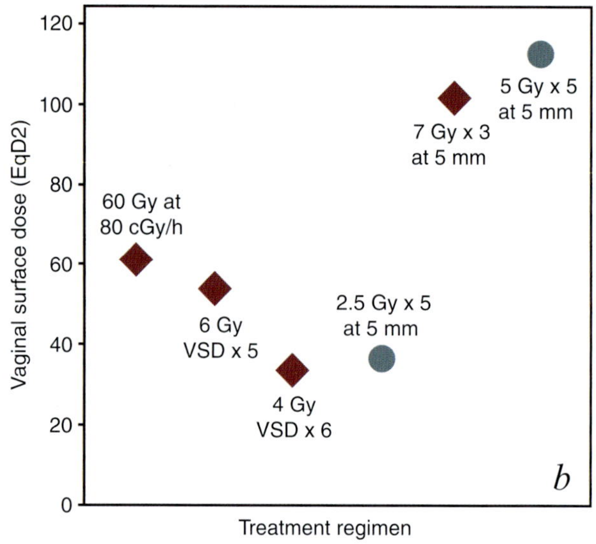

FIGURE 8.14 A variety of dose schedules have been used to treat the vaginal cuff prophylactically after hysterectomy for endometrial cancer. In 2005, Sorbe et al. compared two schedules—5 Gy × 5 and 7 Gy × 5, prescribed in each case at 5 mm depth. These schedules were found to yield similar tumor control rates, but patients treated with the higher dose schedule had dramatically higher rates of severe vaginal shortening than those treated with the lower-dose schedule *(a)*. In *b*, some of the more common schedules are compared in terms of the ~2 Gy per fraction equivalent dose (EqD2) delivered to the vaginal surface (VSD), assuming a 3-cm-diameter cylinder. Note that the effective surface dose delivered with Sorbe's high-dose schedule of 5 Gy × 5 at 5 mm is very similar to that of 7 Gy × 5 at 5 mm, a popular schedule used in the United States. (*a*, adapted from Sorbe B, Straumits A, Karlsson L. Intravaginal high-dose-rate brachytherapy for stage I endometrial cancer: a randomized study of two dose-per-fraction levels. *Int J Radiat Oncol Biol Phys.* 2005;62(5):1385-1389.)

length than patients treated with the lower dose regimen (6.3 vs. 8.3 cm).[24] The commonly used regimen in the United States, three treatments of 7 Gy prescribed to 5 mm, delivers an effective dose similar to the higher-dose regimen used in the Sorbe et al. trial (**Fig. 8.14b**). High rates of intravaginal control have been reported after lower-dose-per-fraction treatment, which should be associated with lower toxicity.[25] At MD Anderson, we use five treatments of 6 Gy prescribed to the vaginal surface for women who require prophylactic vaginal treatment for endometrial cancer.

References

1. Viswanathan AN, Thomadsen B; American Brachytherapy Society Cervical Cancer Recommendations Committee, American Brachytherapy Society. American Brachytherapy Society consensus guidelines for locally advanced carcinoma of the cervix. Part I: general principles. *Brachytherapy.* 2012;11:33–46.
2. Petereit DG, Sarkaria JN, Chappell R, et al. The adverse effect of treatment prolongation in cervical carcinoma. *Int J Radiat Oncol Biol Phys.* 1995;32:1301–1307.
3. Mould R. Radium tubes, radium needles & radium bombs. *Nowotwory J Oncol.* 2007;57(suppl. 4):151–200.
4. Price MJ, Horton JL, Gifford KA, et al. Dosimetric evaluation of the Fletcher-Williamson ovoid for pulsed-dose-rate brachytherapy: a Monte Carlo study. *Phys Med Biol.* 2005;50: 5075–5087.
5. Klopp AH, Mourtada F, Yu ZH, et al. Pilot study of a computed tomography-compatible shielded intracavitary brachytherapy applicator for treatment of cervical cancer. *Pract Radiat Oncol.* 2013;3:115–123.
6. Nomden CN, de Leeuw AA, Moerland MA, et al. Clinical use of the Utrecht applicator for combined intracavitary/interstitial brachytherapy treatment in locally advanced cervical cancer. *Int J Radiat Oncol Biol Phys.* 2012;82:1424–1430.
7. Katz A, Eifel PJ. Quantification of intracavitary brachytherapy parameters and correlation with outcome in patients with carcinoma of the cervix. *Int J Radiat Oncol Biol Phys.* 2000;48: 1417–1425.
8. Swanick CW, Castle KO, Rechner LA, et al. Optimizing packing contrast for MRI-based intracavitary brachytherapy planning for cervical cancer. *Brachytherapy.* 2015;14:385–389.
9. Haie-Meder C, Potter R, Van Limbergen E, et al. Recommendations from Gynaecological (GYN) GEC-ESTRO Working Group (I): concepts and terms in 3D image based 3D treatment planning in cervix cancer brachytherapy with emphasis on MRI assessment of GTV and CTV. *Radiother Oncol.* 2005;74: 235–245.
10. Grover S, Harkenrider MM, Cho LP, et al. Image Guided Cervical Brachytherapy: 2014 Survey of the American Brachytherapy Society. *Int J Radiat Oncol Biol Phys.* 2016;94:598–604.
11. Logsdon MD, Eifel PJ. Figo IIIB squamous cell carcinoma of the cervix: an analysis of prognostic factors emphasizing the balance between external beam and intracavitary radiation therapy. *Int J Radiat Oncol Biol Phys.* 1999;43:763–775.
12. Eifel PJ, Thoms WW Jr, Smith TL, et al. The relationship between brachytherapy dose and outcome in patients with bulky endocervical tumors treated with radiation alone. *Int J Radiat Oncol Biol Phys.* 1994;28:113–118.
13. Eifel PJ, Morris M, Oswald MJ, et al. Adenocarcinoma of the uterine cervix. Prognosis and patterns of failure in 367 cases. *Cancer.* 1990;65:2507–2514.
14. Fletcher G. *Female Pelvis. Textbook of Radiotherapy.* Philadelphia, PA: Lea & Febiger; 1980:720–851.
15. International Commission on Radiation Units and Measurements. *Dose and Volume Specification for Reporting Intracavitary*

Therapy in Gynecology. Bethesda, MD: International Commission on Radiation Units and Measurements; 1985.

16. Pelloski CE, Palmer M, Chronowski GM, et al. Comparison between CT-based volumetric calculations and ICRU reference-point estimates of radiation doses delivered to bladder and rectum during intracavitary radiotherapy for cervical cancer. *Int J Radiat Oncol Biol Phys.* 2005;62:131–137.
17. Dimopoulos JC, Potter R, Lang S, et al. Dose–effect relationship for local control of cervical cancer by magnetic resonance image-guided brachytherapy. *Radiother Oncol.* 2009;93:311–315.
18. Potter R, Georg P, Dimopoulos JC, et al. Clinical outcome of protocol based image (MRI) guided adaptive brachytherapy combined with 3D conformal radiotherapy with or without chemotherapy in patients with locally advanced cervical cancer. *Radiother Oncol.* 2011;100:116–123.
19. Viswanathan AN, Szymonifka J, Tempany-Afdhal CM, et al. A prospective trial of real-time magnetic resonance-guided catheter placement in interstitial gynecologic brachytherapy. *Brachytherapy.* 2013;12:240–247.
20. Viswanathan AN, Dimopoulos J, Kirisits C, et al. Computed tomography versus magnetic resonance imaging-based contouring in cervical cancer brachytherapy: results of a prospective trial and preliminary guidelines for standardized contours. *Int J Radiat Oncol Biol Phys.* 2007;68:491–498.
21. Charra-Brunaud C, Harter V, Delannes M, et al. Impact of 3D image-based PDR brachytherapy on outcome of patients treated for cervix carcinoma in France: results of the French STIC prospective study. *Radiother Oncol.* 2012;103:305–313.
22. Christensen EN, Yu HZ, Klopp AH, et al. Variable impact of intracavitary brachytherapy fractionation schedule on biologically effective dose to organs at risk in patients with cervical cancer. *Brachytherapy.* 2014;13:240–249.
23. Viswanathan AN, Creutzberg CL, Craighead P, et al. International brachytherapy practice patterns: a survey of the Gynecologic Cancer Intergroup (GCIG). *Int J Radiat Oncol Biol Phys.* 2012; 82:250–255.
24. Sorbe B, Straumits A, Karlsson L. Intravaginal high-dose-rate brachytherapy for stage I endometrial cancer: a randomized study of two dose-per-fraction levels. *Int J Radiat Oncol Biol Phys.* 2005;62: 1385–1389.
25. Townamchai K, Lee L, Viswanathan AN. A novel low dose fractionation regimen for adjuvant vaginal brachytherapy in early stage endometrioid endometrial cancer. *Gynecol Oncol.* 2012;127: 351–355.

CHAPTER 9

Posttreatment Monitoring

INTRODUCTION

Posttreatment monitoring is an important phase of every gynecologic cancer patient's care. Many patients will continue to have some treatment-related or tumor-related symptoms after treatment is completed; the anxiety caused by these symptoms is lessened if patients know what to expect and are counseled about which symptoms may require acute intervention. Also, close monitoring allows early detection of locoregional recurrences, increasing the likelihood of cure with salvage treatment.

The completion of treatment can be a jarring experience, particularly for patients who have been coming to the clinic daily for radiation treatments and who have developed close, supportive relationships with their caregivers. It is important for patients' sense of well-being that they feel a sense of continuity between the care provided during treatment and the care provided after treatment. Even when the prognosis is excellent, most patients struggle with the uncertainties attached to a cancer diagnosis.

THE SURVIVORSHIP CARE PLAN

In its 2006 report, *From Cancer Patient to Cancer Survivor: Lost in Transition*, the Institute of Medicine recommended a series of measures for the quality of care delivered to cancer survivors (**Table 9.1**).[1] The first measure was "provision of a written posttreatment summary outlining the proposed follow-up plan." The report also emphasized the importance of communication and coordination between oncologists and primary care providers. A well-articulated survivorship care plan that involves the patient and her providers promotes patient engagement and compliance with posttreatment recommendations and reduces the likelihood of duplicative care.[2] However, despite these recommendations, surveys suggest that most oncologists and primary care providers do not provide written summaries or even discuss the follow-up care plan with their patients.[1]

Every patient should have a clearly defined plan for posttreatment monitoring. Patients and their providers should understand who will be responsible for various aspects of the patient's care and how monitoring for recurrence ("cancer surveillance") will be integrated with other aspects of the patient's overall medical care needs. In the final phases of treatment, every patient should meet with members of her oncology care team to discuss the following questions:

- Which provider (gynecologic oncologist, medical oncologist, radiation oncologist, other specialist, or the primary care provider) will be responsible for each aspect of the patient's care, including posttreatment cancer surveillance, management of treatment-related adverse effects, pain management, management of non–cancer-related medical problems, and routine cancer screening (e.g., screening for breast and colorectal cancer)?
- What will be the frequency of surveillance visits and why?
- What methods will be used for cancer surveillance?
- When should the patient expect lingering treatment-related symptoms to resolve?
- What symptoms should cause the patient to contact her provider before scheduled visits?
- Assuming the patient does not develop recurrence or adverse effects that require special interventions, how long will she require monitoring by an oncologist, and how much of her cancer surveillance can be shared with her primary care provider?

TABLE 9.1 Potential Survivorship Quality of Care Measures (2006)

Processes of care • Provision of a survivorship care plan, a written posttreatment summary outlining the proposed follow-up plan • Assessment of psychosocial distress, referral to mental health providers • Assessment of employment, insurance, and financial issues, referral to rehabilitation and social work providers • Provision of written information on available community support services
Screening guidelines • Adherence to evidence-based follow-up and surveillance guidelines, where available
Survivorship interventions • Adherence to adjuvant therapy • Assessment and management of pain • When appropriate, referral to enterostomal care • When appropriate, referral for lymphedema management • When appropriate, assessment of sexual function and referral to sexuality counseling • When appropriate, referral to genetic counseling • Recommendation of exercise for fatigue • Smoking cessation counseling, if necessary
Survivor assessments of care • Ratings by survivors of their satisfaction with care, coordination of care, and quality of care

From Hewitt M, Greenfield S, Stovall E. From Cancer Patient to Cancer Survivor: Lost In Transition. Washington, DC: National Academies Press; 2006.

At the conclusion of treatment, the patient and her care providers (including her primary care provider) should be given a written summary of the treatment that the patient received and the plan for posttreatment monitoring.

The frequency and nature of follow-up visits should be customized to the patient's specific problem list and informed by an understanding of the risks of tumor recurrence and treatment-related adverse effects. The following sections of this chapter address these aspects of follow-up care.

MONITORING FOR CANCER RECURRENCE

Early detection of locoregional recurrences that are potentially curable with salvage treatment is one of the most important goals of posttreatment surveillance. The most common types of locoregional recurrence potentially amenable to successful salvage treatment include the following:

- *Central recurrence after initial definitive surgical treatment.* Radiation therapy (RT) or chemoradiation is the usual treatment for isolated central recurrence after definitive surgery unless definitive surgical resection can be accomplished without major organ compromise (CS 12.3, 13.8, 13.9).
- *Regional nodal recurrence after initial definitive surgical treatment.* Isolated nodal recurrences are usually treated with chemoradiation (CS 12.10, 13.6, 13.7).
- *Nodal recurrence near the margin of RT fields.* Depending on the size of the recurrence and its relationship with previous RT fields, marginal nodal recurrences after RT may be treated with RT or surgical resection followed by RT (CS 13.5, 15.3).
- *Isolated central uterine, cervical, vaginal, or vulvar recurrence near the margin of RT fields* (CS 10.8, 12.9). Depending on the size and extent of the recurrence and its relationship with previous RT fields, isolated central recurrences after RT may be treated with radical surgery, radiation, or palliative chemotherapy.
- *Oligometastasis.* Because most patients with distant metastases are incurable, the focus of their treatment is usually palliative (Chapter 16). However, in rare cases, isolated metastases in surgical scars, lungs, or other sites may be amenable to definitive targeted treatments (CS 13.9).

Specific approaches to the treatment of isolated locoregional recurrences are discussed in greater detail in individual disease-site chapters. This section focuses on studies of the time course of locoregional recurrence and recommendations for the monitoring of patients for recurrence after definitive treatment of gynecologic cancers.

How Long Are Patients at Risk for Developing Recurrent Disease?

In all cases of locoregional recurrence, the success of treatment depends on early detection. For this reason, the intensity of surveillance is greatest during the immediate posttreatment period when the risk of recurrence is greatest.

Central Recurrence

For most locally advanced gynecologic cancers treated with definitive RT, the risk of central disease recurrence is greatest during the first posttreatment year and then declines sharply; few recurrences occur after the 3rd year. However, patients who have been treated for human papillomavirus (HPV)-related cancers of the lower genital tract are at risk throughout their lifetime for developing intraepithelial neoplasia or new invasive cancers of the vulva, vagina, or cervix (if the cervix has not been removed).

In a 2006 MD Anderson Cancer Center study of 2,997 patients treated with definitive RT for stages I and II cervical cancer, Eifel et al.[3] described the biphasic time course of central recurrences. In that study, the hazard rate peaked at about 8 months after treatment and then declined rapidly to a baseline of <1% per year by the 3rd year (Fig. 9.1a). After the 4th year, there was a low but continuous risk of between 0.2% and 0.5% per year that persisted beyond 30 years of follow-up. Most

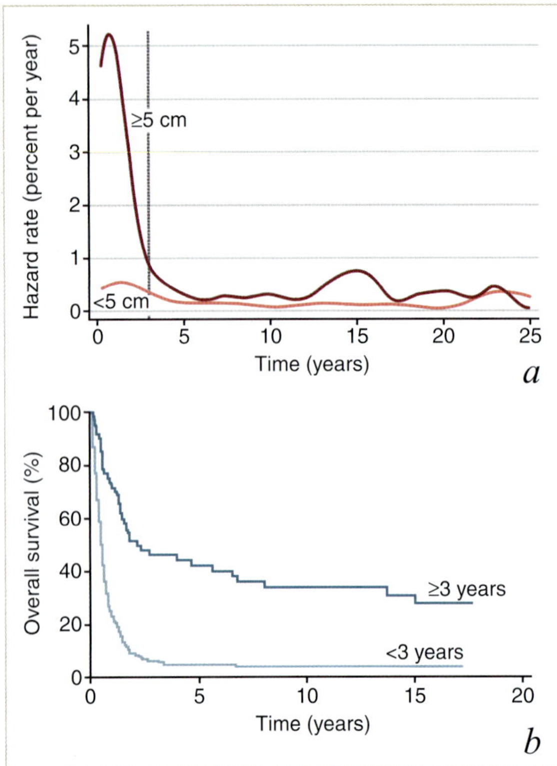

FIGURE 9.1 Time course of central disease recurrence *(a)* and overall survival after central disease recurrence *(b)* in 2,997 patients treated with definitive RT for stage I or stage II squamous carcinoma of the cervix between 1960 and 2001. All occurrences of invasive squamous carcinoma involving the cervix, paracervix, or vagina were scored as events. For patients with tumors ≥5 cm in diameter, the risk of recurrence was greatest in the first year and then declined rapidly *(a)*. After 3 years (*dotted line*), the risk of recurrence was approximately constant, at a rate of 0.3% to 0.5% per year. For patients with smaller tumors, the risk of central recurrence averaged about 0.2% per year throughout the follow-up period, with only a small peak in the first 2 years. Patients who had recurrence 3 years or more after the completion of treatment had significantly better overall survival than patients who had recurrence before 3 years *(b)*. The median follow-up duration for patients in this study was 104 months. Most patients did not have concurrent chemotherapy, which would be expected to decrease the central recurrence rate by 30% to 40%. (From Eifel PJ, Jhingran A, Brown J, et al. Time course and outcome of central recurrence after radiation therapy for carcinoma of the cervix. *Int J Gynecol Cancer.* 2006;16:1106-1111.)

of the recurrences occurring more than 3 years after treatment undoubtedly reflected the development of new HPV-related cancers. These late recurrences were the ones most likely to be treated successfully with surgery (usually pelvic exenteration) (**Fig. 9.1b**). These data suggest that patients who have been cured of locally advanced cervical cancer continue to have a greater risk of developing new preinvasive and invasive cancers of the lower genital tract than does the general population.

The time course for central recurrence of vaginal or vulvar cancers treated with RT appears to be similar to that for central recurrence of cervical cancers treated with RT.[4,5]

Patients who are treated with radiation for small cancers or with primary surgery for early invasive disease tend to have a constant very low annual risk of recurrence because treatment of the initial lesion is usually successful and most "recurrences" are actually new cancers. This pattern is reflected in the constant low risk of recurrence in patients with small cervical cancers treated with RT (**Fig. 9.1a**) and patients with early vulvar cancers treated with surgery (Fig. 12.2).

Because patients in the MD Anderson study mentioned above[3] were treated between 1960 and 2001, most did not receive concurrent chemotherapy with RT, and none had follow-up positron emission tomography (PET) scans. These 21st-century advances in diagnosis and treatment would be expected to reduce the peak hazard rate and may shorten the mean time to recurrence if central recurrences are detected earlier by PET than by physical examination.

Most vaginal recurrences of endometrial cancer also occur within the first 3 years after hysterectomy. However, vaginal recurrences have been diagnosed as late as 5 to 10 years after hysterectomy, particularly in patients treated for low-grade adenocarcinoma (Fig. 13.3).[6,7]

Nodal Recurrence

Although nodal recurrences are occasionally diagnosed more than 5 years after definitive treatment of gynecologic cancers, such late nodal recurrences are very rare. Of 2,949 patients treated for invasive cervical or vaginal cancers between 1985 and 2006 at MD Anderson, 289 had paraaortic or pelvic wall recurrences without evidence of central disease recurrences. Of these 289 nodal recurrences, 63% were diagnosed within the first year after diagnosis, 84% were diagnosed within 3 years, and 97% were diagnosed within 5 years (unpublished data). Most of these patients did not undergo routine surveillance imaging, and most were symptomatic at the time their nodal recurrences were detected.

The use of modern imaging, particularly PET–computed tomography (PET–CT), for diagnosis and surveillance is likely to alter these statistics. Retrospective studies suggest that regional recurrences are less frequent when RT plans are guided by PET imaging.[8,9] Evidence also suggests that patients who have routine surveillance imaging are more likely to have nodal recurrences detected at an earlier, more treatable stage than are patients with nodal recurrence diagnosed only after symptoms develop.[10,11]

Nodal recurrences tend to occur in sites of initial disease and at the upper margins of pelvic or extended pelvic RT fields.[12,13] Factors that are associated with a high risk of regional involvement are discussed in detail in Chapters 10 to 14.

Recommendations for Evaluation for Possible Tumor Recurrence

Both the Society of Gynecologic Oncologists (SGO) and the National Comprehensive Cancer Network (NCCN) have published guidelines for cancer surveillance in patients with gynecologic cancers.[14–16] Their recommendations regarding the frequency of surveillance visits are similar

TABLE 9.2 Suggested Guidelines for Posttreatment Surveillance[14–16]

Diagnosis, evaluation	Years after completion of treatment 1	2	3	4–5	>5
Endometrial cancer					
Physical examination and symptom review					
Low risk of recurrence	Every 6 mo	Yearly	Yearly	Yearly	Yearly
Intermediate risk of recurrence	Every 3 mo	Every 6 mo	Every 6 mo	Every 6 mo	Yearly
High risk of recurrence	Every 3 mo	Every 3 mo	Every 6 mo	Every 6 mo	Yearly
Papanicolaou test	Not indicated				
CA-125 measurement	SGO: "insufficient data to support routine use"; NCCN: "optional"				
Diagnostic imaging					
No recurrence suspected	SGO: "insufficient data to support routine use"; NCCN: "optional"				
Recurrence suspected	CT or PET ± CA-125				
Cervical, vulvar, or vaginal cancer					
Physical examination and symptom review					
Low risk of recurrence, treated with surgery only	Every 6 mo	Every 6 mo	Yearly	Yearly	Yearly
High risk of recurrence, treated with primary or adjuvant RT	Every 3 mo	Every 3 mo	Every 6 mo	Every 6 mo	Yearly
Papanicolaou test	Yearly	Yearly	Yearly	Yearly	Yearly
Diagnostic imaging					
No recurrence suspected	SGO: "insufficient data to support routine use"; NCCN: not recommended for routine surveillance[a]				
Recurrence suspected	CT or PET (MRI in selected cases of suspected central recurrence)				

[a]Per NCCN, "A single PET-CT scan performed at 3–6 months after chemoradiation for locally advanced cervical cancer can be used to suggest early or asymptomatic persistence or recurrence. Other imaging studies (such as chest x-ray, CT scan, MRI, and subsequent PET-CT) may also be used to assess or follow recurrence when clinically indicated but are not recommended for routine surveillance."

mo, months; SGO, Society of Gynecologic Oncologists; NCCN, National Comprehensive Cancer Network; CT, computed tomography; PET, positron emission tomography; MRI, magnetic resonance imaging; CA-125, cancer antigen-125.

National Comprehensive Cancer Network. Uterine Neoplasms (Version 2.2016). Available at http://www.nccn.org/professionals/physician_gls/pdf/uterine.pdf. Accessed February 23, 2016; National Comprehensive Cancer Network. Cervical Cancer (Version 2.2016). Available at http://www.nccn.org/professionals/physician_gls/pdf/cervical.pdf. Accessed February 23, 2016; Salani R, Backes FJ, Fung MF, et al. Posttreatment surveillance and diagnosis of recurrence in women with gynecologic malignancies: Society of Gynecologic Oncologists recommendations. Am J Obstet Gynecol. 2011;204:466–478.

and reflect the need for closer surveillance during the initial posttreatment period, when the risk of recurrence is highest (Table 9.2).

Physical Examination and Symptom Review

For detection of recurrent disease, both the SGO and NCCN place their greatest emphasis on physical examination and symptom review. For most gynecologic cancers, the hallmark symptoms for recurrence are bleeding, pain, and palpation of a new mass, although metastatic disease can present with a variety of symptoms according to the site of involvement. At the end of treatment and at each follow-up visit, patients should be counseled about symptoms that should prompt patients to schedule an appointment with their oncologist. Follow-up pelvic examinations should include careful inspection of the vulva, vagina, and cervix; bimanual examination; and rectovaginal examination, as discussed in Chapter 4.

Surveillance Imaging

Any patient who has symptoms or clinical findings that suggest possible recurrence should have an appropriately focused diagnostic imaging study, usually CT or PET–CT, although magnetic resonance imaging (MRI) is sometimes particularly valuable for assessment of vaginal or paravaginal abnormalities (Chapter 4).

The indications for imaging of asymptomatic patients are more controversial. Both the SGO and NCCN leave their recommendations vague, although they agree that routine imaging of every gynecologic cancer patient is inappropriate (Table 9.2).[14–16]

Several studies have suggested that patients who have persistent or recurrent cervical cancer are more likely to be cured by salvage treatments if their disease is detected before it becomes symptomatic.[10] These findings led the NCCN to suggest that patients with locoregionally advanced cervical cancer undergo a single PET scan at 3 to 6 months after completion of treatment to allow early detection of potentially treatable recurrences (Table 9.2).[15] Because many insurers do not support more than one follow-up PET scan, the timing of the study is crucial. Ideally, the study should be done when it allows early detection of persistent disease without a high rate of false-positive findings due to post-RT tumor necrosis and inflammation. A modest delay after treatment increases the likelihood that early recurrences near the margins of pelvic RT fields will be detected. However, an overly long delay could miss the optimal window for definitive treatment. Investigators at Washington University, who have done much of the work evaluating the value of PET surveillance, have focused on follow-up PET scans obtained 3 months after RT. Their studies demonstrated that patients who had persistent fluorodeoxyglucose (FDG) uptake in initial sites of involvement were much more likely to have recurrence than were patients who had complete resolution of abnormal FDG uptake.[17] However, in their study, about 30% of patients with persistent FDG uptake failed to have confirmation of progressive disease, and about 20% of patients who had negative findings on PET at 3 months did subsequently develop progressive cervical cancer (Fig. 9.2). We usually recommend performing PET 3 to 5 months after the end of treatment. However, more detailed studies are needed to determine the best timing of this study.

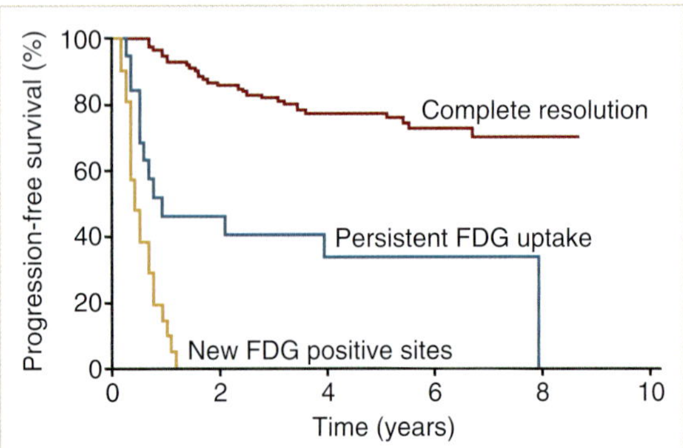

FIGURE 9.2 Relationship between progression-free survival and PET–CT findings 3 months after completion of definitive RT for cervical cancer. Patients who had no residual FDG uptake had significantly better survival than patients who had persistent FDG uptake. All patients who developed new FDG uptake after completion of RT had confirmed progression of their disease. The mean follow-up duration for the 92 patients in this study was 70 months. (Adapted from Schwarz JK, Siegel BA, Dehdashti F, et al. Association of posttherapy positron emission tomography with tumor response and survival in cervical carcinoma. *JAMA*. 2007;298:2289–2295.)

Neither the SGO nor the NCCN recommends routine imaging in any other setting. However, we believe there are a number of other situations that warrant routine surveillance imaging. The arguments for surveillance imaging of patients with locally advanced cancers involving the vagina are similar to those for follow-up imaging of patients with locally advanced cervical cancer, although MRI may play a more important role in patients with asymptomatic vaginal cancer than in patients with asymptomatic cervical cancer. Patients who have a significant risk of recurrence in unirradiated pelvic or paraaortic nodes are also good candidates for posttreatment imaging. This group includes patients treated with chemotherapy alone for stage IIIC endometrial cancer or with pelvic RT for stage IIIC1 endometrial cancer. These patients are frequently curable if nodal progression is caught early.[13] On the other hand, there is probably less justification for routine surveillance imaging in patients who have already had full extended-field irradiation, because in-field recurrences can only very rarely be treated successfully. Ultrasound surveillance of groins that may be at risk for nodal recurrence may also be helpful in selected cases (CS 12.10).

Cytologic Screening

Papanicolaou (Pap) screening is no longer recommended for detection of recurrent endometrial cancer. This change followed several reports indicating that fewer than 5% of vaginal recurrences were detected by Pap screening in asymptomatic patients.[18,19] For similar reasons, Pap tests are no longer recommended for detection of recurrent cervical or vaginal cancer.[20,21] The current recommendation for women who have been treated for HPV-positive cervical or vaginal cancer is for cytologic screening only once a year, in keeping with general cervical cancer screening guidelines. Pap screening should never be performed sooner than 4 months after RT because studies performed before this time are likely to show postradiation cytologic changes that can be misinterpreted as cancer or dysplasia.

As discussed earlier, there is a low but significant rate of locoregional recurrence of gynecologic cancer even after 5 years. By this time, patients are usually being followed by their primary care providers. For this reason, patients and their primary care providers should be reminded about the possibility of late recurrence and the continued need to evaluate any incidence of vaginal bleeding or protracted pelvic pain. Because of the increased risk of second gynecologic cancers, patients who have been treated for an HPV-related cancer should have annual Pap screening for life (Table 9.2).

MONITORING AND MANAGEMENT OF LATE ADVERSE EFFECTS OF TREATMENT

Because many patients with gynecologic cancer are cured, many survive to potentially experience late sequelae of cancer treatments. Most late radiation-related adverse effects occur during the first 3 years after RT; however, in some cases, symptoms do not begin until many years later, when patients are no longer routinely followed by oncologic specialists. For this reason, it is important to use the first several years of more intensive surveillance to educate patients about the possible late adverse effects of RT and to encourage them to seek specialized care if symptoms develop.

The long-term adverse effects of surgery and chemotherapy are summarized in Chapter 3, and acute adverse effects of RT are described in Chapter 7. In this chapter, the symptoms, pathophysiology, frequency, and management of some of the more important late adverse effects of RT for gynecologic cancer are discussed.

Sexual Dysfunction and Menopausal Symptoms

Recent literature reviews have concluded that research into the causes, incidence, and severity of sexual dysfunction in gynecologic cancer survivors is still in its infancy, with many unanswered questions remaining.[22,23] However, it is clear that many psychological and physical factors contribute to decreased sexual satisfaction in gynecologic cancer survivors and that these problems can affect patients' overall quality of life in important ways.

In the course of infrequent surveillance visits, the radiation oncologist cannot adequately address psychosocial issues related to sexual dysfunction. However, as part of routine review of symptoms, patients should be questioned about overall sexual satisfaction and specifically about any problems with dyspareunia or decreased libido. Those who describe symptoms should be offered referral to a therapist who specializes in cancer-related sexual disorders.

Risk Factors for Sexual Dysfunction

Before and during treatment, tumor- and treatment-associated symptoms often inhibit normal sexual activity for a protracted period of time. In the posttreatment period, depression and anxiety, fatigue, altered body image, grief over the loss of fertility, and fears about possible sexual transmission of cancer to a partner can all inhibit return to normal function even if there are no physical barriers. Hypoestrogenism after oophorectomy or pelvic irradiation may cause hot flashes, emotional lability, decreased libido, and vaginal dryness and atrophy.[23,24] Scarring or vaginal shortening caused by tumor destruction, surgery, and RT can contribute to dyspareunia and decreased sexual satisfaction.[23] All of these factors can cause or exacerbate strain in relationships.

Most studies indicate that patients with cervical or vulvar cancer who receive RT have a higher rate of sexual dysfunction than those treated with surgery alone.[22,25] However, because patients treated with RT tend to have relatively advanced disease, direct comparisons between patients treated with surgery alone and those treated with RT are difficult to interpret. Also, radiation technique may play an important role. For example, an MD Anderson survey study that included 269 patients with endometrial cancer failed to identify adjuvant RT as a major factor contributing to subsequent sexual dysfunction.[25] However, other studies have reported problems with sexual function after vaginal brachytherapy.[22] These variations may reflect differences in brachytherapy technique and schedule that are known to influence the likelihood of vaginal injury (Chapters 8 and 13).[26,27]

Vaginal Dilator Treatment

Many clinicians believe that frequent use of a vaginal dilator can improve vaginal capacity and sexual function of patients who have had pelvic RT. However, the data supporting this are weak. A 2014 Cochrane meta-analysis[28] concluded, "There is no reliable evidence to show that routine, regular vaginal dilation during RT prevents stenosis or improves quality of life." The authors noted that although observational studies report an association between frequent dilator use and lower rates of self-reported stenosis, this may be because patients with a healthy vagina are more likely to comply with dilation therapy than are those with strictures. Although it is reasonable to recommend dilator use to young motivated patients, the evidence may not be strong enough to justify a very forceful recommendation to patients who are elderly or who have a personal aversion to dilator therapy.

Hormone Replacement Therapy

Hypoestrogenism can play a major role in sexual dysfunction. For women <40 to 45 years of age who undergo premature menopause after treatment of squamous carcinoma, estrogen replacement therapy is usually recommended unless there is a major contraindication (e.g., a strong family history or personal history of breast cancer or venous thrombosis). If the uterus is in situ, combined treatment with estrogen and progesterone is usually recommended to prevent intrauterine bleeding from residual endometrium; a starting daily dose of 0.3 mg of estrogen and 1.5 mg of progesterone is usually recommended. Randomized trials showing an increased risk of heart disease with hormone replacement therapy probably cannot be generalized to women who undergo treatment-related premature menopause; however, such women should be counseled carefully about the risks and benefits of treatment. Young women who do not have a uterus may be treated with estrogen alone. In both cases (estrogen plus progesterone or estrogen alone), treatment should be discontinued when the patient reaches the age of 45 to 50 years.

Hormone replacement therapy is more controversial in patients who have adenocarcinomas, particularly endometrial cancers, which may be hormone responsive. Hormone therapy is usually denied to these patients, although it has never been proven that relapse rates are higher in endometrial cancer survivors who receive estrogen replacement therapy.[29] A number of nonestrogenic treatments for hot flashes have been used with varying success rates.[30,31]

Radiation Proctitis

Rectal bleeding due to radiation proctitis is one of the more common adverse effects of definitive treatment of cervical

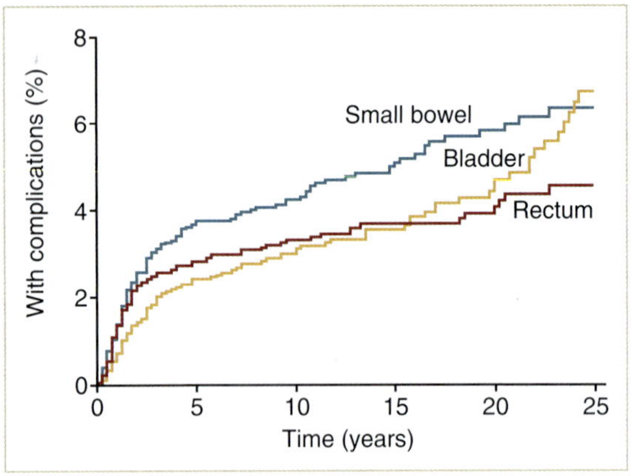

FIGURE 9.3 Incidence of major late complications of the rectum, bladder, or bowel after definitive RT for International Federation of Gynecology and Obstetrics stage I or II carcinoma of the cervix. Any complication occurring or persisting more than 3 months after treatment that required hospitalization, transfusion, or operation or caused severe symptoms such as fistula or the patient's death was considered a major complication. All patients were treated at MD Anderson between 1960 and 1995. Of the 3,499 patients in this analysis, 99% were followed for more than 3 years or to death, and 1,623 were followed more than 10 years. (Previously unpublished figure from data reported in Eifel PJ, Jhingran A, Bodurka DC, et al. Correlation of smoking history and other patient characteristics with major complications of pelvic radiation therapy for cervical cancer. *J Clin Oncol.* 2002;20:3651–3657.)

cancer. In a series of 3,489 patients treated with definitive RT for cervical cancer, about 25% reported at least one episode of rectal bleeding during the first 5 years after treatment; most of these were minor and resolved spontaneously or after a short course of steroid enemas. Severe radiation proctitis requiring transfusion or leading to fistula was rare, with an actuarial rate of ~3% at 10 years; most cases occurred within 6 months to 2 years after RT (**Fig. 9.3**).[32,33]

Acutely, radiation causes crypt cell depletion, breakdown of mucosal barriers, infiltration of bacterial products, and inflammation. Although most patients receiving RT have some degree of acute radiation proctitis, this often causes only minimal symptoms or cannot be differentiated from resolving small bowel effects of radiation. Symptoms of mucous discharge, tenesmus, and urgency during the several months immediately after RT suggest more severe acute radiation proctitis. Although these symptoms typically resolve shortly after RT, mucosal injury that occurs during this period may contribute to so-called consequential late effects.

The more chronic phase of radiation proctitis begins 3 to 6 months after RT and is characterized by connective tissue fibrosis and neoangiogenesis. On proctoscopy, the classic appearance of chronic radiation proctitis is a pale mucosa punctuated by multiple angioectasias (**Fig. 9.4**). Defecation may cause sufficient trauma to these abnormally fragile vessels to cause rectal bleeding. In severe cases, there may be ulceration of the mucosa; in rare cases, fistulization of the rectovaginal septum may occur.

Risk Factors for Chronic Radiation Proctitis

In gynecologic oncology patients, most cases of symptomatic radiation proctitis occur in patients who have received high-dose brachytherapy for definitive management of cervical or vaginal cancer; radiation-related hematochezia is rare in patients who receive only external pelvic RT unless the rectum receives a dose of 60 Gy or more. In general, the recommendation is to avoid treating a rectal volume of more than 2 cc to 70 Gy or more. The advent of image-guided brachytherapy promises to reduce the rate of rectal complications by allowing greater control of the dose to the rectum (Chaper 8).[34] Thin body habitus (body mass index <22) and heavy smoking (≥1 pack per day) are significant risk factors for radiation proctitis.[33]

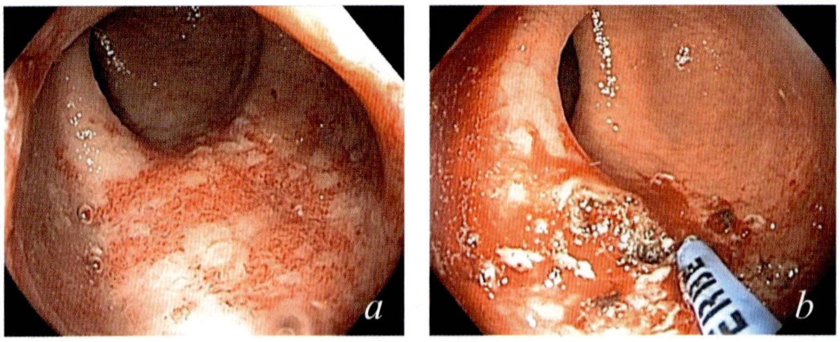

FIGURE 9.4 Radiation proctitis in a patient who was treated with definitive RT for recurrent adenocarcinoma at the vaginal apex 1 year after undergoing hysterectomy and vaginal cuff brachytherapy. Details of this patient's treatment are described in **CS 13.8**. Eight months after treatment, the patient had onset of intermittent, apparently mild rectal bleeding. However, at 20 months, she complained of increased bleeding and required a transfusion because of a hemoglobin level of 6 g/dL. Proctoscopy showed diffuse colonic angioectasias *(a)*. The patient was initially treated successfully with steroid suppositories but subsequently underwent three treatments with argon plasma coagulation *(b)*. At 5 years after RT, she continued to have hematochezia several times per month but had not required additional transfusions.

Management of Radiation Proctitis

The management of chronic radiation proctitis depends on the severity and duration of the bleeding. It is always wise to have patients with rectal bleeding undergo rectal endoscopy to rule out causes other than proctitis. *However, biopsies of the irradiated area should be avoided* because they can exacerbate symptoms and could serve as a nidus for ulceration or even fistula formation. The patient's hemoglobin level should be checked to ensure that the bleeding is not more severe than is suggested by the history.

Most cases of minor bleeding are self-limited and require no intervention other than reassurance and optimization of stool consistency.[35] Steroid or sucralfate enemas have been used, although the evidence of benefit from either one of these treatments is weak.[36,37]

Argon plasma coagulation is frequently favored by gastroenterologists as the treatment of choice for radiation proctitis. Although retrospective studies suggest that this treatment has helped to achieve control in some cases of refractory bleeding, there have been no randomized trials evaluating its use in this setting, and the treatment is not without risk: reported complication rates range from 7% to 26%.[36] In addition to being associated with rare catastrophic complications (e.g., explosive events occurring during treatment of inadequately prepared bowel), argon plasma coagulation has been implicated as the cause of deep ulceration, fistula, stricture, and perforation.[36] Although technical modification may reduce the complication rate, this has not been proven.[36] Also, many of the studies of argon plasma coagulation have addressed its use in men with proctitis following RT for prostate cancer; women may have a different risk of complications when ablative treatments are used in the region of the thin rectovaginal septum. For all these reasons, ablative treatments should be limited to patients who have severe, persistent bleeding.

Hyperbaric oxygen has been used as a treatment for severe radiation proctitis for many years.[36,38] Although many practitioners have been convinced of its effectiveness, a recent randomized trial failed to demonstrate any significant benefit of the use of hyperbaric oxygen in patients with chronic bowel injury, including radiation proctitis.[39]

Although rectal bleeding is the most common symptom of radiation-related rectal injury, patients who receive a very high rectal dose (usually >70 Gy) or who have had damage to the rectovaginal septum by infiltrative tumor may develop a rectovaginal fistula. Most patients experience a short period of rectal urgency, tenesmus, or fever before the fistula becomes apparent. Rectovaginal fistulas that occur within a heavily irradiated field cannot be repaired surgically; attempts to do so can set off a cascade of events leading to catastrophic pelvic complications. For this reason, the treatment is usually colostomy.

Most cases of radiation proctitis occur in patients who have had vaginal brachytherapy and therefore involve primarily the anterior rectal wall. However, patients who receive high-dose external beam RT (usually >60 Gy) to the entire circumference of the rectum or sigmoid are at risk for developing a rectal stricture. If a severe stricture develops, colostomy may be necessary to relieve symptoms.

Sigmoid perforation is a catastrophic complication that is fatal in about 50% of cases. Sigmoid perforation can present as an acute abdomen, although in some cases, the perforation may form a walled-off abscess with symptoms of fever, pain, and failure to thrive. Fortunately, sigmoid perforation is usually a rare complication in most series; for example, it occurred in fewer than 0.2% of patients treated definitively for cervical cancer at MD Anderson.[32,33] However, sigmoid perforation is an expected complication of brachytherapy if a radiation source is placed in a tandem or interstitial needle that has entered the peritoneal cavity and, thus, come into direct contact with the sigmoid (Chapter 8).

Radiation Enteropathy

RT for gynecologic cancers usually requires irradiation of some small bowel. During treatment, most patients experience at least mild symptoms of diarrhea, crampy abdominal pain, and fatigue caused by depletion of the rapidly dividing intestinal crypt epithelium, breakdown of the mucosal barrier, and mucosal inflammation.[40] These acute symptoms usually resolve within 1 to 3 months after the end of RT. Depending on the dose of radiation, volume irradiated, previous surgery, and other patient characteristics, patients may also develop late symptoms of small bowel injury.

Symptoms and Incidence of Radiation Enteropathy

Chronic radiation enteropathy tends to arise because of treatment of a relatively large volume of bowel with a moderately high dose of radiation. Symptoms can include diarrhea, frequency, flatulence, pain, malabsorption, urgency, and incontinence. Symptoms usually develop within the first 2 years after RT, although in some patients the onset is more delayed. The reported incidence varies widely with the method of assessment and probably varies with the radiation techniques used and predisposing patient characteristics. Quality-of-life studies suggest that the incidence of enteropathy is higher than has previously been suggested. Nout et al.[41] reported results of a quality-of-life study of patients treated for endometrial cancer in the PORTEC-1 trial; patients responded via questionnaire a median of 13 years (range, 9 to 18 years) after treatment. Compared with patients who received no adjuvant RT, patients who received pelvic RT after hysterectomy reported significantly higher rates of fecal urgency, leakage, and diarrhea (**Fig. 9.5**).

If a fixed loop of small bowel has received a high dose of radiation (usually >60 Gy), a small bowel obstruction or perforation may occur. This typically presents with acute onset of nausea, vomiting, and pain. Although some small bowel obstructions respond to medical management, radiation-related obstructions usually require surgical intervention. If adjacent bowel is healthy, a localized obstruction can often be corrected by surgical resection of the site of obstruction, and the patient may return to having normal bowel function.

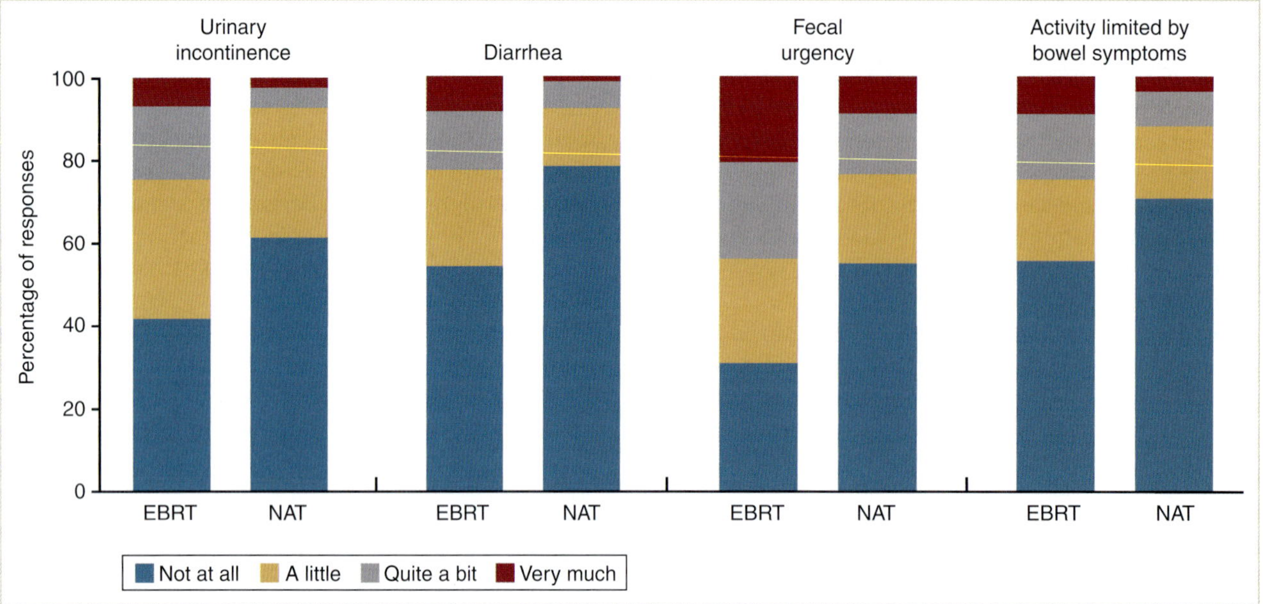

FIGURE 9.5 Selected quality-of-life scores from a 10-year follow-up study of 715 patients entered on the PORTEC-1 trial. Patients in the trial were randomly allocated to receive external beam radiation therapy (EBRT) to the pelvis (46 Gy at 2 Gy per fraction) or no adjuvant treatment (NAT). Quality of life was evaluated using the European Organization for Research and Treatment of Cancer PR25 module for bowel and bladder symptoms. (Adapted from Nout RA, van de Poll-Franse LV, Lybeert ML, et al. Long-term outcome and quality of life of patients with endometrial carcinoma treated with or without pelvic radiotherapy in the post operative radiation therapy in endometrial carcinoma 1 (PORTEC-1) trial. *J Clin Oncol.* 2011;29:1692–1700.)

Most major small bowel injuries (e.g., obstructions, perforations, or severe chronic diarrhea) occur during the first 2 to 3 years after treatment (**Fig. 9.3**).[32] However, about one-third of the actuarial risk is after 5 years, with late occurrences often associated with pelvic surgical procedures performed for other reasons.

Risk Factors for Radiation Enteropathy

The risk of complications rises steeply with external beam doses over 40 to 50 Gy.[42] Patients who have had a transperitoneal lymph node dissection have a significantly increased risk of developing radiation-related enteric complications, but lymph node dissections that are performed laparoscopically appear to pose less risk.[43] Patients who have a history of peritonitis, pelvic inflammatory disease, or thin body habitus (body mass index <22) are at significantly increased risk of bowel obstruction.[32,33] Smokers, particularly those who smoke one pack or more of cigarettes per day, have several times the risk of bowel complications that nonsmokers have (**Fig. 9.6**).[32]

Pathogenesis and Treatment

The pathogenesis of late radiation enteropathy is complex and is still not fully understood. The probability of late enteropathy is poorly correlated with the severity of acute symptoms. Late symptoms appear to result from combinations of primary cytocidal effects, changes in the intracellular environment, and secondary effects of cytokine release and tissue inflammation.[40] Recent research has uncovered changes in the bowel microbiota that begin during RT and may persist long after treatment is over.[44] The extent to which these changes contribute to symptoms of radiation enteropathy is uncertain; however, early studies suggest that bacterial overgrowth and dysbiosis may contribute to dysmotility and diarrhea. Studies of bacteriobiotherapy before or during RT have yielded inconsistent results. The success of fecal microbiota transplant has not yet been tested in patients with radiation enteropathy, but the success of this procedure in treatment of *Clostridium difficile* infection **(CS 12.1)** suggests an interesting possible avenue for future research.[44]

Many cases of late radiation enteropathy can be improved with dietary modification, antidiarrheal medications, or other treatments; however, no single treatment can be expected to work for all patients. In many cases, radiation enteropathy is complicated by or potentiates an underlying dietary intolerance. Andreyev et al.[35] have created an extremely detailed guide to the symptoms, causes, and treatment of radiation-related bowel disease. As emphasized in their manuscript, the first step in the evaluation and treatment of suspected radiation enteropathy should always be to obtain an accurate history of the patient's gastrointestinal symptoms; this should include the following:

- *The frequency and consistency of stools.* Tools like the Bristol stool chart[45] may be helpful for obtaining accurate descriptions.[35]

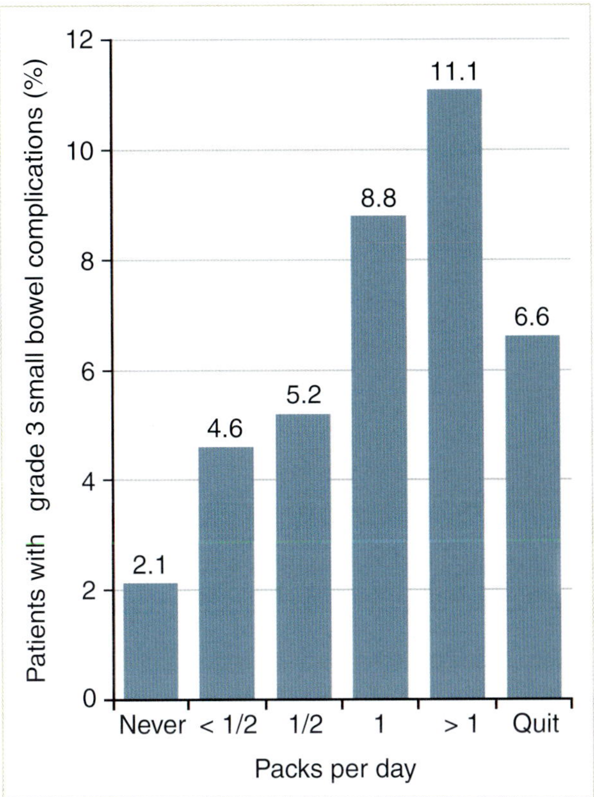

FIGURE 9.6 Relationship between smoking intensity and the actuarial rate of major small bowel complications at 10 years in 3,489 patients treated with definitive RT for stage I or II carcinoma of the cervix. Complications were scored as grade 3 or higher if they required hospital admission, required surgical intervention, or caused the death of the patient. (Eifel PJ, Jhingran A, Bodurka DC, et al. Correlation of smoking history and other patient characteristics with major complications of pelvic radiation therapy for cervical cancer. *J Clin Oncol.* 2002;20:3651–3657.).

- *Evidence of change in bowel habits*. Did the patient have symptoms before RT? If so, how have they evolved over time? Was the onset of symptoms sudden or gradual?
- *Steatorrhea*. Steatorrhea, an important clue to bile acid malabsorption, can be easily missed unless the patient is specifically queried about the presence of an oily film in the toilet water or stool that floats or is difficult to flush.
- *A detailed dietary history*. How does the quantity of fiber, lactose, gluten, or alcohol influence symptoms? A food diary correlated with monitoring of stool consistency can help to reveal a specific dietary intolerance.
- *Correlation between changes in medications and onset or worsening of symptoms*. Some common medications that can cause diarrhea include metformin, proton pump inhibitors, and beta-blockers. A history of recent intravenous antibiotics and a sudden onset of symptoms can suggest *C. difficile* infection **(CS 12.1)**.

If the symptoms are severe or do not resolve promptly, the patient should be referred to a gastroenterologist experienced in the management of radiation-related bowel disease for detailed evaluation and treatment.

Duodenal Injury

The C loop of the duodenum typically crosses over the aorta and vena cava just below the renal vessels in a location that is a common site of metastasis from gynecologic cancers. The relatively fixed retroperitoneal location of this portion of the duodenum makes it particularly vulnerable to the effects of high-dose RT; for this reason, duodenal injury is typically the most important factor limiting the radiation dose deliverable to the paraaortic nodes.

Radiation may cause bleeding, ulceration, or stricture. Duodenal ulcers may cause symptoms of nausea, bloating, gnawing epigastric pain, or early satiety. Patients may specifically complain of difficulty swallowing red meat. A bleeding ulcer may cause anemia or melena. Patients in whom radiation-related duodenal injury is suspected should be referred immediately for evaluation by a gastroenterologist.

The most catastrophic duodenal complication is perforation. Duodenal perforation typically presents suddenly with symptoms of peritonitis, although small perforations may initially be walled off by the omentum and cause more gradual onset of pain, nausea, and weight loss. The treatment is surgical, but the mortality rate is high.

The best approach is prevention. Recent studies suggest that the risk of serious duodenal injury is low if the volume of duodenum receiving 55 Gy or more is <15 cc and if the volume receiving 60 Gy is <2 cc.[46,47]

Radiation Cystitis

The most common late adverse effect of irradiation of the bladder is bleeding. Most cases occur in patients who have received brachytherapy or who have received more than 50 Gy to the bladder from external beam RT.[32]

In a large retrospective review of patients treated at MD Anderson with definitive RT for carcinoma of the cervix, ~10% of patients followed for 5 years had experienced at least one episode of gross hematuria.[32] Most of these cases were minor, often associated with bladder infections, and resolved spontaneously with no treatment or with a short course of antibiotic therapy. However, a smaller percentage of patients had a more severe episode of bleeding requiring transfusion or bladder irrigation. About two-thirds of these complications consisted of a major bleeding episode that responded to treatment and did not recur.[32,33,48] However, about one-third (about 1% of patients followed 10 years) developed very severe complications of intractable bleeding, vesicovaginal fistula, or severe bladder contraction that required surgical intervention with urinary diversion or, rarely, cystectomy. Although the risk of fistula formation should be very low for patients treated for stage I or II cervical cancer, patients with massive disease, particularly those who have extensive destruction of the vesicovaginal septum by tumor, have a higher risk. Many patients with stage IVA disease have evidence of fistula at diagnosis (**CS 10.11**); others develop a fistula as tumor responds, removing the only remaining barrier between the bladder and the vagina.

Time Course and Risk Factors

The time course of radiation cystitis is very different from that of bowel complications. Although most minor bleeding episodes occur within the first 2 to 3 years after RT, major bladder complications can have their symptomatic onset many years after RT.[32,33,48] In the MD Anderson series,[32] only about one-third of the 25-year actuarial risk was manifest in the first 5 years of follow-up (**Fig. 9.3**). Although some of the later events were associated with pelvic surgical procedures, late-onset, uncontrolled diabetes mellitus, or infections, some cases of radiation cystitis had no discernable explanation for their late onset.

The bladder seems to tolerate radiation doses equivalent to 80 to 90 Gy at 2 Gy per fraction if <2 cc of the bladder receives that dose.[49] However, the larger the volume of bladder irradiated, the lower the tolerated dose. Patients who receive 60 Gy or more to the entire bladder have a significant risk of hemorrhagic cystitis and are also at high risk for developing fibrosis and contractures causing severely diminished bladder capacity. Patient factors also contribute to the risk of major bladder complications, particularly smoking one pack of cigarettes or more per day.[32]

Treatment of Radiation Cystitis

Patients who have hematuria should always be evaluated for infection, and those with confirmed infection or who have other symptoms and findings suspicious for infection should be treated promptly with appropriate antibiotic therapy. Because most episodes of minor hematuria resolve spontaneously, potentially traumatic interventions should be avoided. However, if no infection is found, cystoscopy is usually indicated to rule out bladder cancer. Typical late findings of radiation change include pale mucosa and telangiectasia, usually of the posterior bladder wall; these areas should not be biopsied unless there are findings suggestive of cancer. Biopsies of heavily irradiated bladder mucosa are usually slow to heal, can exacerbate bleeding and other symptoms, and may lead to ulceration and fistula formation.

The focus of care for patients with more severe hemorrhagic cystitis is relief of symptoms.[50] This includes blood transfusion to correct severe anemia and bladder catheterization followed by continuous or intermittent bladder irrigation with saline until the urine is clear. More aggressive measures, including intravesical instillation of silver nitrate or formalin, should be reserved for refractory cases that do not respond to other measures because these treatments can cause bladder contracture with symptoms of chronic urgency, frequency, or urine retention. Fulguration of persistent bleeding points may help in some cases, but poor healing may lead to chronic ulceration and dysuria. In very rare cases of severe, relapsing hemorrhagic cystitis, fistula, or severe bladder contractures, cystectomy or urinary diversion may be required. Hyperbaric oxygen may be effective in some refractory cases but is not a treatment for acute bleeding.[50]

Ureteral Stenosis

Ureteral stenosis is very rarely seen as a complication of definitive RT.[33] The ureters, which are at the approximate location of point A, appear to tolerate 2-Gy equivalent doses of 90 Gy or more with little risk of injury. However, doses of more than 120 Gy may cause stricture with resulting hydronephrosis. In an MD Anderson study of patients treated with definitive RT for early cervical cancer, McIntyre et al.[51] reported no ureteral strictures in 261 patients who received 40 Gy to the pelvis followed by ~45 Gy of intracavitary brachytherapy; in contrast, 210 patients who received their entire central dose of RT from brachytherapy and had external RT delivered using a 4-cm midline block had an actuarial risk of developing hydronephrosis of 5% at 15 years. It was hypothesized that the ureters may, in some cases, have been exposed to the external beam irradiation as well as the more heavily weighted brachytherapy, causing them to receive doses of 120 Gy or more.

Hydronephrosis is a frequent presenting symptom of locally advanced cervical or vaginal cancer. The initial management of tumor-related hydronephrosis is discussed in Chapter 7. However, posttreatment management can be particularly challenging, particularly for patients who have persistent bilateral obstruction. Long-term indwelling nephrostomy tubes are a source of infection, require frequent exchanges, and degrade quality of life. Stents can cause pain and are also a source of infection. Patients with indwelling stents or nephrostomy tubes should be tested 2 to 4 months after treatment to determine whether adequate ureteral flow has been reestablished. Although successful treatment may relieve the obstruction, in many cases, scarring from tumor and treatment causes a permanent occlusion. If possible, patients who have bilateral ureteral stenosis and who, after thorough evaluation, have no evidence of cancer 1 to 2 years after treatment should be evaluated for a more permanent bypass solution such as an ileal loop diversion.

Any patient who develops hydronephrosis after treatment must be carefully evaluated for recurrence. Nearly all instances developing in the first few years after RT are due to cancer (**Fig. 9.7**).[51]

Pelvic Insufficiency Fractures

With the increased use of CT and MRI in the follow-up of patients treated with RT for gynecologic cancers has come a greater appreciation of the effects of RT on bone. In particular, it has become apparent that the incidence of treatment-related pelvic insufficiency fractures is greater than had been previously thought. The most frequent sites of insufficiency fractures are the sacral alae, although fractures may also be seen in the pubis. Femoral fractures are rarely seen as a result of standard pelvic irradiation but are a major concern when larger fields encompassing the groin are used; femoral fractures are a particular concern in vulvar cancer patients, who are often elderly and osteoporotic (**CS 12.9**).[52]

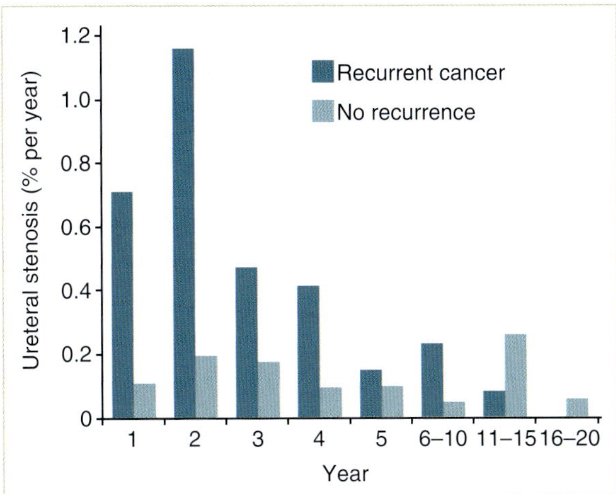

FIGURE 9.7 The average percentage of surviving patients per year of follow-up who had a diagnosis of ureteral stenosis caused by tumor or treatment among 1,784 patients with stage IB carcinoma of the cervix treated at MD Anderson between 1960 and 1989. Surviving patients in this study were followed for a median of 12.4 years. (From McIntyre JF, Eifel PJ, Levenback C, et al. Ureteral stricture as a late complication of radiotherapy for stage IB carcinoma of the uterine cervix. *Cancer.* 1995;75:836–843.)

Early diffuse bone marrow edema has been described during the course of RT; within a few weeks after the completion of treatment, the marrow begins to be replaced by fat, causing increased signal intensity on T1-weighted images (Fig. 4.1). In contrast, the edema associated with insufficiency fractures is seen as patchy areas of depressed signal intensity on T1-weighted MRI, often contrasting starkly with the fatty post-RT marrow, and high signal intensity on T2-weighted MRI (**Fig. 9.8a, b**).[53] On CT, there can be patchy sclerosis and displaced or nondisplaced fractures (**Fig. 9.8c**). Because insufficiency fractures can cause increased FDG uptake on PET, care must be taken not to misinterpret insufficiency fractures as metastasis on PET.

The mechanism of radiation-induced insufficiency fractures is not fully understood. However, animal studies indicate that radiation causes a dose-dependent increase in cortical bone density and a corresponding loss of trabecular bone, causing a decrease in bone strength despite an increase in bone mass.[54]

The first signs of fracture are usually seen 3 to 24 months after RT.[53,55] The reported incidences of pelvic insufficiency fracture after pelvic RT vary widely, from 2% to as high as 89%, in part due to variations in the method and frequency of imaging.[55] One of the most consistently identified risk factors for insufficiency fracture is low body mass index; this may in part explain why studies in Asian women tend to suggest higher rates of fracture than studies in US women.[55] Fractures are also more common in postmenopausal women and in women with generalized osteoporosis. The risk of fracture undoubtedly increases with increasing radiation dose, although there are many reports in patients who received doses of 40 to 45 Gy. The contribution of concurrent or sequential chemotherapy to the development of fractures is unknown, as is the contribution of radiation-induced menopause or hormone replacement therapy.

In a retrospective study of 300 cervical cancer patients treated at MD Anderson, Schmeler et al.[55] reported a fracture rate of 10%. Of the patients with fractures, 45% had symptoms, but none had serious complications associated with the fractures. When symptoms do occur, they are usually palliated by rest and nonnarcotic analgesic drugs. Surgical intervention is rarely, if ever, indicated.

Soft Tissue Effects

Unless the vulva or groins are included in the treatment field, modern RT techniques usually do not cause long-term skin changes. The long-term effects of vulvar treatment depend on the dose, fractionation, and volume irradiated and on the degree of tissue damage from tumor and previous surgery (Chapter 12). However, patients who receive 60 Gy or more

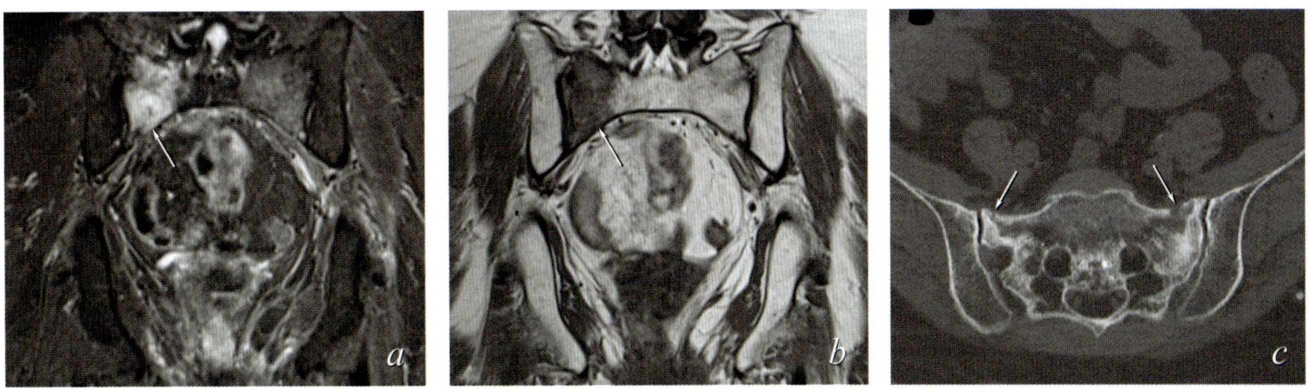

FIGURE 9.8 Pelvic insufficiency fractures in a 78-year-old woman treated with chemoradiation for vulvar cancer. The patient had a long-standing history of severe osteoporosis. One year after treatment, MRI showed early signs of pelvic insufficiency, with marrow edema characterized by high signal intensity on T2 *(arrow, a)* and depressed signal intensity on T1 *(arrow, b)*; findings involved both sacral alae but were greater on the right side than the left side of the body. Several nondisplaced fracture lines were noted. Six months later, CT showed progression with patchy areas of sclerosis and bilateral minimally displaced sacral alar fractures *(arrows, c)*.

to the skin surface and subcutaneous tissues may develop late changes that include hyperpigmentation, telangiectasia, or subcutaneous fibrosis (**CS 12.9**). Prepubic edema is a common late side effect of comprehensive RT of the groins and vulva, particularly if the patient has also had an inguinal lymph node dissection.

Radiation-related neurologic complications are also rare unless patients receive a very high effective dose to the sacral plexus. In an informal review based on a database of ~7,500 patients treated with RT for cervical or vaginal cancer at MD Anderson between 1960 and 2012, we found 18 patients who developed lower extremity weakness that was not clearly explained by cancer or other non–radiation-related causes. Half of these patients received 60 Gy or more to the central pelvis for treatment of stage III disease during the 1960s and 1970s. Most others received usual doses of 40 to 45 Gy. In general, it is wise to avoid exposing the sacral plexus to more than 60 Gy whenever possible (**CS 15.1**). Stereotactic techniques that use very high doses per fraction should also be used with great caution in this region (**Fig. 9.9**).

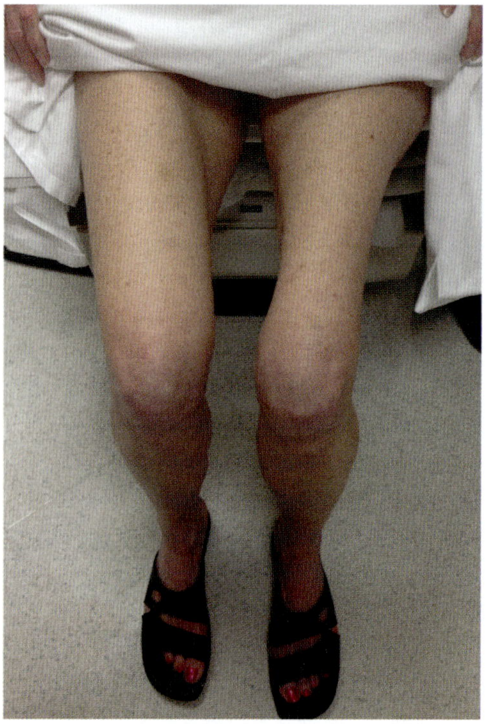

FIGURE 9.9 Photograph of a 59-year-old woman who was treated with CyberKnife RT for ovarian cancer recurrent on the left pelvic side wall. She received a prescribed dose of 30 Gy in three fractions to the gross tumor volume only. She had marked improvement in her pain and returned to normal activity, but ~8 months after completion of RT, she began to develop progressive hypoesthesia, weakness, and atrophy of the left leg. Five years after completion of RT, she developed new buttock pain and was referred after she was discovered to have a 2-cm recurrence of her disease at the distal margin of the CyberKnife treatment. At the time of referral, the patient had persistent numbness and weakness of the left leg but was able to walk with a cane.

RISK OF AND SURVEILLANCE FOR SECOND MALIGNANCIES

The diagnosis of cancer should not be allowed to interfere with a patient's routine cancer screening program. In fact, patients treated for gynecologic cancer frequently are at greater risk for developing a new cancer than the general population for several reasons, including environmental factors, genetic factors, and the treatment for the gynecologic cancer.

Patients who have one HPV-related or smoking-related cancer are at increased risk for developing another. In a large population-based study, Chaturvedi et al. reported that patients who were treated for cervical cancer had an increased risk of developing other HPV-related cancers (cancers of the vagina, vulva, anus, and pharynx) or smoking-associated cancers (cancers of the pharynx, lung, pancreas, and bladder) whether or not they had received RT as part of their cervical cancer treatment.[56] In particular, compared with the general population, patients treated for cervical cancer had five times the risk of developing second lower genital tract cancers, whether or not they had received RT. When irradiated and nonirradiated patients were compared with each other, the irradiated patients appeared to have a greater risk of second cancers than those treated with surgery alone.[56] However, this may be difficult to interpret because MD Anderson data suggest that patients with cervical cancer treated with RT have a greater risk of second vaginal cancers if they were initially treated for locally advanced disease (**Fig. 9.1a**).[3] There are several potential explanations for this MD Anderson finding, including the possibility that patients who present with more advanced cancers are less likely to seek regular preventative care and are, therefore, less likely to have second cancers detected at a preinvasive stage.[3]

Several studies have suggested that patients treated with radiation for cervical or endometrial cancer have an increased risk of developing bladder or colorectal cancer.[56,57] Other studies have failed to detect an increased risk of these cancers.[58] Interestingly, several studies have suggested that the risk of breast cancer is actually decreased in cervical cancer survivors.[56] In the study by Chaturvedi et al.,[56] patients treated with radiation for cervical cancer did not have significantly increased risks of second cancers of the ovary and uterus. However, when endometrial cancers do occur in previously irradiated patients, they tend to be high-grade cancers.[59]

As discussed in Chapter 1, some patients with uterine or ovarian cancers may also have genetic syndromes that increase their risks of second cancers. However, there is as yet no evidence that pelvic irradiation increases these patients' risk of developing second cancers.

For all these reasons, patients who have been treated for gynecologic cancers should be discharged from treatment with an appropriate risk-stratified plan for routine cancer surveillance. All patients, particularly those treated for HPV-related cancers should have annual pelvic examinations and Pap testing for lower genital tract cancers. All patients should have screening colonoscopy at least every 10 years and routine mammograms. For patients with genetic syndromes that increase the risk of cancer, genetic counseling should be obtained to determine the optimal schedule for cancer surveillance.

References

1. Hewitt M, Greenfield S, Stovall E. *From Cancer Patient to Cancer Survivor: Lost in Transition*. Washington, DC: National Academies Press; 2006.
2. Blanch-Hartigan D, Forsythe LP, Alfano CM, et al. Provision and discussion of survivorship care plans among cancer survivors: results of a nationally representative survey of oncologists and primary care physicians. *J Clin Oncol.* 2014;32:1578–1585.
3. Eifel PJ, Jhingran A, Brown J, et al. Time course and outcome of central recurrence after radiation therapy for carcinoma of the cervix. *Int J Gynecol Cancer.* 2006;16:1106–1111.
4. Frank SJ, Jhingran A, Levenback C, et al. Definitive radiation therapy for squamous cell carcinoma of the vagina. *Int J Radiat Oncol Biol Phys.* 2005;62:138–147.
5. Koay EJ, Jhingran A, Klopp AH, et al. Factors associated with long-term survival in locally-advanced squamous cell carcinoma of the vulva treated with definitive radiation therapy. *Int J Radiat Oncol Biol Phys.* 2013;87:S129.
6. Vargo JA, Kim H, Houser CJ, et al. Definitive salvage for vaginal recurrence of endometrial cancer: the impact of modern intensity-modulated-radiotherapy with image-based HDR brachytherapy and the interplay of the PORTEC 1 risk stratification. *Radiother Oncol.* 2014;113:126–131.
7. Scholten AN, van Putten WL, Beerman H, et al. Postoperative radiotherapy for Stage 1 endometrial carcinoma: long-term outcome of the randomized PORTEC trial with central pathology review. *Int J Radiat Oncol Biol Phys.* 2005;63:834–838.
8. Grigsby PW. PET/CT imaging to guide cervical cancer therapy. *Future Oncol.* 2009;5:953–958.
9. Osborne E, Klopp A, Jhingran A, et al. Definitive extended-field radiation therapy for cervical cancer patients with para-aortic lymph node metastases. *Int J Radiat Oncol Biol Phys.* 2015;93:S202–S203.
10. Brooks RA, Rader JS, Dehdashti F, et al. Surveillance FDG-PET detection of asymptomatic recurrences in patients with cervical cancer. *Gynecol Oncol.* 2009;112:104–109.
11. Sironi S, Picchio M, Landoni C, et al. Post-therapy surveillance of patients with uterine cancers: value of integrated FDG PET/CT in the detection of recurrence. *Eur J Nucl Med Mol Imaging.* 2007;34:472–479.
12. Beadle BM, Jhingran A, Yom SS, et al. Patterns of regional recurrence after definitive radiotherapy for cervical cancer. *Int J Radiat Oncol Biol Phys.* 2010;76(5):1396–1403.
13. Shirvani SM, Klopp AH, Likhacheva A, et al. Intensity modulated radiation therapy for definitive treatment of paraaortic relapse in patients with endometrial cancer. *Pract Radiat Oncol.* 2013;3:e21–e28.
14. National Comprehensive Cancer Network. *Uterine Neoplasms (Version 2.2016)*. Available at http://www.nccn.org/professionals/physician_gls/pdf/uterine.pdf. Accessed February 23, 2016.
15. National Comprehensive Cancer Network. *Cervical Cancer (Version 2.2016)*. Available at http://www.nccn.org/professionals/physician_gls/pdf/cervical.pdf. Accessed February 23, 2016.
16. Salani R, Backes FJ, Fung MF, et al. Posttreatment surveillance and diagnosis of recurrence in women with gynecologic malignancies: Society of Gynecologic Oncologists recommendations. *Am J Obstet Gynecol.* 2011;204:466–478.
17. Schwarz JK, Siegel BA, Dehdashti F, et al. Association of posttherapy positron emission tomography with tumor response and survival in cervical carcinoma. *JAMA.* 2007;298:2289–2295.
18. Hunn J, Tenney ME, Tergas AI, et al. Patterns and utility of routine surveillance in high grade endometrial cancer. *Gynecol Oncol.* 2015;137:485–489.
19. Salani R, Nagel CI, Drennen E, et al. Recurrence patterns and surveillance for patients with early stage endometrial cancer. *Gynecol Oncol.* 2011;123:205–207.
20. Bodurka-Bevers D, Morris M, Eifel PJ, et al. Posttherapy surveillance of women with cervical cancer: an outcomes analysis. *Gynecol Oncol.* 2000;78:187–193.
21. Zanagnolo V, Minig LA, Gadducci A, et al. Surveillance procedures for patients for cervical carcinoma: a review of the literature. *Int J Gynecol Cancer.* 2009;19:306–313.
22. Mirabeau-Beale KL, Viswanathan AN. Quality of life (QOL) in women treated for gynecologic malignancies with radiation therapy: a literature review of patient-reported outcomes. *Gynecol Oncol.* 2014;134:403–409.
23. Abbott-Anderson K, Kwekkeboom KL. A systematic review of sexual concerns reported by gynecological cancer survivors. *Gynecol Oncol.* 2012;124:477–489.
24. Frumovitz M, Sun CC, Schover LR, et al. Quality of life and sexual functioning in cervical cancer survivors. *J Clin Oncol.* 2005;23:7428–7436.
25. Westin SN, Sun CC, Tung CS, et al. Survivors of gynecologic malignancies: impact of treatment on health and well-being. *J Cancer Surviv.* 2016;10:261–270.
26. Park HS, Ratner ES, Lucarelli L, et al. Predictors of vaginal stenosis after intravaginal high-dose-rate brachytherapy for endometrial carcinoma. *Brachytherapy.* 2015;14:464–470.
27. Sorbe B, Nordstrom B, Maenpaa J, et al. Intravaginal brachytherapy in FIGO stage I low-risk endometrial cancer: a controlled randomized study. *Int J Gynecol Cancer.* 2009;19:873–878.
28. Miles T, Johnson N. Vaginal dilator therapy for women receiving pelvic radiotherapy. *Cochrane Database Syst Rev.* 2014;(9):CD007291.
29. Barakat RR, Bundy BN, Spirtos NM, et al.; Gynecologic Oncology Group Study. Randomized double-blind trial of estrogen replacement therapy versus placebo in stage I or II endometrial cancer: a Gynecologic Oncology Group Study. *J Clin Oncol.* 2006;24:587–592.
30. Morrow PK, Mattair DN, Hortobagyi GN. Hot flashes: a review of pathophysiology and treatment modalities. *Oncologist.* 2011;16:1658–1664.
31. Loprinzi CL, Barton DL, Qin R. Nonestrogenic management of hot flashes. *J Clin Oncol.* 2011;29:3842–3846.
32. Eifel PJ, Jhingran A, Bodurka DC, et al. Correlation of smoking history and other patient characteristics with major complications of pelvic radiation therapy for cervical cancer. *J Clin Oncol.* 2002;20:3651–3657.
33. Eifel PJ, Levenback C, Wharton JT, et al. Time course and incidence of late complications in patients treated with radiation therapy for FIGO stage IB carcinoma of the uterine cervix. *Int J Radiat Oncol Biol Phys.* 1995;32:1289–1300.
34. Vargo JA, Beriwal S. Image-based brachytherapy for cervical cancer. *World J Clin Oncol.* 2014;5:921–930.

35. Andreyev HJ, Muls AC, Norton C, et al. Guidance: the practical management of the gastrointestinal symptoms of pelvic radiation disease. *Frontline Gastroenterol.* 2015;6:53–72.
36. Andreyev HJ, Davidson SE, Gillespie C, et al. Practice guidance on the management of acute and chronic gastrointestinal problems arising as a result of treatment for cancer. *Gut.* 2012;61:179–192.
37. Sanguineti G, Franzone P, Marcenaro M, et al. Sucralfate versus mesalazine versus hydrocortisone in the prevention of acute radiation proctitis during conformal radiotherapy for prostate carcinoma. A randomized study. *Strahlenther Onkol.* 2003;179:464–470.
38. Laterza L, Cecinato P, Guido A, et al. Management of radiation-induced rectal bleeding. *Curr Gastroenterol Rep.* 2013;15:355.
39. Glover M, Smerdon GR, Andreyev HJ, et al. Hyperbaric oxygen for patients with chronic bowel dysfunction after pelvic radiotherapy (HOT2): a randomised, double-blind, sham-controlled phase 3 trial. *Lancet Oncol.* 2016;17:224–233.
40. Hauer-Jensen M, Denham JW, Andreyev HJ. Radiation enteropathy—pathogenesis, treatment and prevention. *Nat Rev Gastroenterol Hepatol.* 2014;11:470–479.
41. Nout RA, van de Poll-Franse LV, Lybeert ML, et al. Long-term outcome and quality of life of patients with endometrial carcinoma treated with or without pelvic radiotherapy in the post operative radiation therapy in endometrial carcinoma 1 (PORTEC-1) trial. *J Clin Oncol.* 2011;29:1692–1700.
42. Logsdon MD, Eifel PJ. Figo IIIB squamous cell carcinoma of the cervix: an analysis of prognostic factors emphasizing the balance between external beam and intracavitary radiation therapy. *Int J Radiat Oncol Biol Phys.* 1999;43:763–775.
43. Ghezzi F, Cromi A, Serati M, et al. Radiation-induced bowel complications: laparoscopic versus open staging of gynecologic malignancy. *Ann Surg Oncol.* 2011;18:782–791.
44. Ferreira MR, Muls A, Dearnaley DP, et al. Microbiota and radiation-induced bowel toxicity: lessons from inflammatory bowel disease for the radiation oncologist. *Lancet Oncol.* 2014;15:e139–147.
45. Bristol stool form scale. Available at http://bowelcontrol.nih.gov/bristol.aspx. Accessed March 1, 2016.
46. Verma J, Sulman EP, Jhingran A, et al. Dosimetric predictors of duodenal toxicity after intensity modulated radiation therapy for treatment of the para-aortic nodes in gynecologic cancer. *Int J Radiat Oncol Biol Phys.* 2014;88:357–362.
47. Yoon H, Oh D, Park HC, et al. Predictive factors for gastroduodenal toxicity based on endoscopy following radiotherapy in patients with hepatocellular carcinoma. *Strahlenther Onkol.* 2013;189: 541–546.
48. Levenback C, Eifel PJ, Burke TW, et al. Hemorrhagic cystitis following radiotherapy for stage Ib cancer of the cervix. *Gynecol Oncol.* 1994;55:206–210.
49. Viswanathan AN, Yorke ED, Marks LB, et al. Radiation dose–volume effects of the urinary bladder. *Int J Radiat Oncol Biol Phys.* 2010;76:S116–S122.
50. Zwaans BM, Chancellor MB, Lamb LE. Modeling and treatment of radiation cystitis. *Urology.* 2016;88:14–21.
51. McIntyre JF, Eifel PJ, Levenback C, et al. Ureteral stricture as a late complication of radiotherapy for stage IB carcinoma of the uterine cervix. *Cancer.* 1995;75:836–843.
52. Grigsby PW, Roberts HL, Perez CA. Femoral neck fracture following groin irradiation. *Int J Radiat Oncol Biol Phys.* 1995;32:63–67.
53. Blomlie V, Rofstad EK, Talle K, et al. Incidence of radiation-induced insufficiency fractures of the female pelvis: evaluation with MR imaging. *AJR Am J Roentgenol.* 1996;167: 1205–1210.
54. Wernle JD, Damron TA, Allen MJ, et al. Local irradiation alters bone morphology and increases bone fragility in a mouse model. *J Biomech.* 2010;43:2738–2746.
55. Schmeler KM, Jhingran A, Iyer RB, et al. Pelvic fractures after radiotherapy for cervical cancer: implications for survivors. *Cancer.* 2010;116:625–630.
56. Chaturvedi AK, Engels EA, Gilbert ES, et al. Second cancers among 104,760 survivors of cervical cancer: evaluation of long-term risk. *J Natl Cancer Inst.* 2007;99:1634–1643.
57. Onsrud M, Cvancarova M, Hellebust TP, et al. Long-term outcomes after pelvic radiation for early-stage endometrial cancer. *J Clin Oncol.* 2013;31:3951–3956.
58. Wiltink LM, Nout RA, Fiocco M, et al. No increased risk of second cancer after radiotherapy in patients treated for rectal or endometrial cancer in the randomized TME, PORTEC-1, and PORTEC-2 trials. *J Clin Oncol.* 2015;33:1640–1646.
59. Pothuri B, Ramondetta L, Eifel P, et al. Radiation-associated endometrial cancers are prognostically unfavorable tumors: a clinicopathologic comparison with 527 sporadic endometrial cancers. *Gynecol Oncol.* 2006;103:948–951.

PART III

SITE-SPECIFIC INDICATIONS AND TECHNIQUES

CHAPTER 10

Cervical Cancer

INTRODUCTION

Invasive cervical cancer is relatively rare in developed countries, and only about 12,000 new cases are diagnosed each year in the United States.[1] However, invasive cervical cancer remains a major public health problem in medically underserved communities and is the most common cause of cancer death for women in many developing countries. The high frequency of cervical cancer in young mothers contributes to a disproportionate socioeconomic impact of the disease.

As discussed in Chapter 1, more than 99% of cervical carcinomas arise as a direct result of sexual transmission of human papillomavirus (HPV), which in some cases leads to the development of intraepithelial neoplasia and ultimately invasive cervical cancer. The long preinvasive phase of most cervical cancers has enabled successful prevention programs based on cytologic screening, screening for high-risk HPV, and treatment of high-grade squamous intraepithelial lesions. Primarily because of differences in access to screening and treatment, there are large socioeconomic, racial, and national disparities in the incidence rates of invasive cervical cancer. For example, in the United States, the incidence of invasive cervical cancer in non-Hispanic White women is about half that in Black women and about 70% that in Hispanic women; the incidence in women whose family income is at least twice the poverty threshold is one-third to one-half the incidence in women who have lower family incomes.[2]

Although safe sexual practices reduce the risk of HPV infection, recent development of an effective HPV vaccine offers the greatest chance for achieving a major reduction in the incidence of cervical cancer (Chapter 1). However, to be effective, the vaccine must be administered before infection occurs. Because of the long latent period from HPV infection to development of invasive cervical cancer and because of low vaccination rates in the United States and elsewhere, it will be many years before introduction of the HPV vaccine has a major impact on cervical cancer incidence.

Cervical cancer was one of the first cancers to be treated successfully with radiation therapy (RT); the first encouraging reports of cervical cancer treatment with radiation came within 5 years of the discovery of radium. There remain few diseases for which the radiation oncologist plays a more central role in treatment and few diseases that pose more difficult management challenges.

Because the close proximity of the cervix to the bladder, ureters, and rectum limits the resectability of bulky cervical cancers, RT is usually the treatment of choice for locoregionally advanced disease. Definitive RT is highly effective in the treatment of such cancers; however, the best results are achieved with combinations of external beam irradiation, brachytherapy, and chemotherapy that are technically complex and have significant acute adverse effects. This complicated multimodality treatment makes the management of this disease particularly challenging. Cure of locoregionally advanced cervical cancer requires control of local disease. Distant metastases are rarely present at diagnosis, and even cancers that are locoregionally extensive can often be cured if locoregional control can be achieved **(CS 10.6 to 10.10)**. The salvage options for most recurrences of locoregionally advanced disease are poor, and thus, the success of initial treatment is particularly crucial. However, patients who have localized recurrences in unirradiated sites can sometimes be cured with definitive chemoradiation **(CS 10.7 and 10.9)**.

For patients treated with initial hysterectomy, adjuvant RT reduces pelvic recurrences and probably improves survival **(CS 10.1 and 10.2)**.

The demographics of cervical cancer can limit access to high-quality care in two major ways. First, most cases occur in regions of the world that are medically underserved and have limited access to the diagnostic tools and treatments that may yield the best results. Second, in developed countries, the rarity of cervical cancer cases makes it difficult for most clinicians to maintain the specialized technical skills required for optimal disease management. In particular, in the United States, where RT has become increasingly decentralized, most nonacademic practices treat fewer than two to three cases of intact cervical cancer per year. Surveys have revealed that patients treated in nonacademic practices are, on average, more likely to have protracted or incomplete treatment and less likely to receive brachytherapy than those treated in academic centers.[3] These disparities, the reasons for which are probably multifactorial, highlight some of the challenges faced by radiation oncologists and their cervical cancer patients.

This chapter focuses on the factors used to guide treatment choices for cervical cancer and the strategies used to combine multiple modalities to deliver treatment optimally. Technical details of external beam irradiation and brachytherapy are discussed in greater detail in Chapters 6 and 8, respectively.

PRETREATMENT EVALUATION AND STAGING

Thorough and accurate pretreatment evaluation is a critical step in the curative treatment of cervical cancer. The goals of pretreatment evaluation are as follows:

- *To determine the extent of the primary tumor.* Although even large cervical tumors may remain grossly confined to the cervix, tumors also may infiltrate the adjacent supporting ligaments (Chapter 5), vagina, uterine body, and, rarely, bladder or rectum. The size and distribution of cancer in the cervix and uterus and the presence and pattern of paracervical tumor infiltration influence the design of external beam RT fields and the details of subsequent brachytherapy.
- *To determine whether hydronephrosis is present.* Locally advanced tumors can cause ureteral compromise that influences the stage of disease and, if untreated, can affect chemotherapy tolerance (Chapter 7).
- *To determine the extent of regional disease.* Cervical cancers generally follow a fairly orderly pattern of regional spread to pelvic and, secondarily, paraaortic nodes (Chapter 5). Even extensive nodal disease can often be cured if it is detected and treated with an adequate radiation dose.
- *To determine whether distant metastases are present.* Although extremely rare in patients with early-stage squamous carcinomas of the cervix, distant metastases are sometimes present at diagnosis in patients who have very extensive local disease or high-risk histologic types, such as small cell neuroendocrine cancer. For patients who have distant metastases, chemotherapy is rarely, if ever, curative; distant metastases should always be confirmed histologically before a decision is made not to administer potentially curative local treatment.
- *To determine the patient's overall medical condition.* All patients require a detailed history and physical examination to evaluate their level of pain and distress and to identify any medical conditions that could affect their ability to tolerate treatment.
- *To assign an FIGO (International Federation of Gynecology and Obstetrics) stage.* All patients should have a stage assigned, using the FIGO clinical staging system (**Table 10.1**).

All patients with cervical cancer require standard laboratory studies, including complete blood cell count, measurement of electrolyte levels, and renal and liver function studies, to determine their fitness for treatment.

The following studies are particularly useful in the evaluation of patients with cervical cancer:

- *Physical examination.* Even advanced imaging techniques do not obviate the need for a careful physical examination. The size, morphology, and mobility of the tumor and the presence of paracervical and vaginal extension should be carefully noted and described. If there is more than minimal vaginal involvement, fiducial markers can be placed at the distal extent of disease to help with treatment planning for external beam irradiation and subsequent brachytherapy. Pelvic examination is discussed in more detail in Chapter 4.
- *Magnetic resonance imaging (MRI).* The excellent soft tissue detail provided by MRI makes it the most useful study for the evaluation of the cervix and paracervical tissues.[6,7] However, it should be remembered that there are few published studies on the accuracy of MRI findings (particularly those regarding early paracervical involvement) in patients with locally advanced cervical cancer (Chapter 4). For patients with early-stage disease, MRI can be used to estimate the extent of cervical stromal involvement and may be helpful in determining whether patients should be treated with primary surgery or primary RT. For patients with adenocarcinoma involving the cervix, MRI can be used to evaluate the distribution of disease in the cervix and uterus and suggest the most likely primary tumor site. MRI can also yield important information about the extent of paracervical involvement, the position of the uterus, and the conformation of the cervicouterine canal—details that are particularly important for brachytherapy treatment planning. MRI can also provide information about the disease status of regional nodes and clarify the nature of fluorodeoxyglucose (FDG)-avid pelvic wall lesions (e.g., differentiate involved nodes from physiologically active ovaries). As discussed in

TABLE 10.1 FIGO Clinical Staging System for Carcinoma of the Uterine Cervix (2009)

FIGO stage		TNM categories
	Primary tumor cannot be assessed	TX
I	The carcinoma is strictly confined to the cervix (extension to the uterine corpus should be disregarded)	T1
IA[a]	Invasive cancer identified only microscopically (all macroscopically visible lesions—even with superficial invasion—are stage IB/T1b). Invasion is limited to measured stromal invasion with a maximum depth of 5 mm and no wider than 7 mm	T1a
IA1	Stromal invasion no more than 3.0 mm in depth and 7.0 or less in horizontal spread	T1a1
IA2	Stromal invasion more than 3.0 mm and not more than 5.0 mm with a horizontal spread 7.0 mm or less	T1a2
IB[b]	Clinically visible lesion confined to the cervix or microscopic lesion greater than IA2/T1a2	T1b
IB1	Clinically visible lesion 4.0 cm or less in greatest dimension	T1b1
IB2	Clinically visible lesion more than 4.0 cm in greatest dimension	T1b2
II	Tumor invades beyond the uterus but not to the pelvic wall or to the lower third of the vagina	T2
IIA	Without parametrial extension	T2a
IIA1	Tumor size no more than 4 cm with involvement of less than the upper two-thirds of the vagina	T2a1
IIA2	Tumor size more than 4 cm with involvement of less than the upper two-thirds of the vagina	T2a2
III[c]	Tumor extends to the pelvic wall and/or involves the lower third of the vagina and/or causes hydronephrosis or nonfunctioning kidney	T3
IIIA	Tumor extends to the lower third of the vagina; no extension to the pelvic wall	T3a
IIIB	Tumor extends to the pelvic wall and/or causes hydronephrosis or nonfunctioning kidney	T3b
IVA[d]	Tumor involves mucosa of the bladder or rectum and/or extends beyond the true pelvis	T4
IVB	Distant metastasis	M1

FIGO notes about clinical staging:

[a]The diagnosis of both stages Ia1 and Ia2 should be based on microscopic examination of removed tissue, preferably a cone biopsy, which must include the entire lesion. The depth of invasion should not be more than 5 mm measured from the base of the epithelium, either surface or glandular, from which it originates. The depth of invasion is defined as the measurement of the tumor from the epithelial-stromal junction of the adjacent most superficial epithelial papilla to the deepest point of invasion. Vascular space involvement, venous or lymphatic, does not affect classification. Larger lesions should be staged as IB.

[b]As a rule, it is impossible to clinically estimate if a cancer of the cervix has extended to the corpus. Extension to the corpus should therefore be disregarded.

[c]A patient with a growth fixed to the pelvic wall by a short and indurated, but not nodular, parametrium should be allotted to stage IIB. It is impossible at clinical examination to decide whether a smooth and indurated parametrium is truly cancerous or only inflammatory. Therefore, the case should be placed in stage III only if the parametrium is nodular to the pelvic wall or if the growth itself extends to the pelvic wall.

[d]The presence of bullous edema is not sufficient to classify a tumor as T4.

From Pecorelli S, Zigliani L, Odicino F. Revised FIGO staging for carcinoma of the cervix. Int J Gynaecol Obstet. 2009;105:107–108; Benedet JL, Bender H, Jones H III, et al. FIGO staging classifications and clinical practice guidelines in the management of gynecologic cancers. FIGO Committee on Gynecologic Oncology. Int J Gynaecol Obstet. 2000;70:209–262. Refs.[4,5]

Chapter 8, MRI is also increasingly being used for image-guided brachytherapy (**CS 10.4 and 10.5**).

- *Cystoscopy and proctoscopy*. Any patient who has findings suggesting bladder or rectal involvement on MRI or physical examination should have cystoscopy to confirm or rule out bladder involvement or proctoscopy to confirm or rule out rectal involvement. Biopsy proof of bladder or rectal mucosal involvement is required to classify cervical cancer as stage IVA (**Table 10.1**).

- *Positron emission tomography–computed tomography (PET–CT).* PET–CT is currently the most accurate noninvasive method for detecting nodal metastases from cervical cancer.[8,9] PET–CT can also detect hydronephrosis and is a sensitive method for detecting distant disease. PET–CT is extremely helpful in treatment planning for patients with extensive nodal disease. For these reasons, PET–CT is recommended for most patients with greater than stage IB1 cervical cancer. PET–CT is also useful in the evaluation of response to treatment (Chapter 7). For further discussion of the advantages and limitations of PET, see Chapter 4.

- *Contrast-enhanced CT.* If PET is unavailable, contrast-enhanced CT of the chest, abdomen, and pelvis can be used for detection of nodal and distant metastases, although the sensitivity of this technique is lower than that of PET–CT. Contrast-enhanced CT can also provide some useful information about the size of cervical tumors, although the soft tissue detail is far inferior to that of MRI.

For patients who are to have surgical treatment for stage IA or IB1 cancers, physical examination, chest radiography, and laboratory studies are usually sufficient for preoperative evaluation; in selected cases, MRI may help to select the best initial treatment by delineating the extent and distribution of tumor in the cervix and uterus. For patients with more advanced lesions, the ideal evaluation probably includes pelvic examination, MRI of the pelvis, and PET–CT, with endoscopic studies reserved for patients who have radiologic evidence of organ involvement. All patients who have neuroendocrine tumors should be evaluated for the presence of metastatic disease; this evaluation usually includes CT or MRI of the brain, although the yield is low for patients who do not have other evidence of distant disease.

In low-resource settings, CT of the chest, abdomen, and pelvis may be performed in place of MRI or MRI and PET–CT as a less sensitive but still useful method of detection of locoregional and distant disease.

Although nodal findings from tomographic imaging studies do not influence stage in the current FIGO clinical staging system, some form of imaging to rule out gross nodal involvement should always be performed because the incidence of nodal involvement in cervical cancer is high and failure to deliver a sufficient dose of radiation to sites of gross disease is likely to lead to fatal infield disease recurrences. Patients with locoregionally advanced disease also require some form of imaging to rule out the presence of hydronephrosis.

RISK ASSESSMENT

Before the clinician can offer informed treatment recommendations or counsel the patient about her prognosis, a thorough analysis of important risk factors for pelvic disease recurrence, nodal and distant metastases, and death from cervical cancer is necessary. Although all newly diagnosed cancers are classified in terms of FIGO stage, treatment decisions and assessment of prognosis are heavily influenced by factors not reflected in or incompletely addressed in the FIGO staging system.

FIGO Stage

The internationally accepted FIGO clinical staging system is based primarily on findings from physical examination, plain film radiography, and, where appropriate, cystoscopy, proctoscopy, and cone biopsy (**Table 10.1**). Although FIGO stage is correlated with outcome, it does not take into account many of the most important prognostic indicators, most notable among them the presence of nodal metastases. In the FIGO clinical staging system, most findings that are detectable by modern tomographic imaging studies, including distant metastases, cannot be used to alter the clinical stage unless these findings are also detectable by physical examination or other approved studies.

Since its inception in the early 20th century, the FIGO clinical staging system has had the same four major categories. However, the system has been amended a number of times, most notably to refine the definition of stage IA in 1994 and to subdivide the stage IB and IIA categories according to tumor diameter in 1994 and 2009, respectively. Also in 2009, FIGO for the first time permitted tomographic imaging findings to influence primary tumor classifications, stating, "The use of diagnostic imaging techniques to assess the size of the primary tumor is encouraged but is not mandatory. Other investigations (i.e., examination under anesthesia, cystoscopy, sigmoidoscopy, intravenous pyelography) are optional and no longer mandatory."[4] Presumably, the "other investigations" can only be excluded if some other method is used to assess for bladder, ureteral, and rectal involvement.

Under the 2009 FIGO clinical staging system, regional metastases detected by CT, MRI, or PET still cannot be used to alter the FIGO stage; as a result, only rare patients who have palpable pelvic lymphadenopathy can have their stage increased (to stage IIIB) on the basis of nodal metastases. This policy has been maintained by FIGO for several reasons:

- Most cervical cancers are diagnosed in underdeveloped countries that have limited access to advanced imaging methods.

- Most locally advanced cervical cancers are not surgically staged.

- Because the methods used to evaluate nodal involvement (CT, MRI, PET, lymphadenectomy, etc.) have widely varying sensitivities and specificities, their incorporation into the staging system would cause hidden inconsistencies that would confound outcome comparisons.

FIGO has defined a supplemental pathologic staging system for patients who undergo primary treatment with radical hysterectomy and lymphadenectomy (**Table 10.2**).

TABLE 10.2 FIGO/UICC Stage Grouping for Patients Treated with Radical Hysterectomy and Lymphadenectomy[a]

Stage	T	N	M
IA1	T_{1a1}	N_0	M_0
IA2	T_{1a2}	N_0	M_0
IB1	T_{1b1}	N_0	M_0
IB2	T_{1b2}	N_0	M_0
IIA1	T_{2a1}	N_0	M_0
IIA2	T_{2a2}	N_0	M_0
IIB	T_{2b}	N_0	M_0
IIIa	T_{3a}	N_0	M_0
IIIB	T_1 T_2 T_{3a} T_{3b}	N_1 N_1 N_1 Any N	M_0 M_0 M_0 M_0
IVA	T_4	Any N	M_0
IVB	Any T	Any N	M_1

FIGO, International Federation of Gynecology and Obstetrics; UICC, International Union Against Cancer; T, tumor; N, nodes; M, metastasis.

[a]*This pathologic staging system can only be applied to patients whose initial treatment is radical hysterectomy (or radical trachelectomy) with pelvic lymphadenectomy. Assignment of a pathologic TNM stage to such patients is reasonable. However, we do not recommend the use of the Roman numeral stage assignments, which are too easily confused with the very different FIGO clinical stage categories.*

From Pecorelli S, Zigliani L, Odicino F. Revised FIGO staging for carcinoma of the cervix. Int J Gynaecol Obstet. 2009;105:107–108. Ref.[4]

This system is meant only for patients who undergo primary surgical treatment; it should never be applied in other cases. Unfortunately, the FIGO pathologic staging system is often published without the rules for its application, causing it to be misapplied in various ways to cases of intact cervical cancer and resulting in considerable confusion. The fact that the same stage labels (I, II, III, and IV) are used for the clinical staging system, which ignores evidence of nodal involvement, and the pathologic staging system, which places all surgically treated patients with nodal metastases in the stage IIIB category, has compounded the potential for misunderstanding.

Clinical Characteristics of the Primary Tumor

Tumor Diameter

For patients treated with definitive RT, primary tumor diameter is probably the most important single predictor of central disease recurrence (**Fig. 10.1**)[10]; when the analysis is fully corrected for tumor diameter, other clinical features, such as paracervical involvement, appear to have little influence on local recurrence risk. Tumor diameter is also correlated with the presence of nodal metastases and with overall survival. For patients treated with primary surgery, both clinical tumor diameter and histologic measurement of tumor size are strong predictors of nodal metastasis and of disease recurrence.

Parametrial Involvement

Tumor can infiltrate the paracervical supporting ligaments by direct extension or the parametrial nodes by lymphatic spread. Ever since the FIGO staging system was devised in the early 20th century, that system has included the clinical impression of parametrial involvement as a dominant feature, at least in part because the presence of parametrial involvement has been considered a relative contraindication to primary surgical management. Parametrial involvement should probably still be considered a contraindication to surgery today. However, clinical assessment of parametrial involvement is notoriously inaccurate.[11–13] For example, in a large Austrian series of patients who had radical hysterectomy

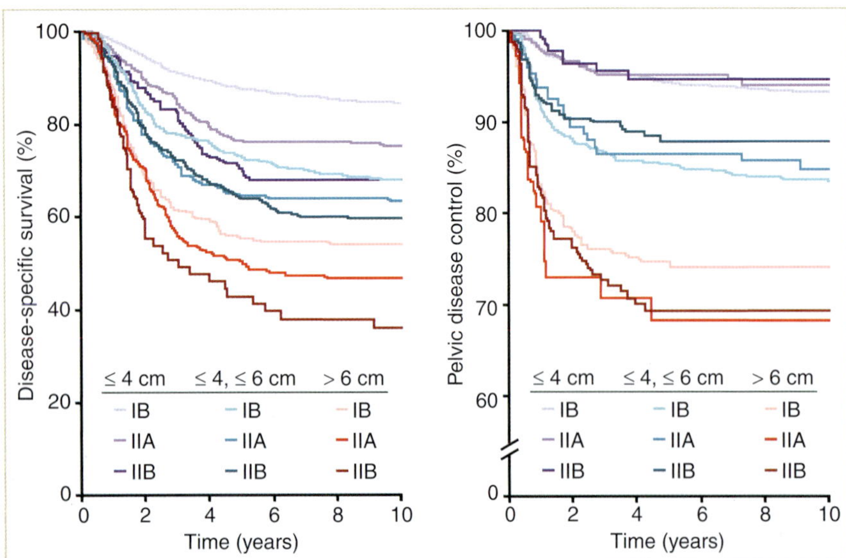

FIGURE 10.1 Disease-specific survival and pelvic disease control rates of 4,490 consecutive patients treated for FIGO stage IB, IIA, or IIB carcinoma of the cervix between 1960 and 2001 at MD Anderson Cancer Center. Primary treatment included RT or hysterectomy; about 6% of the patients who had RT during these years received concurrent chemotherapy. Although both tumor size and FIGO stage influenced disease-specific survival, tumor diameter was the most important predictor of pelvic disease recurrence. (From Eifel PJ, Jhingran A, Levenback CF, et al. Predictive value of a proposed subclassification of stages I and II cervical cancer based on clinical tumor diameter. *Int J Gynecol Cancer.* 2009;19:2–7.)

for stage I to IIB cancer,[11] only 30% of patients diagnosed by physical examination as having "stage IIB" disease actually had histologic evidence of paracervical involvement; this was only slightly more than the 14% rate of parametrial involvement in patients with stage IB disease. Nodular endovaginal disease is commonly confused with parametrial involvement (Chapter 4). Also, large tumors are more likely than smaller tumors to be labeled as stage IIB, confounding the correlation between parametrial involvement and survival. In a large study from MD Anderson,[10] the clinical impression of parametrial involvement did appear to be independently correlated with disease-specific survival but was a poor predictor of pelvic disease control (**Fig. 10.1**). FIGO recently permitted MRI findings of parametrial involvement to be considered in the staging system. It is unclear whether MRI is more accurate than clinical examination in the evaluation of parametrial involvement, but MRI findings are likely to be somewhat more reproducible than findings on clinical examination.

Morphology

As cervical tumors enlarge, they may exhibit a predominantly exophytic, endocervical ("barrel-shaped"), or infiltrative growth pattern. MD Anderson studies have suggested that exophytic tumors are more responsive to RT and tend to have a lower rate of central disease recurrence than do endocervical tumors. In a 1994 study of patients with stage IB cancers, Eifel et al.[14] reported central disease recurrence rates of 3% for exophytic tumors 5 to 7.9 cm in diameter and 9% for predominantly endocervical tumors of similar size, although there was no difference in the overall rate of pelvic disease recurrence. This study predated the use of concurrent chemotherapy and RT (chemoradiation), which has reduced the overall incidence of central disease recurrence and may have blunted or eliminated the independent prognostic impact of morphology.

Pelvic Wall Involvement

Tumors that are fixed to pelvic wall structures are considered stage IIIB. These tend to be large, infiltrative cancers with a relatively poor prognosis. At MD Anderson, the prognosis of patients with stage IIIB disease is very similar to that of patients with earlier-stage cancers that measure 7 cm or more in diameter[10,15]; both groups have 5-year disease-specific survival rates of 50% to 60%.

However, clinical assessment of pelvic wall fixation tends to be highly inaccurate. On the other hand, hydronephrosis, the second criterion for diagnosing stage IIIB disease, is a relatively objective finding. This provides a means for estimating physicians' relative thresholds for interpreting physical findings as pelvic wall involvement—a relatively low proportion of stage IIIB patients having hydronephrosis suggests that physicians are more likely than others to diagnose a patient with questionable findings as having stage IIIB disease. For example, in a 2009 South Korean review, only 44 (11%) of 388 patients treated with radiation for stage IIIB disease between 1986 and 2004 had hydronephrosis.[16] In contrast, 165 (57%) of 287 patients with stage IIIB disease diagnosed at MD Anderson during these same years had hydronephrosis (unpublished data). Unfortunately, the rate of hydronephrosis is rarely reported in reports of locally advanced cervical cancer, making it difficult to estimate the pervasiveness of this cause of stage migration.

A number of factors contribute to overdiagnosis of pelvic wall involvement. Large tumors can fill the lower pelvis without extensively infiltrating adjacent tissues; these may seem immobile until initial response to treatment reveals that the paracervical tissues are free of gross disease. Also, prior pelvic infection can affect the mobility of the uterus. In our experience, MRI rarely demonstrates true direct invasion of lateral pelvic structures. Occasionally, cancer is seen directly invading from the cervix to the piriform muscle via the uterosacral ligaments; this is a poor prognostic sign, usually associated with very advanced disease.

Vaginal Involvement

Unless it is very minimal, vaginal involvement is a relative contraindication to primary surgical treatment because the chance of a positive margin is high. However, involvement of the upper two-thirds of the vagina generally has little independent influence on the prognosis of patients treated with radiation[10] (**Fig. 10.1**). Most patients who have distal vaginal involvement also have massive primary tumors. Stage IIIA cancers that involve the distal vagina without pelvic fixation or hydronephrosis are rare. Some of these cancers are undoubtedly primary vaginal cancers that involved the cervix secondarily but are by convention classified as cervical cancers. Discontinuous involvement of the vagina is a poor prognostic sign,[17] but even patients with this finding can sometimes be cured **(CS 10.8)**.

Hydronephrosis

The finding of hydronephrosis is a poor prognostic sign because it is a sign of extracervical involvement associated with locoregionally advanced cervical cancer and because secondary renal failure can complicate treatment of cervical cancer. Although the relationship between hydronephrosis and prognosis is heavily confounded by other adverse findings, most investigators have found hydronephrosis to be an independent predictor of poor outcome. In our experience, patients with bilateral hydronephrosis do not have a worse prognosis than patients with unilateral hydronephrosis if outcome is corrected for other factors.[15]

Ureteral obstruction usually occurs at the base of the bladder as a result of local tumor infiltration. However, the ureters are also vulnerable to secondary involvement by lymph nodes, particularly in the region just distal to the common iliac bifurcation, where the ureters cross into the pelvis (Fig. 5.2).

Acute or chronic renal compromise and, if treatment does not relieve the ureteral obstruction, long-term adverse effects of urinary diversion can have a significant negative impact on quality of life and long-term survival.

Histologic Type

Squamous Carcinoma

Most primary cervical cancers are squamous carcinomas. Although squamous carcinomas are frequently subclassified according to the cell size, presence or absence of keratin, or degree of cell differentiation, these characteristics are poorly correlated with the likelihood of lymph node metastases and the likelihood of recurrence.[18]

Adenocarcinoma

In the United States and most other economically advanced countries, ~20% to 25% of cervical cancers are adenocarcinomas. This proportion has increased by about 30% since the 1970s, and the proportion of adenocarcinomas relative to squamous carcinomas has about doubled during that time.[19] The increase in adenocarcinomas relative to squamous carcinomas is in large part due to the fact that methods for detection of preinvasive adenocarcinomas are worse than methods for detection of squamous carcinomas.[20] Also, adenocarcinomas are significantly more likely to be associated with HPV-18 than are squamous carcinomas, and some studies have suggested that cytologic screening is less effective in the detection of HPV-18–positive cancers than in the detection of HPV-16–positive cancers.[20]

In general, although adenocarcinomas exhibit a number of morphologic patterns, the pattern does not appear to have a major independent influence on outcome.[21] However, adenocarcinomas differ from squamous carcinomas in that grade appears to be strongly correlated with the risk of recurrence for adenocarcinomas but not for squamous carcinomas. Adenosquamous cancers, which have both glandular and squamous elements, tend to have a particularly poor prognosis,[22] reflecting their high cytologic grade. Whether their prognosis is poorer than that of other high-grade adenocarcinomas is unclear. Serous cancers are rare but, in our experience, tend to exhibit an aggressive behavior similar to that of uterine serous cancers (Chapter 13).

In a 1990 MD Anderson review of more than 367 patients treated with definitive radiation for cervical adenocarcinoma,[23] patients with stage II or III disease were found to have a much higher rate of pelvic and distant recurrence than was typical for squamous carcinomas treated at that institution; remarkably, 73% of patients with stage II adenocarcinoma in that study developed distant metastases. In a separate study of patients treated with radiation only for stage I cervical cancer, adenocarcinoma was found to be an independent risk factor for distant metastases, although the rates of pelvic disease recurrence were similar for squamous carcinoma and adenocarcinoma.[24] Adenocarcinoma may also to be a risk factor for local recurrence after radical hysterectomy, particularly for tumors of high grade with lymphovascular space invasion (LVSI).[23,25]

The prognostic differences between adenocarcinoma and squamous carcinoma appear to be blunted by the use of adjuvant treatments after hysterectomy[26] and by the use of concurrent chemoradiation.[27] For example, a subset analysis of the GOG-92 study suggested that patients with adenocarcinoma received a disproportionate benefit from adjuvant pelvic RT after radical hysterectomy.[26] However, in our experience, concurrent chemoradiation has not eliminated adenocarcinoma as a risk factor for recurrence of locoregionally advanced cervical cancer.[28]

Although the median time to recurrence of adenocarcinoma tends to be short,[22,23] in some cases, the disease can be very indolent, with pelvic disease recurrences not diagnosed until 5 years or more after RT.[23] In our experience, such late recurrences are extremely rare for squamous carcinoma.

Small Cell Neuroendocrine Cancer

Small cell neuroendocrine cancer is a rare subtype of cervical cancer that has a very high rate of distant metastasis and a poor prognosis even after aggressive multimodality treatment.[29,30] It should not be confused with small cell squamous carcinoma.

Lymph Node Metastasis

Lymph node metastasis is a common finding in patients with cervical cancer; 50% or more of patients with locally advanced disease have PET evidence of nodal metastases at diagnosis. The likelihood of lymph node involvement is correlated with tumor size, stage, and depth of invasion, and in surgically treated patients, the presence of LVSI is a strong predictor of lymph node involvement.[31]

The presence of lymph node metastases is correlated with increased rates of pelvic disease recurrence, distant metastases, and death from disease.[10,28,31] However, most patients with lymph node metastases at the time of their initial diagnosis of cervical cancer do not have evidence of synchronous distant metastases. The pattern of nodal metastasis tends to be orderly: paraaortic node metastases are rarely seen in the absence of iliac node metastases. The presence of paraaortic node metastases is associated with a poorer prognosis, although even patients with this finding can be cured in up to 50% of cases[32,33] **(CS 10.5 to 10.10)**.

In a study of 256 patients with node-positive cervical cancer treated with radical hysterectomy and pelvic RT,[34] the rates of relapse and survival were independently correlated with the number of positive lymph nodes and with the presence of extracapsular extension but not with the size of the largest metastatic deposit; the authors did not specifically report the rates of pelvic disease recurrence.

FIGO stage remains only a very crude predictor of prognosis. Although the rigid rules for FIGO staging, if applied correctly, promote some level of international consistency in staging, these rigid rules are also a source of considerable frustration. Ultimately, FIGO stage, although somewhat useful for reporting and comparison of results, is of limited value for treatment planning. The reporting of clinical findings according to the FIGO clinical staging system should always be supplemented with more detailed descriptions of clinical and tumor characteristics.

Risk Factors for Patients Undergoing Radical Hysterectomy

For patients undergoing radical hysterectomy, the finding of any type of extracervical involvement—lymph node metastases, parametrial involvement, or positive surgical margins—is associated with a high risk of pelvic disease recurrence.[12,13,31,35] However, because patients with such findings usually receive adjuvant treatment, the magnitude of the recurrence risk for patients with untreated extracervical involvement is difficult to estimate.

Local cervical tumor features are predictive of both lymph node involvement and outcome. In the GOG-49 study, a classic prospective registry study of patients undergoing radical hysterectomy for FIGO clinical stage I squamous carcinoma, depth of invasion, LVSI, and parametrial involvement were all strongly correlated with lymph node involvement.[36] For patients with involvement of the inner, middle, and outer thirds of the cervical stroma, the risks of lymph node involvement were 5%, 13%, and 26%, respectively; lymph node metastases were found in 25% of patients with LVSI versus 8% of patients without LVSI and 43% of patients with parametrial involvement versus 13% of patients without parametrial involvement. In a second analysis of the GOG-49 results,[31] the authors reported that clinical tumor diameter, depth of invasion, and LVSI were the most powerful predictors of relapse. The results of GOG-49 were refined such that various categories of tumor diameter, depth of invasion, and LVSI were combined to define a group of patients with an intermediate risk for recurrence after radical hysterectomy; these so-called Sedlis criteria were subsequently used to define eligibility for the GOG-92 study of adjuvant pelvic RT (Table 10.3).

More recently, in a large Korean study, Ryu et al.[37] evaluated a variety of potential predictive models using development and validation groups. These authors confirmed the predictive value of the GOG-92 criteria but proposed a different model that was somewhat simpler and appeared to more accurately predict recurrence. In this model, patients who had any two of four findings—tumor diameter >3 cm, invasion of the outer third of the cervical stroma, LVSI, or adenocarcinoma—had a relative risk of recurrence 3.1 times that of patients without none or only one of those findings.

TABLE 10.3 Eligibility Criteria for GOG-92 Study

LVSI	Stromal invasion	Tumor size
Positive	Deep third	Any
Positive	Middle third	≥2 cm
Positive	Superficial third	≥5 cm
Negative	Deep or middle third	≥4 cm

GOG, Gynecologic Oncology Group; LVSI, lymphovascular space invasion.

From Sedlis A, Bundy BN, Rotman MZ, et al. A randomized trial of pelvic radiation therapy versus no further therapy in selected patients with stage IB carcinoma of the cervix after radical hysterectomy and pelvic lymphadenectomy: a Gynecologic Oncology Group Study. Gynecol Oncol. 1999;73:177–183.

MULTIDISCIPLINARY TREATMENT

Today, most patients with cervical cancer are treated with more than one modality. Optimal multidisciplinary management requires close collaboration between radiation oncologists and other care providers. To make informed recommendations about the role of RT, the radiation oncologist must understand the indications for surgery and chemotherapy and the evidence supporting various treatment approaches.

Role of Surgery

Hysterectomy as Initial Treatment of the Primary Tumor

The preferred local treatment for most patients with early-stage cervical cancer (stage IA or IB1) is hysterectomy, and the preferred treatment for most patients with locally advanced cervical cancer is RT. However, a number of factors should be weighed before a final recommendation is made:

- *Is surgical resection possible? If so, how radical a surgical procedure would be needed to remove the cancer?* Stage IA and IB1 cancers generally can be removed with at most a type II radical hysterectomy. For larger cancers, resection with negative surgical margins may be possible, but removal of such cancers usually requires more extensive procedures that are associated with higher rates of bladder atony, fistula, chronic constipation, and other adverse effects (Chapter 3).
- *What is the probability that adjuvant RT would be required after primary surgical treatment?* In the past, the morbidity of open radical hysterectomy followed by pelvic RT was generally believed to exceed that of primary RT alone.[38] For this reason, definitive RT was often preferred if preoperative evaluation revealed high-risk features. Modern laparoscopic techniques and highly conformal RT techniques have reduced the morbidity of combined surgery and RT (Chapter 3). However, the probability that adjuvant RT will be required should be considered when the risks and benefits of different treatment strategies are considered.
- *What is the likelihood that surgical resection would result in a positive surgical margin?* When preoperative evaluation suggests that surgical resection would most likely result in a positive surgical margin, definitive RT is usually the preferred treatment. Because the most common sites for positive margins after hysterectomy are typically beyond the reach of vaginal intracavitary brachytherapy, adjuvant RT after hysterectomy must be delivered with high-dose

external beam RT (**CS 10.2**), which confers a significant risk of late adverse effects.

- *What is the patient's age and medical condition?* For young women with early-stage tumors that would not require adjuvant RT after primary surgical treatment, hysterectomy is nearly always preferred because it preserves ovarian function and avoids the risk of radiation-related adverse effects. In contrast, for elderly women with serious medical comorbidities, definitive RT is often preferred over a major surgical procedure (**CS 10.3**).

For stage IA1 cervical cancer, simple (type I) hysterectomy is usually sufficient treatment; lymphadenectomy is not required because of the very low risk of lymph node metastases. For patients who desire to retain fertility, a cone biopsy with negative margins may be sufficient treatment, but close follow-up is necessary.

For patients with stage IA2 disease, the risk of lymph node involvement is about 5%, and the standard treatment is radical (type II) hysterectomy and pelvic lymphadenectomy. If fertility preservation is desired, radical trachelectomy is an alternative; this procedure has been used without apparent compromise of cure rates.[39] More conservative fertility-sparing procedures, such as cone biopsy and simple trachelectomy with surgical lymph node evaluation, have been explored for patients with stage IA2 disease, but data are insufficient to permit meaningful comparisons between outcomes of these procedures and outcomes of radical hysterectomy.

Radical trachelectomy has also been used to treat selected patients with small stage IB1 cancers who desire fertility preservation. Most experts agree that this surgery should be limited to patients whose tumors are <2 cm in diameter; for these patients, the overall recurrence rate after radical trachelectomy is 3% to 6%, and survival rates are similar to those achieved with radical hysterectomy.[39] Although fertility can be impaired after radical trachelectomy because of cervical stenosis, scarring, and decreased mucous production, 40% to 80% of women attempting to conceive after radical trachelectomy are successful.[39] The rates of preterm delivery, however, are increased; about 12% of third-trimester deliveries occur at <32 weeks.[40] Ongoing studies are exploring the use of simple hysterectomy with lymphatic mapping for patients with low-risk stage IB1 cervical cancers.

Some investigators have attempted to expand the criteria for fertility preservation to tumors more than 2 cm in diameter by using neoadjuvant chemotherapy to reduce the volume of disease. This approach is more controversial, but preliminary results are encouraging.[41]

Today, radical hysterectomy is increasingly being performed laparoscopically with or without robotic assistance, and the laparoscopic approach is associated with significant reduction in operating times, hospital stays, and complications. Several studies are also currently exploring the use of less radical, type I hysterectomy for selected patients with small stage IB1 cancers.

The adverse effects of hysterectomy and lymphadenectomy are discussed in Chapter 3.

Adjuvant Hysterectomy after RT

In the mid-1970s, results of a retrospective review of MD Anderson data suggested that the risk of central disease recurrence might be reduced if patients who had bulky endocervical tumors were treated with adjuvant extrafascial hysterectomy after administration of a slightly reduced dose of pelvic RT and brachytherapy.[42] This approach rapidly gained popularity, particularly in the United States. However, by the 1980s, the approach was no longer routinely used at MD Anderson, and a reexamination of the earlier data suggested that selection bias accounted for the apparent advantage of adding adjuvant hysterectomy after RT.[43] A subsequent randomized trial (GOG-123) showed no difference in overall survival rates between combined treatment and definitive RT only.[44] With concurrent chemoradiation, central disease control rates are high even for patients with stage IB2 disease, and thus, extrafascial hysterectomy is rarely indicated today.

That said, RT followed by extrafascial hysterectomy may be appropriate for certain patients. These include patients who have very extensive uterine body involvement that cannot be adequately treated with brachytherapy because of fundal extension. However, if there is also extensive paracervical extension, such patients are generally still better treated with RT only. In rare cases, RT followed by extrafascial hysterectomy may be used for patients with stage IB2 disease who have massive fibroids that need to be removed because of symptoms, particularly if the fibroids have compromised the quality of brachytherapy coverage (Fig. 8.1d–f).

It is important to remember that combined treatment requires a compromise in the RT and in the surgery to avoid an unacceptable risk of fistula and other complications. The dose of RT must be decreased; in general, the dose to point A should not exceed 75 Gy (equivalent dose at 2 Gy/fraction), and the bladder and rectal doses (minimum dose to the 2 mL receiving the highest dose) should not exceed 65 and 60 Gy, respectively. Also, the recommended surgery after these radiation doses is a type I extrafascial hysterectomy because radical hysterectomy after high-dose RT confers a high risk of fistula. Because of these necessary treatment compromises, combined treatment is not usually recommended for cancers of stage greater than IB2.

Lymphadenectomy for Locally Advanced Cancers

Two possible roles have been proposed for preradiation lymphadenectomy in patients with locally advanced cancer: debulking of grossly enlarged lymph nodes and paraaortic lymph node dissection to determine whether extended radiation fields are needed. Lymphadenectomy has not been clearly demonstrated to be of benefit in either role.[45] In practice, we rarely recommend nodal debulking in patients with cervical cancer, for reasons discussed in Chapter 3. Whether paraaortic lymphadenectomy adds sufficiently to the information gained from PET to justify the added morbidity of invasive surgery is unknown but is currently the subject of an ongoing prospective randomized trial.[46] Because skip metastases are extremely rare, dissection of the supramesenteric nodes is rarely indicated.[47]

The use of somewhat extended fields for patients at high risk for paraaortic node metastases is an alternative approach that we tend to favor over staging lymphadenectomy; however, more study is needed to determine the most accurate, lowest risk method of defining the nodal target volume.

Role of Chemotherapy

Concurrent Chemotherapy

In 1999, after a series of prospective randomized trials demonstrated consistent improvements in survival with the addition of concurrent chemotherapy to RT, chemoradiation was rapidly adopted as the standard of care for most patients with locoregionally advanced cervical cancer. Meta-analyses indicate that concurrent chemotherapy reduces the risks of recurrence and death by 50% to 70%[48,49] (**Fig. 10.2**). Although trials suggest that patients with stage IB2 or II disease achieve the greatest benefit from concurrent chemotherapy, meta-analyses and subset analyses of individual trials indicate that patients with stage III and IVA pelvic-confined disease also benefit from such treatment (**Fig. 10.3**).[49,50] A large population-based Canadian study that demonstrated a significant improvement in national survival rates following the 1999 adoption of concurrent chemotherapy as standard treatment confirmed the benefit of concurrent chemotherapy even outside the controlled environment of clinical trials.[51]

Most randomized trials of concurrent chemotherapy used platinum-based regimens. Most of the trials of cisplatin-based chemotherapy used either weekly cisplatin (at a dose of 40 mg/m^2) or combinations of cisplatin (usually 70 to 75 mg/m^2) and 5-fluorouracil given at 3-week intervals. Both approaches were beneficial, but because weekly cisplatin was easier to deliver and tended to cause fewer acute adverse effects (Chapter 7),[52] it became the favored regimen in most practices. Other concurrent chemotherapy regimens, most notably combinations of mitomycin C and 5-fluorouracil, have also been demonstrated to be of benefit.[48,49]

Although investigators have investigated a number of strategies to improve on the 1999 trial results, no alternative has yet been clearly proven to be superior to weekly cisplatin. A 2011 trial by Duenas-Gonzalez et al.[53] suggested that multiagent chemotherapy may be more effective than weekly cisplatin. In a multinational randomized trial, these authors compared a combination of concurrent weekly cisplatin and gemcitabine followed by adjuvant cisplatin and gemcitabine with a control standard of concurrent weekly cisplatin. The authors reported 3-year progression-free survival rates of 74% and 65% for the combined regimen and single-drug regimen, respectively ($p = 0.03$). Although these results were

Trial	Patients	Eligibility (FIGO stages)	Chemotherapy: Cisplatin-based	Chemotherapy: Comparison
GOG 85	388	IIB-IVA	Cisplatin, 5-FU	HU
GOG 120 (a)	384	IIB-IVA	Weekly cisplatin	HU
GOG 120 (b)	383	IIB-IVA	Cisplatin, 5-FU, HU	HU
GOG 123	369	IB ≥4 cm	Weekly cisplatin	None
RTOG 90-01	403	IB ≥4 cm, IIB-IVA or pelvic N+	Cisplatin, 5-FU	None
NCIC (Pearcey)	259	IB ≥5 cm, IIB-IVA or pelvic N+	Weekly cisplatin	None
SWOG 87-97	268	IA2–IIA, RH with high-risk features	Cisplatin, 5-FU	None
GOG 165	316	IIB-IVA	Weekly cisplatin	5-FU

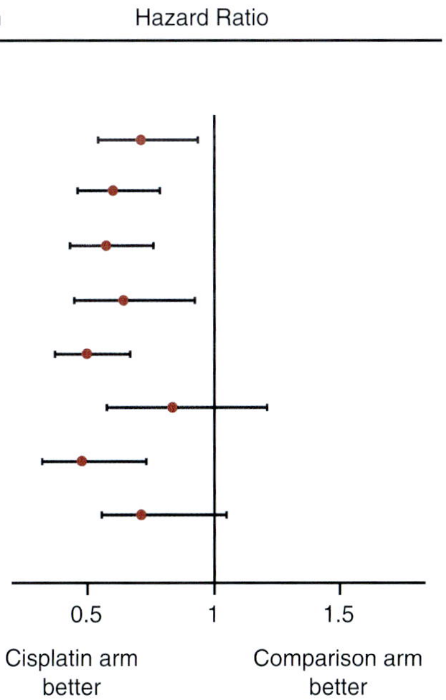

FIGURE 10.2 Prospective randomized trials that investigated the role of cisplatin-based concurrent radiation therapy and chemotherapy for patients with locoregionally advanced cervical cancer. This figure only includes trials that had more than 200 eligible patients. (FIGO, International Federation of Gynecology and Obstetrics; GOG, Gynecology Oncology Group; 5-FU, 5-fluorouracil; HU, hydroxyurea; RTOG, Radiation Therapy Oncology Group; SWOG, Southwest Oncology Group; NCIC, National Cancer Institute of Canada Clinical Trials Group.) (From Green J, Kirwan J, Tierney J, et al. Concomitant chemotherapy and radiation therapy for cancer of the uterine cervix. *Cochrane Database Syst Rev.* 2005:CD002225; Lanciano R, et al. *J Clin Oncol.* 2005;23:8289–8295.)

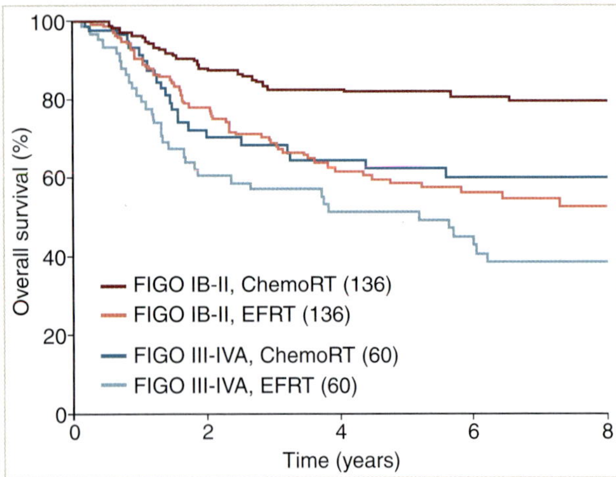

FIGURE 10.3 Kaplan-Meier estimates of overall survival for patients who received extended field radiation therapy (EFRT) or concurrent chemotherapy and pelvic radiation therapy (ChemoRT) on Radiation Therapy Oncology Group Trial 90-01. Survival rates are shown stratified by FIGO stage. (From Eifel PJ, Winter K, Morris M, et al. Pelvic irradiation with concurrent chemotherapy versus pelvic and para-aortic irradiation for high-risk cervical cancer: an update of radiation therapy oncology group trial (RTOG) 90-01. *J Clin Oncol.* 2004;22:872–880.)

encouraging, the trial had incomplete follow-up, particularly of late complications, which were reported with only 1 year of monitoring. Because of this and other concerns about the trial and because combination chemotherapy was associated with worse adverse effects, the addition of gemcitabine to cisplatin has not gained wide acceptance.

Not all patients who receive radiation for cervical cancer require concurrent chemotherapy. In particular, patients who received definitive RT for clinically node-negative stage IB1 or IIA1 disease have pelvic disease control rates of better than 95% with RT alone[14]; for elderly or medically inoperable patients with these small cancers, the adverse effects of concurrent chemotherapy undoubtedly outweigh any potential benefit **(CS 10.3)**. Also, it is not certain whether chemotherapy is needed for patients with intermediate-risk disease after hysterectomy (i.e., patients with negative nodes and negative surgical margins who have high-risk primary tumor features); this question is the subject of an ongoing clinical trial.

Nearly all the prospective trials of concurrent chemotherapy excluded patients who had known extrapelvic nodal disease. However, the combination of weekly cisplatin and extended field irradiation for extrapelvic nodal disease is generally well tolerated.[54,55] Despite the lack of level 1 evidence supporting this approach, concurrent weekly cisplatin is usually recommended for patients with paraaortic nodal disease to optimize locoregional control and, hopefully, survival **(CS 10.6, 10.8 to 10.10)**. For similar reasons, concurrent chemotherapy is usually recommended for patients who are candidates for potentially curative RT for recurrent disease **(CS 10.7 and 10.9)**, although experience with advanced recurrent disease suggests that initial cisplatin treatment may reduce the effectiveness of cisplatin at the time of recurrence.[56]

Some patients have insufficient renal function to tolerate cisplatin. Acute renal failure due to ureteral obstruction often resolves within 1 to 2 weeks of stent or nephrostomy placement. However, for patients who have not yet achieved normal renal function before they begin RT, other concurrent chemotherapy may be used. Although the evidence supporting the use of carboplatin is not as strong as the evidence supporting the use of cisplatin, weekly carboplatin is a reasonable alternative that can be considered if cisplatin is contraindicated **(CS 10.8)**.

Chemotherapy after RT

There is currently no direct evidence that adjuvant chemotherapy after RT improves outcome (Chapter 3).

Adjuvant chemotherapy was included in the experimental arms of several trials of chemoradiation. One large randomized trial demonstrated no benefit when adjuvant single-agent 5-fluorouracil was added after concurrent chemoradiation.[57] Results of a post hoc analysis of the SWOG 87-97 trial have been interpreted as evidence of benefit from adjuvant chemotherapy.[58] In the experimental arm of that trial, surgically treated patients who had high-risk features were supposed to receive four courses of cisplatin and 5-fluorouracil, two during pelvic RT and two after. However, 34 patients failed to complete more than two courses of chemotherapy; these patients were found to have a poorer outcome than the 90 who received at least three courses of chemotherapy (i.e., at least one adjuvant treatment). However, many of the patients who did not receive adjuvant treatment also did not complete the two concurrent chemotherapy courses; this combined with the possibility that adverse patient or tumor factors influenced patients' ability to complete treatment limited the significance of the findings of this post hoc analysis.

Ongoing trials that are comparing chemoradiation alone versus chemoradiation followed by adjuvant chemotherapy should yield valuable information about adjuvant chemotherapy's potential benefit. In the meantime, we generally do not recommend adjuvant chemotherapy, particularly for patients with squamous cancers.

Neoadjuvant Chemotherapy before RT

Multiagent chemotherapy can produce response rates of 60% or higher in previously untreated patients with locally advanced cervical cancer. This has fostered the hope that a course of neoadjuvant chemotherapy before RT could improve the outcome of patients with locally advanced disease. However, review of the many randomized trials that have addressed this question reveals little evidence of benefit and some evidence suggesting that administration of chemotherapy before RT may actually be harmful.

A 2004 meta-analysis summarized data from 18 trials that evaluated RT with or without neoadjuvant chemotherapy in more than 1,000 patients with locally advanced cervical cancer[59]; this analysis showed no improvement in overall survival with administration of neoadjuvant chemotherapy (odds ratio [OR], 1.05; 95% confidence interval [CI], 0.94 to 1.19) (**Fig. 10.4**). Separate analysis of the seven trials that used relatively short treatment cycles of 14 or fewer days suggested that there may have been a modest benefit from these more intensive regimens (OR, 0.83; 95% CI, 0.69 to 1.00); however, this analysis was dominated by the results of the three positive trials reported by Sardi et al.[59] Separate analysis of the 11 trials that involved longer neoadjuvant treatment cycles actually demonstrated a significant decrement in survival with neoadjuvant chemotherapy (OR, 1.25; 95% CI, 1.07 to 1.46). It is also important to recognize that these trials, all of which were conducted before 1999, used RT alone, as opposed to chemoradiation, in their control arms. A strong argument against the use of neoadjuvant chemotherapy before RT is the risk that such treatment could compromise the delivery or effectiveness of concurrent chemoradiation (Chapter 3).

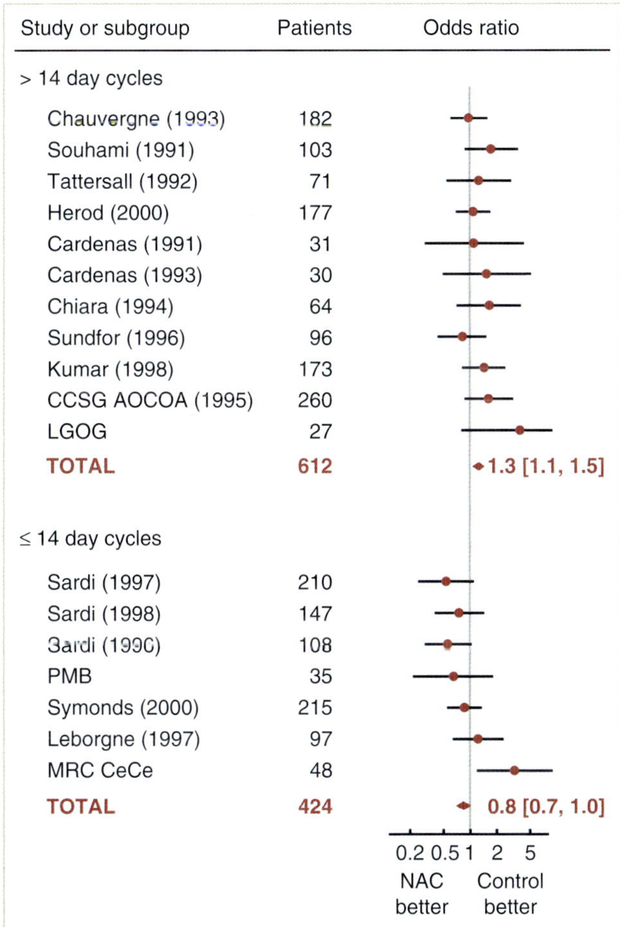

FIGURE 10.4 Meta-analysis of 18 clinical trials evaluating the role of cisplatin-based neoadjuvant chemotherapy for patients with locally advanced cervical cancer. Most trials evaluated the use of definitive radiation therapy with or without neoadjuvant chemotherapy. However, two trials, Sardi (1997) and MRC CeCe, included some patients who had local treatment with radical hysterectomy followed by pelvic radiation therapy. CCSG AOCOA, LGOG, PMB, and MRC CeCe represent unpublished trials that were included in the analysis by the Neoadjuvant Chemotherapy for Cervical Cancer Meta-analysis Collaboration. (NAC, neoadjuvant chemotherapy.) (From Neoadjuvant Chemotherapy for Cervical Cancer Meta-Analysis Collaboration. Neoadjuvant chemotherapy for locally advanced cervix cancer. *Cochrane Database Syst Rev.* 2004;CD001774.)

Neoadjuvant Chemotherapy before Radical Surgery

Several trials have compared cisplatin-based neoadjuvant chemotherapy followed by radical hysterectomy (with or without postoperative pelvic RT) versus RT alone in patients with locally advanced cervical cancer. A 2004 meta-analysis included five of these trials and 872 patients; more than half of the patients came from one large multi-institutional Italian trial.[60] The overall survival results favored patients treated with neoadjuvant chemotherapy (OR, 0.65; 95% CI, 0.53 to 0.80). However, patients in the control arms of these five trials were treated with pelvic RT only rather than the current more effective standard of concurrent chemoradiation. Also, the definitive RT used in the Italian trial may have been suboptimal, with relatively low doses and protracted treatment courses.

The meta-analysis did not include a subsequent trial, GOG-141,[61] which compared radical hysterectomy with or without neoadjuvant chemotherapy for patients with stage IB2 disease; this trial demonstrated no significant survival benefit and no reduction in the need for postoperative RT for patients who had neoadjuvant chemotherapy.

The ability to cure relatively advanced cancers with neoadjuvant chemotherapy followed by surgery is intriguing, particularly for patients in underdeveloped countries where brachytherapy may not be available. However, this approach needs to be compared with high-quality chemoradiation; several ongoing trials should provide additional insights in the near future.

RT after Hysterectomy

RT after hysterectomy for cervical cancer is used to treat three major groups of patients: patients who undergo radical hysterectomy and have findings suggesting a high risk of recurrence, patients who undergo radical hysterectomy and have findings suggesting an intermediate risk of recurrence, and patients who have invasive cervical cancer treated with inappropriate simple (rather than radical) hysterectomy.

RT after Radical Hysterectomy in Patients with High Risk of Recurrence

Posthysterectomy chemoradiation is recommended for patients who have positive lymph nodes, positive surgical margins, or parametrial involvement. These recommendations are based on the results of the SWOG 87-97 trial,[58] which demonstrated a 50% reduction in the risk of death when chemotherapy was added to pelvic RT (**Fig. 10.5**). The regimen used in that trial was four 3-week cycles of cisplatin and 5-fluorouracil, two during and two after RT. As discussed earlier in this chapter, the benefit of the adjuvant

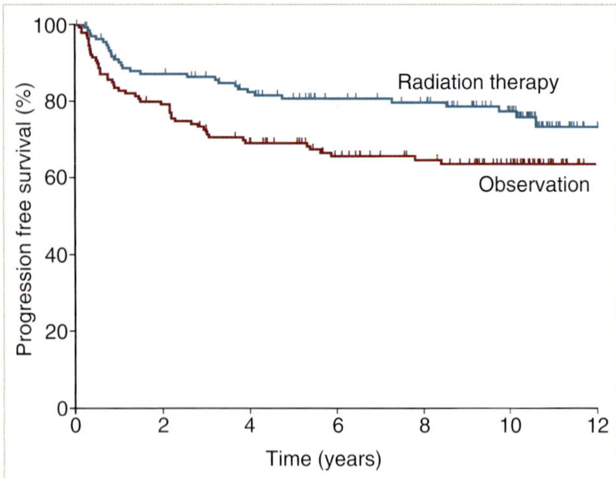

FIGURE 10.5 Progression-free survival (PFS) of 277 patients entered on Gynecologic Oncology Group trial GOG-92 after having radical hysterectomy and pelvic lymphadenectomy for cervical cancer. Patients were eligible for the trial if they had risk factors suggesting an intermediate risk of recurrence (**Table 10.3**). Patients who received adjuvant RT had a significantly better PFS than patients who were observed after hysterectomy (HR = 0.58; CI = 0.40 to 0.85, *p* = 0.019). (From Rotman M, Sedlis A, Piedmonte MR, et al. A phase III randomized trial of postoperative pelvic irradiation in Stage IB cervical carcinoma with poor prognostic features: follow-up of a gynecologic oncology group study. *Int J Radiat Oncol Biol Phys.* 2006;65:169–176.)

portion of this treatment is uncertain; on the basis of trials of chemoradiation in other settings, many practitioners substitute concurrent weekly cisplatin for the regimen used in SWOG 87-97.

RT after Radical Hysterectomy in Patients with Intermediate Risk of Recurrence

The results of the GOG-92 trial[26,62] demonstrated that patients who had an intermediate risk of recurrence (**Table 10.3**) had a 46% reduction in recurrence risk and a 30% reduction in the risk of death when adjuvant pelvic RT was administered after radical hysterectomy. Although postoperative RT can be recommended for all patients who meet the eligibility criteria for GOG-92, that trial included patients with varying risk of recurrence, and certain subgroups appeared to derive greater benefit from RT. For example, subset analysis suggested that the benefit was greatest for patients with adenocarcinoma or adenosquamous carcinoma; among the 59 patients with these histologic types, delivery of adjuvant pelvic RT reduced the risk of recurrence by 77%, from 44% to 9%.[26] Although results of unplanned subset analyses must be interpreted with caution, the less dramatic benefit of RT for patients with squamous cancers in this trial raises the question whether somewhat more restrictive criteria could be used for squamous cancers; certainly for patients whose cancers barely meet the criteria used for GOG-92, the potential benefit of RT should be very carefully weighed against the risks of adjuvant treatment. On the other hand, for a patient whose cancer falls in the highest risk end of the spectrum (e.g., a high-grade adenocarcinoma with close but negative surgical margins, LVSI, and primary tumor >4 cm), we believe it is reasonable to offer concurrent chemotherapy with adjuvant pelvic RT because the results of GOG-92 suggest that the risk of recurrence for such a patient approaches that of patients entered in SWOG 87-97. The GOG is currently addressing this question in a prospective trial, although the eligibility criteria for this trial (which are similar to those for GOG-92) suggest that only a minority of patients entered will have such high intermediate-risk features.

RT after Inappropriate Simple Hysterectomy for Invasive Cervical Cancer

As discussed above, several trials are evaluating the possible role of simple hysterectomy for patients with stage IA2 or small stage IB1 cancers. However, the appropriate procedure for most IB1 cancers is radical hysterectomy and bilateral pelvic lymphadenectomy. Unfortunately, invasive cervical cancer is sometimes unexpectedly discovered only after inappropriate simple hysterectomy has been performed.[63] Depending on the hysterectomy findings, treatment options may include a second surgery to perform a parametrectomy and pelvic lymphadenectomy or adjuvant RT. For relatively early-stage cancers, either treatment can be recommended, depending on the patient's wishes and comorbidities. However, if the hysterectomy findings or postoperative imaging suggests that adjuvant RT would be required even after additional surgery, RT alone or RT with concurrent chemotherapy is usually recommended. In this setting, additional surgery usually delays adjuvant RT and probably does not add significantly to the probability of local disease control, which is usually excellent with postoperative RT alone.[64]

Dose, Technique, and Timing of RT after Hysterectomy

For patients who have negative margins, no extracapsular extension, and no evidence of residual disease on postoperative imaging, 45 Gy in 25 fractions is usually an adequate dose to control microscopic disease. For patients who have positive margins (**CS 10.2**) or extracapsular nodal extension, a higher dose (usually 60 Gy) is recommended for the treatment of the high-risk clinical target volume. For patients who have close margins or very extensive nodal involvement, intermediate doses of 50 to 56 Gy may be given. Postoperative tomographic imaging should always be carefully scrutinized before treatment planning, particularly for patients who have extensive regional involvement or inadequate lymphadenectomy. When doses higher than 45 Gy are used, intensity-modulated RT (IMRT) is strongly recommended to minimize the dose to critical structures (Chapter 6).

Although it is desirable to begin adjuvant RT several weeks after hysterectomy to permit postoperative recovery and resolution of acute inflammation, the goal should always be to start postoperative pelvic RT within 4 to 6 weeks of surgery. Longer delays permit regrowth of residual clonogens and may be an indication for delivery of a somewhat higher radiation dose (**CS 10.1**). Intratreatment delays should always be avoided because they cannot improve and probably diminish the probability of tumor control from a given dose of radiation (Chapter 7).

RT FOR INTACT CERVICAL CANCER

The successful treatment of locally advanced cervical cancer requires careful planning and implementation of a comprehensive treatment strategy. As illustrated in the appended case studies, treatment often involves many components that must be integrated to assure delivery of an adequate radiation dose to multiple targets without exceeding normal tissue tolerance limits. Brachytherapy, a key component of treatment for locally advanced disease, contributes to the complexity of cervical cancer treatment, requiring skill and advance preparation. Excellent multidisciplinary collaboration is necessary to optimize delivery and minimize adverse effects of concurrent chemotherapy.

In this section, the factors that need to be considered in development of an overall treatment strategy will be discussed. The technical aspects of external beam irradiation and brachytherapy planning and delivery are discussed in greater detail in Chapters 4 to 8.

Determining the Overall Treatment Goals

After the diagnostic evaluation and simulation have been completed (Chapter 4), the next step should be to define and list the target volume(s) and desired radiation doses. The potential target volumes include the following:

- *Central clinical target volume.* Whether or not there is evidence of gross involvement, the cervix (if intact), uterus, upper half of the vagina, and paracervical (broad and uterosacral) ligaments should be considered at risk for at least microscopic involvement. An internal target volume (ITV) should always be designated to allow for internal organ motion of the uterus, cervix, and vagina, particularly if highly conformal treatment planning techniques such as IMRT are used (Chapter 5).
- *Central gross target volume.* The size and distribution of gross central disease should be clearly documented as this information will be used to design the final boost treatment, which is usually delivered with brachytherapy. All sites of initial gross disease require a boost even if they are no longer detectable after initial chemoradiation (Chapter 8). Fiducial markers should be used to demarcate the distal extent if there is extensive vaginal disease.
- *Regional clinical target volume.* At a minimum, it is recommended that fields extend cephalad to include all external and internal iliac nodes up to and including the bifurcation of the common iliac vessels. In cases of locally advanced disease or pelvic node involvement, we typically extend fields to include the common iliac nodes to the level of the aortic bifurcation (Chapter 5). If there is common iliac or paraaortic nodal disease, a proximal margin of at least 6 cm above the highest gross disease is recommended. If the distal vagina is involved, at least the medial inguinal nodes should be treated. In the absence of gross disease, 40 to 45 Gy is usually sufficient to prevent regional recurrence. However, a somewhat higher dose (usually 50 Gy) may be prescribed to treat possible in-transit metastases in areas between sites of gross disease, particularly if such areas contain smaller, nonspecific nodes (**CS 10.9**).
- *Regional gross target volume(s).* At the start of treatment, all sites of gross nodal involvement should be catalogued, and the desired total radiation dose to each site should be determined. In general, all suspicious or grossly involved nodes should be treated to a minimum dose of 60 Gy; a higher dose (e.g., 64 to 66 Gy) may be indicated, particularly for large nodes, when it can be delivered without exceeding normal tissue tolerance limits (Chapter 6). In patients receiving definitive RT, because the distal pelvic nodes usually receive a significant dose from brachytherapy, pelvic node boosts are usually planned after the first implant, which can be used to estimate the total contribution from brachytherapy. However, at the time of initial pelvic treatment planning, all involved nodes should be contoured, and space should be designated in the prescription for any possible nodal boosts; this provides a clear record of the initial treatment plan and assures that required boosts will not be forgotten.

External beam treatment fields should be designed to cover the entire central and regional target volumes as described above. As discussed in Chapter 6, these volumes can be treated using a three-dimensional conformal technique (**CS 10.3 to 10.5, 10.7**) or IMRT (**CS 10.8 and 10.10**). However, adequate margin must be included to account for internal motion of the central targets and daily setup variation; once these factors are considered, IMRT frequently holds little advantage over a four-field technique. However, for patients with extensive nodal disease, IMRT of the paraaortic and common iliac nodes can significantly reduce the dose to bowel, kidneys, duodenum, spinal cord, and other critical structures. In some cases, the optimal solution may be to treat the pelvis using a conformal technique while treating proximal nodal targets with IMRT (**CS 10.6**). Methods for integrating external beam irradiation, including nodal boosts, with brachytherapy are discussed below.

Role of Brachytherapy

Brachytherapy plays a critical role in the treatment of cervical cancer, permitting safe delivery of high doses to central disease in most cases. Several factors make brachytherapy, and particularly intracavitary brachytherapy, particularly well suited to the treatment of cervical cancer:

- *Anatomy.* Of all the cancers treated with radiation, probably none has a more fortuitous location than cervical cancer. The uterus, which is no longer a critical structure once child bearing is complete, serves as a vessel allowing radiation sources to be positioned in the midst of the tumor; meanwhile, the uterine wall and vaginal packing usually displace adjacent bladder and bowel away from the sources. In most cases, this anatomic advantage permits safe delivery of central tumor doses of at least 85 Gy, contributing to remarkably high central tumor control rates even for very large cancers.[10,15]

- *The fixed relationship between the target and brachytherapy source(s).* Because brachytherapy sources are fixed in their relationship to the primary target, no margins need to be added to the cervical target volume to compensate for variations in the position of the uterus. In contrast, most external beam techniques require margins of 2 cm or more to accommodate uterine motion and daily setup uncertainties (Chapters 5 and 6).
- *The inverse square law.* The rapid falloff in dose from intracavitary sources—which are commonly located at the highest risk, central portion of the target volume—to peripheral critical structures contributes to a favorable therapeutic ratio.
- *The dose rate effect and fractionation.* Traditional low-dose rate cervical cancer brachytherapy exploited the dose–rate effect to maximize the ratio between the effective dose to tumor and critical structures. Today, brachytherapy is more often delivered at high dose rates, with treatment fractionated to reduce the dose per fraction to proximate critical structures.

Cervical brachytherapy is a subspecialized form of treatment requiring skills that are very specific to RT for cervical cancer; it is likely that some minimum number of cases is required to optimize and maintain these brachytherapy skills. Population-based studies suggest that, in the United States, 20% or more of patients treated with definitive RT for cervical cancer do not receive brachytherapy.[3,65] The likelihood of receiving brachytherapy is lowest for patients treated at small, nonacademic facilities that treat fewer than three cases per year.[3] In contrast, at MD Anderson, 99.5% of patients treated with radiation for stage I to IVA intact cervical cancer receive intracavitary brachytherapy; the only major group of patients not routinely treated with brachytherapy are those with stage IVA disease complicated by a fistula **(CS 10.11)**.

Although the central role of brachytherapy in the treatment of intact cervical cancer is generally accepted, a wide variety of brachytherapy techniques have been used. These include variations in brachytherapy dose rate, schedule, applicator types, and method of dose specification. Because few data are available from comparisons of these different approaches, clinical practices tend to be based on first principles, observational studies, and experience. See Chapter 8 for a critical evaluation of various intracavitary techniques and detailed discussion of recommended methods.

Integration of External Beam Irradiation and Brachytherapy

In cases of locally advanced cervical cancer, an initial course of pelvic RT with concurrent chemotherapy is recommended to reduce the diameter of the cervix, shrink exophytic disease, and reduce the volume of vaginal disease. This facilitates placement of intracavitary applicators and, by reducing the distance between radiation sources and the tumor periphery, increases the dose deliverable to central targets.

In most cases, 40 to 45 Gy of chemoradiation produces sufficient response to optimize intracavitary brachytherapy; higher external doses to the central pelvis tend to severely limit the dose of brachytherapy deliverable within normal tissue tolerance limits and are, therefore, rarely recommended. Brachytherapy can be initiated before central pelvic RT is completed if the cervical diameter is <4 cm. For patients who have early-stage (IA or IB1) disease and narrow vaginal anatomy, it may be desirable to begin brachytherapy early, even at the start of treatment, before external irradiation causes any additional vaginal narrowing that would limit brachytherapy options **(CS 10.3)**.

If brachytherapy is interdigitated within the initial course of RT, care should be taken to ensure that this does not cause protraction of regional treatment, particularly treatment of common iliac and paraaortic nodes, which typically receive a negligible dose from brachytherapy. *Schedules that deliver radiation at an average rate of <850 to 900 cGy per week to any part of the target volume are not recommended.*

The interdigitation of pelvic node boosts with brachytherapy can pose special challenges. An AP–PA boost technique may be used if boost fields are small and if less than an additional 8 to 10 Gy is needed to increase the combined external beam and brachytherapy dose to a minimum of 60 to 66 Gy. When higher boost doses are required, more complex techniques are recommended (Chapter 6); however, to avoid compromising subsequent brachytherapy, care must be taken to minimize the dose to the rectum and bladder from lateral fields or IMRT **(CS 10.4 and 10.5)**. Any dose that is delivered to rectosigmoid or bladder must be included in calculations of the total combined doses delivered to these structures from external beam and brachytherapy.

Because the paraaortic and common iliac nodes typically receive a negligible dose from brachytherapy, integrated boosts are often used to increase the dose to involved nodes in these regions to 50 Gy during initial extended field treatment **(CS 10.6)**. This usually reduces the total number of boost treatments and facilitates integration of boost treatments with pelvic boosts and brachytherapy.

External Beam Boosts to Paracervical Tissues

The volume of tissue included in so-called parametrial boost fields varies widely. Some clinicians supplement initial pelvic radiation for several fractions using AP–PA fields that treat most of the pelvis but shield midline tissues with blocks of varying widths. Radiation doses of more than 45 Gy to the whole pelvis have been associated with an increased risk of small bowel complications[15]; because 40 to 45 Gy is generally sufficient to control microscopic nodal disease, we do not recommend routine use of large boost fields that treat low-risk pelvic tissues to higher external beam doses. Some clinicians insert a midline block early in the treatment course (i.e., before 40 Gy) and increase the central dose given with brachytherapy; when this is done, care must be taken not to exceed the tolerance of the ureters, which are often located 2.5 cm or more from midline.[66]

The benefit of and indications for smaller parametrial boosts that target only the broad and uterosacral ligaments are unclear. Typically, the medial borders of such fields are placed 2 to 3 cm from the cervical canal, avoiding the high-dose portion of the brachytherapy distribution; the proximal borders are usually placed at or just above the level of the uterine fundus (CS 10.7). It has long been our practice to boost the paracervical tissues, usually for an additional 6 to 8 Gy, only if there is residual induration or nodular disease fixed to the pelvic wall at the time of brachytherapy (CS 10.7); with this policy, isolated parametrial recurrences were very rare, even before routine use of concurrent chemotherapy.

However, with chemoradiation, central disease usually responds rapidly and MRI rarely demonstrates gross disease extending more than 2 cm from the internal cervical os, even when induration is still palpable in the cardinal ligament. Whether the additional dose delivered with brachytherapy is sufficient to control residual microscopic disease in the adjacent parametrium may depend on the type of brachytherapy applicator used and the distribution of radiation sources (or dwell times). Compact applicators like the ring and tandem tend to deliver a lower dose to parametrial tissues than, for example, a 6- to 8-cm tandem with 2-cm shielded ovoids; also, the lower nominal dose delivered with HDR brachytherapy tends to result in a lower effective dose to the lateral parametrium than PDR or LDR brachytherapy (Chapter 8). Selective placement of interstitial parametrial needles can make up for this shortcoming in selected cases (discussed below).

Rarely, tumors may infiltrate the uterosacral ligaments to invade the mesorectal fascia and piriformis muscle. In such cases, because AP–PA fields cannot treat the residual disease without overlapping midline critical structures, IMRT or multifield conformal techniques are recommended to bring the total dose to 66 Gy or more.

Role of Interstitial Brachytherapy

To improve central disease control rates for patients with locally advanced cervical cancer, a number of groups have investigated the use of interstitial brachytherapy as an alternative to intracavitary brachytherapy. Most of these groups have used interstitial templates to guide transperineal insertion of needles; in some cases, interstitial needles were combined with an intrauterine tandem inserted through a narrow vaginal obturator. Enthusiasm for interstitial template brachytherapy has waxed and waned over the past 40 years or more. Most reported experiences have involved fewer than 50 patients, the results have generally not been superior to those achieved with intracavitary treatment, and some investigators have reported disturbingly high complication rates.[67,68] One of the recommended indications for interstitial brachytherapy has been the "inability" to perform intracavitary therapy; however, when brachytherapy is attempted by experienced clinicians with ultrasound guidance, this indication should be extremely rare. Also, in the chemoradiation era, it is uncommon for patients to have massive residual disease at the time of brachytherapy, and image guidance usually demonstrates that the target volume can be covered with less invasive techniques.

More recently, several groups have explored the use of much more restricted supplementation of intracavitary brachytherapy with three or four interstitial needles placed in the parametrium through channels in a specially adapted ring applicator or ovoids (Fig. 8.5). These channels are relatively close to the tandem, so this technique provides only modest additional lateral coverage. However, interstitial needles may be helpful in selected patients, particularly those with asymmetrical parametrial extension.

In our practice, the most frequent indication for interstitial brachytherapy is to treat gross disease in the distal vagina than cannot be adequately treated with intracavitary brachytherapy alone (CS 10.8).

Image guidance, ideally with MRI, is recommended for any treatment that involves placement of interstitial needles, particularly if needles are placed in locations that cannot be monitored under direct palpation.

TREATMENT OF RECURRENT DISEASE

Most patients who develop recurrence after initial definitive treatment for cervical cancer are incurable. However, selected patients who have localized recurrences may be curable, depending on the site of the disease and the nature of their previous treatment.

Central Recurrence after Definitive Radiation Therapy

Patients who have a central recurrence after pelvic RT and who have no other evidence of disease can sometimes be candidates for curative surgery. In most cases, some form of pelvic exenteration is required. In rare cases, a radical hysterectomy may be curative; however, the rate of fistula and other major complications is high when radical hysterectomy is attempted after definitive RT.[69] In a large review from MD Anderson, patients who had a central recurrence 36 months or more after definitive RT had a significantly better survival than patients who had recurrence within 3 years (Fig. 9.1b).

Recurrences in Nodes Marginal to Radiation Therapy Fields

Nodal recurrences occurring above the upper margin of radiation fields pose particularly difficult management challenges because they are usually located immediately above the field.[70] By the time patients present with symptoms, most patients are incurable because they have either distant metastases or massive disease extending retrograde into the previously treated radiation fields.[70,71] Recently, routine PET surveillance has permitted some of these recurrences to be detected before symptoms have developed (**CS 10.7**); Singh et al.[71] reported encouraging survival rates for patients who have asymptomatic recurrences treated with IMRT and concurrent chemotherapy.

Vaginal Recurrence after Hysterectomy

The treatment of choice for patients who have a localized vaginal recurrence after hysterectomy is definitive RT. The techniques used to treat recurrent disease are identical to those used to treat vaginal cancers of similar extent and disease distribution (Chapters 8 and 11). The overall prognosis is good if there is no evidence of metastatic disease at the time of first recurrence.[72,73] Although reported survival rates are very good even with RT alone, concurrent chemoradiation is usually recommended, particularly if there is more than superficial vaginal disease.

Pelvic Nodal Recurrence after Hysterectomy

Today, few patients are diagnosed with pelvic node recurrence after initial treatment with hysterectomy only because most patients who are found to have high-risk features receive adjuvant RT. Historical data indicated that the prognosis for patients who had pelvic node recurrence after hysterectomy was poor even if they had not received adjuvant RT.[73] However, modern imaging methods with improved target definition, conformal radiation techniques, and the use of concurrent chemoradiation have probably improved the outlook for these patients. Definitive treatment with curative intent should be considered for any patient having pelvic or paraaortic node recurrence (**CS 10.9**).

Recurrent or Metastatic Disease That Is Not Amenable to Definitive Local Treatments

About 30% to 50% of patients can be expected to respond to platinum-based chemotherapy. Response rates are lower for patients who have recurrence inside a previous radiation field and for patients who received concurrent cisplatin with their initial radiation treatment. Overall, the median progression-free survival rates for patients entered in phase III trials of chemotherapy for recurrent and metastatic disease range between 3 and 6 months; median overall survival rates for most studies have been <12 months. Recent studies have demonstrated a 3-month increase in overall survival (from 14 to 17 months) when bevacizumab was added to chemotherapy; however, patients who received bevacizumab also had a higher incidence of bleeding, thromboembolism, and gastrointestinal fistulae than patients who received only cytotoxic chemotherapy.

Although patients with distant metastatic disease are generally considered to be incurable, patients who have oligometastatis occasionally enjoy prolonged disease-free survival after definitive treatment of their metastasis. We have seen several patients cured of isolated supraclavicular metastases (**CS 10.10**) and a few patients who have had prolonged disease-free intervals after isolated mediastinal recurrences (**CS 10.8**). Patients who have pulmonary parenchymal lesions may benefit from wedge resection or stereotactic RT.[74] However, aggressive treatment of oligometastatic disease is recommended only for patients who have a good performance status and a single site of metastatic disease that can be treated without significant toxicity. Each case must be considered carefully, weighing the potential benefit against the side effects, cost, and inconvenience of ablative treatment.

References

1. Siegel R, Naishadham D, Jemal A. Cancer statistics, 2013. *CA Cancer J Clin.* 2013;63:11–30.
2. Clegg LX, Reichman ME, Miller BA, et al. Impact of socioeconomic status on cancer incidence and stage at diagnosis: selected findings from the surveillance, epidemiology, and end results: National Longitudinal Mortality Study. *Cancer Causes Control.* 2009;20:417–435.
3. Eifel PJ, Ho A, Khalid N, et al. Patterns of radiation therapy practice for patients treated for intact cervical cancer in 2005 to 2007: a quality research in radiation oncology study. *Int J Radiat Oncol Biol Phys.* 2014;89:249–256.
4. Pecorelli S, Zigliani L, Odicino F. Revised FIGO staging for carcinoma of the cervix. *Int J Gynaecol Obstet.* 2009;105:107–108.
5. Benedet JL, Bender H, Jones H III, et al. FIGO staging classifications and clinical practice guidelines in the management of gynecologic cancers. FIGO Committee on Gynecologic Oncology. *Int J Gynaecol Obstet.* 2000;70:209–262.
6. Lakhman Y, Akin O, Park KJ, et al. Stage IB1 cervical cancer: role of preoperative MR imaging in selection of patients for fertility-sparing radical trachelectomy. *Radiology.* 2013;269:149–158.
7. Bhosale P, Peungjesada S, Devine C, et al. Role of magnetic resonance imaging as an adjunct to clinical staging in cervical carcinoma. *J Comput Assist Tomogr.* 2010;34:855–864.
8. Haie-Meder C, Morice P, Castiglione M, et al. Cervical cancer: ESMO Clinical Practice Guidelines for diagnosis, treatment and follow-up. *Ann Oncol.* 2010;21(suppl 5):v37–v40.
9. Grigsby PW. PET/CT imaging to guide cervical cancer therapy. *Future Oncol.* 2009;5:953–958.
10. Eifel PJ, Jhingran A, Levenback CF, et al. Predictive value of a proposed subclassification of stages I and II cervical cancer based on clinical tumor diameter. *Int J Gynecol Cancer.* 2009;19:2–7.
11. Burghardt E, Pickel H, Haas J, et al. Prognostic factors and operative treatment of stages IB to IIB cervical cancer. *Am J Obstet Gynecol.* 1987;156:988–996.
12. Inoue T, Okumura M. Prognostic significance of parametrial extension in patients with cervical carcinoma stages IB, IIA, and IIB. A study of 628 cases treated by radical hysterectomy and

lymphadenectomy with or without postoperative irradiation. *Cancer.* 1984;54:1714–1719.
13. Kamura T, Tsukamoto N, Tsuruchi N, et al. Multivariate analysis of the histopathologic prognostic factors of cervical cancer in patients undergoing radical hysterectomy. *Cancer.* 1992;69:181–186.
14. Eifel PJ, Morris M, Wharton JT, et al. The influence of tumor size and morphology on the outcome of patients with FIGO stage IB squamous cell carcinoma of the uterine cervix. *Int J Radiat Oncol Biol Phys.* 1994;29:9–16.
15. Logsdon MD, Eifel PJ. Figo IIIB squamous cell carcinoma of the cervix: an analysis of prognostic factors emphasizing the balance between external beam and intracavitary radiation therapy. *Int J Radiat Oncol Biol Phys.* 1999;43:763–775.
16. Kim YB, Lee IJ, Kim SY, et al. Tumor heterogeneity of FIGO stage III carcinoma of the uterine cervix. *Int J Radiat Oncol Biol Phys.* 2009;75:1323–1328.
17. Kavadi VS, Eifel PJ. FIGO stage IIIA carcinoma of the uterine cervix. *Int J Radiat Oncol Biol Phys.* 1992;24:211–215.
18. Zaino RJ, Ward S, Delgado G, et al. Histopathologic predictors of the behavior of surgically treated stage IB squamous cell carcinoma of the cervix. A Gynecologic Oncology Group study. *Cancer.* 1992;69:1750–1758.
19. Smith HO, Tiffany MF, Qualls CR, et al. The rising incidence of adenocarcinoma relative to squamous cell carcinoma of the uterine cervix in the United States—a 24-year population-based study. *Gynecol Oncol.* 2000;78:97–105.
20. Sherman ME, Wang SS, Carreon J, et al. Mortality trends for cervical squamous and adenocarcinoma in the United States. Relation to incidence and survival. *Cancer.* 2005;103:1258–1264.
21. Alfsen GC, Kristensen GB, Skovlund E, et al. Histologic subtype has minor importance for overall survival in patients with adenocarcinoma of the uterine cervix: a population-based study of prognostic factors in 505 patients with nonsquamous cell carcinomas of the cervix. *Cancer.* 2001;92:2471–2483.
22. dos Reis R, Frumovitz M, Milam MR, et al. Adenosquamous carcinoma versus adenocarcinoma in early-stage cervical cancer patients undergoing radical hysterectomy: an outcomes analysis. *Gynecol Oncol.* 2007;107:458–463.
23. Eifel PJ, Morris M, Oswald MJ, et al. Adenocarcinoma of the uterine cervix. Prognosis and patterns of failure in 367 cases. *Cancer.* 1990;65:2507–2514.
24. Eifel PJ, Burke TW, Morris M, et al. Adenocarcinoma as an independent risk factor for disease recurrence in patients with stage IB cervical carcinoma. *Gynecol Oncol.* 1995;59:38–44.
25. Eifel PJ, Burke TW, Delclos L, et al. Early stage I adenocarcinoma of the uterine cervix: treatment results in patients with tumors less than or equal to 4 cm in diameter. *Gynecol Oncol.* 1991; 41:199–205.
26. Rotman M, Sedlis A, Piedmonte MR, et al. A phase III randomized trial of postoperative pelvic irradiation in Stage IB cervical carcinoma with poor prognostic features: follow-up of a gynecologic oncology group study. *Int J Radiat Oncol Biol Phys.* 2006;65:169–176.
27. Rose PG, Java JJ, Whitney CW, et al. Locally advanced adenocarcinoma and adenosquamous carcinomas of the cervix compared to squamous cell carcinomas of the cervix in gynecologic oncology group trials of cisplatin-based chemoradiation. *Gynecol Oncol.* 2014;135:208–212.
28. Bishop AJ, Allen PK, Klopp AH, et al. Relationship between low hemoglobin levels and outcomes after treatment with radiation or chemoradiation in patients with cervical cancer: has the impact of anemia been overstated? *Int J Radiat Oncol Biol Phys.* 2015;91:196–205.
29. Satoh T, Takei Y, Treilleux I, et al. Gynecologic Cancer InterGroup (GCIG) consensus review for small cell carcinoma of the cervix. *Int J Gynecol Cancer.* 2014;24:S102–S108.
30. Viswanathan AN, Deavers MT, Jhingran A, et al. Small cell neuroendocrine carcinoma of the cervix: outcome and patterns of recurrence. *Gynecol Oncol.* 2004;93:27–33.
31. Delgado G, Bundy B, Zaino R, et al. Prospective surgical-pathological study of disease-free interval in patients with stage IB squamous cell carcinoma of the cervix: a Gynecologic Oncology Group study. *Gynecol Oncol.* 1990;38:352–357.
32. Macdonald OK, Chen J, Dodson M, et al. Prognostic significance of histology and positive lymph node involvement following radical hysterectomy in carcinoma of the cervix. *Am J Clin Oncol.* 2009;32:411–416.
33. Osborne E, Klopp A, Jhingran A, et al. Definitive extended-field radiation therapy for cervical cancer patients with para-aortic lymph node metastases. *Int J Radiat Oncol Biol Phys.* 2015;93:S202–S203.
34. Horn LC, Hentschel B, Galle D, et al. Extracapsular extension of pelvic lymph node metastases is of prognostic value in carcinoma of the cervix uteri. *Gynecol Oncol.* 2008;108:63–67.
35. Burghardt E, Baltzer J, Tulusan AH, et al. Results of surgical treatment of 1028 cervical cancers studied with volumetry. *Cancer.* 1992;70:648–655.
36. Delgado G, Bundy BN, Fowler WC Jr, et al. A prospective surgical pathological study of stage I squamous carcinoma of the cervix: a Gynecologic Oncology Group Study. *Gynecol Oncol.* 1989;35:314–320.
37. Ryu SY, Kim MH, Nam BH, et al. Intermediate-risk grouping of cervical cancer patients treated with radical hysterectomy: a Korean Gynecologic Oncology Group study. *Br J Cancer.* 2014;110:278–285.
38. Landoni F, Maneo A, Colombo A, et al. Randomised study of radical surgery versus radiotherapy for stage Ib-IIa cervical cancer. *Lancet.* 1997;350:535–540.
39. Pareja R, Rendon GJ, Sanz-Lomana CM, et al. Surgical, oncological, and obstetrical outcomes after abdominal radical trachelectomy—a systematic literature review. *Gynecol Oncol.* 2013;131:77–82.
40. Covens AL, Dodge JE, Lacchetti C, et al. Surgical management of a suspicious adnexal mass: a systematic review. *Gynecol Oncol.* 2012;126:149–156.
41. Plante M, Lau S, Brydon L, et al. Neoadjuvant chemotherapy followed by vaginal radical trachelectomy in bulky stage IB1 cervical cancer: case report. *Gynecol Oncol.* 2006;101:367–370.
42. Jampolis S, Andras J, Fletcher GH. Analysis of sites and causes of failures of irradiation in invasive squamous cell carcinoma of the intact uterine cervix. *Radiology.* 1975;15:681–685.
43. Thoms WW, Eifel PJ, Smith TL, et al. Bulky endocervical carcinomas: a 23-year experience. *Int J Radiat Oncol Biol Phys.* 1992;23:491–499.
44. Keys HM, Bundy BN, Stehman FB, et al. Radiation therapy with and without extrafascial hysterectomy for bulky stage IB cervical carcinoma: a randomized trial of the Gynecologic Oncology Group. *Gynecol Oncol.* 2003;89:343–353.
45. Dornhofer N, Hockel M. New developments in the surgical therapy of cervical carcinoma. *Ann NY Acad Sci.* 2008;1138: 233–252.

46. Frumovitz M, Querleu D, Gil-Moreno A, et al. Lymphadenectomy in locally advanced cervical cancer study (LiLACS): phase III clinical trial comparing surgical with radiologic staging in patients with stages IB2-IVA cervical cancer. *J Minim Invasive Gynecol.* 2014;21:3–8.
47. Leblanc E, Katdare N, Narducci F, et al. Should systematic infrarenal para-aortic dissection be the rule in the pretherapeutic staging of primary or recurrent locally advanced cervix cancer patients with a negative preoperative para-aortic PET imaging? *Int J Gynecol Cancer.* 2016;26:169–175.
48. Green J, Kirwan J, Tierney J, et al. Concomitant chemotherapy and radiation therapy for cancer of the uterine cervix. *Cochrane Database Syst Rev.* 2005:CD002225.
49. Chemoradiotherapy for Cervical Cancer Meta-Analysis Collaboration. Reducing uncertainties about the effects of chemoradiotherapy for cervical cancer: a systematic review and meta-analysis of individual patient data from 18 randomized trials. *J Clin Oncol.* 2008;26:5802–5812.
50. Eifel PJ, Winter K, Morris M, et al. Pelvic irradiation with concurrent chemotherapy versus pelvic and para-aortic irradiation for high-risk cervical cancer: an update of radiation therapy oncology group trial (RTOG) 90-01. *J Clin Oncol.* 2004;22:872–880.
51. Pearcey R, Miao Q, Kong W, et al. Impact of adoption of chemoradiotherapy on the outcome of cervical cancer in Ontario: results of a population-based cohort study. *J Clin Oncol.* 2007;25:2383–2388.
52. Likhacheva A, Jhingran A, Bodurka DC, et al. Prospective study of symptom assessment among patients with cervical cancer during concurrent chemoradiotherapy with weekly cisplatin or every-3-week cisplatin and 5-fluorouracil. *Int J Gynecol Cancer.* 2013;23:1520–1527.
53. Duenas-Gonzalez A, Zarba JJ, Patel F, et al. Phase III, open-label, randomized study comparing concurrent gemcitabine plus cisplatin and radiation followed by adjuvant gemcitabine and cisplatin versus concurrent cisplatin and radiation in patients with stage IIB to IVA carcinoma of the cervix. *J Clin Oncol.* 2011;29:1678–1685.
54. Klopp A, Jhingran A, Pardeshi V, et al. Chemoradiation followed by adjuvant chemotherapy for management of stage IIIC2 endometrial cancer. *Int J Radiat Oncol Biol Phys.* 2011;81:S191.
55. Malfetano JH, Keys H, Cunningham MJ, et al. Extended field radiation and cisplatin for stage IIB and IIIB cervical carcinoma. *Gynecol Oncol.* 1997;67:203–207.
56. Long HJ III. Management of metastatic cervical cancer: review of the literature. *J Clin Oncol.* 2007;25:2966–2974.
57. Lorvidhaya V, Chitapanarux I, Sangruchi S, et al. Concurrent mitomycin C, 5-fluorouracil, and radiotherapy in the treatment of locally advanced carcinoma of the cervix: a randomized trial. *Int J Radiat Oncol Biol Phys.* 2003;55:1226–1232.
58. Peters WA III, Liu PY, Barrett RJ II, et al. Concurrent chemotherapy and pelvic radiation therapy compared with pelvic radiation therapy alone as adjuvant therapy after radical surgery in high-risk early-stage cancer of the cervix. *J Clin Oncol.* 2000;18:1606–1613.
59. Neoadjuvant Chemotherapy for Cervical Cancer Meta-Analysis Collaboration. Neoadjuvant chemotherapy for locally advanced cervix cancer. *Cochrane Database Syst Rev.* 2004:CD001774.
60. Benedetti-Panici P, Greggi S, Colombo A, et al. Neoadjuvant chemotherapy and radical surgery versus exclusive radiotherapy in locally advanced squamous cell cervical cancer: results from the Italian multicenter randomized study. *J Clin Oncol.* 2002;20: 179–188.
61. Eddy GL, Bundy BN, Creasman WT, et al. Treatment of ("bulky") stage IB cervical cancer with or without neoadjuvant vincristine and cisplatin prior to radical hysterectomy and pelvic/para-aortic lymphadenectomy: a phase III trial of the gynecologic oncology group. *Gynecol Oncol.* 2007;106: 362–369.
62. Sedlis A, Bundy BN, Rotman MZ, et al. A randomized trial of pelvic radiation therapy versus no further therapy in selected patients with stage IB carcinoma of the cervix after radical hysterectomy and pelvic lymphadenectomy: a Gynecologic Oncology Group Study. *Gynecol Oncol.* 1999;73:177–183.
63. Roman L, Morris M, Eifel P, et al. Reasons for inappropriate simple hysterectomy in the presence of invasive cancer of the cervix. *Obstet Gynecol.* 1992;79:485–489.
64. Roman LD, Morris M, Mitchell MF, et al. Prognostic factors for patients undergoing simple hysterectomy in the presence of invasive cancer of the cervix. *Gynecol Oncol.* 1993;50:179–184.
65. Smith GL, Eifel PJ. Trends in the utilization of brachytherapy in cervical cancer in the United States. In regard to Han et al. *Int J Radiat Oncol Biol Phys.* 2014;88:459–460.
66. McIntyre JF, Eifel PJ, Levenback C, et al. Ureteral stricture as a late complication of radiotherapy for stage IB carcinoma of the uterine cervix. *Cancer.* 1995;75:836–843.
67. Hughes-Davies L, Silver B, Kapp D. Parametrial interstitial brachytherapy for advanced or recurrent pelvic malignancy: the Harvard/Stanford experience. *Gynecol Oncol.* 1995;58:24–27.
68. Monk BJ, Tewari K, Burger RA, et al. A comparison of intracavitary versus interstitial irradiation in the treatment of cervical cancer. *Gynecol Oncol.* 1997;67:241–247.
69. Coleman RL, Keeney ED, Freedman RS, et al. Radical hysterectomy for recurrent carcinoma of the uterine cervix after radiotherapy. *Gynecol Oncol.* 1994;55:29–35.
70. Beadle BM, Jhingran A, Yom SS, et al. Patterns of regional recurrence after definitive radiotherapy for cervical cancer. *Int J Radiat Oncol Biol Phys.* 2010;76:1396–1403.
71. Singh AK, Grigsby PW, Rader JS, et al. Cervix carcinoma, concurrent chemoradiotherapy, and salvage of isolated paraaortic lymph node recurrence. *Int J Radiat Oncol Biol Phys.* 2005; 61:450–455.
72. Grigsby PW. Radiotherapy for pelvic recurrence after radical hysterectomy for cervical cancer. *Radiat Med.* 2005;23:327–330.
73. Ijaz T, Eifel PJ, Burke T, et al. Radiation therapy of pelvic recurrence after radical hysterectomy for cervical carcinoma. *Gynecol Oncol.* 1998;70:241–246.
74. Bodurka-Bevers D, Morris M, Eifel PJ, et al. Posttherapy surveillance of women with cervical cancer: an outcomes analysis. *Gynecol Oncol.* 2000;78:187–193.

Case Studies

The following case studies illustrate various features of cervical cancer treatment. All of these cases were complex and involved multiple treatment components. However, these cases are representative of the types of challenges routinely faced in the multidisciplinary treatment of cervical cancer. The cases were also selected to demonstrate a range of treatment methods; while some of the treatment plans were designed using three-dimensional conformal techniques, others demonstrate how IMRT can be used to optimize the therapeutic ratio, particularly for patients with regionally advanced disease. Several patients with longer follow-up received brachytherapy that was planned using two-dimensional techniques; more recent cases were planned with image guidance using CT or MRI. Additional discussion of brachytherapy and external beam irradiation techniques is included in Chapters 6 and 8.

List of Case Studies for Chapter 10:

CS 10.1. Stage IB1 cervical cancer in a patient treated with hysterectomy who had high-risk features and a treatment delay

CS 10.2. Stage IB1 cervical cancer in a patient treated with radical hysterectomy who had a positive parametrial margin

CS 10.3. Stage IB1 cervical cancer in an elderly woman

CS 10.4. Stage IB2 cervical cancer with bilateral pelvic node metastases

CS 10.5. Stage IB2 squamous carcinoma with bilateral pelvic node metastases

CS 10.6. Stage IIB cervical cancer with pelvic and aortic node metastases

CS 10.7. Stage IIB cervical cancer with bilateral pelvic nodes and a marginal PAN recurrence

CS 10.8. Stage IIIB squamous carcinoma with a skip lesion in the distal vagina

CS 10.9. Adenocarcinoma of the cervix recurrent in pelvic nodes after radical hysterectomy

CS 10.10. Stage IB2 cervical cancer with extensive lymphadenopathy, including supraclavicular metastasis

CS 10.11. Stage IVA squamous carcinoma with vesicovaginal fistula

Abbreviations used in the case studies:

AP	Anterior–posterior
CI	Common iliac
CT	Computed tomography
CTV	Clinical target volume
CXR	Chest x-ray
D_{2cc}	Minimum dose to the 2 cc receiving the highest dose
D_{90}	Dose received by 90% of the target volume
DM	Distant metastases
EBRT	External beam radiation therapy
ECE	Extracapsular extension
EI	External iliac
EqD2	Equivalent dose at 2 Gy/fraction
EUA	Examination under anesthesia
FDG	Fluorodeoxyglucose
FIGO	International Federation of Gynecology and Obstetrics
GTV	Gross target volume
HDR	High-dose rate
HPV	Human papillomavirus
HRCTV	High-risk clinical target volume
HSIL	High-grade squamous intraepithelial lesion
ICRU	International Commission on Radiation Units and Measurements
IMRT	Intensity-modulated radiation therapy
ITV	Internal target volume
KPS	Karnofsky performance status
LEEP	Loop electrosurgical excision procedure
LND	Lymph node dissection
LVSI	Lymphovascular space invasion
MRI	Magnetic resonance imaging
NED	No evidence of disease
PA	Posterior–anterior
PAN	Paraaortic node
PDR	Pulsed-dose rate
PET	Positron emission tomography
PTV	Planning target volume
RT	Radiation therapy

CS 10.1 • Stage IB1 Cervical Cancer in a Patient Treated with Hysterectomy Who had High-Risk Features and a Treatment Delay

History: A 36-year-old woman with stage IB1 squamous carcinoma of the cervix had robotic radical hysterectomy and bilateral pelvic LND at an outside facility. Her recovery was uneventful, but social problems delayed each stage of treatment. Eleven weeks after surgery, the patient was referred to gynecologic oncology for a second opinion regarding the need for adjuvant therapy.

Pathology (Hysterectomy): Squamous carcinoma invading 15 mm; closest deep margin 5.5 mm; extensive LVSI; early parametrial involvement; 1 of 12 pelvic lymph nodes involved with microscopic disease; no ECE.

Evaluation at Diagnosis: *PET*: NED outside the cervix.

Evaluation Before RT: *Exam, abdominopelvic CT, and CXR*: NED

Treatment Plan: The deep invasion, parametrial involvement, and lymph node metastasis suggested a >25% risk of pelvic disease recurrence without further treatment. The use of adjuvant chemoradiation was strongly supported by level 1 evidence. However, the effectiveness of standard-dose RT could be compromised by the long interval between surgery and RT. Also, the patient's treatment start date was mid-December, which meant that several holidays would fall during her treatment. We anticipated that her social situation could cause additional delays. For these reasons, the pelvis was treated using IMRT with a slightly higher-than-usual dose and dose per fraction, and the vaginal cuff was boosted using brachytherapy.

Several other steps were taken to minimize the total time from surgery to the end of RT. Immediately upon learning the patient's history, the gynecologic oncologist requested urgent RT consultation; the patient was seen and simulation was performed that day. Treatment was started on the subsequent Monday (12 weeks after surgery); b.i.d. treatments (with a 6-hour interfraction interval) were scheduled to make up for holidays. The risks of additional treatment protraction were discussed with the patient, and she was supported in her efforts to keep on schedule. Social services were consulted to provide assistance as needed. When the patient missed 5 days because of personal issues, 2 more days of b.i.d. treatment were arranged.

Pelvic IMRT (*a to c*): Nodal CTV and vaginal ITV + 7 mm: 50 Gy in 25 fractions (completed in 46 days). The vaginal ITV was derived from fused CT scans, one with a full bladder and very full rectum (***a***, ***c***) and the other after the patient had evacuated the bladder and rectum. The apex was located using radiopaque marker seeds that had been inserted adjacent to the vaginal scar.

Brachytherapy: HDR: 5 Gy × 2 prescribed to the surface of apical vagina.

Chemotherapy: Concurrent weekly cisplatin was discontinued after two cycles because of severe migraines and tinnitus.

Outcome: At 3 months, NED on active surveillance.

Comment: Because the indications for treatment were compelling, adjuvant treatment was recommended despite the long interval between surgery and RT. The impact of treatment delay was minimized through proactive management of the RT schedule to compensate for holidays and other impediments. A background of close multidisciplinary collaboration meant that the gynecologic oncologist understood the urgency of prompt RT consultation and avoided added delays in the initiation of adjuvant treatment.

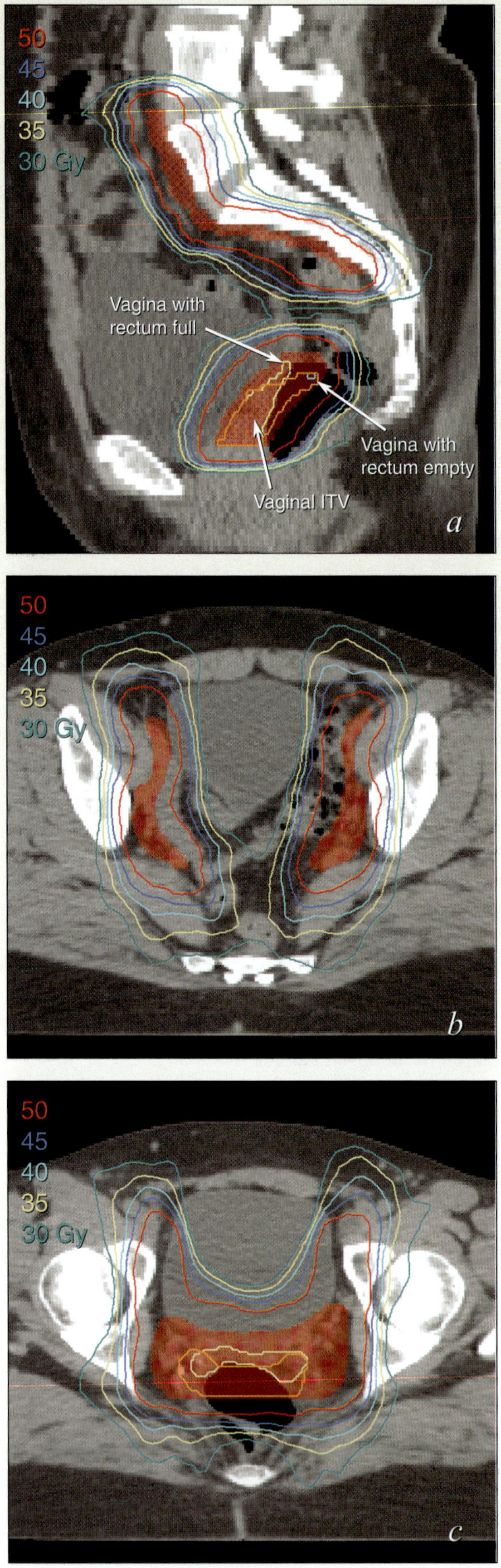

CS 10.2 • Stage IB1 Cervical Cancer in a Patient Treated with Radical Hysterectomy Who had a Positive Parametrial Margin

History: A 40-year-old woman with 3 to 4 months of intermenstrual bleeding had a Pap test showing HSIL and high-risk HPV. Endocervical curettage showed invasive squamous carcinoma, and an LEEP biopsy had widely positive margins. The patient was referred for evaluation and treatment. She smoked one pack of cigarettes per day but was otherwise in good health.

Evaluation: *Exam*: Expected sequelae of LEEP biopsy; the cervix otherwise appeared normal without palpable lesions. *Chest radiography*: NED.

Initial Surgical Treatment: Laparoscopic radical hysterectomy and bilateral pelvic LND. After the uterine specimen was removed, nodularity was noted at the right vaginal margin; frozen section evaluation showed a positive margin, which was re-excised.

Pathology: Squamous carcinoma involving the entire cervix with 19.5 mm of invasion; extensive LVSI; perineural invasion; positive right parametrial margin; positive margin of the vaginal re-excision; only four nodes found in the lymphadenectomy specimens, all negative.

Treatment Plan: With a positive parametrial margin and other high-risk features, this patient was at very high risk for local recurrence. In addition, with very few nodes in the surgical specimen, the risk of undetected lymph node involvement was high. PET would not have been helpful during the immediate postoperative period because there were no abnormal nodes on planning CT with good visualization of the node-bearing regions; thus, no additional staging was obtained.

A minimum dose of 60 Gy is recommended to prevent recurrence in the region of a positive margin. After hysterectomy, the retracted parametrial tissues are unlikely to be close enough to the vaginal apex to be adequately treated with intracavitary brachytherapy. Instead, integrated and sequential IMRT boosts were used to treat the HRCTV-ITV in the right vagina and parametrium to a total dose of 60 Gy. The HRCTV was designated after detailed review of the operative findings and discussion with the surgeon and examining pathologist.

The patient was counseled that her heavy smoking would increase the risk of major treatment-related complications, and she enrolled in a smoking cessation program.

Radiation Therapy (IMRT):

Setup: Supine in a custom cradle. Bladder volume was monitored with sonography, and the locations of vaginal fiducial markers (***c***, *arrows*) were monitored on daily KV imaging.

*Fractions 1 to 25 (**a, b**)*:

Nodal CTV and vaginal ITV + 7 mm: 45 Gy (1.8 Gy/fraction)

HRCTV + 5 mm: 50 Gy (2 Gy/fraction)

*Fractions 26 to 30 (**c**)*:

HRCTV + 6 mm: 10 Gy (2 Gy/fraction), increasing the total dose to 60 Gy (***d***, ***e***)

Treatment was completed in 39 days.

Chemotherapy: Weekly cisplatin × 5.

Outcome: At 6 months, NED by CT and exam. At 2 years, NED by CT and exam, under active surveillance. No gastrointestinal or urinary tract symptoms.

Comment: In general, primary surgical treatment is not recommended if there is a high likelihood of positive surgical margins because the risk of bladder and bowel complications increases steeply with central external beam doses >50 to 55 Gy. Occasionally, apparently early-stage cancers are more infiltrative than expected. In such cases, IMRT can be used to reduce the doses to critical structures from postoperative RT, but boost volumes should be sufficiently generous to fully cover the paracervical region and account for organ motion (Chapter 5).

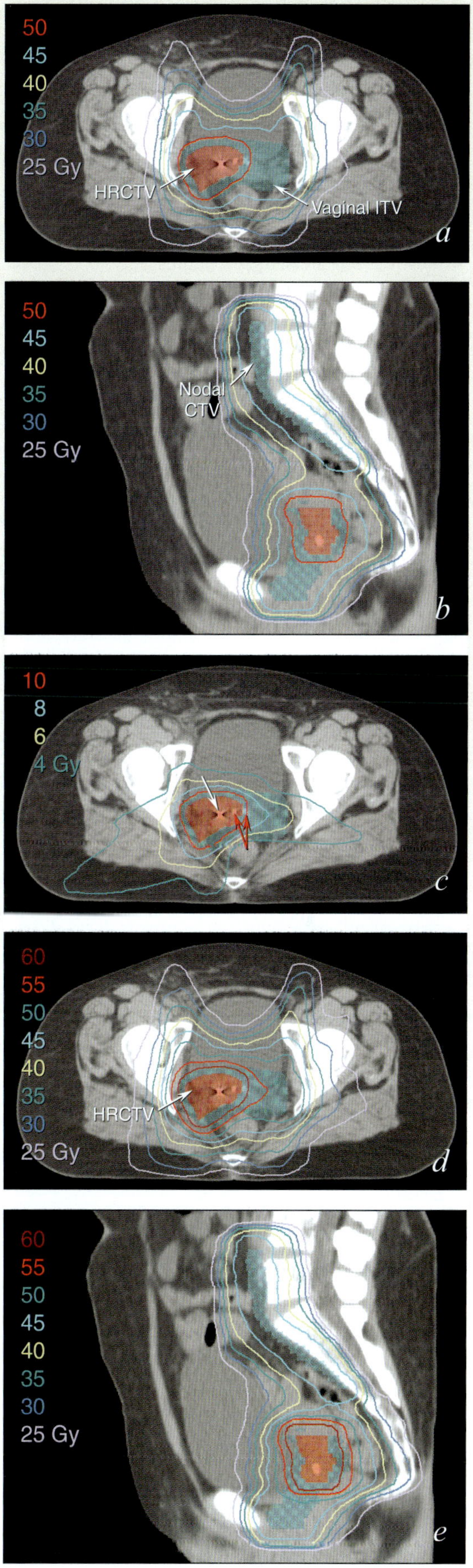

CS 10.3 • Stage IB1 Cervical Cancer in an Elderly Woman

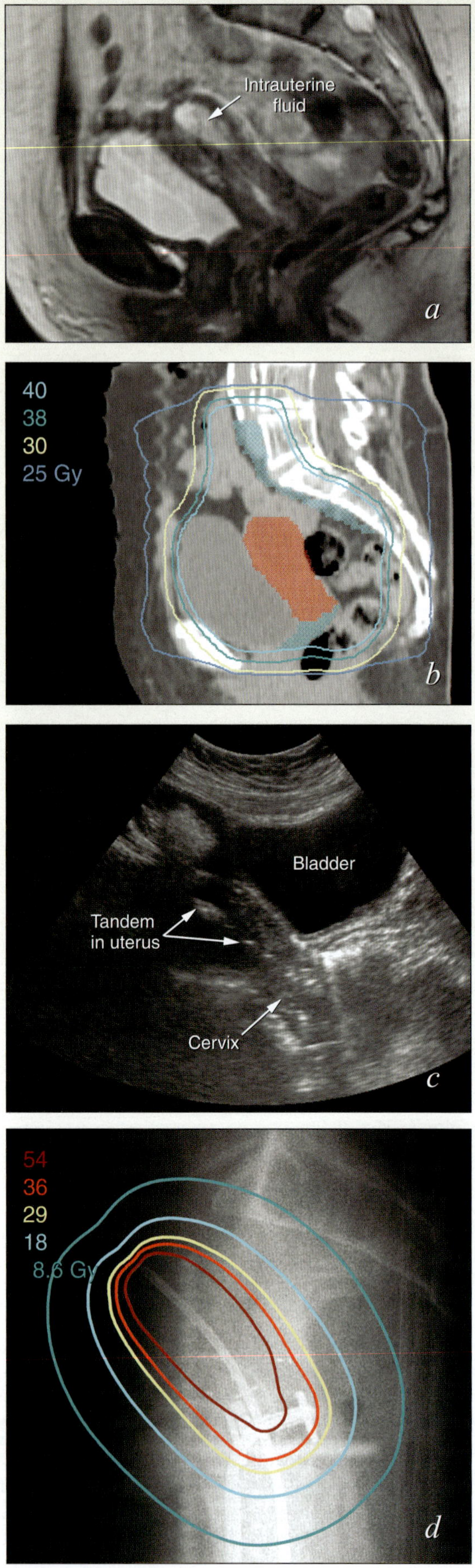

History: An 84-year-old woman with postmenopausal bleeding had had an endocervical curettage, which revealed squamous carcinoma. After undergoing a cold knife cone biopsy, she was referred for further evaluation and treatment. She was in good health for her age, with treated hypertension and hypercholesterolemia.

Evaluation: *Exam*: Sequelae of cone biopsy and a suspicious 2-cm lesion on the remaining anterior cervix. *KPS*: 90. *MRI (**a**)*: Fluid in the uterine cavity and cervical canal consistent with hematometra; changes within the cervix were interpreted as nonspecific; no parametrial involvement or lymphadenopathy. *Chest radiography*: NED. *Cone biopsy*: Poorly differentiated squamous carcinoma involving the full thickness of the cone (>5 mm) with LVSI. *Biopsy (anterior cervix)*: Squamous carcinoma.

Treatment Plan: Radical hysterectomy would have been a reasonable option; however, with widely positive cone margins and LVSI, the patient would have had a significant chance of requiring adjuvant RT. After discussion with the patient, definitive RT was recommended.

According to MD Anderson data, the pelvic control rate after definitive RT for a small stage IB1 squamous carcinoma with negative nodes is 98%.[14] Patients with such cancers were not included in the randomized chemoradiation trials. Given the narrow margin for improvement with chemotherapy over RT alone, the risks of chemotherapy were judged to outweigh any theoretical benefit, particularly for a woman of this advanced age.

It was decided to begin treatment with brachytherapy for several reasons. First, for a small tumor like this, the vaginal anatomy is typically more accommodating prior to EBRT than after. Second, elderly women who have had a cone biopsy can develop severe occlusion of the endocervical canal, complicating uterine sounding for brachytherapy after EBRT. In this case, initial sounding of the uterus released 10 to 15 mL of pus, indicating that the patient had a pyometra. The planned brachytherapy was aborted. The endocervical canal was dilated to 12 mm to facilitate drainage, the patient was started on a 10-day course of antibiotics, EBRT was started, and intracavitary brachytherapy was rescheduled for 2 weeks later.

Radiation Therapy:

Setup: Supine in a fixed immobilization device.

EBRT: The pelvis was treated using a four-field technique with 18-MV photons to a dose of 40 Gy in 20 fractions (***b***). The nodal target volume included the external and internal iliac nodes proximally to about 1 cm above the common iliac bifurcation.

Brachytherapy: After the 2nd week of EBRT, the patient had a single PDR intracavitary treatment. Sonography of the uterus (***c***) revealed no residual intrauterine fluid. The dose to point A was 36 Gy (at 50 cGy per hourly pulse) for a total dose of 76 Gy (***d***). Based on the size of the cervix documented on pretreatment MRI and sonography, the HRCTV was treated to >85 Gy (including EBRT); the total doses to ICRU bladder and rectal points were 59 Gy and 63 Gy, respectively.

Treatment was completed in 28 days.

Outcome: At 5 years, NED by exam. No gastrointestinal or urinary tract symptoms.

Comment: The dose of brachytherapy should be based on the size of the target volume rather than on a rigidly prescribed dose to point A; direct image guidance is ideal, although reference to pretreatment imaging can be used to determine the dose, as was done in this case. Ultrasound guidance is particularly helpful when there is evidence of endocervical obstruction.

CS 10.4 • Stage IB2 Cervical Cancer with Bilateral Pelvic Node Metastases

History: A 30-year-old woman, gravida 3, para 3, had a routine Pap test showing HSIL. At follow-up evaluation 4 months later, she had an abnormal 4- to 4.5-cm cervix and was 8 weeks pregnant. She was referred for evaluation and treatment.

Evaluation (3 Weeks After Follow-up Evaluation): *Exam*: 5- to 6-cm cervical tumor; no parametrial or vaginal lesions. *MRI* (***a***): 5 × 6 cm cervical mass; bilateral EI nodes (*red arrows*), 2.8 × 2 cm on the right and 1.6 × 3 cm on the left. *Sonography*: Intrauterine pregnancy, 10 to 11 weeks' gestation. *Biopsy (cervix)*: Invasive squamous carcinoma.

Chemotherapy can often be used as a temporizing measure to bring a pregnancy to near term. However, this patient's locoregionally extensive tumor appeared to be progressing rapidly; a minimum 5-month delay would have been required to bring the fetus to 32 weeks. After counseling and discussion of options, the patient elected to terminate her pregnancy.

Subsequent PET–CT (***b***) showed FDG avidity in the cervix, bilateral EI nodes, and a small right CI node anterior to S1; otherwise, the patient had NED.

Treatment Plan: Chemoradiation with EBRT and PDR brachytherapy.

EBRT: The proximal border of the CTV (***d***) was placed at the aortic bifurcation, 10 cm above the suspicious CI node. The CTV was treated using four fields of 18-MV photons to 45 Gy in 25 fractions (***c***, ***d***).

Brachytherapy: At EUA, the cervix was 3.5 cm in diameter. The doses from the first 44-hour PDR brachytherapy administration were as follows: *HRCTV* D_{90}, 25 Gy; *point A*, 20 Gy; *bladder* D_{2cc}, 18 Gy; *rectum* D_{2cc}, 8.6 Gy (***e***, ***f***). A second, similar treatment was performed 2 weeks later but planned without MRI guidance.

Boosts to Nodal GTVs: Nodal GTVs were boosted (***g***, ***h***) between the first and second implants. The minimum total doses from brachytherapy were estimated to be about 9 Gy to the right EI, 7 Gy to the left EI, and 6 Gy to the CI node.

These nodes were then boosted using IMRT to 12 Gy in 6 fractions. Using AP–PA fields, an additional 2 Gy was given to the left EI GTV. The planning dosimetrist was instructed to minimize the doses to central structures (***h***).

Total doses (including all treatments): *point A*, 87 Gy; HRCTV, 95 Gy; *right and left EI nodes*, 66 Gy; *left CI node*, 63 Gy.

Treatment was completed in 53 days.

Chemotherapy: Weekly cisplatin × 6.

Outcome: At 4 months, NED by PET and exam. At 2 years, Pap showed HSIL; cervical biopsies showed foci of CIN2 in a background of CIN1. At 3 years, NED with no gastrointestinal or urinary complaints.

Comments: Although the total dose to the ICRU bladder point was 62 Gy, the estimated bladder D_{2cc} was 85 to 87 Gy. Guidelines for balancing doses to tumor and critical structures are evolving, but today, we would reduce the HRCTV somewhat and would attempt to keep the bladder D_{2cc} below 80 Gy. This requires careful consideration of the doses from each component, including nodal boosts.

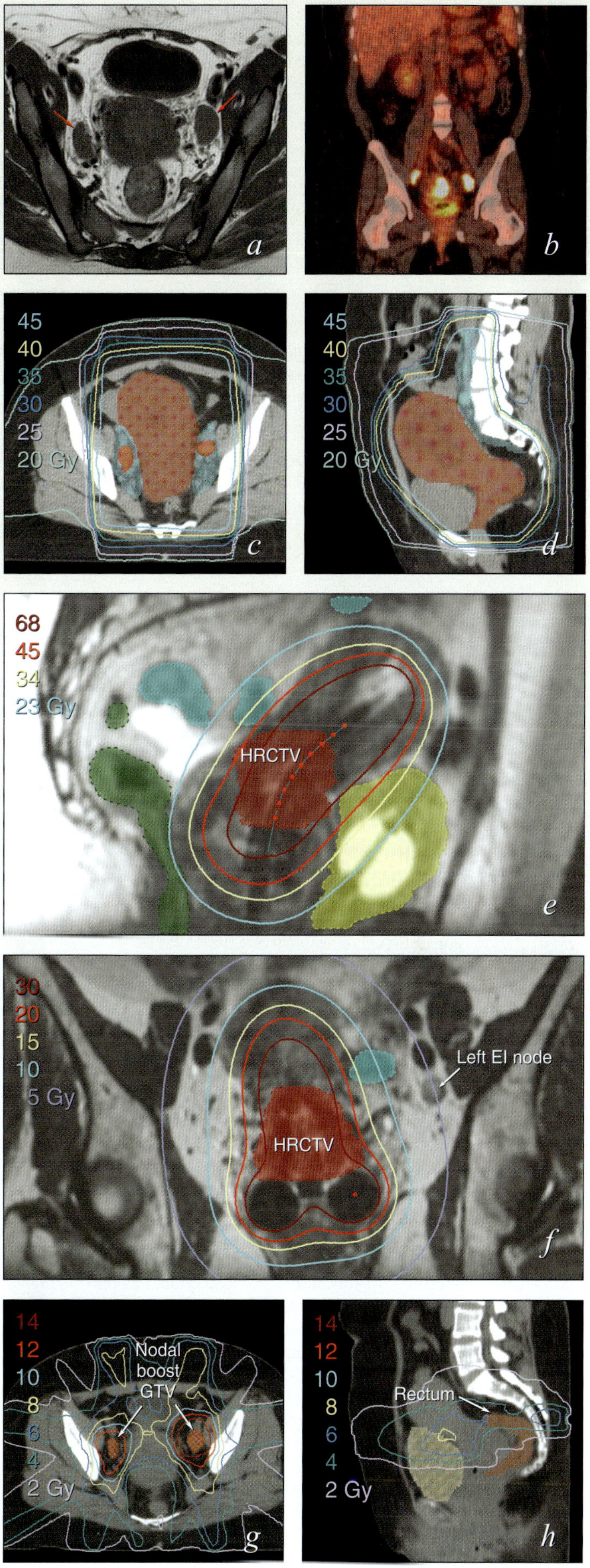

CS 10.5 • Stage IB2 Squamous Carcinoma with Bilateral Pelvic Node Metastases

History: A 30-year-old woman with a 6-month history of intermenstrual bleeding had a Pap test showing poorly differentiated squamous carcinoma. Exam revealed an abnormal cervix, and the patient was referred for evaluation and treatment.

Evaluation: *Exam*: Expanded, barrel-shaped cervix 5 cm in diameter; no parametrial or vaginal involvement. *KPS*: 100. *MRI*: 5 × 4.5 × 3.5 cm cervical mass involving the right parametrium (***a***, *arrows*); 1.7 × 1 cm right internal iliac node; 1.3 × 1 cm left EI node (***b***). *PET–CT*: FDG-avid cervical mass and bilateral iliac nodes; no DM. *Biopsy (cervix)*: Squamous carcinoma. *Extraperitoneal PAN dissection*: 15 PANs, all negative.

Treatment Plan: Definitive chemoradiation using a combination of EBRT and brachytherapy. The target volume included the external, internal, and common iliac nodes. The bladder was empty during the simulation (***c***); however, the MRI (***a***) showed a shift of at least 3 cm with bladder filling. IMRT would have provided limited sparing in this situation.

Radiation Therapy:

Setup: Supine in a custom cradle.

Fractions 1 to 25 (***c***, ***d***): Using a four-field technique and 18-MV photons, the whole pelvis was treated to a total dose of 45 Gy in 25 fractions.

Fractions 26 to 32: Using IMRT with a noncoplanar technique (***g***, ***h***; composite EBRT, ***i***, ***j***):

Right and left nodal GTV + 6 mm: 14 Gy (total dose including brachytherapy, 65 to 67 Gy)

Brachytherapy:

After pelvic EBRT, the cervix was friable and measured 3.5 cm. PDR brachytherapy was performed in two sessions using a tandem and 2-cm shielded ovoids. Doses from the first brachytherapy are shown in ***e*** and ***f***.

The combined doses from EBRT and brachytherapy were point A (mean), 88 Gy; D_{90} HRCTV (cervix), 95 Gy; ICRU rectum, 65Gy; D_{2cc} rectum, <60 Gy; ICRU bladder, 56 Gy; and D_{2cc} bladder, 68 Gy.

Treatment was completed in 48 days.

Chemotherapy: Weekly cisplatin × 4. The patient declined chemotherapy in her 3rd week after an allergic reaction to cisplatin. Chemotherapy was subsequently resumed using a desensitization protocol.

Outcome: At 3 months, NED by exam; minimal residual FDG uptake in the cervix (SUV, 3.8). At 5 months, NED by PET. At 14 months, intermittent mild hematuria for several weeks; cystoscopy showed inflammation of the posterior bladder wall. At 3 years, NED in active follow-up; no gastrointestinal or genitourinary symptoms; no dyspareunia.

Comment: The role of staging lymphadenectomy has not yet been clearly established; in this case, PAN dissection was performed as part of an investigational trial.

AP–PA techniques are not recommended for boost doses >8 to 10 Gy. Coplanar IMRT techniques frequently contribute unacceptable doses to central critical structures, potentially requiring compromises in the central brachytherapy dose. The noncoplanar technique used here contributed 2 Gy or less to the rectosigmoid (***j***).

This patient was treated during our transition to image-guided brachytherapy. Today, we would probably give a slightly lower dose of 85 to 90 Gy to the D_{90}, which would have reduced the dose to small bowel in the cul-de-sac.

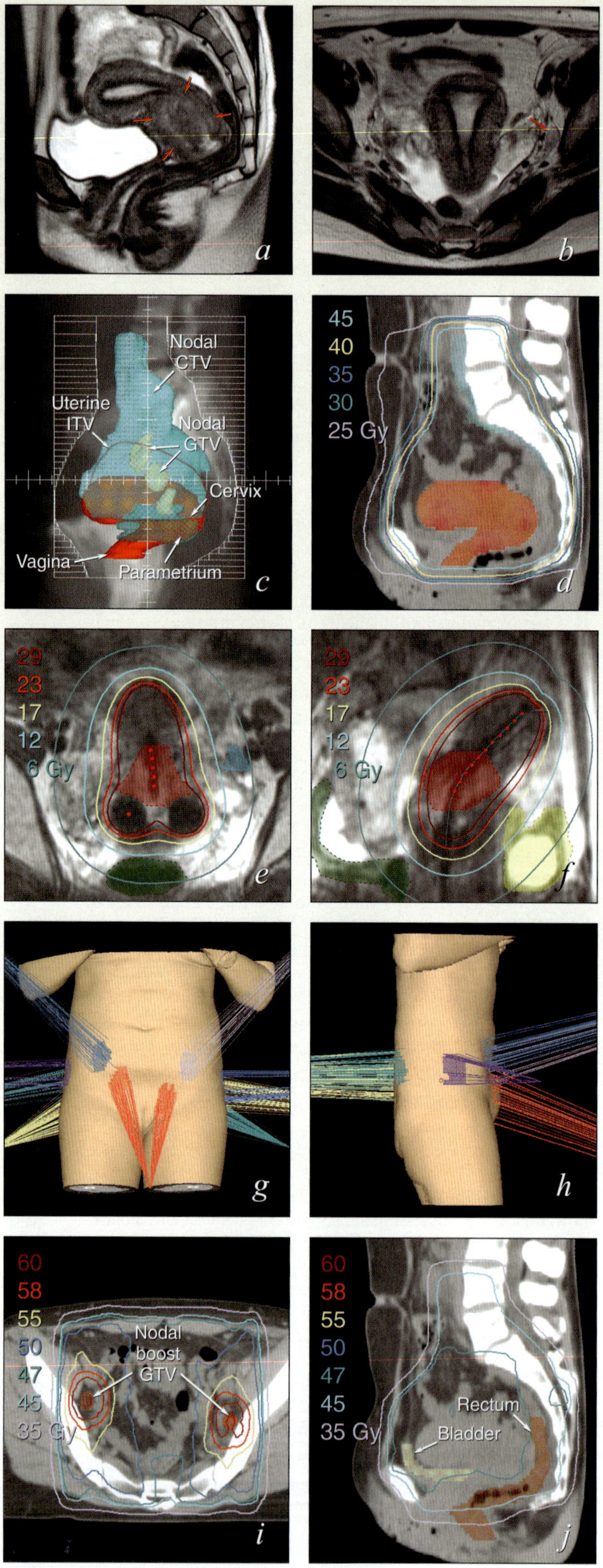

CS 10.6 • Stage IIB Cervical Cancer with Pelvic and Aortic Node Metastases

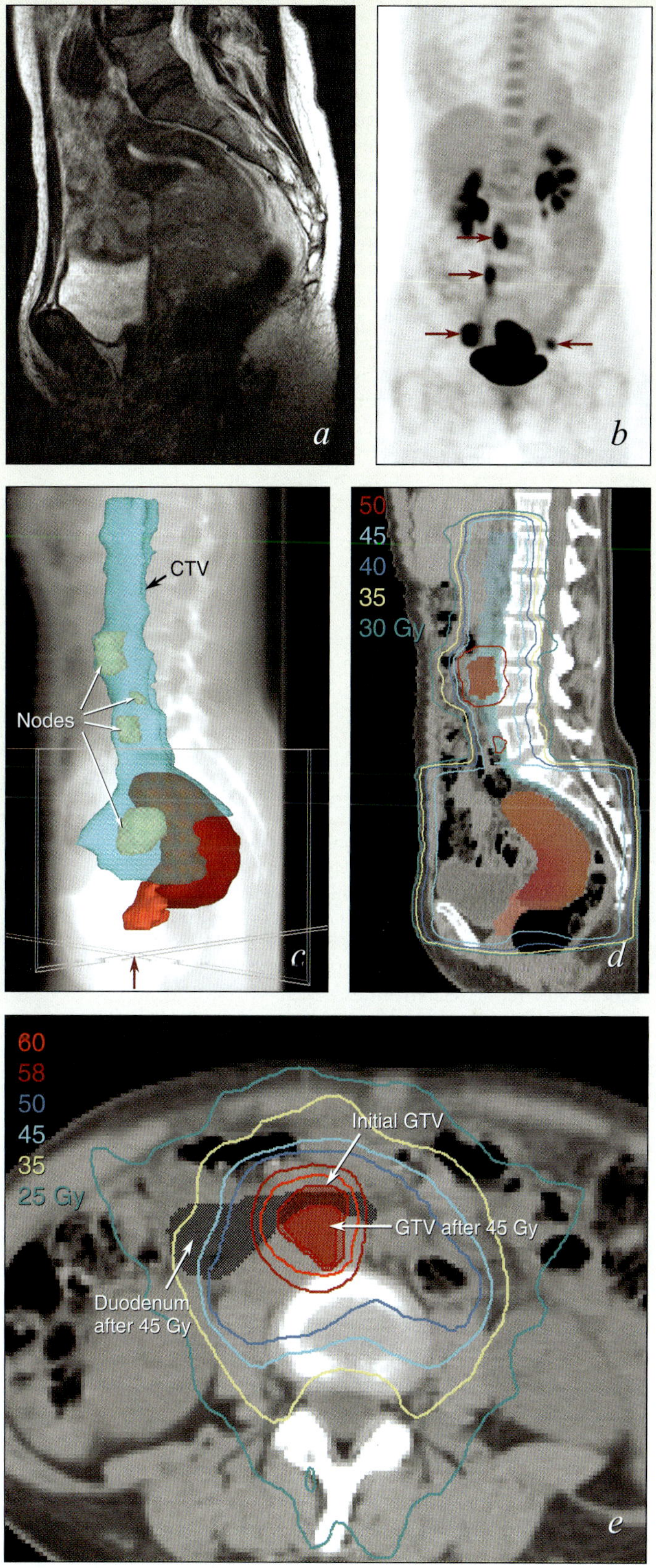

History: A 49-year-old with metrorrhagia and pelvic pain.

Evaluation: *Exam*: 7-cm endocervical tumor involving the left vaginal fornix and parametrium; *KPS*: 80. *MRI* (***a***): 6.5-cm cervix with left parametrial nodule and enlarged pelvic nodes; *PET* (***b***): FDG-avid cervix; bilateral external iliac, right common iliac, and distal PANs up to 3 cm in diameter (*red arrows*); *Biopsy (cervix)*: Squamous carcinoma.

Treatment Plan: Definitive chemoradiation using EBRT and brachytherapy. Treatment options for the nodes included RT alone (≥60 Gy) or resection of enlarged nodes followed by RT. The largest nodes were considered marginally resectable with a high probability of at least ECE. Also, the size of the primary tumor and the risk of DM were believed to be greater obstacles to cure than the enlarged nodes, and the decision was made to treat with chemoradiation only.

EBRT: *Setup* (***c***): Supine in upper and lower cradles with arms above the head. The isocenter was placed above the uterus between involved nodes. Distal field lengths were adjusted to match the distal vaginal target (*red arrow*).

The PTV nearly filled the pelvis in this thin patient (***c***). Because lateral fields or IMRT would have contributed very little tissue sparing once organ motion was considered, the distal pelvis was treated using AP–PA 18-MV fields. The CTV extended 7 cm above the highest PET-positive node.

*Fractions 1 to 25 (**d**)*:

Distal pelvis (AP–PA): 45 Gy (1.8 Gy/fraction)

CI and PAN CTV + 7 mm: 45 Gy

CI and PAN GTV + 5 mm: 50 Gy (2.0 Gy/fraction)

Fractions 26 to 30 (between brachytherapy applications):

CI and PAN boost GTV + 6 mm: 50 Gy (2.0 Gy/fraction)

In addition, the bilateral PET-positive distal iliac nodes were boosted using AP–PA fields to increase the total dose to 63 to 64 Gy (including the brachytherapy contribution).

GTVs for the nodal boosts were based on repeat CT (***e***) showing marked tumor response. In particular, the PAN had decreased significantly (*solid red*), allowing an accompanying shift in the position of the duodenum (***e***, *black*). The duodenal $D_{55\ Gy}$ was <15 cc.

Brachytherapy (not shown): After 45 Gy of pelvic RT, the cervix was about 4 cm in diameter. The patient was then treated using PDR in two treatments 2 weeks apart. Both treatments were given using a 6-cm tandem and 2-cm shielded Fletcher-style ovoids. With this, the total dose (EqD2) to the cervix GTV/HRCTV was ≥90 Gy (88 Gy to point A). Bladder and rectal reference doses were ≤66 Gy.

All treatment was completed in 42 days.

Chemotherapy: Weekly cisplatin was discontinued after four courses because of neutropenia.

Outcome: At 4 months, NED on PET and physical exam. At 5 years, NED with normal bowel and bladder function, occasional postcoital spotting, and no dyspareunia.

Comments: While advanced imaging and IMRT have contributed to improved survival rates for patients with PAN metastases, the radiation dose to the duodenum must be monitored closely. Today, we would reimage in the 3rd week to consider an earlier plan adjustment.

CS 10.7 • Stage IIB Cervical Cancer with Bilateral Pelvic Nodes and a Marginal PAN Recurrence

History: A 56-year-old woman with postmenopausal bleeding.

Evaluation: *Exam*: 7-cm exophytic mass; left parametrial involvement tethered but not definitely fixed to pelvic wall. *KPS*: 90. *MRI*: 7 × 5 × 5 cm mass replacing the cervix and involving most of the uterine body (***a**, arrows*); parametrial involvement; 1.8 × 2 cm left external iliac node; 1.9 × 0.7 cm right external iliac node. *PET* (***b***): FDG-avid mass replacing the cervix and uterine body and bilateral EI nodes; several FDG-negative subcentimeter retroperitoneal nodes; no DM. *Biopsy (cervix)*: Squamous carcinoma.

Treatment Plan: Definitive chemoradiation using EBRT and intracavitary brachytherapy. The fields were extended to L2/3 to include equivocal PET-negative distal PANs (***c***, ***d***). EUA at the first brachytherapy application revealed residual left parametrial thickening tethered to the pelvic wall. Between brachytherapy applications, this region and the initially involved nodes were boosted; doses were selected to increase the total doses to 62 to 64 Gy, including the contribution from brachytherapy (estimated from the first implant).

EBRT: *Setup*: Supine in a fixed device.

Fractions 1 to 25: The pelvis and distal PANs were initially treated using a four-field technique to a total dose of 45 Gy in 25 fractions.

Fractions 26 to 29 (***g***, ***h***):

Right EI node (AP-PA, 18-MV photons): 6 Gy in 3 fractions

Left parametrium and external iliac GTV (AP-PA, 18-MV photons): 8 Gy in 4 fractions

Brachytherapy: After 45 Gy of pelvic RT, the cervix was 4 cm in diameter. Central disease was then treated using PDR in two treatments 2 weeks apart. The tandem length was adjusted to cover the entire uterine cavity, with correct positioning verified intraoperatively using sonography (***e***). The total dose (EqD2) to the cervix GTV/HRCTV was ≥85 Gy (86 Gy to point A). Bladder and rectal reference doses were 70 Gy and 68 Gy, respectively. Dwells were activated along the full length of the uterine tandem to provide adequate coverage of intrauterine disease (first application shown in ***f***).

Treatment was completed in 40 days.

Chemotherapy: Weekly cisplatin × 6.

Outcome: Treatment was well tolerated, although high glucose levels after chemotherapy-associated steroids revealed the patient to be diabetic. At 5 months, PET showed complete resolution of pelvic disease, but there was a new 1-cm FDG-avid lymph node near the left renal vein, just above the previous RT fields. The patient was retreated definitively with chemoradiation; IMRT was used to treat the PAN GTV + 5 mm to 60 Gy and PAN CTV + 5 to 6 mm to 45 to 47 Gy (***i***). Composite plan (***j***) showed a small region of 70 Gy where the fields overlapped but the duodenal D_{2cc} was <60 Gy. Four years after her recurrence, the patient had NED.

Comments: Marginal recurrences can sometimes be cured if detected early, but composite doses to critical structures must be monitored closely. The high paraaortic recurrence in this case may have been a secondary metastasis or a rare direct metastasis from her extensive uterine body disease.

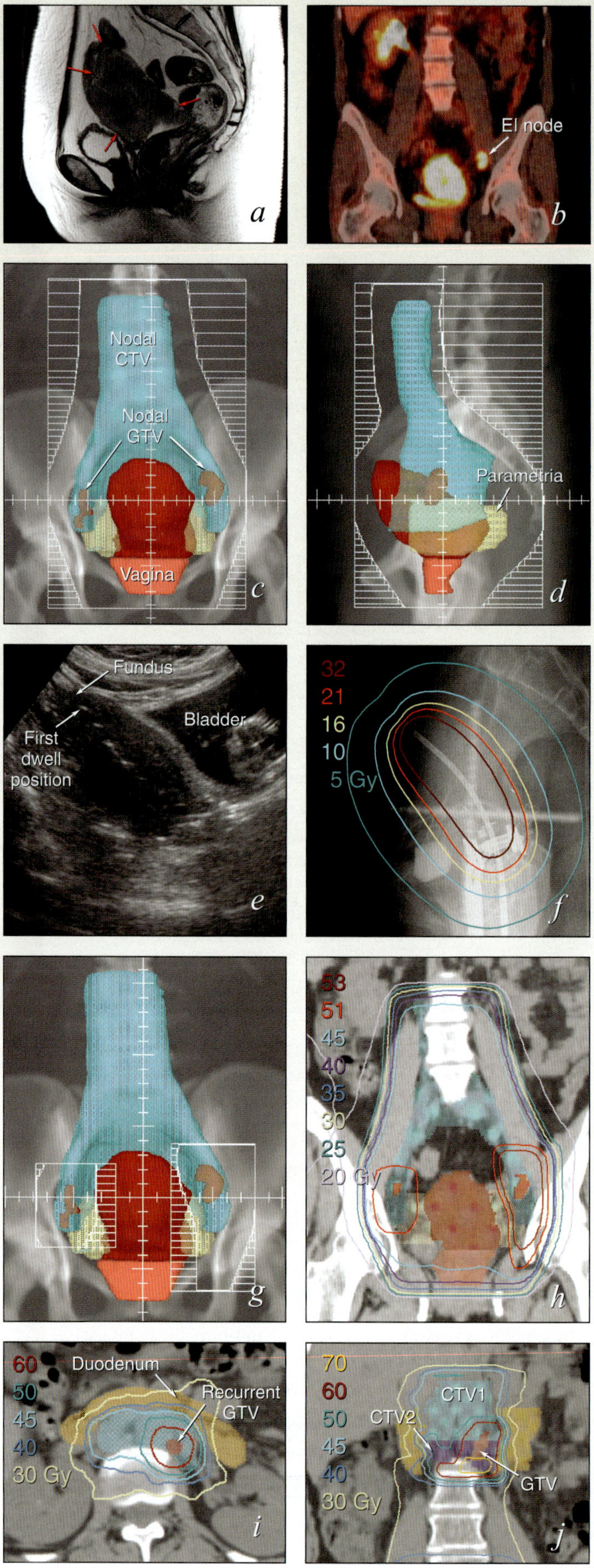

CS 10.8 • Stage IIIB Squamous Carcinoma with a Skip Lesion in the Distal Vagina

History: A 60-year-old woman with 1 year of vaginal spotting and an abnormal cervix.

Evaluation: *Exam*: 6-cm mass replacing the cervix and infiltrating the upper vagina with a separate 2-cm distal suburethral vaginal mass. *KPS*: 90. *Creatinine*: 7 mg/dL. *CT, MRI*: 6 × 5 × 4 cm cervical mass involving the anterior vaginal wall and bilateral parametria (***a***); distal 2.7 × 2.3 cm anterior vaginal nodule displacing the urethra and possibly involving the right levator anus (***b***, *red arrows*); bilateral iliac nodes; bilateral hydronephrosis. *PET–CT*: FDG-avid masses in the cervix and distal vagina; multiple bilateral pelvic nodes up to 2 cm in diameter, including a distal right CI node; small (5- to 6-mm) bilateral PET-avid inguinal nodes; no DM. *Biopsy (cervix)*: Squamous carcinoma.

Treatment Plan: Definitive chemoradiation using a combination of EBRT and brachytherapy. Following placement of bilateral percutaneous nephrostomies, renal function began to improve. However, creatinine levels did not return to normal for 4 weeks, so concurrent weekly carboplatin was given in place of cisplatin. Deeply infiltrating disease in the right periurethral sulcus would have been inadequately covered with intracavitary brachytherapy; consequently, this region was treated with an integrated IMRT boost and was further treated using interstitial brachytherapy.

Radiation Therapy (IMRT):

Setup: Supine in frog-leg position with arms above the head.

Fractions 1 to 25 (***e***) (fractions 1 to 4 were delivered using a four-field technique):

Nodal CTV + 7 mm: 45 Gy (1.8 Gy/fraction)

Distal vaginal GTV + 5 mm: 48.6 Gy

Fractions 26 to 33 (not shown):

PET-positive pelvic nodes (***c,d***) were boosted using IMRT to increase the total dose (including brachytherapy) to ≥64 Gy; equivocal nodes in the bilateral groins were boosted to 54 Gy using electrons.

Brachytherapy:

After pelvic EBRT, the cervix measured 3 cm, and there was minimal residual thickening in the anterior fornix and parametrium; residual distal vaginal disease measured 8 to 10 mm. PDR brachytherapy was performed using a tandem and 3-cm intravaginal cylinders. During the first of two PDR treatments (***e,f***), two interstitial needles (***g***) were inserted in the right periurethral sulcus.

The combined doses from EBRT and brachytherapy were as follows: D_{90} HRCTV (cervix, upper vagina), 90 Gy; distal vaginal nodule GTV, 70 Gy; D_{2cc} rectum, 69 Gy; D_{2cc} bladder, 65.5 Gy; and point A (mean), 77 Gy.

Treatment was completed in 54 days.

Chemotherapy: Weekly carboplatin × 5.

Outcome: At 2 months, the nephrostomies were successfully removed. At 4 months, NED by PET–CT and MRI (***h***). At 1 year, PET showed a new, solitary 1.5-cm PET-avid lesion in the mediastinum (arrow, ***i***). Biopsy showed metastatic squamous carcinoma. After some discussion, the recurrence was treated definitively with chemoradiotherapy (***j***). At 2.5 years (1.5 years after recurrence), the patient has NED in active surveillance.

Comment: This is an uncommon disease presentation that has historically had a poor prognosis. However, modern image-guided techniques improve control over the radiation dose distribution, which may lead to improved local disease control. The decision to treat mediastinal oligometastasis definitively is controversial, but we have seen prolonged disease-free survival in some patients.

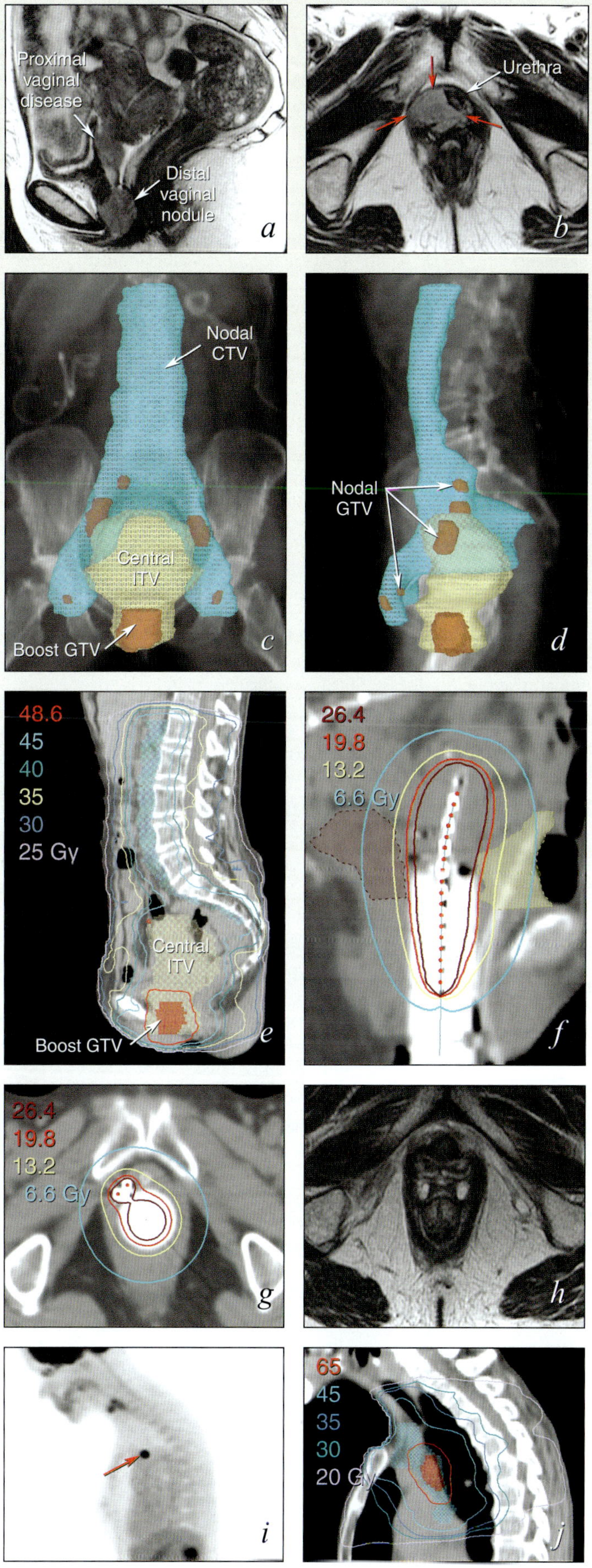

CS 10.9 • Adenocarcinoma of the Cervix Recurrent in Pelvic Nodes After Radical Hysterectomy

History: A 32-year-old woman had a radical hysterectomy, left oophorectomy, and bilateral LND for adenocarcinoma of the cervix, villoglandular type. There was 4 mm of stromal invasion and no LVSI; 15 right and 9 left pelvic nodes had NED. Imaging findings in the first year of follow-up were reportedly negative. Four years later, the patient had onset of left thigh and buttock pain.

Initial Evaluation (Before Referral): *CT, PET–CT*: FDG-avid 4 × 2 cm right CI mass; 5 × 5.8 cm left pelvic mass (***a, c****, white arrows*) and several smaller left iliac nodes (***c****, red arrows*); right iliac lymphocyst (***a***); cystic right ovary. *Laparoscopic right oophorectomy*: NED. *Biopsy of left iliac mass*: Villoglandular adenocarcinoma.

The patient was treated with three cycles of carboplatin and Taxotere and then sought a second opinion regarding the possible role of RT.

Postchemotherapy Evaluation: *PET–CT*: Marked improvement (***b***) with >50% response and minimal residual FDG avidity.

Treatment Plan: Although this patient had a very good early response, chemotherapy alone is rarely if ever curative for patients with cervical cancer. Although continuation of chemotherapy for several more cycles was considered, there is no evidence that prolonged neoadjuvant chemotherapy improves the outcome of definitive RT for cervical cancer. Additional chemotherapy also would have compromised the ability to give full-dose concurrent cisplatin with extended field RT. For this reason, immediate chemoradiation was recommended. Even after a good chemotherapy response, doses of at least 60 Gy are recommended for initial areas of gross disease. The most difficult question was how to treat several 6- to 7-mm nodes noted on the original imaging. Although the nodes were PET negative, their location just proximal to bulky nodal disease was concerning. It was decided to designate this region an HRCTV (***d***) to receive 55 Gy. The proximal border of the CTV was placed 10 cm above the highest originally FDG-avid node. The vagina was not treated because of the long interval with NED in this site.

Radiation Therapy (IMRT):

Setup: Supine in custom cradles with arms above the head.

*Fractions 1 to 25 (**e, f**)*:

Nodal CTV + 7 mm: 45 Gy (1.8 Gy/fraction)

Nodal boosts:

*Fractions 26 to 30 (**g, h**)*:

Nodal GTV and HRCTV + 7 mm: 10 Gy (2 Gy/fraction)

Fractions 31 to 33:

Nodal GTV + 5 mm: 6 Gy (2 Gy/fraction)

Treatment was completed in 44 days.

Chemotherapy: Weekly cisplatin × 5. After RT, the patient returned home, where she completed two more courses of chemotherapy for a total of six.

Outcome: At 1 year, NED by PET and exam. At 3 years, NED with moderate left leg edema.

Comment: Although we usually recommend initial treatment with concurrent chemoradiation (Chapter 3), this patient had a very good outcome with combined sequential and concurrent chemotherapy. Integration of a portion of the GTV boost from the start of RT would have permitted somewhat tighter PTV margins; however, because the arrival of complete DICOM files from prechemotherapy PET was delayed, the boosts were planned sequentially.

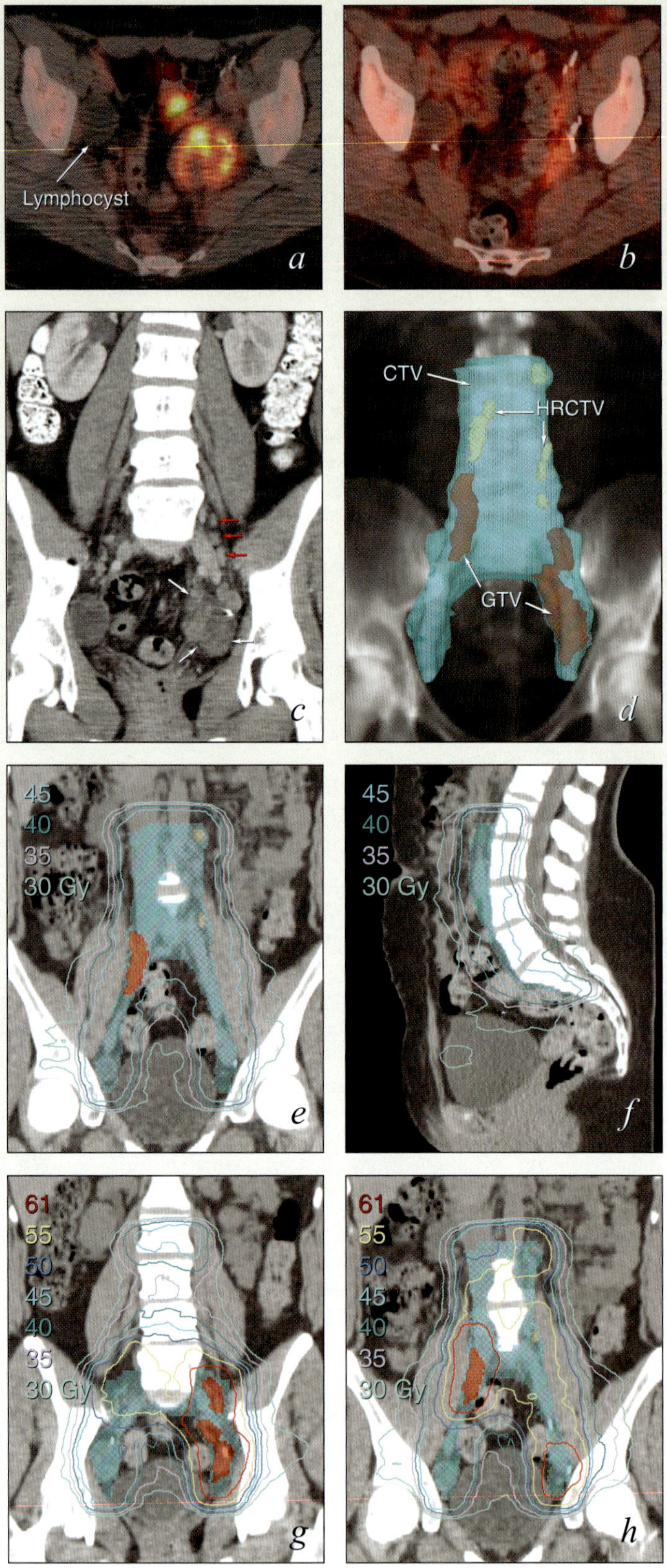

CS 10.10 • Stage IB2 Cervical Cancer with Extensive Lymphadenopathy, Including Supraclavicular Metastasis

History: A 55-year-old woman with recent onset of postmenopausal bleeding and a cervical mass.

Evaluation: *Exam*: Friable cervix, 4 to 5 cm in diameter. No involvement of the vagina or parametria; no palpable lymphadenopathy. *PET*: Numerous hypermetabolic EI, CI, and PANs up to 2 cm in diameter and extending to the renal vessels (contoured on ***a, b***); mildly increased uptake in two 0.5-cm left supraclavicular nodes; no hematogenous metastases. *CT with contrast*: Confirmed PET findings. *Biopsy (cervix and left supraclavicular node)*: Squamous carcinoma.

Treatment Plan: Definitive chemoradiation. Although the risk of distant recurrence is high, some patients with supraclavicular metastases have been cured with RT. This patient had some features increasing the likelihood of cure: the primary tumor and PAN metastases were relatively small, and the neck involvement was early. Concurrent cisplatin is usually well tolerated, even with extended fields. Because of the high risk of DM, the patient's gynecologic oncologist also recommended adjuvant chemotherapy although there is no proof of benefit.

EBRT:

IMRT (***c** to **f***): In 29 fractions:

Central ITV + 7 mm: 43 Gy (1.5 Gy/fraction)

Nodal CTV + 7 mm: 48 Gy (1.6 Gy/fraction)

Nodal GTV + 7 mm: 60 Gy (2.06 Gy/fraction)

Nodal GTV + 5 mm: 62.5 Gy (2.15 Gy/fraction)

The left neck was treated to 50 Gy followed by a 10-Gy electron boost to the GTV (***g***).

Less than 6 mL of duodenum (***c, d, f***) received >55 Gy.

Brachytherapy (not shown): At the end of EBRT, the cervix was <2 cm in diameter. It was then treated with a boost dose delivered using intracavitary brachytherapy (not shown).

All RT was completed in 56 days.

Chemotherapy: Weekly cisplatin × 6; adjuvant carboplatin and paclitaxel × 4.

Outcome: At 7 years, NED without treatment-related complaints.

Comments: Technically, because the patient's metastases were not detectable by FIGO-approved methods, this patient had stage IB2 disease.

In this case, because most high paraaortic disease was on the right and because the patient had generous visceral fat displacing critical structures, tolerance limits were met despite modest hypofractionation. However, in most cases, a combination of integrated and sequential boosts is recommended to decrease the effective dose to critical structures and to reduce protraction of the central pelvic dose. A slightly lower dose of 60 Gy should have been effective for the smaller nodes and would have decreased the dose to the duodenum.

Contouring for such cases is very labor intensive; if even one abnormal node is excluded from the boost volume, recurrence is likely.

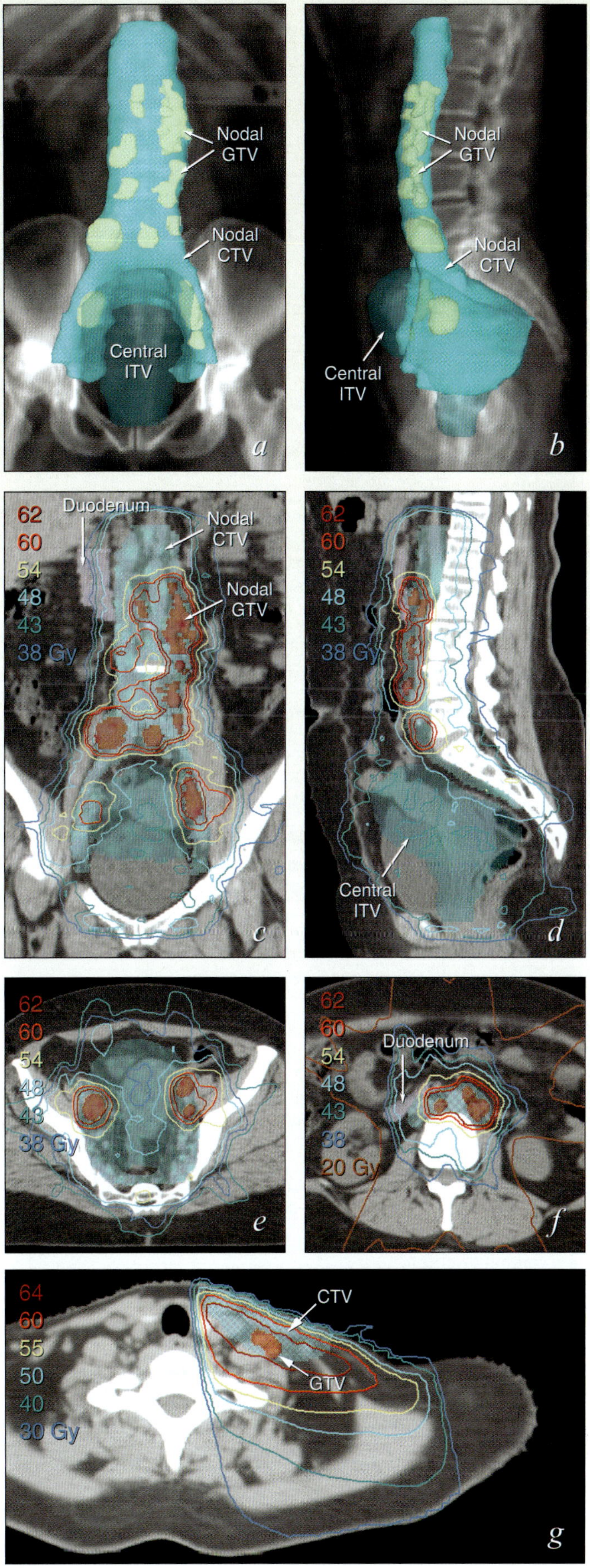

CS 10.11 • Stage IVA Squamous Carcinoma with Vesicovaginal Fistula

History: A 33-year-old woman had a distant history of cervical dysplasia with subsequent negative Pap tests; 6 months of progressive hip and pelvic pain leads to the discovery of a cervical mass on pelvic examination. CT also revealed bilateral hydronephrosis, and the serum creatinine level was 4.4 mg/dL. Bilateral percutaneous nephrostomies were placed, and the patient was referred for further evaluation and treatment.

Evaluation: *Exam*: Large, ulcerating cervical tumor infiltrating the proximal half of the anterior and lateral vaginal walls; palpable vesicovaginal fistula with urine in the vagina; bilateral parametrial infiltration with fixation. *KPS*: 80. *MRI* (***a***) and *PET–CT* (***b***): 3.5 × 4.5 cm poorly defined, irregular FDG-avid mass replacing the cervix and involving the proximal vagina, bilateral parametria, and bladder (***a***, *red arrows*); probable vesicovaginal fistula. No lymphatic or distant metastases. *Renal Lasix scan*: 72% of renal function from the left kidney. *Biopsy (cervix)*: Squamous carcinoma.

Treatment Plan: The patient was referred to the supportive care department for management of refractory pain. Because her creatinine level rapidly returned to normal after nephrostomy placement, it was believed that the patient could tolerate weekly cisplatin concurrent with definitive RT. The initial plan was for pelvic EBRT with a reevaluation after 4 weeks of treatment. However, because of the fistula and extensive infiltration of the posterior bladder, it was believed that intracavitary brachytherapy would likely not be feasible. For this reason, treatment was begun using IMRT, and arrangements were made for reimaging in time to permit IMRT boost planning without a break in treatment.

Radiation Therapy (IMRT):

Set up: Supine in a custom cradle.

Fractions 1 to 25 (***c***):

Nodal CTV and central pelvic CTV/ITV + 7 mm: 45 Gy (1.8 Gy/fraction)

Cervix GTV/ITV + 5 mm: 50 Gy (2.0 Gy/fraction)

At 4 weeks, repeat MRI showed an excellent tumor response but enlargement of the vesicovaginal fistula.

Fractions 26 to 33 (***d***): (positioning verified with daily CT on rails):

HRCTV + 5 mm: 14.4 Gy (1.8 Gy/fraction)

GTV + 5 mm: 16 Gy (2 Gy/fraction)

GTV + 0 mm: 16.8 Gy (2.1 Gy/fraction)

From these plans, the combined doses were 65 to 68 Gy to the GTV and ≥60 Gy to the HRCTV (***e***).

Treatment was completed in 45 days.

Chemotherapy: Weekly cisplatin × 5.

Outcome: Treatment was well tolerated, pain lessened, and the patient had only mild diarrhea. However, 3 days after her last treatment, she required admission for sudden-onset, refractory diarrhea. *Clostridium difficile* enteritis was diagnosed and responded swiftly to oral vancomycin. At 4 months, NED by MRI (***f***) and exam; PET findings were difficult to evaluate locally because of urine contamination but showed no DM. At 1 year, NED by exam and MRI; large vesicovaginal fistula (***g***) but no GI symptoms; undergoing evaluation for ileal conduit diversion.

Comment: Although brachytherapy can sometimes be used to treat stage IVA disease, intracavitary applicators typically provide inadequate coverage of extensive bladder infiltration and are poorly adapted to treatment when a large fistula is present. Although some have recommended volume interstitial implants in this situation, we favor IMRT, which provides a more homogeneous distribution to fixed tumor that is infiltrating critical structures. Nested target volumes enabled delivery of a high central dose without exceeding rectal tolerance.

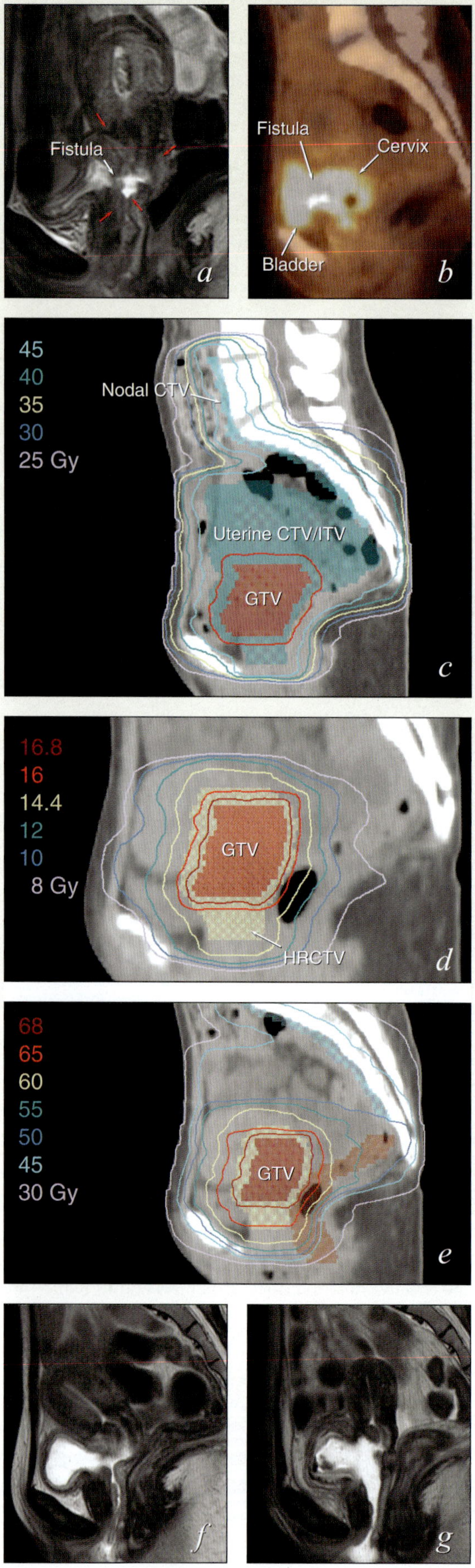

CHAPTER 11

Vaginal Cancer

INTRODUCTION

Among the gynecologic malignancies treated with radiation therapy, vaginal cancers pose some of the greatest management challenges. Several factors contribute to this:

- *Vaginal cancer is rare.* Fewer than 3,000 cases are diagnosed per year in the United States. Less than 5% of gynecologic cancers referred for radiation therapy are primary vaginal cancers, and physicians who have nonspecialized radiation oncology practices are likely to see fewer than 10 to 15 cases during their careers.
- *Vaginal cancers are typically located within millimeters of critical structures.* Because most tumors cannot be removed surgically without sacrificing the bladder or rectum, definitive radiation therapy is usually the treatment of choice.
- *The intimate relationship between the vagina and adjacent structures also means that the therapeutic window for radiation therapy is very narrow.* To obtain the best results, clinicians must customize radiation treatment to the specific clinical situation using physical examination and high-quality imaging to accurately define target volumes and avoidance structures for each stage of treatment.
- *The technical aspects of treatment are highly specialized.* Depending on the precise location of the target *vis-à-vis* adjacent critical structures, external beam and brachytherapy techniques can vary widely. Many of these techniques are very specific to the management of tumors in the vagina.
- *Treatments often have many components, including intensity modulated radiation therapy (IMRT), concurrent chemotherapy, and brachytherapy.* Advance planning for each component helps to minimize delays that could compromise the effectiveness of treatment.

For all these reasons, vaginal cancers are often best treated in large centers by radiation oncologists who have specialized expertise in the management of gynecologic cancers. In any setting, careful planning, attention to detail, and close multidisciplinary collaboration are likely to produce the best outcomes.

Because there have been no randomized trials specific to treatment of vaginal cancers, treatment choices are often guided at least in part by the results of cervical cancer trials. In many ways, vaginal cancers are similar to cervical cancers. Like cervical cancers, vaginal cancers rarely have evidence of distant metastasis at presentation. Nodal metastases follow patterns that reflect the different regional anatomy of the vagina (Chapter 5), but even extensive lymph node metastases can often be cured with chemoradiotherapy. However, with a mean age of 60 to 65 years, women with vaginal cancer tend to be, on average, about 20 years older than cervical cancer patients. About 70% of vaginal cancers are associated with human papillomavirus (HPV) infection (vs. more than 99% of cervical cancers). Also, different anatomical relationships dictate somewhat different approaches to local treatments of cervical and vaginal cancers.

PRETREATMENT EVALUATION AND STAGING

The goals of pretreatment evaluation are also similar to those for cervical cancer:

- *To determine whether the treatment intent should be curative or palliative.* Patients who have hematogenous or peritoneal metastases from vaginal cancer are rarely curable, but even patients who have extensive locoregional disease may do well if they are treated with definitive intent.

- *To define and document the extent of primary disease.* This is particularly critical for patients with vaginal cancer because even small variations in the extent and location of mucosal and paravaginal disease can have a major influence on the choice of treatment modality. Documentation of the initial extent of mucosal involvement is extremely important because the final boost must take into consideration the pretreatment disease extent.
- *To determine the extent of regional disease.* Curative treatment depends on an accurate assessment of the volume at risk for regional microscopic disease and accurate identification of enlarged nodes that require an extra dose of radiotherapy.
- *To rule out second primary cancers or precancers.* Women with HPV-positive vaginal cancers are at increased risk for having other HPV-related neoplasia.
- *To determine the patient's overall medical condition.* It is particularly important to identify any conditions that would influence the patient's ability to tolerate external beam radiotherapy (EBRT), brachytherapy, or chemotherapy.
- *To assign a FIGO stage.* Although the FIGO classification of vaginal cancers (**Table 11.1**) has limited value in the selection of treatment or even determination of prognosis, it provides an important means for comparing results in different clinical settings.

Clinical Evaluation

The patient's initial evaluation should be designed to address these goals as efficiently and accurately as possible. The following studies are particularly useful for assessing the extent of disease in women with primary vaginal cancers:

TABLE 11.1	FIGO Staging of Vaginal Cancer
Stage I	The carcinoma is limited to the vaginal wall
Stage II	The carcinoma has involved the subvaginal tissue but has not extended to the pelvic wall
Stage III	The carcinoma has extended to the pelvic wall
Stage IV	The carcinoma has extended beyond the true pelvis or has involved the mucosa of the bladder or rectum; bullous edema as such does not permit a case to be allotted to stage IV
Stage IVA	The tumor invades bladder and/or rectal mucosa and/or direct extension beyond the true pelvis
Stage IVB	The tumor has spread to distant organs

From Hacker NF, Eifel PJ, van der Velden J. Cancer of the vagina. Int J Gynaecol Obstet. 2012;119(suppl 2):S97–S99.

Physical examination

Although modern diagnostic imaging methods are very useful, physical examination is still the best method for evaluating the extent of vaginal mucosal disease. The size, morphology, and location of vaginal lesions should always be carefully documented (see Chapter 4 for more discussion of vaginal examination). If there are multiple lesions, any of uncertain nature should be biopsied to clarify the extent of the gross tumor volume (GTV).

Fiducial markers should be placed at the periphery of the tumor to assist in initial planning, to facilitate monitoring of vaginal motion, and to record the initial extent of disease for subsequent EBRT or brachytherapy boost planning. Because patient comfort and bleeding often limit the quality of examination and accuracy of marker placement, examination under anesthesia is recommended for most cases.

To rule out second cancers, physical examination should always include a careful examination of the vulva, anal margin, and cervix (if present) and biopsy of any suspicious lesions.

MRI

Pelvic MRI, by far the best imaging study for visualization of tumors involving the vagina, is recommended for most cases. To optimize the study, the radiologist must be given detailed information about the clinical situation and region of interest (Chapter 4). Distension of the vagina with aqueous gel optimizes evaluation of the vaginal walls and tumor contours (**CS 11.2, 11.9, and 11.10**). When combined with the information from physical examination, MRI can provide a detailed understanding of the extent of vaginal disease that is critical for accurate delineation of target volumes.

PET–CT

PET is the preferred method for evaluating the extent of regional metastasis and for ruling out distant disease that would change the intent of treatment. Although there are few data specific to vaginal cancer, clinical experience and the similarities between vaginal and cervical cancer suggest that the sensitivity and specificity are probably similar for these two cancers.

Contrast-enhanced CT

If PET or MRI is unavailable or contraindicated for medical reasons, contrast-enhanced CT should be obtained to evaluate the extent of nodal disease. However, even high-resolution CT with digital reconstruction frequently fails to provide useful detail about the extent of disease in the vagina.

In addition, all patients require standard laboratory studies, including CBC, electrolytes, and renal and liver function studies to determine their fitness for treatment.

In summary, detailed pelvic examination is still the most important part of the pretreatment evaluation of vaginal cancer. Modern imaging, including PET and MRI, improves the accuracy of local and regional target definition, potentially allowing safe delivery of more effective doses to gross disease. However, these studies cannot replace a thorough understanding of the regional anatomy, potential paths of local and regional microscopic disease spread, and the influence of internal organ motion (Chapter 5).

RISK ASSESSMENT

Because most patients are treated with definitive radiotherapy, prognostic assessment is usually based on the histologic type of cancer and clinical findings.

Histologic Type

Squamous Carcinoma

Eighty to ninety percent of vaginal cancers are squamous, and at least two-thirds of these are HPV related. Squamous cancers are usually locoregionally confined at the time of diagnosis, and the potential for cure is high. Even before the use of advanced imaging modalities and concurrent chemotherapy, favorable outcomes could be achieved with definitive radiotherapy. For example, from a review of 193 consecutive women with squamous carcinomas treated at MD Anderson Cancer Center between 1970 and 2000,[1] the 5-year disease-specific survival rates were 81% for stages I–II and 58% for stages III–IVA (**Fig. 11.1**).

DES-Related Clear Cell Adenocarcinoma

In 1971, Herbst and Scully first reported the association between maternal use of diethylstilbestrol (DES) and the subsequent development of clear cell adenocarcinomas of the cervix and vagina in daughters who had been exposed in utero.[2] That same year, alerts were disseminated recommending that DES, which had been given to prevent miscarriage in high-risk pregnancies, no longer be administered to pregnant women; registries were established to follow women who had in utero DES exposure or a diagnosis of clear cell carcinoma. Analyses of the resulting data indicated that the peak risk period for development of clear cell carcinoma after DES exposure was between ages 20 and 30; however, case reports and analyses of cancer incidence suggest that an increased risk persists beyond age 40. Exposed women also appear to have a somewhat increased risk of breast cancer after the age of 40. Clear cell carcinomas in the context of DES exposure tended to be diagnosed at an early stage and to have a better prognosis than non–DES-related adenocarcinomas of the vagina.[3] Today, women in the exposed cohort are generally aged 45 to 75, so the history of exposure may be difficult to obtain from their mothers.

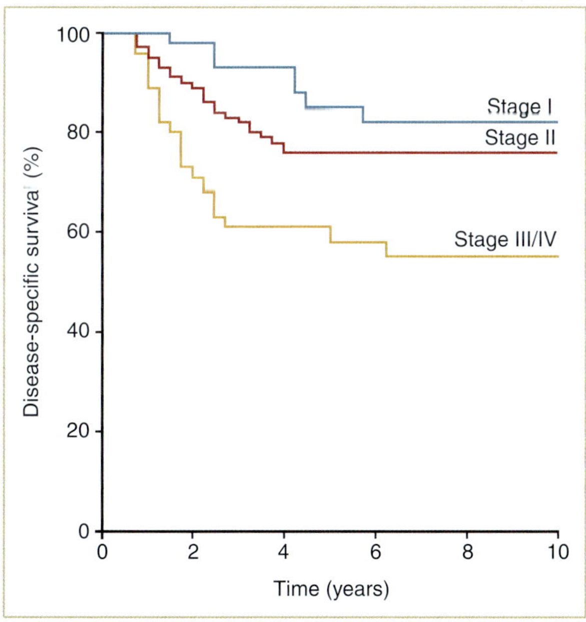

FIGURE 11.1 Disease-specific survival by disease stage for 193 patients with squamous cell carcinoma of the vagina treated between 1970 and 2000 at MD Anderson Cancer Center. Patients with stage III and IVA diseases were combined for the analysis because of the small number of patients ($n = 7$) with stage IVA disease ($p < 0.01$). Numbers in parentheses indicate the number of patients at risk 5 or 10 years after treatment. (From Frank SJ, Deavers MT, Jhingran A, et al. Primary adenocarcinoma of the vagina not associated with diethylstilbestrol (DES) exposure. *Gynecol Oncol.* 2007;105:470–474.)

Non-DES-Related Adenocarcinoma

Primary adenocarcinomas of the vagina are exceedingly rare. Most adenocarcinomas involving the vagina are metastases from other sites (e.g., endometrium, ovary, bowel) that must be excluded before a diagnosis of primary vaginal adenocarcinoma is established. Women with non–DES-related adenocarcinomas are, on average, about 10 years younger than those with squamous cancers. Unlike women with DES-related adenocarcinomas, they appear to have a poor prognosis. Frank et al.[4] reported results of radiation therapy for 20 confirmed cases of primary non–DES-related vaginal adenocarcinomas treated at MD Anderson; these women had significantly higher local and distant failure rates and poorer survival rates than women with squamous cancers treated during the same period (**Figs. 11.2 and 11.3**). However, most patients treated during the years of

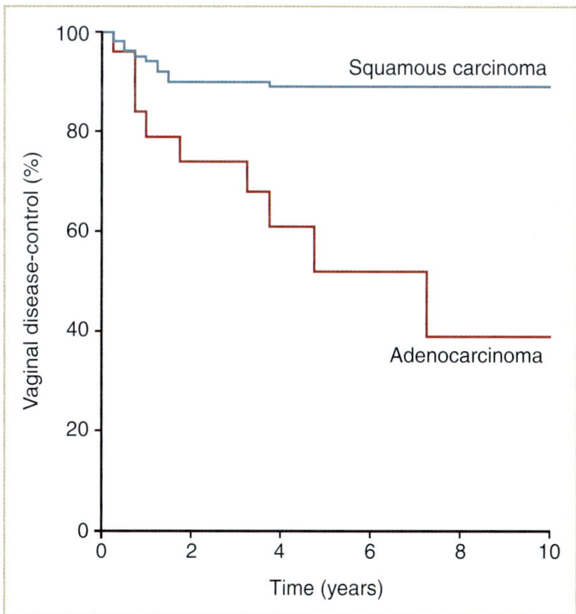

FIGURE 11.2 The vaginal disease control rates for 193 patients with squamous cell carcinoma of the vagina and 26 patients with non-DES-related adenocarcinoma of the vagina treated at MD Anderson Cancer Center between 1970 and 2000. (From Frank SJ, Deavers MT, Jhingran A, et al. Primary adenocarcinoma of the vagina not associated with diethylstilbestrol (DES) exposure. *Gynecol Oncol.* 2007;105:470–474.)

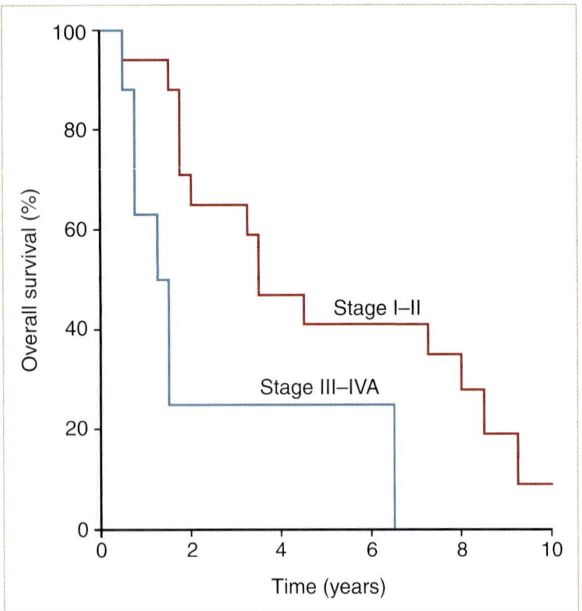

FIGURE 11.3 Overall survival for 26 patients with early-stage (stages I–II) and advanced-stage (stages III–IVA) primary non–DES-related adenocarcinoma of the vagina (*p* = 0.01) treated at MD Anderson Cancer Center between 1970 and 2000. (From Frank SJ, Deavers MT, Jhingran A, et al. Primary adenocarcinoma of the vagina not associated with diethylstilbestrol (DES) exposure. *Gynecol Oncol.* 2007; 105:470–474.)

their study did not receive chemotherapy; its potential influence on outcome is unknown. Although it is difficult to draw broad generalizations about such a rare cancer, analysis of recurrence patterns suggests that these cancers may require somewhat higher radiation doses and possibly more generous clinical target volume (CTV) margins for treatment of primary disease as well as effective chemotherapy to reduce the risk of metastatic disease.

FIGO Stage, Tumor Size, and Location

The FIGO staging system for vaginal cancer is based on clinical findings (**Table 11.1**).[5] Patients with FIGO stage III or IV cancers tend to have a poorer outcome than those with stage I or II. However, in two of the largest single-institutional studies,[1,6] little difference in outcome was detected between stages I and II. In fact, the distinction between carcinoma "limited to the vaginal wall" and "involving subvaginal tissue" is nearly impossible to make on clinical examination and is difficult even on MRI. As a result, the stage designation tends to be highly subjective and likely difficult to reproduce.

The correlation between stage and outcome reflects at least in part the larger size of higher stage tumors. Several authors[1,6] have concluded that tumors larger than 4 cm in diameter have a poorer prognosis than smaller cancers. Frank et al.[1] found this correlation to be independent of FIGO stage.

Although, as discussed elsewhere in this chapter, the management approach varies considerably according to the location of tumors within the vagina, there is little evidence of an independent correlation between the tumor site and outcome.[1,6] However, as discussed in Chapter 5, the pattern of regional metastasis is strongly correlated with the site of involvement. The tumor site may also influence the pattern of distant metastasis; for example, isolated liver metastasis seems to be more frequent in patients who have extensive involvement of the *cul-de-sac* or rectovaginal septum **(CS 11.6)**.

Lymph Node Metastasis

Because most patients are treated with radiation alone and only the more recent cases have been evaluated with advanced imaging, there are remarkably few data concerning the incidence of lymph node metastases in women with vaginal cancer. Small lymphadenectomy series suggest that at least 30% of patients have lymph node involvement.[7,8] None of the large retrospective studies of radiation therapy for vaginal cancer have addressed lymph node involvement as a risk factor. Although this finding undoubtedly influences the risk of recurrence, even patients who have extensive node metastases can often be cured if they receive adequate doses of radiation to all regions of gross disease **(CS 11.2)**.

MULTIDISCIPLINARY CONSIDERATIONS

The Role of Surgery

Initial primary surgical resection is rarely considered for patients who have vaginal cancer. Small stage I cancers that involve the apical posterior vagina (above the peritoneal reflection) have occasionally been treated with radical hysterectomy, upper vaginectomy, and lymphadenectomy.[9] Very small superficial tumors at the apex of a posthysterectomy vagina can occasionally be removed with an upper vaginectomy. However, patients must be carefully chosen; surgery that leaves a positive or close margin complicates subsequent radiation therapy because the region of the positive margin is often beyond the range of intravaginal brachytherapy treatment once the apical vagina has been removed.

The volume and dose of regional treatment are usually based on clinical imaging findings. The arguments for and against lymph node staging or resection of enlarged nodes are similar to those made for patients with other lower genital tract cancers and are discussed in detail in Chapter 3.

The Role of Chemotherapy

Because of the similarities between vaginal and cervical cancers, it is probably reasonable to apply the results from randomized trials of chemotherapy in patients with cervical cancer to patients with vaginal cancers. Unless there is a medical contraindication, concurrent chemotherapy is generally recommended for all patients with stages II to IVA, some bulky stage I cancers, any patient with evidence of lymph node metastasis, and most adenocarcinomas. The most commonly used regimen is weekly cisplatin. Although there are no randomized studies documenting the advantage of concurrent chemotherapy in patients with vaginal cancer, retrospective studies and analyses of national databases suggest that chemotherapy does benefit these patients[10–12] (**Fig. 11.4**).

There is as yet no proven benefit for adjuvant chemotherapy in patients with lower genital tract cancer. However, because

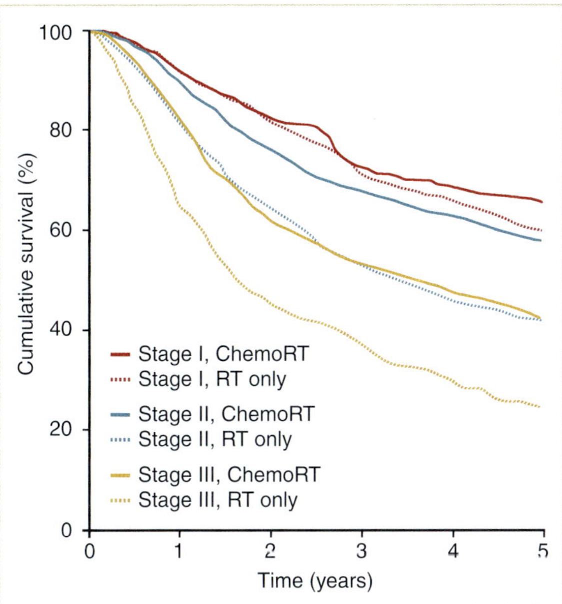

FIGURE 11.4 Overall survival rates for patients with stage I, II, or III vaginal cancer treated between 1998 and 2011 with radiation alone or with concurrent chemoradiation. The analysis, which was drawn from the National Cancer Database, included 8,086 of 13,689 patients who were classified as having vaginal cancers. A large number of patients were excluded from this study because of inadequate treatment information and a much higher than expected proportion of patients (28%) had nonsquamous histologic types, suggesting that the study may have included some patients who did not have primary vaginal cancers. However, the significantly higher overall survival rates, particularly for stages II and III disease, provide important evidence of benefit of concurrent chemotherapy in the treatment of vaginal cancer. The survival curves in this figure have been redrawn from the original manuscript to emphasize outcome during the first 5 years, when most disease-related events would have occurred. (From Rajagopalan MS, Xu KM, Lin JF, et al. Adoption and impact of concurrent chemoradiation therapy for vaginal cancer: A National Cancer Data Base (NCDB) study. *Gynecol Oncol.* 2014;135:495–502.)

of the high rate of distant metastasis observed for adenocarcinomas of the vagina, we have sometimes offered adjuvant chemotherapy (usually carboplatin and paclitaxel for 4 to 6 cycles) to these patients (CS 11.3). However, the potential side effects of adjuvant chemotherapy and the fact that there are currently no data proving the efficacy of this treatment must be discussed in detail with the patient. Adjuvant chemotherapy is generally not recommended for women with squamous lesions because the margin for improvement over chemoradiotherapy alone is small and the potential benefit uncertain.

DEVELOPING A RADIATION TREATMENT STRATEGY

Most treatments consist of at least two phases: (1) several weeks of EBRT encompassing the primary site, paravaginal tissues, and appropriate regional lymph nodes and (2) boost treatment focused on regions of gross disease (GTVs) or other high-risk areas (high-risk CTVs).

A well-articulated treatment strategy for the second phase should always be developed before the first phase is begun. In many cases, the best method for boosting vaginal disease cannot be determined until the patient is re-examined in the 4th or 5th week of pelvic treatment. However, *preparations should be made at the beginning of treatment to enable any treatment option(s) that might be considered for the boost*. The importance of this cannot be overemphasized. Potentially harmful interruptions in treatment are inevitable if the end of pelvic radiotherapy is reached without any arrangements having been made for repeat imaging, IMRT planning, operating room time, or other requirements (CS 11.7).

If brachytherapy is being considered, the physician who will perform the procedure must be consulted and given an opportunity to examine the patient before treatment and at least once during initial pelvic radiotherapy. MRI or written descriptions of a physical examination performed by someone else a month before the procedure do not provide sufficient information for the brachytherapist to plan treatment. Any misunderstanding of the initial distribution of disease can result in a recurrence; conversely, unnecessary side effects may result if an overly large volume is treated to compensate for inadequate description of the initial disease extent.

Serial clinical examinations are a particularly important part of treatment planning for patients with vaginal cancer. The initial extent of mucosal involvement can easily be obscured by bulky intravaginal tumor but is often made clear as the tumor begins to regress in the 3rd or 4th week of treatment. For boost planning, almost all patients require a detailed re-evaluation after about 40 Gy of pelvic treatment (CS 11.2–11.10). In some cases, physical examination is sufficient to provide an accurate sense of the disease extent. However, if there is any remaining uncertainty about the extent of residual disease, repeat MRI may be helpful.

The goal of radiotherapy is to eliminate gross disease in the primary site and involved nodes, to sterilize microscopic disease in grossly uninvolved nodal and paravaginal sites, and to minimize the dose to normal tissues without compromising local disease control. The balance between the probability of local control and the likelihood of complications is what drives the decision to treat using EBRT only or a combination of EBRT and intracavitary or interstitial brachytherapy.

Planning the Initial Phase of Pelvic Treatment

An initial course of EBRT is recommended for all patients who have invasive disease. In general, the vagina and paravaginal tissues should be treated with at least a 3-cm distal margin on gross disease. For bulky lesions, a small integrated boost to the vagina can be used to supplement the vaginal GTV–internal target volume (ITV) to a dose of 50 Gy, while the rest of the pelvic CTV is treated to 45 Gy in 25 fractions (CS 11.2, 11.3, 11.5, 11.6, 11.9, and 11.10). However, if brachytherapy is planned, the external dose to the vagina rarely exceeds 50 Gy.

As discussed below and in Chapter 5, the initial nodal treatment volume is determined by the sites of involvement within the vagina and by the presence or absence of gross lymph node involvement. The recommended dose for at-risk nodes that are not grossly involved is typically 43–45 Gy in 24–25 fractions. Tissues between or immediately surrounding extensively involved nodal compartments may be treated to somewhat higher doses (CS 11.2). Grossly involved nodes are usually treated to at least 60 Gy, but large nodes, particularly those not closely approximating critical structures, may be treated to higher doses.

Excellent results can be achieved using standard conformal external beam techniques. However, IMRT holds several advantages for the treatment of vaginal cancers:

- IMRT reduces the dose to the central pelvis, which is often filled with bowel in patients who have had a previous hysterectomy.
- For distal lesions, treatment of the inguinal nodes can be accomplished with relative sparing of the femoral heads.
- If the final boost is to be given using EBRT, IMRT provides a more conformal plan than standard four-field conformal techniques with less collateral high-dose exposure of critical structures.
- IMRT permits integration of boosts, thereby shortening the overall duration of treatment. However, large doses per fraction that could close the already narrow therapeutic window should be avoided.

Although IMRT is a very useful tool in the treatment of vaginal cancers, as discussed in Chapter 6, great care must be taken to provide sufficient margin to account for patient setup errors and internal organ motion.

For patients who have bulky tumors that are displacing bowel or other critical structures, repeat imaging at about 3 weeks may already reveal significant tumor shrinkage. Although infiltrated structures must continue to be included in the target, in some cases, there is enough tumor regression and shift of displaced structures to permit a revision of the GTV–ITV and spare additional normal tissue (particularly bowel).

As a rule, stereotactic body radiotherapy (SBRT) is contraindicated in the definitive management of vaginal cancer because the very close relationship between the vagina and surrounding critical structures makes it impossible to avoid sensitive structures without risking marginal recurrence.

Some authors have recommended treatment with brachytherapy alone for selected patients with stage I cancers. However, in the series by Frank et al.,[1] three of the nine patients who were treated with brachytherapy alone for small, superficial, stage I cancers developed vaginal or paravaginal recurrence. Although this group of patients was small, this number of recurrences in patients who had very favorable cancers was too high. In contrast, the combined overall vaginal recurrence rate for patients with stage I or II disease was only 9%. For this reason, an initial course of EBRT is recommended even for patients with early stage I cancers, although a reduced field size may be used in some very early cases (CS 11.1).

Brachytherapy versus EBRT for the Boost to Gross Disease

Methods for boosting gross nodal disease are discussed in Chapter 6.

The selection of EBRT or brachytherapy to boost primary disease is based on a careful analysis of pre- and intratreatment physical examinations and imaging. Because brachytherapy sources have a relatively fixed relationship to the target, little or no planning target volume (PTV) margin is required. The radiation dose also declines rapidly with increasing distance from the sources. This can be very advantageous, particularly for relatively small or superficial lesions that are well defined (CS 11.1–11.5). For such small, discreet lesions, a higher dose often can be delivered with greater sparing of normal tissues using brachytherapy than with EBRT (Chapter 8).

However, the steep falloff and heterogeneous dose distribution of brachytherapy can be a disadvantage if they lead to underdosage of a portion of the target or excessive dose to critical structures in close contact with a radiation source. In general, when a large volume needs to be treated, particularly when tumor is extensively involving a critical structure (e.g., rectovaginal or vesicovaginal septum), EBRT provides broader, more homogeneous coverage than brachytherapy (CS 11.8–11.10). For this reason, external beam techniques are often preferred for very large, extensively infiltrating lesions or for tumors that have poorly defined margins, particularly if they are fixed to pelvic structures. In these situations, the benefit of a homogeneous dose distribution may outweigh the disadvantages of EBRT; with daily image guidance and IMRT, treatment is more conforming and the PTV margin can be somewhat reduced (but not eliminated), adding to the advantages of EBRT in these situations.

Ultimately, this means that higher doses of radiation can often be delivered to relatively small tumors, accounting for the very low local recurrence rates of stage I and II tumors reported in some large single-institution series.[1] Large tumors that require lower-dose volume implants or external beam boosts tend to have somewhat higher local recurrence rates. However, even before the routine use of concurrent chemotherapy, advanced imaging methods, or IMRT, Frank et al.[1] reported a vaginal control rate of 83% for patients with stage III or IVA squamous carcinomas of the vagina, many of whom were treated without brachytherapy.

MANAGEMENT CONSIDERATIONS ACCORDING TO TUMOR LOCATION

Cancers Involving the Apex of the Vagina

At least 75% of proximal vaginal cancers occur in women who have had a prior hysterectomy. There are several explanations for this. If the uterus is still in place, some proximal cancers grow to involve the cervix before detection and are therefore classified as cervical cancers. Also, patients who have had a hysterectomy as treatment for cervical intraepithelial neoplasia (CIN) or vaginal intraepithelial neoplasia (VAIN) are at increased risk for developing subsequent invasive vaginal cancers.

Laser ablations and other treatments for VAIN can cause mucosal injuries that sometimes result in fusion of the vaginal walls with significant vaginal foreshortening. Consequently, the apex of the vagina, as appreciated clinically, may actually represent the mid or even distal vagina anatomically; it is important to consider this when the paths of potential regional spread are being determined for treatment planning. Scarring also can make it difficult to appreciate invasive lesions at an early stage; even if the patient is being closely followed, an invasive lesion may escape detection until it is quite advanced (**CS 11.2**). This can be a source of considerable frustration for the patient and her physician.

Regional Treatment

The nodal target volume for apical cancers is usually similar to that for cervical cancers, requiring coverage of the internal and external iliac nodes (Table 5.1). For small, extremely superficial cancers, a smaller field covering the primary target and distal nodes may be sufficient, although the data supporting this approach are limited.[1] If there is infiltration of the posterior vagina, uterosacral ligaments, or cul-de-sac, the presacral or even perirectal nodes may be at risk (**CS 11.6**). Depending on the extent of distal involvement and degree of foreshortening of the vagina, the inguinal nodes may also be at risk for metastatic involvement.

Treatment of the Primary Lesion

Apical cancers may appear as superficial granular lesions or mucosal plaques, as primarily exophytic growths, or as infiltrating tumors that penetrate paravaginal tissues.

In all cases, the initial target volume should include the vagina and paravaginal tissues with margins of at least 1 to 2 cm proximal to the apex and 3 cm beyond the most distal gross disease. Fiducial markers inserted in the apex can help to define the proximal extent of the target volume; however, if the upper vagina has fused for the reasons described above, some additional proximal margin should be included in the CTV (**CS 11.1**). Internal organ motion can cause variations in the location of the upper vagina of as much as 2 to 3 cm, and this must be carefully considered in treatment planning (**CS 11.1–11.7 and CS 11.10**). See Chapter 5 for additional discussion of vaginal ITV designation.

The weighting of EBRT versus brachytherapy and the type of brachytherapy depend on the initial extent of disease and the degree of response:

- For small superficial lesions confined to the apex, an initial dose of 40–45 Gy in 20–25 fractions is usually followed by intracavitary brachytherapy using a domed cylinder with a central channel (**CS 11.1**). An EqD2 of 40 to 45 Gy prescribed to the vaginal surface should be sufficient to achieve a local control rate of >95%.
- Exophytic lesions that respond well to initial chemoradiotherapy may also be treated with intracavitary brachytherapy alone if the residual disease is <4 to 5 mm thick (**CS 11.2**). If there is any doubt about the physical findings or if irregularities in the apical anatomy could distance the mucosa from an intracavitary applicator, high-quality imaging (preferably MRI) should be obtained with the cylinder in place to confirm that the deepest portion of the target volume will receive a total dose (including 45 to 50 Gy of EBRT) of at least 70 Gy. The vaginal surface dose should generally not exceed a total EqD2 of 90 to 95 Gy (**CS 11.1**). If there is localized extension to the walls of the vagina, peripheral channels or interstitial needles may be added to treat these areas (**CS 11.2**). See Chapter 8 for further discussion of typical dose constraints, dose rate, and high-dose rate (HDR) fractionation.
- If after about 40 Gy of EBRT the thickness of apical disease exceeds 4 to 5 mm, preparations should be made for an interstitial or EBRT boost. Interstitial implantation of the vaginal apex requires a template to stabilize the needles and must be performed under laparoscopic or direct image guidance to avoid overdose of overlying intestines, adjacent bladder, or rectum. Several investigators have reported good results with this approach.[13] At MD Anderson, interstitial templates have occasionally been used to treat discrete apical lesions that have responded poorly to initial EBRT. However, as a rule, we have preferred to boost such lesions with IMRT using daily image guidance and careful monitoring of internal organ motion.
- In particular, if the patient had a simple hysterectomy prior to the diagnosis of vaginal cancer, the cardinal ligament of the uterus (which remains attached to the vaginal apex) can be a route of superolateral spread from the apical vagina toward the pelvic wall (**CS 11.8**). For tumors that have grossly invaded the cardinal or uterosacral ligaments, a carefully designed IMRT boost is usually recommended, bringing the total GTV dose to 64 to 68 Gy.

All of these treatments can be expected to cause some shortening of the vagina. The amount and its effect on sexual function depend on the dose delivered to the distal vagina with EBRT and brachytherapy as well as the patient's age, hormonal status, and other factors.

Cancers Involving the Lateral Walls

Regional Treatment

Treatment should include the external and internal iliac nodes; if there is infiltration of the distal one-third, the CTV should include at least the medial inguinal lymph nodes (**CS 11.4**).

Treatment of the Primary Lesion

For lateralized lesions, it is particularly important to accurately define and record the initial GTV, ideally by placing fiducial markers during examination under anesthesia

(CS 11.4 and 11.5). Initially, the vaginal ITV should extend from the apex proximally to include at least 3 cm of mucosa beyond the most distal gross disease. If tumor approaches the distal one-third of the vagina, the patient should be treated in a frog-leg position to reduce vulvar skin reactions (Chapter 4). An initial course of 45 to 50 Gy of EBRT usually results in flattening of exophytic disease and should in most cases be sufficient treatment for uninvolved vaginal mucosa.

The ideal boost technique provides excellent coverage of initial sites of disease without excessively treating uninvolved vagina. Intracavitary techniques that use a cylinder with a single central channel are not well suited to lateralized midvaginal lesions because the entire circumference of the vagina and most of the length receive the same dose as the target. Adequate treatment of the primary lesion will almost always cause severe vaginal narrowing if brachytherapy is given using a single channel. Cylinders that contain peripheral channels can be used to treat very superficial lesions **(CS 11.2)**, but the short distance between sources and vaginal mucosa makes this approach less useful to more deeply penetrating lesions.

Lateral wall lesions are particularly well suited to treatment with interstitial brachytherapy using a free-hand technique **(CS 11.4 and 11.5)**. With this approach, needles are positioned under direct palpation, optimizing control of the relationship between the sources, the tumor, the vaginal mucosa, and the rectum. Interstitial needles are usually combined with a vaginal cylinder; in some cases, peripheral channels in the cylinder are used to achieve a more homogeneous dose to the tumor and to treat superficial disease at the margin, particularly posteriorly **(CS 11.5)**.

Although some clinicians favor the use of interstitial templates, the fixed obturator diameter (which is too narrow for many vaginas) and inability to palpate the lesion during needle insertion are relative disadvantages of this technique. See Chapter 8 for further discussion of interstitial techniques and dose rate in vaginal interstitial brachytherapy.

Periurethral Cancers

Regional Treatment

The primary target volume includes at least the internal and external iliac nodes and, because of the distal location, the inguinal nodes.

Treatment of the Primary Lesion

Because it is usually necessary to treat at least the anterior perineum, patients should be treated in an open leg position to minimize local skin reactions. In most cases, the entire vagina should be included in the initial target volume to achieve adequate margin on proximal disease.

Several unique aspects of tumors in this location influence the choice of boost options:

- Because of their distal location and because deep invaginations in the periurethral sulci (**Fig. 5.16a**) distance the mucosa from the surface of a vaginal cylinder, tumors in this location are usually unsuitable for treatment with intracavitary brachytherapy alone.
- Tumors involving the periurethral region tend to be relatively immobile and are subject to relatively small changes in location with variations in bladder and rectal filling.
- Tumors in this location sometimes cause urethral obstruction **(CS 11.9)**; tumor infiltration or treatment-related injury to the urethra–vaginal septum or urethral sphincters can result in fistula or incontinence.

Relatively small periurethral tumors and tumors that extend from the lateral wall to involve the periurethra can be effectively boosted with interstitial brachytherapy **(CS 11.3)**. Although we successfully performed interstitial implants of this region before the advent of advanced imaging, MRI guidance is strongly recommended to ensure adequate coverage, particularly deep in the sulci, regions that can be difficult to reach with interstitial needles. Although the urethra can usually tolerate doses of 65 to 70 Gy, care must be taken to avoid heterogeneities that could expose portions of the urethra to much higher doses during brachytherapy. See Chapter 8 for further discussion of volumetric dose guidelines.

Free-hand techniques permit excellent control of the relationship between needles, urethra, and vaginal mucosa. We have found templates to be less well suited to the treatment of tumors in this location. In particular, the slope of the periurethral sulci, which is steeper than that of the vaginal walls, may be difficult to accommodate to the parallel arrangement of template needles; also, the fixed needle spacing of templates permits less control of the relationship between needles and the urethra than free-hand techniques performed under direct palpation.

In our view, large tumors that extensively involve the periurethral spaces, vagina, and paravagina are more effectively treated with IMRT than with large volume implants **(CS 11.9)**. Although this is controversial, we feel that for these cases, IMRT provides a more homogeneous dose distribution and better coverage of tumor and minimizes heterogeneities to critical structures such as urethra and bladder neck that often must be included in the target volume. Because these cancers are generally fixed, usually, relatively little accommodation needs to be made for internal organ motion, although great care should be taken not to underestimate the volume at risk for microscopic infiltration and, as always, an adequate PTV margin must be added to account for set-up uncertainties.

Tumors Involving the Posterior Vagina Wall

Regional Treatment

In addition to the external and internal iliac nodes, the presacral and perirectal nodes are at particularly high risk for involvement with tumor and should be included in the target volume.

Treatment of the Primary Lesion

Superficial cancers, exophytic lesions that regress during EBRT to less than 4 to 5 mm in thickness, and tumors that extend superficially to involve the posterior vagina can usually be boosted with intracavitary therapy, although image guidance is strongly recommended to verify adequate coverage of the target **(CS 11.6)**. Early placement of fiducial markers guides conformal treatment, avoiding unnecessary high-dose treatment of the rectum. Low-dose rate (LDR), pulsed-dose rate (PDR), or heavily fractionated HDR techniques are recommended to avoid delivery of large fractional doses to the rectum.

Lesions involving the distal 1 to 2 cm of the posterior vagina can sometimes be treated with interstitial implants if the perineum is sufficiently thick **(CS 11.4)**. In general, there should be sufficient tissue to support needles with at least 4 to 5 mm of tissue between the needles and the vaginal and anal mucosae. Some women, particularly those who have a history of fourth-degree obstetrical lacerations, have insufficient perineal tissue to accommodate needles even in the distal vagina.

Tumors that extensively involve the rectovaginal septum pose particularly difficult management problems. Target volumes that penetrate further than 4 to 5 mm from the vaginal surface usually cannot be adequately covered with intracavitary therapy without delivering an unacceptably high dose to the vaginal mucosa. Patients who have extensive invasion of this region are already at high risk for fistula because of damage to the rectovaginal septum. The local heterogeneities of interstitial brachytherapy and the injury caused by placement of needles in a delicate structure can add significantly to this risk. Because, in most cases, interstitial implants of this region would be expected to deliver a higher maximum dose to rectum than the minimum dose to tumor, they do not provide a favorable therapeutic ratio.

For these reasons, we favor the use of EBRT alone, preferably using IMRT, for tumors in this region that have extensive residual disease after 40 to 50 Gy. Typically, the total dose prescribed to the target is between 64 and 68 Gy, depending on the size of the target.

Massive Tumors Involving the Entire Vagina or Adjacent Critical Structures

Regional Treatment

All the principles of regional treatment described apply to these cancers.

Treatment of the Primary Lesion

For the reasons described above, we favor the use of IMRT to treat massive tumors **(CS 11.8–11.10)**. In general, EBRT provides a more homogeneous distribution than interstitial brachytherapy for the treatment of large volumes that intimately involve critical structures. In general, fraction sizes >2 to 2.2 Gy per fraction should be avoided, and even mild hypofractionation should be used sparingly if critical structures are included in the target. SBRT is not recommended for these or any other vaginal cancers because critical structures cannot be safely excluded from the target volume.

References

1. Frank SJ, Jhingran A, Levenback C, et al. Definitive radiation therapy for squamous cell carcinoma of the vagina. *Int J Radiat Oncol Biol Phys.* 2005;62:138–147.
2. Smith EK, White MC, Weir HK, et al. Higher incidence of clear cell adenocarcinoma of the cervix and vagina among women born between 1947 and 1971 in the United States. *Cancer Causes Control.* 2012;23:207–211.
3. Waggoner SE, Mittendorf R, Biney N, et al. Influence of in utero diethylstilbestrol exposure on the prognosis and biologic behavior of vaginal clear-cell adenocarcinoma. *Gynecol Oncol.* 1994;55:238–244.
4. Frank SJ, Deavers MT, Jhingran A, et al. Primary adenocarcinoma of the vagina not associated with diethylstilbestrol (DES) exposure. *Gynecol Oncol.* 2007;105:470–474.
5. Hacker NF, Eifel PJ, van der Velden J. Cancer of the vagina. *Int J Gynaecol Obstet.* 2012;119(suppl 2):S97–S99.
6. Kirkbride P, Fyles A, Rawlings GA, et al. Carcinoma of the vagina—experience at the Princess Margaret Hospital (1974–1989). *Gynecol Oncol.* 1995;56:435–443.
7. Al Kurdi M, Monagham JM. Thirty-two years experience in management of primary tumors of the vagina. *Br J Obstet Gynaecol.* 1981;88:1145–1150.
8. Stock RG, Chen ASJ, Seski J. A 30 year experience in the management of primary carcinoma of the vagina: analysis of prognostic factors and treatment modalities. *Gynecol Oncol.* 1995;56:45–52.
9. Hacker NF. Vaginal cancer. In: Berek JS, Hacker NF, eds. *Gynecologic Oncology.* Philadelphia, PA: Wolters Kluwer/Lippincott Williams & Wilkins; 2010:576–592.
10. Rajagopalan MS, Xu KM, Lin JF, et al. Adoption and impact of concurrent chemoradiation therapy for vaginal cancer: A National Cancer Data Base (NCDB) study. *Gynecol Oncol.* 2014;135:495–502.
11. Miyamoto DT, Viswanathan AN. Concurrent chemoradiation for vaginal cancer. *PLoS One.* 2013;8:e65048.
12. Ghia AJ, Gonzalez VJ, Tward JD, et al. Primary vaginal cancer and chemoradiotherapy: a patterns-of-care analysis. *Int J Gynecol Cancer.* 2011;21:378–384.
13. Viswanathan AN, Szymonifka J, Tempany-Afdhal CM, et al. A prospective trial of real-time magnetic resonance-guided catheter placement in interstitial gynecologic brachytherapy. *Brachytherapy.* 2013;12:240–247.

Case Studies

The case studies for this chapter were selected to illustrate the variety of vaginal cancer presentations and the reasoning behind various treatment selections. In particular, the selection of regional target volume and the reasons for choosing intracavitary, interstitial, or external beam boost treatments are emphasized. The discussions also emphasize the importance of advance planning and careful delineation of the mucosal tumor extent prior to the initiation of treatment. Additional discussion of external beam and brachytherapy techniques is included in Chapters 6 and 8.

List of Case Studies for Chapter 11

CS 11.1. Superficial stage I squamous cancer of the vaginal apex

CS 11.2. Stage II squamous carcinoma of the upper vagina with extensive lymph node involvement

CS 11.3. Stage II adenocarcinoma of the distal anterior and lateral vagina

CS 11.4. Stage II squamous carcinoma of the lateral and posterior wall

CS 11.5. Stage II cancer of the distal lateral vagina

CS 11.6. Stage II cancer involving the rectovaginal septum

CS 11.7. Stage III vaginal cancer referred after incomplete response to initial pelvic radiotherapy

CS 11.8. Stage III squamous carcinoma of the vaginal apex

CS 11.9. Locally extensive cancer of the vagina presenting with urethral obstruction

CS 11.10. Stage IVA squamous carcinoma of the vagina

Abbreviations Used in the Case Studies

AP	Anterior–posterior
CIN	Cervical intraepithelial neoplasia
CTV	Clinical target volume
CI	Common iliac
CT	Computed tomography
D_{2cc}	Minimum dose to the 2 mL receiving the highest dose
D_{90}	Dose received by 90% of the target volume
EBRT	External beam radiotherapy
EI	External iliac
EqD2	Equivalent dose at 2 Gy/fraction
EUA	Examination under anesthesia
FIGO	International Federation of Gynecology and Obstetrics
FDG	Fluorodeoxyglucose
GTV	Gross tumor volume
HDR	High-dose rate
HR CTV	High-risk clinical target volume
IGRT	Image-guided radiation therapy
IMRT	Intensity-modulated radiation therapy
ITV	Internal target volume
KPS	Karnofsky performance status
LEEP	Loop electrosurgical excision procedure
MRI	Magnetic resonance imaging
NED	No evidence of disease
PET	Positron emission tomography
PA	Posterior–anterior
PDR	Pulsed-dose rate
PA	Paraaortic
VAIN	Vaginal intraepithelial neoplasia

CS 11.1 • Superficial Stage I Squamous Cancer of the Vaginal Apex

History: An 80-year-old woman with a history of hysterectomy for dysplasia and laser treatment for VAIN had the recent onset of postmenopausal bleeding and dyspareunia. She had a history of left hip replacement, atrial fibrillation treated with a pacemaker, treated breast cancer, and recent-onset diabetes mellitus.

Evaluation: *Exam*: Alert and oriented. Foreshortened vagina with a 2 cm diameter, superficial, slightly nodular lesion at the apex; no paravaginal abnormality. Fiducial markers were inserted at the margins of the lesion. *KPS*: 90. *CT*: NED but the study was suboptimal because of artifact from the prosthesis. *Chest x-ray*: NED. *Biopsy (vagina)*: Invasive squamous carcinoma.

Treatment Plan: Pelvic radiotherapy and vaginal brachytherapy. Treatment plans calculated with and without heterogeneity correction suggested that, with 18-MV photons, the prosthesis had minimal effect on the radiation dose distribution. Although a treatment plan using four oblique fields would have avoided the hip, it would have considerably increased the volume of bowel irradiated to high dose.

EBRT: The regional nodes (external and internal iliac up to the bifurcation of the CI vessels), vaginal ITV, and paravaginal tissues were treated to a dose of 45 Gy in 25 fractions using a four-field technique with 18-MV photons (***a–d***).

Prebrachytherapy Evaluation: At EUA, there was only mild erythema with no gross residual disease at the apex.

Brachytherapy: A narrow vaginal apex would only accommodate a 2-cm diameter dome and cylinder. Distally, a 2.5-cm cylinder was added, and the applicator was secured with a vulvar suture. A total dose of 45–48 Gy was delivered to the apical vaginal mucosa in 70 hours (***e***), bringing the total mucosal dose to 90 Gy. The total dose at 0.5-cm depth was approximately 24 Gy (69 Gy including EBRT). All radiotherapy was completed within 39 days.

Chemotherapy: None.

Outcome: At 4.5 years, NED on active surveillance; active and alert with stress incontinence, periodic urinary tract infections, and constipation. The patient remained sexually active for several years after radiotherapy but had some decrease in overall activity after a second hip fracture 3 years after treatment.

Comment: Because this patient was treated using a four-field technique, coverage of the proximal vagina was generous. However, it should be noted that the vaginal ITV was extended several centimeters proximal to fiducial markers that had been placed in the apex (***d***, *arrow*). After ablative treatments for VAIN, the apical vagina often fuses so that the apex on examination is distal to the anatomic proximal third of the vagina. Even if the fused portion is not clearly involved (as in this case), it probably should be included in the CTV.

This patient was treated using PDR brachytherapy. A similar EqD2 at the vaginal surface and depth could be achieved with seven HDR fractions of 5 Gy each prescribed at the vaginal surface. Fewer fractions of 5.5 or 6 Gy each could be used but at the expense of a somewhat steeper gradient in effective dose (see Chapter 8).

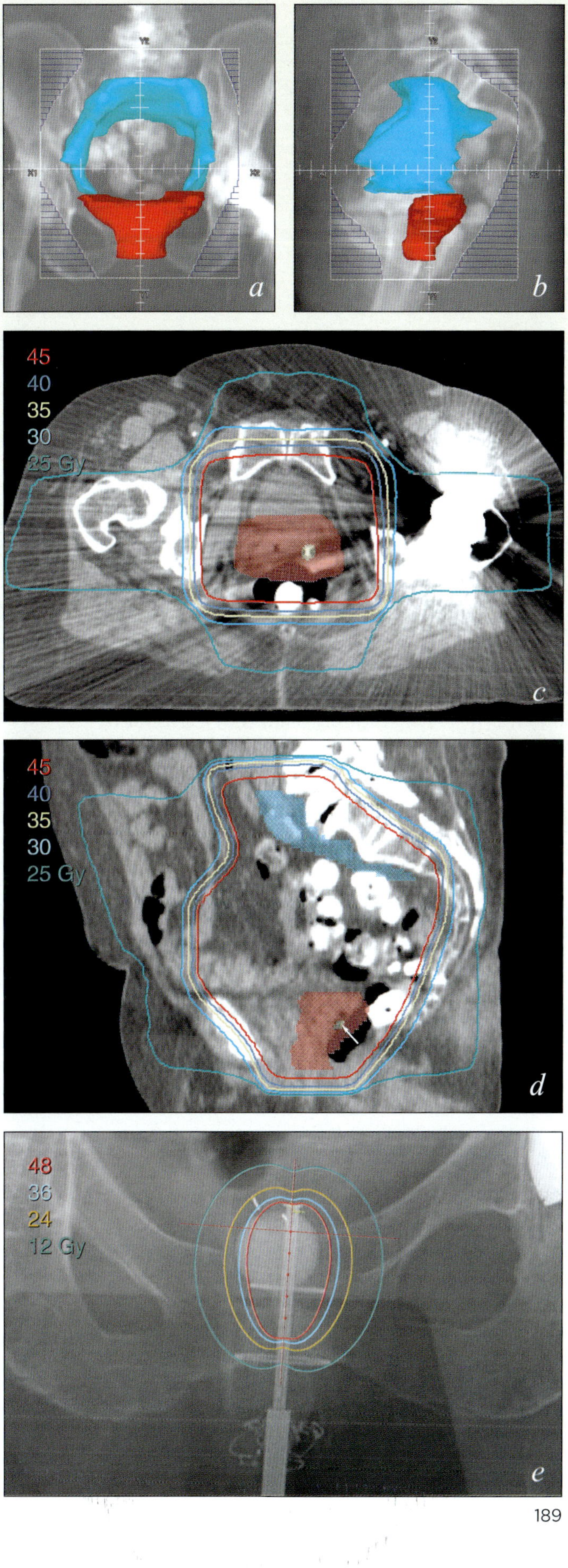

CS 11.2 • Stage II Squamous Carcinoma of the Upper Vagina with Extensive Lymph Node Involvement

History: A 47-year-old woman with a history of hysterectomy for cervical dysplasia and laser vaporization for VAIN was found to have high-grade changes on a routine Pap smear. Colposcopy revealed a lesion in the vaginal apex.

Evaluation: *Exam (EUA)*: A 3 × 2 cm raised lesion involving the apex and proximal right lateral wall of the vagina; fiducial markers were inserted at the tumor periphery. *MRI (**a, b**)*: A lobulated 3 × 2.5 × 2 cm mass involving the proximal right lateral wall and apex (*red arrows*); bulky right CI and EI nodes up to 3.5 cm (*white arrows*). *PET–CT*: Increased FDG uptake in the primary site, right EI and CI nodes, and a small PA node at L2; no distant metastases. *Biopsy (vagina)*: Squamous carcinoma.

Treatment Plan: Chemoradiotherapy to extended fields; reevaluation before planning of GTV boosts.

EBRT: *Setup*: Supine, upper and lower custom cradles with arms above the head.

IMRT (Fractions 1–25)(*c*):

Nodal CTV and vaginal CTV–ITV (+7 mm): 45 Gy

Vaginal GTV–ITV (+7 mm): 50 Gy

Right EI and CI GTVs, intervening high-risk nodal region, and PA GTV (+7 mm): 50 Gy

Interval Evaluation (at 40 Gy): *Exam*: A response of >50% with flattening of the vaginal lesion. *MRI (**e**)*: Right EI node reduced to 2.4 × 1.3 cm; vaginal tumor 1.7 × 0.5 cm.

Brachytherapy: It was felt that intracavitary brachytherapy, using a 3.5-cm diameter cylinder with peripheral channels, would provide sufficient coverage of the residual vaginal disease. However, with the cylinder in place, MRI (***f***) was performed to ensure adequate coverage at depth and to calculate the doses to adjacent critical structures. CT was obtained to ensure coverage of the initial mucosal extent of the tumor (as indicated by fiducial markers; *arrows **g, h***).

Using the central channel and three peripheral channels on the right, a total dose of 45 Gy was delivered to the apical and proximal right lateral vaginal surface in 66 hours. The total dose to the HR CTV was 25–30 Gy; D_{90} for the residual GTV was 27.7 Gy. The D_{2cc} rectum was 28 Gy (total dose, 68 Gy).

IMRT Node Boosts (*d*):

Revised CI, PA GTV (+7 mm): 10 Gy in 5 fractions (total dose, 60 Gy).

EI node GTV (+7 mm): 12 Gy in 6 fractions (total dose with brachytherapy contribution, 66.6 Gy).

All radiotherapy was completed within 48 days.

Chemotherapy: Weekly cisplatin × 3, discontinued due to neutropenia.

Outcome: At 4 months, NED by exam and PET–CT. At 18 months, NED on active surveillance.

Comment: Peripheral channels in the cylinder were used primarily to provide distal mucosal coverage on the right. They also added somewhat to the depth of coverage of the distal GTV but with a disproportionate increase in the dose to the vaginal surface (***h**, dotted line*). For this reason, coverage at depth was provided primarily using the central channel.

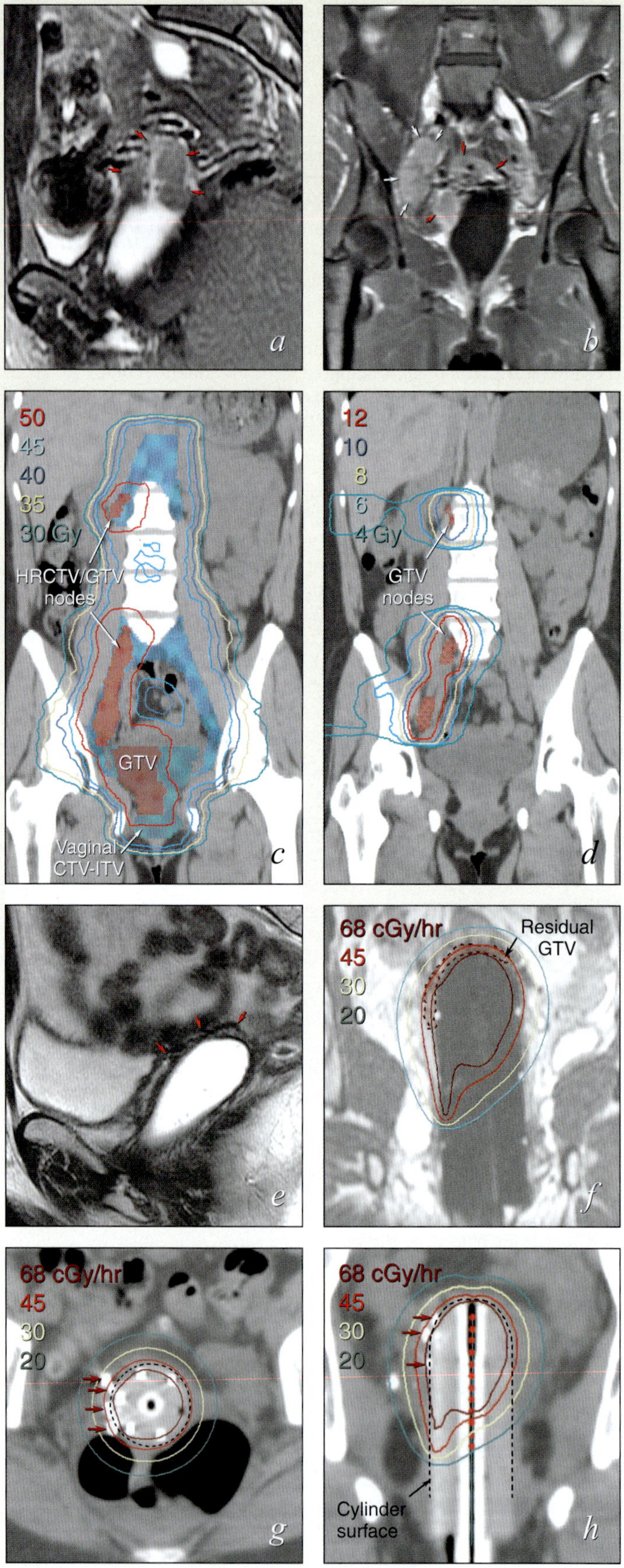

CS 11.3 • Stage II Adenocarcinoma of the Distal Anterior and Lateral Vagina

History: A 35-year-old woman was evaluated for persistent postpartum metrorrhagia. She was scheduled for an endometrial ablation, which was cancelled after a vaginal mass was detected at EUA. The patient was referred for evaluation and treatment.

Evaluation: *EUA*: Nodular 3 × 4 cm mass involving the anterior and right distal one-third of the vagina. *Cystoscopy*: WNL. *MRI* (***a***): Enhancing 3 × 3 × 4 cm mass involving the right and anterior distal vaginal wall, displacing and partially surrounding the urethra and inseparable from the levator ani (*arrows*). *PET–CT*: FDG-avid mass in the vagina; no abnormal nodes or distant metastases. *Biopsy (vagina)*: Poorly differentiated adenocarcinoma.

Treatment Plan: Chemoradiotherapy to the vagina and regional nodes to be followed, after reevaluation, by either an IMRT boost or brachytherapy.

EBRT: *Setup*: Frog-leg position in a custom cradle. Because of the distal vaginal involvement, the CTV included inguinal as well as internal and external iliac nodes (up to mid-L5); the vaginal CTV–ITV extended from 1 cm above the vaginal apex (on full bladder scan) to the urethral meatus. IMRT was delivered in 25 fractions with an integrated boost (***b***):

Inguinal and Iliac Nodal CTV (+7 mm): 45 Gy (1.8 Gy/fraction).

Vaginal GTV and CTV–ITV (+7 mm): 50 Gy (2.0 Gy/fraction).

Interval Evaluation (after 20 fractions): *Exam*: Excellent response; <1 cm residual disease in the right periurethral sulcus; superficial irregularity in the left sulcus and right distal vagina.

Considering the distribution of disease (involving the lateral wall but sparing the rectovaginal septum) and the resistant histologic type, it was felt that brachytherapy would be the safest, most effective central boost method, enabling a higher dose to be delivered over a shorter time than was possible with IMRT.

Brachytherapy: Ten needles were placed approximately 5 mm deep to the vaginal mucosa under direct palpation (***c***). A 3-cm cylinder with peripheral channels was inserted and secured (Chapter 8). The locations of fiducial markers inserted at the tumor margins during preradiotherapy EUA (***c***, *arrows*) were identified on CT and transferred to an MRI for brachytherapy planning (***c***). The final plan (***d***) delivered 20–24 Gy in 66 hours to all regions of initial and persistent disease (as indicated by fiducial markers) with a mucosal margin of about 1 cm (total dose to GTV, 70–74 Gy). The total D_{2cc} to the rectum was <60 Gy. *All radiotherapy was completed in 38 days.*

Chemotherapy: Weekly cisplatin × 3. Additional cisplatin was held because of severe, uncontrollable nausea. Radiotherapy was followed by six courses of carboplatin and paclitaxel.

Outcome: In the final week of EBRT, patchy moist desquamation exacerbated by mild diarrhea caused painful defecation; this was effectively treated using fentanyl lollipops before and sitz baths after each bowel movement. At 4 months, NED by exam and PET–CT. Initial dyspareunia and hot flashes improved with hormone therapy. At 4 years, NED by imaging and exam without GI or GU complaints.

Comment: Vaginal adenocarcinomas have higher local recurrence and distant metastasis rates than squamous carcinomas, with overall survival rates of <50%. Because of the aggressive histologic type and because she received only three courses of cisplatin, the patient was offered the option of adjuvant chemotherapy. However, she was carefully counseled that there was no proof of benefit from chemotherapy in this setting.

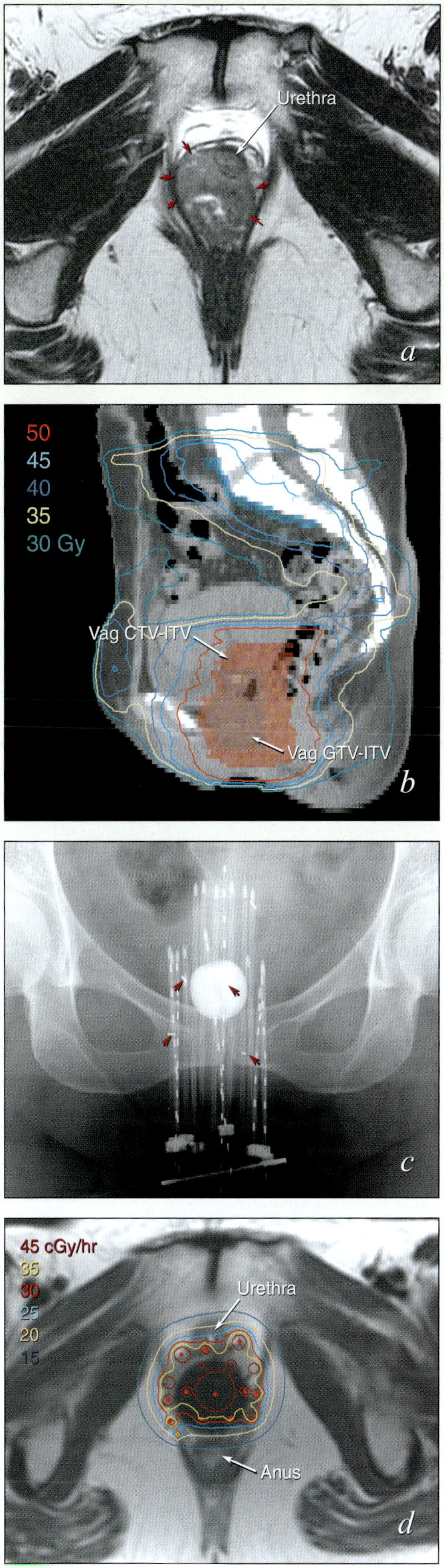

CS 11.4 • Stage II Squamous Carcinoma of the Lateral and Posterior Wall

History: A 76-year-old woman reported 3 months of vaginal bleeding. She had a distant history of hysterectomy for benign disease. Past history was notable for diabetes mellitus and back surgery with lumbar fixation.

Evaluation: *Exam (EUA)*: A 3 × 2 cm partially exophytic mass on the right vaginal wall extended from midvagina to the hymenal ring; anteriorly tumor extended to the urethral sulcus; posteriorly, superficial disease extended to midline. The vagina was very narrow, particularly at the introitus. Fiducial markers were placed at the periphery of the lesion; *PET–CT*: no lymphadenopathy or distant metastases; MRI could not be performed because of orthopedic implants. *Biopsy (vagina)*: Invasive squamous carcinoma.

Treatment Plan: Chemoradiotherapy followed by probable interstitial brachytherapy.

EBRT: *Setup*: (***b***): Supine frog-leg position.

Pelvic treatment was initially planned using a four-field technique (***a, b***). During the first week, after EUA, the vaginal ITV was adjusted to more generously encompass fiducial markers; the treatment plan also was changed to IMRT (***c, d***).

Prebrachytherapy Evaluation: *Exam*: The lesion had flattened, but there was still a plaque of tumor with central ulceration extending on the right from 7 o'clock to 10 o'clock. Because the tumor primarily involved the lateral vaginal wall with only superficial posterior involvement and because of the sluggish response to initial EBRT, it was decided to use interstitial brachytherapy rather than IMRT for the boost. At prebrachytherapy EUA, additional fiducial markers were placed around the residual gross disease. These were distinguished by comparison with preoperative imaging.

Brachytherapy: Seven interstitial needles were inserted transperineally under direct palpation and secured around a 2-cm diameter cylinder as described in Chapter 8 (***e, f***). The two most posterior needles were inserted in the perineum to supplement coverage of distal posterior involvement but were shorter than the lateral needles, avoiding the thinner rectovaginal septum. Orthogonal films taken in the operating room confirmed that the needles had the desired relationship with the fiducial markers (*arrows*, ***g, h***).

The region of palpable residual disease was treated to 30 Gy in 66 hours (45 cGy/h)(***i, j***); adjacent sites of initial mucosal involvement received at least 20 Gy. Including EBRT, the total dose was 65–75 Gy to initial sites of gross disease and 75–78 Gy to the residual gross disease.

All radiotherapy was completed within 40 days.

Chemotherapy: Weekly cisplatin × 4.

Outcome: At 4 months, NED by exam and PET–CT. At 1 year, NED on active surveillance. The vagina was narrow, barely admitting a finger; no change in bowel or bladder habits.

Comment: To encompass the medial inguinal nodes in the initial four-field plan, the AP was wider than the PA field; to reduce the dose to the femoral heads and mons, AP and PA fields were given greater weighting than the lateral fields. Although the initial four-field plan provided adequate sparing of critical structures, IMRT reduced the volumes of bowel, bladder, and subcutaneous tissue treated to high dose.

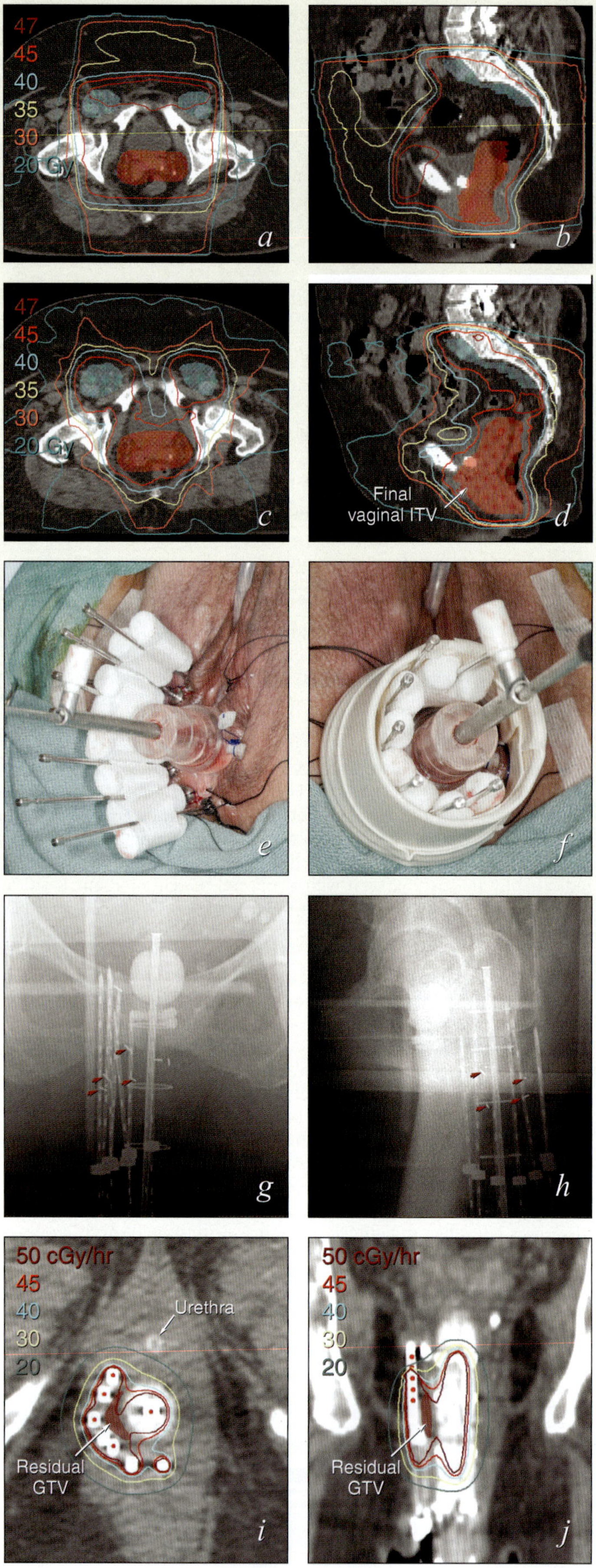

CS 11.5 • Stage II Cancer of the Distal Lateral Vagina

History: A 62-year-old woman with postmenopausal bleeding and discharge was seen by her gynecologist who obtained a negative Pap smear. A year later, the patient noted a lesion on the left side of her vagina, which was cauterized by her gynecologist. When the lesion persisted, a biopsy specimen was obtained and revealed cancer.

Evaluation: *EUA*: A 4 × 3 cm ulcerated, infiltrating lesion involved the distal left vagina from 3 o'clock to 5 o'clock and extended distally to the hymenal ring. Five fiducial markers were inserted at the radial margins of the tumor. *CT (chest, abdomen, pelvis)*: A 3.5 × 2.5 focal area of enhancement along the left lateral aspect of the vagina (***a***). No abnormal nodes or distant metastases were noted. *KPS*: 100. *Biopsy (vagina)*: Poorly differentiated squamous carcinoma.

Treatment Plan: Chemoradiotherapy followed by probable interstitial brachytherapy.

EBRT: *Setup*: Supine, frog-leg position in a custom cradle.

The initial treatment plan included the entire vagina and paravaginal tissues with the distal margin 3 cm beyond the gross disease (***c***); an ITV was determined using full and empty bladder scans. The external and internal iliac nodes were treated up to L5/S1 (just above the bifurcations of the CI vessels). The inguinal nodes were included because of the extent of distal disease immediately adjacent to the vulva.

IMRT (In 25 fractions)(*b, c*):

Nodal CTV and vaginal CTV–ITV (+7 mm): 45 Gy (1.8 Gy/fraction)

Vagina GTV–ITV (+7 mm): 50 Gy (2 Gy/fraction)

Prebrachytherapy Evaluation: *Exam*: Excellent response; flattening and softening of the lesion with residual mucosal irregularity and ulceration of the mucosa. *MRI*: Deformation of the left distal vagina with focal infiltrating soft tissue density.

Brachytherapy (*d*): Five interstitial needles were inserted about 5 mm deep to the mucosa under direct palpation. A 3-cm domed cylinder with peripheral channels was inserted and secured in the vagina. Dwell times in the central channel, in four of the peripheral channels, and in the five needles were optimized to achieve the desired doses and degree of homogeneity. Fiducial markers were used to define the GTV, which received a total dose of 20 Gy in 44 hours at 45 cGy per hour (total dose, 70 Gy). A surrounding margin of tissue (HR CTV) received 10–15 Gy.

All radiotherapy was completed in 37 days.

Chemotherapy: Weekly cisplatin × 4.

Outcome: Treatment was tolerated well with brisk erythema of the vaginal introitus at week 5. At 1 month, a small (0.5-cm) area of residual mucosal ulceration; resolving diarrhea; at 4 months, NED with no bowel or bladder complaints; at 3 years, NED by exam. There was mild atrophy and telangiectasia in a 1 × 2 cm region at the initial site of disease. The patient was not sexually active for social reasons but had good vaginal length, lubrication, and distensibility.

Comment: The region of the distal vagina and vaginal introitus is particularly delicate. To avoid necrosis of the vulvovaginal mucosa, care must be taken to allow sources no closer than 4–5 mm from the mucosal surface.

Lesions of the posterior and distal vagina are easily missed on examination unless the speculum is rotated to view the entire mucosal surface and a careful rectovaginal exam is performed. Suspicious lesions should not be cauterized without biopsy.

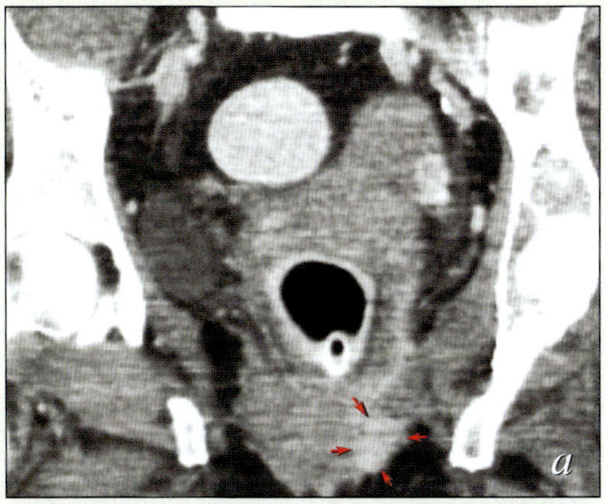

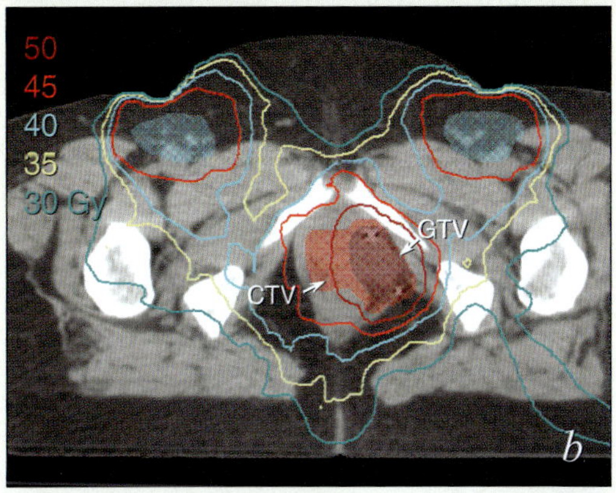

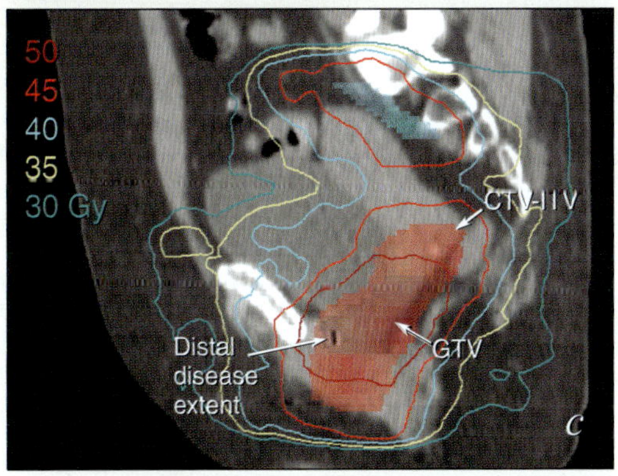

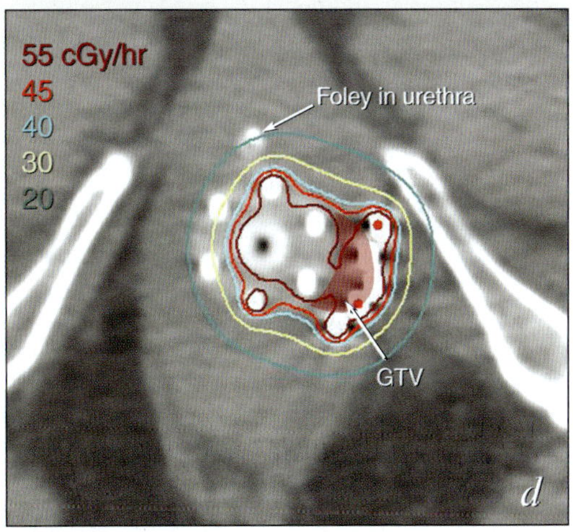

CS 11.6 • Stage II Cancer Involving the Rectovaginal Septum

History: A 40-year-old woman had 2 years of persistently positive Pap smears despite LEEP procedures, a cone biopsy, and a hysterectomy that revealed CIN with negative margins. MRI obtained because of posthysterectomy bleeding was interpreted as showing a possible hematoma in the rectovaginal septum. At EUA, the posterior vaginal wall was incised, revealing suspicious tissue. Biopsy showed squamous carcinoma, and the patient was referred for treatment.

Evaluation: *EUA*: A 4 × 4 × 2 cm mass occupying the posterior distal two-thirds of the vagina with some extension to the right lateral wall. Fiducial markers were inserted at the lesion's margins. *MRI (**a, b**)*: A 5 × 5 × 1.5 to 2 cm mass occupying most of the rectovaginal septum with blurring of the fat plane between the posterior vaginal wall and rectum; also a 2-cm presacral lymph node; PET was not performed because of the patient's recent operations. *Chest x-ray*: WNL. *KPS*: 100.

Treatment Plan: Chemoradiotherapy to the primary site and regional nodes.

EBRT: *Setup*: Supine, frog-leg position. BBs were placed on the clitoris and anal orifice to help determine the distal margin of the CTV (***d***).

The entire presacral space and perirectal nodes were included in the target volume; medial inguinal nodes were included because of the distal disease extent. Full and empty bladder scans were used to designate a vaginal ITV but demonstrated very little movement.

IMRT (Fractions 1–25)(*c, d*):

Nodal CTV and vaginal CTV–ITV (+7 mm): 45 Gy

Vagina GTV–ITV (+7 mm): 50 Gy

Interval Evaluation (at 40 Gy): Dramatic tumor response with no definite evidence of residual disease on exam or MRI (***e***). It was decided to proceed with brachytherapy after 25 treatments of EBRT.

Brachytherapy: A 3.5-cm domed cylinder with peripheral channels was used.

Because there was no palpable residual disease, fiducial markers placed at the initial EUA defined the target volume (***f***). Peripheral channels were used to supplement posterior contribution from the central channel (***g, h***); the posterior target and apical vagina received 20–30 Gy in 48 hours (total dose 70–80 Gy).

IMRT Node Boost: Following brachytherapy, the presacral node was given an additional 16 Gy in 8 fractions.

Chemotherapy: Cisplatin × 5.

All radiotherapy was completed in 45 days.

Outcome: At 4 months, asymptomatic; sexually active with no dyspareunia. *PET–CT*: No residual disease in the vagina but new development of diffuse liver metastases. *Biopsy (liver)*: Metastatic squamous carcinoma. The patient was referred for chemotherapy.

Comment: Had residual disease in the rectovaginal septum been more than 3–4 mm thick, an unacceptably high vaginal surface dose would have been required to treat the tumor with intracavitary brachytherapy; an IMRT boost (possibly with a rectal balloon to control internal motion) would have been used to deliver a boost dose to residual disease.

This pattern of rapid dissemination is uncommon for squamous carcinomas. However, extensive perirectal involvement tends to be a risk factor for development of liver metastases.

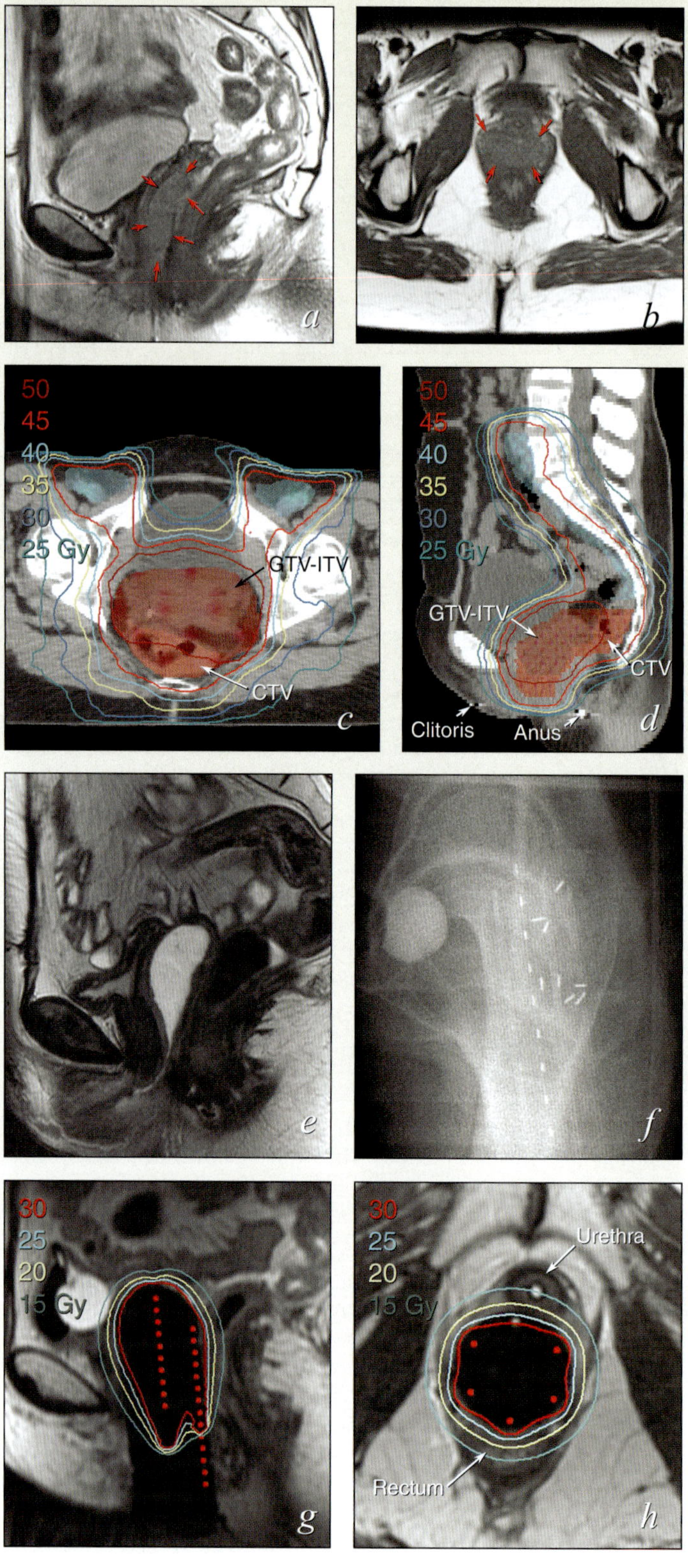

CS 11.7 • Stage III Vaginal Cancer Referred after Incomplete Response to Initial Pelvic Radiotherapy

History: A 36-year-old woman with menorrhagia was scheduled for hysterectomy after no bleeding source was found on exam. When a large vaginal mass was discovered at EUA, the operation was cancelled and the patient was referred for definitive chemoradiotherapy. However, after 45 Gy, the radiation oncologist reexamined the patient, noted large residual disease, and concluded that the cancer could not be cured with radiotherapy alone. The patient returned to her surgeon, who recommended reevaluation in 6 weeks for possible exenteration. The patient sought a second opinion and was seen 3 weeks after completing pelvic radiotherapy.

Evaluation at Diagnosis: *MRI* (***a***): A 6 × 5 × 7 cm tumor in the right vagina filled the paravaginal space to the pelvic wall (*arrows*). *Biopsy*: Squamous carcinoma.

Evaluation before Brachytherapy: *Exam*: A 3 × 3 × 1 cm tumor extending from 7 o'clock to 11 o'clock in the right midvagina. *KPS:* 90–100. *MRI* (***b***): Marked tumor regression with residual thickening of the vaginal wall. *PET*: No metastasis.

Treatment Plan: Brachytherapy.

After a 3-week break, an additional 20–25 Gy of EBRT was unlikely to achieve cure. With interstitial brachytherapy, a higher dose could be delivered over a shorter time with greater sparing of adjacent urethra and anus. Anesthesia assessment was obtained, and the procedure was scheduled for the next day.

Brachytherapy: Platinum marker seeds were inserted to demarcate the margins of the lesion (***e***, *arrows*). Six needles were placed through the perineum and passed 5 mm deep to the vaginal mucosa under direct palpation. A 3-cm cylinder with six peripheral channels was placed in the vagina and secured using the method described in Chapter XX (***c, d***). Adequacy of the implant was determined by palpation and intraoperative x-rays (***e***). Using the six interstitial needles, the central channel, and three of the six peripheral channels of the cylinder, dwell times were adjusted to maximize tumor dose homogeneity while keeping the total maximum rectal dose <70 Gy. A total brachytherapy dose of 3,224 cGy was delivered to the GTV in 62 hours (***f***). The total dose to the GTV was 75–80 Gy delivered in 62 days.

Chemotherapy: Weekly cisplatin with EBRT at an outside facility.

Outcome: At 7 years, NED with no gastrointestinal or urinary symptoms; on hormone replacement therapy; sexually active with occasional dyspareunia relieved with a lubricant.

Comment: Vaginal lesions can be obscured by speculum blades and are easily missed, particularly if no rectovaginal exam is performed.

A full decision tree should always be established at the start of treatment to determine a plan (including possible second opinion from an experienced brachytherapist) to meet different response scenarios. Although this patient appears to be cured, the 3-week delay decreased treatment options and the probability of a good outcome.

Today, we would obtain an MRI with the system in place for brachytherapy planning.

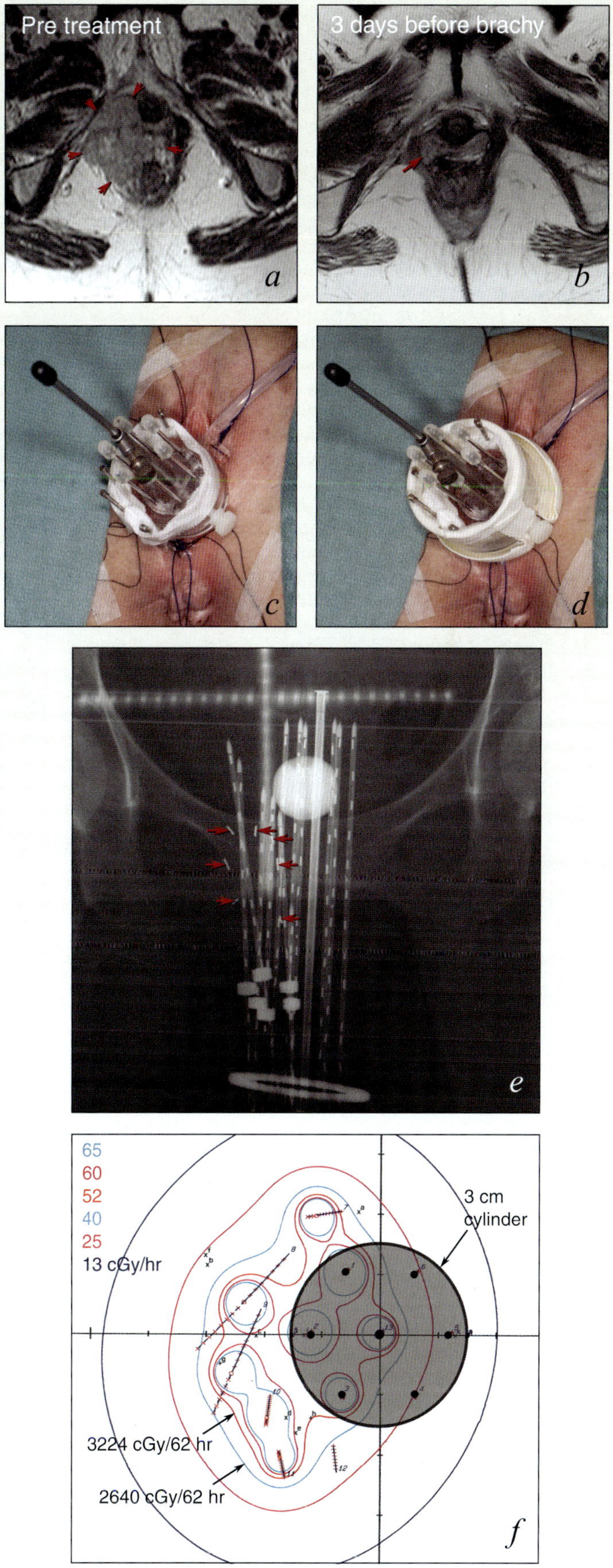

CS 11.8 • Stage III Squamous Carcinoma of the Vaginal Apex

History: A 54-year-old woman with a history of hysterectomy for cervical dysplasia had a recent onset of vaginal bleeding and discharge. A vaginal mass was noted and total pelvic exenteration recommended. The patient requested a second opinion.

Evaluation: *EUA*: A 4- to 5-cm mass replaced the vaginal apex, infiltrated the parametrium, and was tethered to the left pelvic wall. *MRI*: A 4 × 5 cm mass at the vaginal apex with superolateral infiltration of the parametrium (***a, b***); 1.7-cm left CI node (*red arrows*) compressing the CI vein at L5/S1 (***c***). *PET–CT* (***d***): FDG-avid CI node; apical vaginal mass extending toward the left pelvic sidewall (*arrow*); no distant metastases. *Biopsy (vagina)*: Poorly differentiated squamous carcinoma.

Treatment Plan: Pelvic exenteration was contraindicated because of the involved node and probable pelvic wall fixation. Also, chemoradiotherapy had an excellent chance of controlling local disease without sacrificing critical structures.

Because of the positive CI node, the PANs were treated to L1/L2. The plan was to treat with chemoradiotherapy, using IMRT with integrated and sequential boosts to the vagina and nodal GTVs.

EBRT (IMRT): *Setup*: Supine in a custom cradle. Diagnostic studies were digitally fused with the planning CT to assist in target definition. The finding of numerous small FDG-negative nodes led to the use of a somewhat higher than usual nodal CTV dose. Repeat planning CTs in the 3rd and 4th weeks of radiotherapy showed a 40% to 50% reduction in the GTV, permitting some adjustment of the GTVs to improve bowel sparing without excluding any tissues that were initially infiltrated by tumor.

Fractions 1–28 (*e*):

Nodal CTV (+7 mm): 50.4 Gy (1.8 Gy/fraction)

Vaginal ITV (+7 mm): 53.2 Gy (1.9 Gy/fraction)

Vaginal GTV (+7 mm) and CI node GTV (+5 mm): 56 Gy (2.0 Gy/fraction)

Fractions 29–34 (***f***):

Vaginal and nodal GTVs (+7 mm): 10 Gy (2.0 Gy/fraction)

Total GTV dose: 66 Gy in 46 days

Chemotherapy: Weekly cisplatin × 4; discontinued due to neutropenia.

Outcome: Left pelvic deep vein thrombosis during EBRT was treated with anticoagulants. A breast mass noted at initial evaluation was diagnosed as T2N1M0 breast cancer; it was agreed to begin chemotherapy for this after completion of the pelvic treatment. At 2 months, no evidence of vaginal cancer by exam or MRI (***g, h***). At 3 years, on maintenance hormone therapy for breast cancer with no evidence of cancer.

Comment: Venous compression from involved nodes increases the risk of deep vein thrombosis. Patients with this finding should be monitored closely and possibly considered for prophylactic anticoagulation.

This pattern of infiltrative disease cannot receive adequate boost dose with intracavitary treatment even after a good initial response. Because of the extensive superolateral infiltration of the cardinal and uterosacral ligaments, with disease immediately adjacent to bowel and major vessels, it was felt that IMRT could provide more generous and homogeneous coverage of the boost GTV than interstitial brachytherapy.

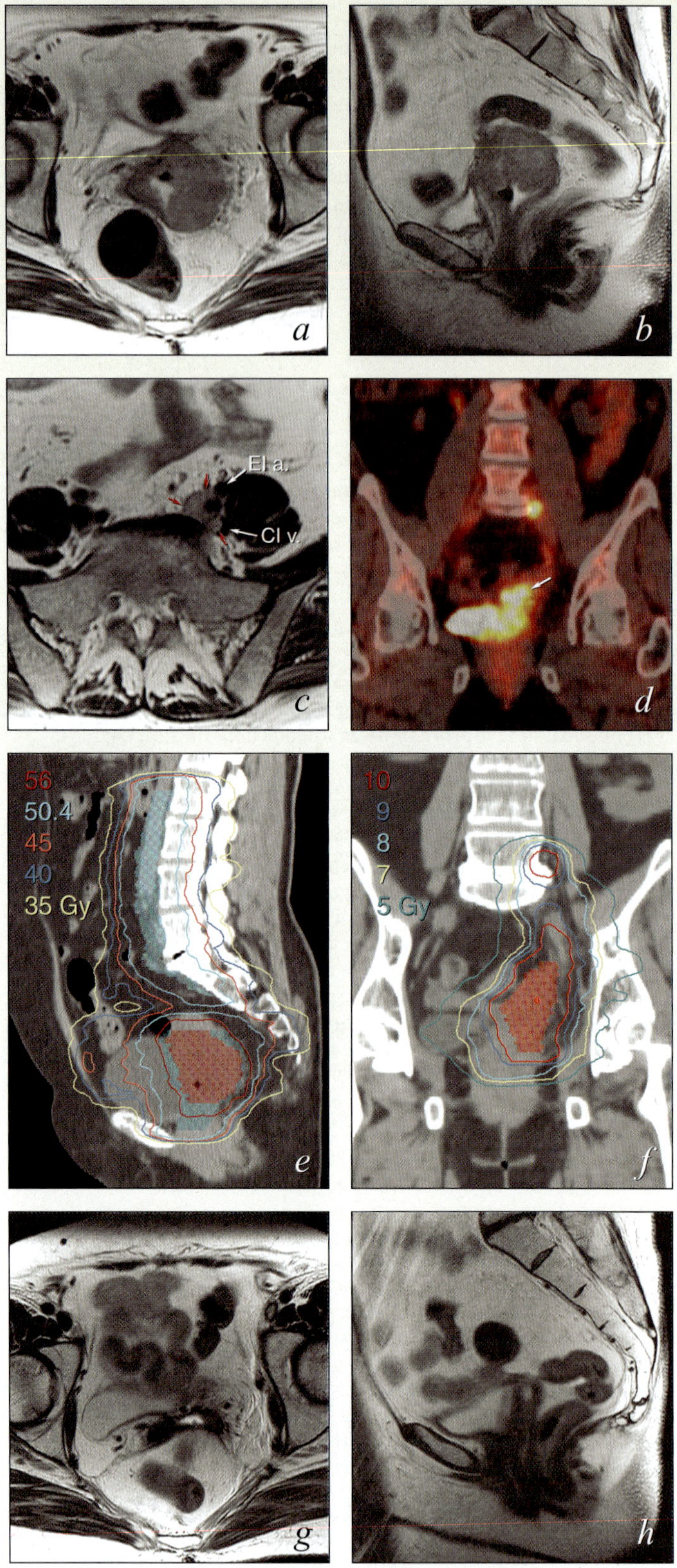

CS 11.9 • Locally Extensive Cancer of the Vagina Presenting with Urethral Obstruction

History: A 79-year-old woman with vaginal bleeding presented to the emergency room with acute inability to void. A suprapubic catheter was inserted after attempts to insert a Foley catheter failed. The patient had a past history of hysterectomy for benign disease. She had no major medical problems.

Evaluation: *Exam*: Friable, infiltrative tumor involving the distal three-fourths of the vagina; tumor was thickest in the suburethral area but also involved lateral and posterior walls. Distally, there was minimal extension to the vestibule of the vagina. Bilateral groin nodes up to 2 cm in diameter. *KPS*: 80. *MRI*: (***a***) An 8 × 4 × 4 cm circumferential vaginal mass encasing urethra and abutting bladder and rectum (*arrows*); bilateral enlarged inguinal nodes; 3-cm left internal iliac node. *CT abdomen, chest*: No extrapelvic disease. *Biopsies of vagina, inguinal node*: Squamous cell carcinoma.

Note: Technically, this patient is classified as having stage IVB vulvar cancer, although 95% of her disease was in the vagina. The choice of treatment was not influenced by this FIGO convention.

Treatment Plan: Definitive chemoradiotherapy with curative intent. Because the primary tumor was unresectable and the enlarged nodes were small relative to the primary tumor, LND was not performed.

Because this large tumor was intimately associated with the urethra and rectovaginal septum, the risk of injury from interstitial brachytherapy would be substantial. In this situation, IMRT can achieve a more homogeneous dose distribution in the interfaces between tumor and critical structures. Because this tumor was fixed and the bladder was continuously drained, only a small posterior expansion was needed to account for apical vaginal motion due to variations in rectal filling.

EBRT: Treatment was delivered using a single IMRT plan with integrated boosts (***b, c***). A nested internal vaginal GTV that excluded the rectum was treated at a slightly higher rate (225 cGy/fraction) than the overall GTV to maximize the effective dose to bulky anterior disease.

Total radiotherapy doses delivered in 30 fractions (completed in 42 days):

GTV–ITV vagina (+7 mm): 64–68 Gy (213–225 cGy/fraction)

GTV nodes (+5 to +7 mm): 60–64 Gy (200–213 cGy/fraction)

CTV groin (+7 mm): 58 Gy (193 cGy/fraction)

CTV pelvic nodes (+7 mm): 52 Gy (173 cGy/fraction)

Chemotherapy: Weekly cisplatin × 5.

Outcome: Treatment was well tolerated with moist desquamation of medial labia at week 5 treated with local care and fluconazole. Urinary tract infection in week 6 responded to antibiotics and removal of the bladder catheter (tumor response was >50%, and the patient was able to void normally by this time).

At 5 months, NED (***d***). At 9 years, NED with rare stress incontinence and normal GI function. As expected after treatment of a tumor this extensive in an elderly woman, the vagina was entirely fused. KPS: 90%–100%.

Comment:

We do not recommend hypofractionation beyond 215–225 cGy per fraction in this region and exceed 200 cGy per fraction only if IMRT and daily IGRT are available, if the tumor response can be monitored during radiotherapy, and if rectal dose constraints can be achieved.

In retrospect, CTV contours extended unnecessarily beyond the levators and into the obturator internus muscle (*arrows*, ***b***).

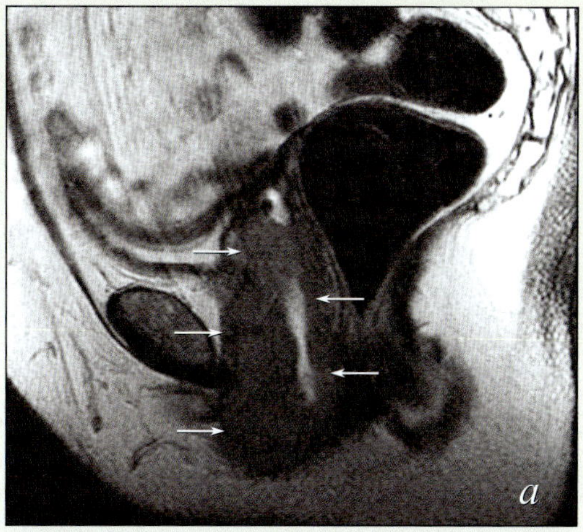

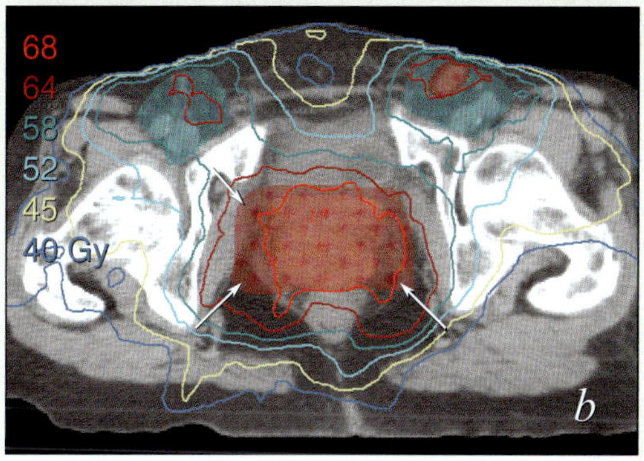

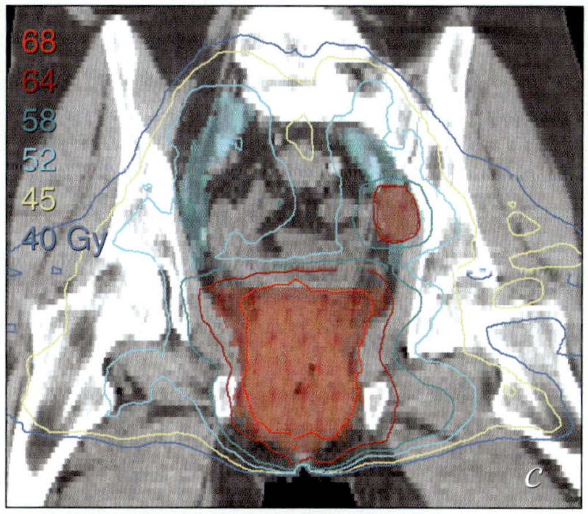

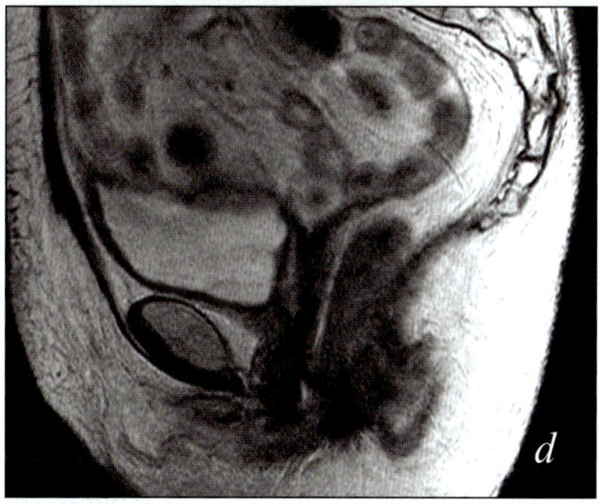

CS 11.10 • Stage IVA Squamous Carcinoma of the Vagina

History: A 53-year-old woman reported several months of recurrent urinary tract infections and intermittent vaginal bleeding. She had a distant history of TAH-BSO for benign disease.

Evaluation: *Exam*: A large infiltrating mass involved the proximal three-fourths of the anterior vagina and was tethered to the left pelvic wall. *KPS*: 90. *Cystoscopy*: Irregular tumor protruding from the trigone. *MRI pelvis (**a, b**)*: A 4.5 × 5 × 5.5 cm vaginal mass invading the posterior bladder wall (arrows). *CT (chest, abdomen)*: No lymphadenopathy or distant metastases.

Pathology (vagina and bladder trigone): Invasive squamous carcinoma.

Treatment Plan: Definitive chemoradiotherapy with curative intent. Because tumor involved the distal vagina, initial EBRT included the medial inguinal as well as iliac nodes. The final boost technique was determined after evaluation of the initial tumor response. Repeat MRI and operating room time were scheduled in advance to prepare for either IMRT or brachytherapy.

Evaluation after 4 Weeks of Radiotherapy: *Exam*: Regression of exophytic tumor with residual thickening and superficial irregularity; no evidence of fistula. *MRI (**c, d**)*: Residual nodularity and focal increased T2 signal in the proximal vagina.

Radiotherapy Boost Plan: To achieve a high rate of local disease control, all areas of initial tumor infiltration should receive at least 65–70 Gy even after an excellent initial response. Intracavitary brachytherapy would not have adequately treated the bladder trigone and paravaginal tissues; dose heterogeneities adjacent to interstitial needles would have increased the risk of fistula through the intact but compromised vesicovaginal septum. It was decided to boost the regions of initial involvement (HR CTV) using IMRT.

EBRT (IMRT): *Setup*: Frog-leg position in a custom cradle. Daily ultrasound was used to verify a bladder volume of 150–250 mL. Locations of fiducial markers placed at the margins of the tumor were monitored daily.

Fractions 1–25 (***e, f***):

Nodal CTV and vaginal ITV (+7 mm): 45 Gy (1.8 Gy/fraction)

Vaginal GTV (+7 mm): 50 Gy (2.0 Gy/fraction)

Fractions 26–34 (***g, h***):

GTV + HR CTV (+7 mm): 16 Gy (2.0 Gy/fraction)

In all, a total dose of 66 Gy was delivered to the GTV in 48 days.

Chemotherapy: Weekly cisplatin × 6.

Outcome: At 3.5 years, NED by imaging and pelvic exam with normal bowel and bladder function. At 3 years, the patient was diagnosed with stage III adenocarcinoma of the lung. Comparison with her initial vaginal biopsies confirmed that this was a new primary cancer.

Comment: A referring physician had recommended pelvic exenteration. This approach may be considered in rare cases of stage IVA disease if the tumor is localized, mobile, and has already caused a fistula. In this case, however, a curative resection would have been unlikely even with total exenteration because of the extensive paravaginal infiltration. Also, because there was no fistula or obvious tumor necrosis, it was felt that there was a chance of retaining both bladder and rectal function with definitive chemoradiotherapy.

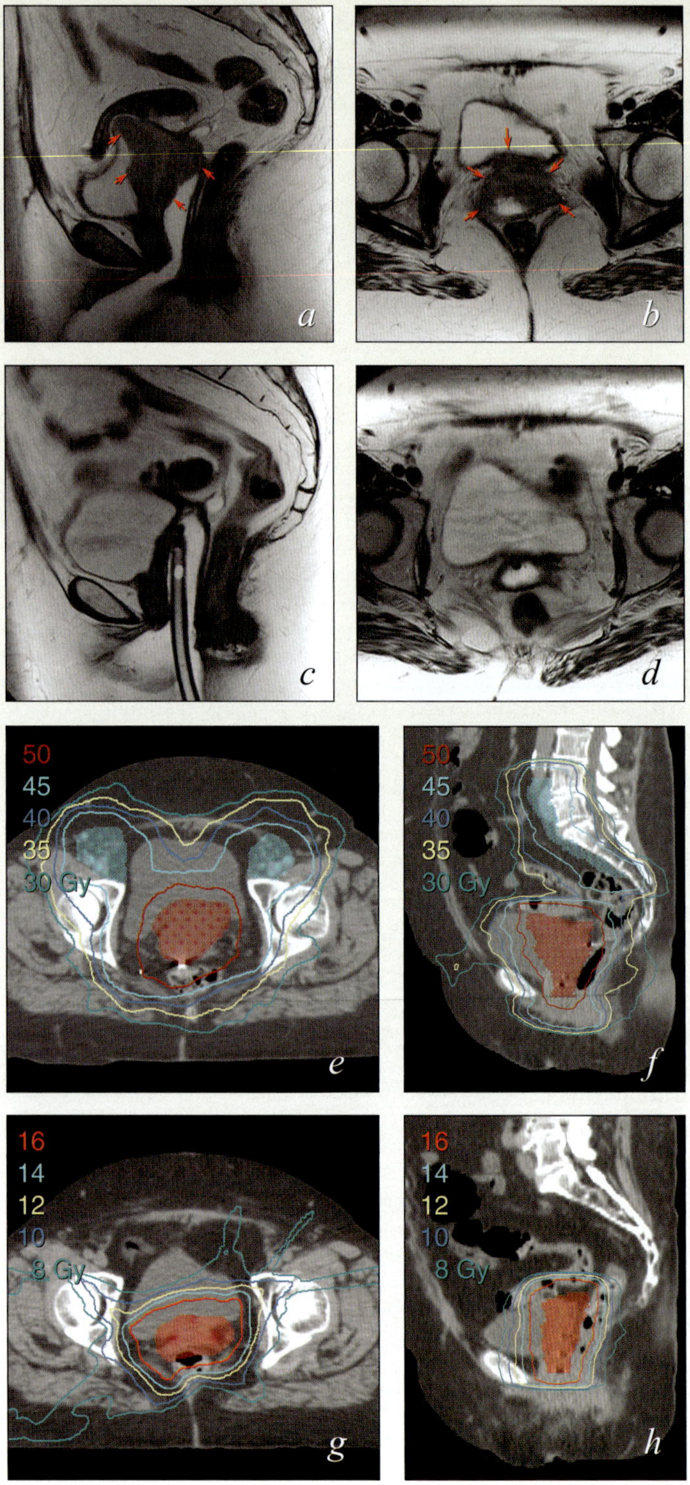

CHAPTER 12

Vulvar Cancer

Before the mid-1980s, it was commonly believed that radiation therapy (RT) had no role in the curative management of vulvar cancer. Then in 1986, Homesley et al.[1] reported the results of a randomized trial that demonstrated improved survival when adjuvant RT was given to patients with node-positive vulvar cancer. Since then, clinicians have sought to refine and, where appropriate, expand the indications for RT. However, there continue to be many sources of controversy concerning the relative roles and optimal treatment guidelines for surgical and radiotherapeutic management. Several features contribute to these management challenges.

- *Vulvar cancer is uncommon.* In the United States, fewer than 6,000 new cases are diagnosed each year. Although multidisciplinary practices vary, generally no more than one-third of patients with vulvar cancer have an indication for RT. This means that vulvar cancer comprises an even smaller proportion of RT practice than vaginal cancer.
- *There is very little level I evidence to guide treatment.* Since the Homesley trial,[1] most studies relevant to the radiotherapeutic management of vulvar cancer have been retrospective. Many of the patients included in these studies were treated before modern diagnostic and therapeutic standards were available, limiting the relevance of their data to current practice.
- *The external beam techniques used to treat vulvar cancer are challenging.* As discussed in this chapter and in Chapter 5, poor visualization of many vulvar tumors on standard diagnostic imaging studies makes accurate target volume definition difficult. The shape and orientation of the targets and close proximity of critical structures also pose special treatment planning challenges.
- *Management of the short-term side effects of surgery and radiation is particularly challenging for patients with vulvar cancer.* Postoperative complications, infection, and radiation effects can all lead to treatment delays that may reduce the effectiveness of RT. Skilled management of treatment-related side effects plays an important role in achieving optimal results.
- *The long-term effects of treatments can be severe.* Many factors, including postoperative complications, radiation effects, infection, and tissue damage caused by the primary vulva cancer, can have lasting effects on the well-being of patients with locoregionally advanced vulvar cancer. These effects can be minimized through careful integration of multidisciplinary treatments. However, clinicians are still searching for the best ways to balance these treatments, particularly for patients with locally advanced disease.

PRETREATMENT EVALUATION

Careful pretreatment evaluation helps to define the extent of disease and to determine whether definitive surgical resection can be accomplished without sacrificing organ function. The primary goals of pretreatment evaluation are as follows:

- *To determine the extent and resectability of local and regional disease.*
- *To rule out metastatic disease that would change the treatment goal from curative to palliative.*
- *To rule out other primary genital tract cancers.* About half of vulvar cancers are human papilloma virus (HPV) related, and these patients are at increased risk for cervical, vaginal, and anal cancers.

- *To determine whether the patient is medically fit for treatment.* All patients require a careful history and complete physical examination before initiation of treatment.

Pretreatment studies should be selected to answer these questions in the most cost-effective way possible. Studies that can help to guide treatment include the following:

- *Physical examination*: Pelvic examination should include careful inspection and palpation of the vulva and perianal region including rectovaginal examination to determine the extent of local disease and proximity of tumor to the urethra, clitoris, anus, and vagina. The cervix and vagina should be carefully examined, ideally with colposcopy, to rule out invasive or preinvasive lesions in those sites. If patient discomfort prevents an adequate assessment in clinic, examination under anesthesia (EUA) should be performed; if there is periurethral disease, cystourethroscopy should be performed. In cases of locally advanced disease, both the gynecologic oncologist and radiation oncologist should be present at EUA if possible. In selected cases (particularly those with vaginal involvement), interstitial placement of fiducial markers can assist in subsequent radiation treatment planning (CS 12.3). All clinical findings should be carefully documented, with detailed descriptions of the location and morphology of abnormal lesions and estimates of tumor diameters and the distances between tumor and perineal structures. Examination should also include an assessment of the groins, although even extensive lymphadenopathy can be missed on physical examination (CS 12.8).
- *Ultrasound*: In experienced hands, ultrasound combined with ultrasound-directed fine needle aspiration (FNA) cytology has a better than 90% sensitivity for detecting nodal metastasis (Chapter 4).[2] In one study of 40 patients, Moskovic et al.[3] correctly identified metastatic nodal disease in 11 of 13 groins; the two false negatives were in nodes with metastatic deposits <3 mm. However, the sensitivity of ultrasound undoubtedly varies with the experience of the ultrasonographer and, even in the most experienced hands, a negative result is insufficient to rule out the need for groin treatment in patients with invasive cancers. Ultrasound-guided FNA may, in selected cases, help to guide the dose of radiation given to equivocal nodes; however, if there is any doubt, suspicious nodes that have not been removed should be treated as if they were positive, because the price for error is high (CS 12.1). Ultrasound is also a noninvasive, inexpensive method for following the groins of patients after negative results for sentinel node biopsy if a complete dissection has not been performed (CS 12.10).
- *Contrast-enhanced computed tomography (CT)*: Although CT is generally superior to physical examination for the detection of lymphadenopathy, it cannot detect micrometastases. Also the infections often associated with vulvar cancers can cause inflammatory nodal enlargement, reducing the specificity of CT. CT can be valuable for detecting extrapelvic metastases but rarely provides useful information about the extent of disease in the vulva.
- *Magnetic resonance imaging (MRI)*: MRI provides much better soft tissue detail than CT and can therefore be very helpful in assessing the extent of disease in the vulva and vagina. It is particularly useful in cases of locally advanced disease, where MRI can assist in the determination of resectability. MRI is often very helpful in radiation treatment planning, particularly if the study can be obtained in the treatment position. *However, MRI cannot replace a careful physical examination.* In particular, MRI frequently underestimates the extent of mucosal involvement in the vagina and, in some cases, fails entirely to detect even fairly extensive vulvar tumors (CS 12.8).
- *Positron emission tomography (PET)*–CT: Studies of the ability of PET–CT to detect inguinal metastases from squamous carcinomas of the vulva have reported sensitivities that range between 50% and 70% and specificities that range from 60% to 90% (Chapter 4).[2] Inflammatory nodes are frequently FDG-avid. PET–CT can sometimes be helpful in the designation of RT target volumes in patients with advanced disease.

To summarize, physical examination is the most important method for clinical evaluation of local disease extent. Most patients with locoregionally advanced disease should also have CT of the chest, abdomen, and pelvis or PET–CT to assess regional nodes and rule out distant disease. MRI may help to determine operability and define disease extent for RT planning. However, in most cases, surgical evaluation determines the stage of disease and the need for adjuvant treatment.

RISK ASSESSMENT

Predictors of Vulvar Recurrence

The most frequent site of recurrence after primary surgical treatment of vulvar cancer is in the vulva.[4] Some vulvar recurrences are true relapses of the initial invasive lesion, whereas others are undoubtedly new cancers arising in areas at high risk for neoplastic transformation because of lichen sclerosis or HPV infection.

One of the most difficult decisions for radiation oncologists is whether and when to give adjuvant radiotherapy to the vulva after surgical excision. Although several investigators have evaluated factors associated with local recurrence after treatment of invasive carcinoma, their results are not always applicable to modern practice because the studies are typically retrospective, span many years of evolving surgical techniques, and are often confounded by the inconsistent delivery of adjuvant radiotherapy. However, any oncologist trying to weigh the risks and benefits of vulvar radiotherapy must consider these data to estimate the probability of vulvar recurrence and whether local recurrence, if it occurs, is likely to be salvageable with additional surgery.

Risk Factors for Vulvar Recurrence after Initial Surgical Treatment

Local tumor characteristics that have been associated with an increased risk of vulvar recurrence include deep stromal invasion,[5–7] large tumor size,[5] multifocal disease,[8] the presence of lichen sclerosis,[8] and the size of the tumor-free surgical margin.[6,7,9,10]

Of these risk factors, margin size has most consistently been found to be predictive of local recurrence. Even after wide excision of a vulvar cancer, final pathologic assessment of the surgical specimen often reveals a smaller than expected tumor-free margin. Several investigators have evaluated the relationship between margin size and recurrence.[6,7,9,10] In the most frequently quoted analysis, Heaps et al.[6] reported a 48% local recurrence rate for 44 patients whose closest margin was <8 mm (after formalin fixation); in contrast, there were no local recurrences among 91 women whose margins were ≥8 mm. For patients whose margins were <4.8 mm, the vulvar recurrence rate was 62%. Other authors have reported similar correlations between margin status and local recurrence, although the relationship is sometimes confounded by the use of adjuvant radiotherapy for patients with very close margins.[7,9–11] Faul et al. demonstrated that patients who had postoperative RT after a vulvar resection with close (≤8 mm) margins had a significantly lower rate of vulvar disease recurrence than patients who did not receive RT. The survival rate was not significantly greater for patients who had adjuvant radiation for close margins, but this comparison is difficult to interpret because the patients who had radiation appeared to have had less favorable tumors with much closer margins. Patients who had positive margins in their study had dramatically better outcome after treatment with adjuvant RT (**Fig. 12.1**).[12]

At least two studies have reported an association between the finding of lymph node metastasis and the risk of local vulvar recurrence.[5,9] Bogani et al.[5] reported that patients with lymph node metastases had a risk of local recurrence that was almost threefold greater than that for patients with negative nodes; multivariate analysis indicated that the risk associated with node involvement was independent of the other risk factors evaluated. This finding has implications for the planning of postoperative adjuvant treatment of patients with lymph node–positive vulvar cancer.

The Outcome of Patients with Recurrence in the Vulva after Vulvectomy

The outcome of salvage surgery for local vulvar recurrence has been the subject of several studies. Woolderink et al.[8] reported a 5-year local recurrence rate of 30% after wide radical excisions of vulvar cancers. The median time to local recurrence was long (40 months, **Fig. 12.2**) with a wide range

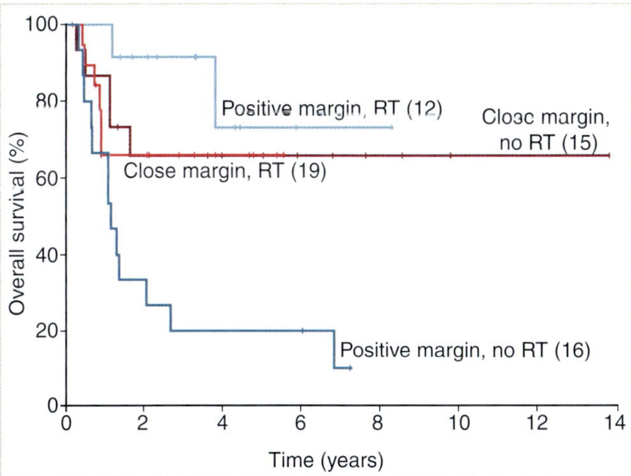

FIGURE 12.1 Overall survival of patients with close (≤8 mm) or positive margins treated with vulvectomy with or without adjuvant vulvar RT. Patients with positive margins had fewer local recurrences (p = 0.005) and better overall survival (p = 0.002) if adjuvant RT was given. Patients who had close margins had fewer local recurrences (p = 0.04) but did not have a better survival outcome than those treated with radiation alone. However, 12 of 19 patients who received radiation had margins ≤4 mm compared with 4 of 15 patients who were observed after excision, suggesting that the patients who had adjuvant radiation had higher risk disease than the patients who were observed. (Faul CM, Mirmow D, Huang Q, et al. Adjuvant radiation for vulvar carcinoma: improved local control. *Int J Radiat Oncol Biol Phys.* 1997;38:381–389.)

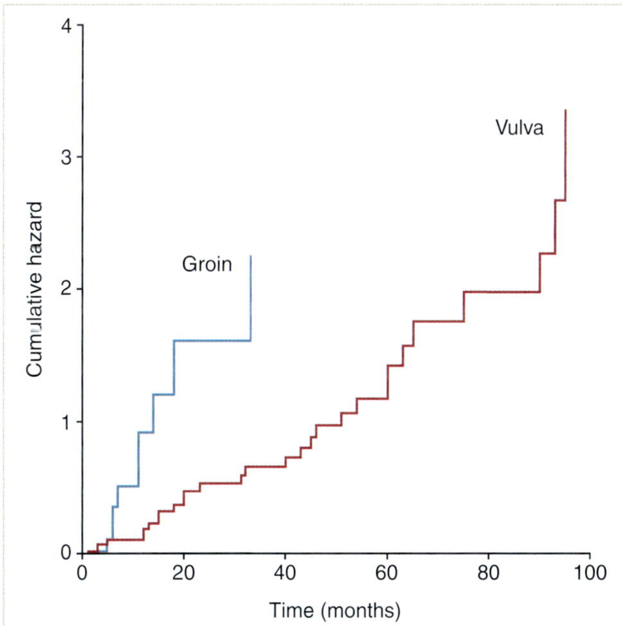

FIGURE 12.2 The time course of 29 vulvar and groin recurrences in 125 patients treated with wide local excision and superficial groin dissection between 1985 and 1999. Most groin recurrences occurred during the first year after surgery. Late vulvar recurrences likely represented new primary lesions associated with lichen sclerosis or HPV. The groin recurrence rate in this series was high, reflecting efforts during the 1990s to reduce the radicality of groin dissection to decrease the rates of perioperative and late side effects. This approach was subsequently abandoned because of the high rate of groin recurrence and death. (Woolderink JM, de Bock GH, de Hullu JA, et al. Patterns and frequency of recurrences of squamous cell carcinoma of the vulva. *Gynecol Oncol.* 2006;103:293–299.)

(3 to 141 months), suggesting that many of these recurrences represented new cancers in a high-risk field. Although recurrences were frequently localized to the vulva, 72% of the 29 patients who were treated for local recurrence had a second recurrence in the vulva. The authors of this study did not discuss the effect of local recurrence on survival.

To summarize, the studies quoted above can be used to suggest some groups that appear to be at particularly high or low risk for local recurrence. The available data are insufficient to provide precise estimates, so the percentages should be considered to be only rough estimates of the risk of recurrence for patients treated with excision without adjuvant RT.

Very high risk (>70%)

- Positive resection margins
- Local recurrence <1 to 2 years after primary resection, particularly if other high-risk features are present.

High risk (about 50% to 60%)

- Margins <5 mm, particularly with tumor >3 cm, deep invasion or positive lymph nodes
- Multifocal disease or local recurrence more than 2 years after resection with other high-risk features

Moderately high risk (about 30% to 40%)

- Margins 5 to 8 mm, particularly with tumor >3 cm, deep invasion or positive lymph nodes

Intermediate risk (<30%)

- Margins >8 mm but tumor >3 cm, deep invasion or positive nodes

Very low risk (<5% to 10%)

- Margins >1 cm, tumor <3 cm, superficially invasive (<2 to 3 mm), negative nodes

Although local recurrences can often be cured with re-excision, the prognosis is not uniformly good. In a review of the outcomes of 47 patients who had isolated local recurrences after initial surgical treatment, Faul et al.[13] reported a 5-year overall survival rate of only 40% (**Fig. 12.3**). In their study, factors associated with a poor outcome after recurrence included short disease-free interval, tumor size >3 cm at the time of recurrence, high initial stage, and lymph-vascular space invasion (LVSI).

As will be discussed later, the risk of postexcision vulvar recurrence is only one factor that must be considered during the formulation of an overall treatment strategy for patients with vulvar cancer.

Predictors of Lymph Node Involvement

The vulva has a rich network of lymphatics that drain primarily to the inguinofemoral nodes (Chapter 5). The rate of lymph node metastasis is strongly correlated with tumor diameter[5,14] (**Fig. 12.4**) and the depth of stromal invasion (as measured from the most superficial dermal papilla adjacent

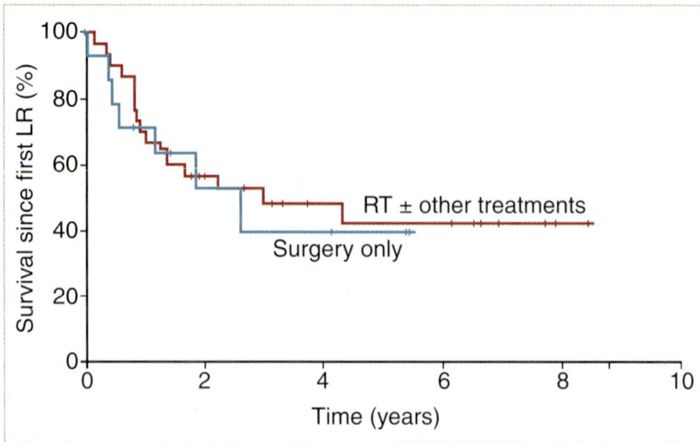

FIGURE 12.3 Survival from the time of first vulvar recurrence for 45 patients who had isolated vulvar recurrences after vulvectomy. Recurrences were treated with re-excision only (31 patients) or with RT with or without chemotherapy or excision (14 patients). The benefits of the two treatment approaches cannot be directly compared because patients who had treatment involving RT had significantly larger recurrent tumors than those treated with excision only. Although many recurrences appear to have been salvaged, the overall survival rate is only about 40%, even after exclusion of patients who had multiple sites of recurrence. (Faul CM, Miramow D, Gerzten K, et al. Isolated local recurrence in carcinoma of the vulva: prognosis and implications for treatment. *Int J Gynecol Cancer.* 1998;8:409–414.)

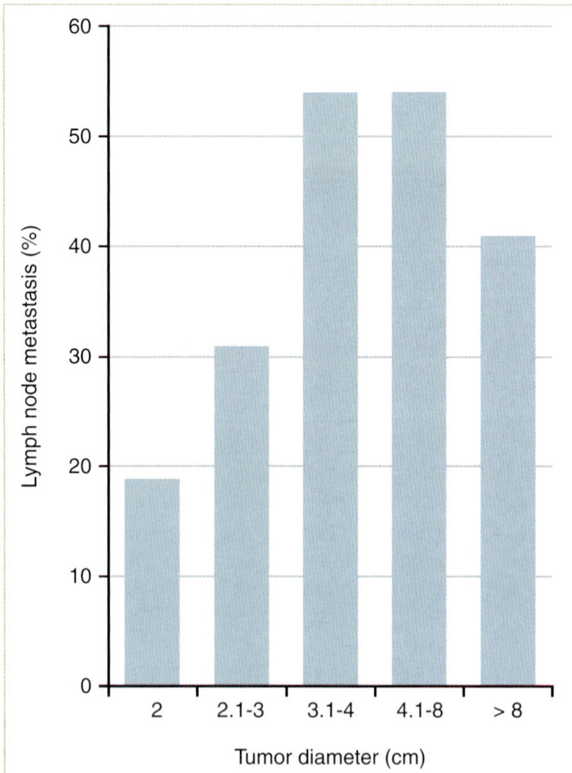

FIGURE 12.4 The relationship between tumor diameter and the incidence of lymph node metastases in 588 patients treated with vulvectomy and lymphadenectomy. (Homesley HD, Bundy BN, Sedlis A, et al. Radiation therapy versus pelvic node resection for carcinoma of the vulva with positive groin nodes. *Obstet Gynecol.* 1986;68:733–740.)

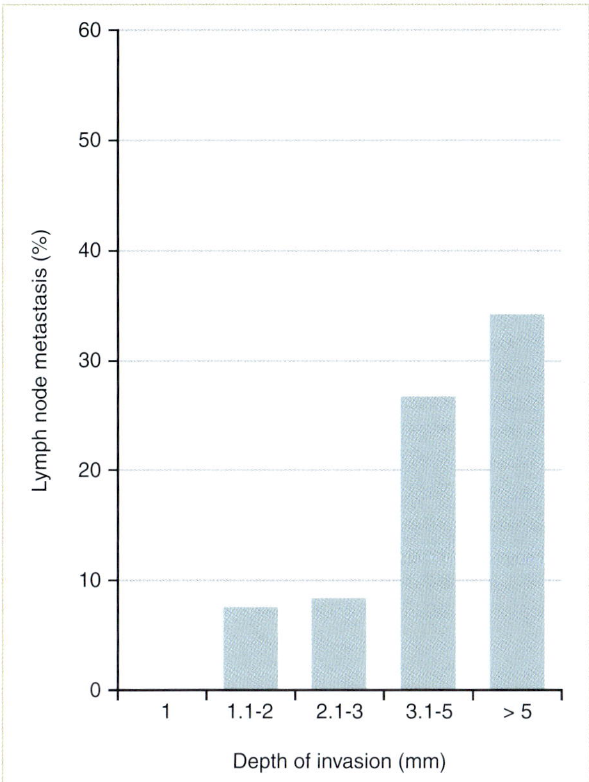

FIGURE 12.5 The relationship between the depth of stromal invasion and the incidence of lymph node metastases. (Hacker NF, Eifel PJ. Vulvar cancer. In: Berek JS, Hacker NF, eds. *Gynecologic Oncology*. Philadelphia, PA: Wolters Kluwer; 2015:560–607.)

to the tumor to the deepest focus of invasion) (**Fig. 12.5**).[2] Only small tumors that invade <1 mm (stage IA) can be considered to have a negligible risk of lymph node metastasis. The risk rises steeply as the depth extends beyond 1 mm.

Other factors that have been associated with lymph node metastasis are high tumor grade[5,14] and the presence of LVSI[14] in the primary tumor.

Predictors of Disease-Related Death

Local or regional recurrence plays a role in most deaths from vulvar cancer; however, distant metastases to lung, bone, or other sites may also occur in isolation or combined with locoregional failure. A number of clinical features can be used to predict outcome.

Inguinal Node Involvement

The most powerful and consistent predictor of outcome is lymph node involvement. The number of positive nodes and the size of the largest focus of intranodal disease are strongly associated with recurrence and death from disease.[14–17] For patients who have a single microscopic nodal metastasis <5 mm, the rate of groin recurrence is <1% *if a radical inguinofemoral lymphadenectomy has been performed.* Patients who have more extensive node involvement or who have had less than a complete lymphadenectomy require adjuvant RT to prevent an unacceptably high rate of groin recurrence.[1,18] For patients who receive adjuvant radiotherapy, the presence of extranodal extension has been consistently found to be an independent predictor of groin recurrence and death from disease.[14,15,17]

The prognosis of patients who have a groin recurrence is very poor. For those whose initial treatment was surgery alone, the survival rate after groin recurrence is <20% in most series, although the doses and techniques used for salvage radiation are rarely mentioned and most reports antedate modern image-based treatment methods.[19] Patients who have a groin recurrence after initial treatment with surgery and radiation can rarely, if ever, be cured.

Pelvic Node Involvement

Historically, pelvic node metastases were associated with poor prognosis with reported survival rates of <20%[1]; patients who have pelvic node metastases are still categorized as having International Federation of Gynecology and Obstetrics (FIGO) stage IVB disease. However, most of the outcome data predate the standard use of adjuvant inguinal and pelvic radiation for node-positive vulvar cancer. In a 2015 review of 20 patients with grossly involved pelvic nodes who were treated with definitive RT, the 5-year overall survival rate was 43%, similar to the rates typically reported for stages IIIB and IIIC disease.[20]

Other Predictors

Most factors that have been associated with an increased risk of vulvar recurrence or lymph node involvement are also correlated with the rates of disease-specific and overall survival. These include tumor size,[5,15,17,21] depth of invasion,[5,15] histologic grade,[5,17,21] and LVSI.[17]

FIGO Stage

The most recent (2009) version of the FIGO staging system incorporates the most powerful predictors of local recurrence, regional involvement, and survival (**Table 12.1**). As such, it will undoubtedly prove to be a strong predictor of outcome. However, it has a few limitations.

- In 1994, FIGO moved to a surgical staging system with categories based on radical local excision and, after 2009, complete inguinal lymphadenectomy. This makes it difficult to categorize patients who are treated with lesser surgical procedures combined with radiotherapy or with radiotherapy alone.
- The grouping of pelvic node metastases and hematogenous metastases together in the stage IVB category underestimates the curability of patients who have pelvic node disease.[20]
- Although the 1994 and 2009 classifications improved the predictive power of the FIGO classifications, the three systems are so radically different that they cannot be readily translated from one to the other. This has made it extremely difficult to interpret stage designations in retrospective studies of vulvar cancer, most of which cross these historical divides (Chapter 2).

TABLE 12.1 Evolution of the FIGO/AJCC Staging System for Vulvar Cancer

	1969–1993	1994–2008	2009–	
AJCC Stage	**(Based on clinical findings)**	**(Based on operative findings)**		**FIGO Stage (2009)**
Primary tumor				
T1	Tumor confined to the vulva ≤2 cm in diameter	$T1_a$ Confined to the vulva or perineum[a]; ≤2 cm diameter and ≤1 mm stromal invasion		IA
		$T1_b$ Confined to the vulva or perineum[a]; ≤2 cm diameter and >1 mm stromal invasion		IB
T2	Tumor confined to the vulva >2 cm in diameter	Tumor confined to the vulva or perineum,[a] >2 cm in diameter	Tumor any size and growing into the anus, lower one-third of the vagina or urethra[b]	II
T3	Tumor any size and growing into the anus, perineum,[a] lower urethra, or vagina	Tumor any size and growing into the anus, lower urethra, or vagina	Tumor any size, growing into the upper urethra, bladder or rectum, upper two-thirds of vagina, or into pubic bone[b]	IVA
T4	Tumor any size, growing into the upper urethra, bladder or rectum, or into pubic bone			
Nodes				
N0	No nodes palpable	No lymph node metastasis	No regional lymph node metastasis	
N1	Nodes palpable in either groin, not enlarged, mobile (not clinically suspect for neoplasm)	Unilateral regional lymph node metastasis	N1a one or two lymph node metastases, each <5 mm	IIIA (i)
			N1b one lymph node metastasis ≥5 mm	IIIA (ii)
N2	Nodes palpable in either or both groins, enlarged, firm, and mobile (clinically suspect for neoplasm)	Bilateral regional lymph node metastasis	N2a three or more lymph node metastases, each <5 mm	IIIB (i)
			N2b two or more lymph node metastases ≥ 5 mm	IIIB (ii)
			N2c Regional lymph node metastasis with extra-capsular spread	IIIC
N3	Fixed or ulcerated nodes		Fixed or ulcerated regional lymph node metastasis	IVA
Distant disease				
M0	No clinical metastases	No distant metastasis		
M1	Palpable deep pelvic lymph nodes	Any distant metastasis including pelvic lymph nodes		IVB
M2	Other distant metastases			

[a]*In 1994, tumors located on the perineum were moved out of the AJCC T3 category and were thereafter grouped with other vulvar cancers according to operative findings.*

[b]*In 2009, tumors involving the anus, distal vagina, or urethra were moved from the AJCC category T3 to T2 and from FIGO stage III to stage II; at the same time, tumors involving the proximal urethra, bladder, rectum, upper vagina, or pubic bone were moved from AJCC T4 to T3 but remained in the FIGO stage IVA category.*

DEVELOPING A MULTIDISCIPLINARY TREATMENT STRATEGY

Locoregionally advanced vulvar cancer requires some of the closest multidisciplinary collaboration of any gynecologic cancer treated with RT. The decision whether to treat with surgery, RT, or a combination of the two treatments requires careful analysis of the role each treatment can play in controlling disease and preserving function. Whenever possible, these uncommon, complex cases should be treated in a center that has an experienced, subspecialized, and closely collaborative multidisciplinary team (Chapter 3).

Once the pretreatment evaluation has been completed, an initial treatment strategy should be developed after considering:

- The risks and benefits of various treatment options for the primary site.
- The risks and benefits of various treatment options for the nodes.
- The combination of approaches to the primary site and groin that will achieve the best overall chance of cure with the least impact on quality of life.

Management of the Primary Site

Surgical Management

A traditional radical vulvectomy involves *en bloc* removal of the entire vulva, including the clitoris, the inguinofemoral nodes, and a "bridge" of intervening tissue. This extensive procedure, which was the standard treatment for most vulvar cancers until at least the late 1980s, had severe psychosexual and physical consequences and is rarely performed today. Vulvectomy and inguinal lymphadenectomy performed through separate incisions is better tolerated than the *en bloc* procedure and is equally effective.[19] Recurrences in the skin bridge are rare after this staged procedure.[19]

Today, most invasive vulvar cancers are treated with an even more limited procedure called a "wide local excision" or "radical local excision." With this procedure, the gross lesion is removed with, whenever possible, a skin margin of 1 to 2 cm; at depth, the dissection is usually carried down to the fascia of the urogenital diaphragm or pubic fascia. If necessary, a portion of the distal urethra can be removed, usually without compromising urethral function. Tumors that involve the perineum are frequently difficult to remove with an optimal margin because of proximity to the anus or rectum. Also, tumors that involve the vagina usually cannot be radically resected without compromising the urethra or rectum.

If preoperative evaluation suggests that organ-sparing surgery is likely to result in a positive resection margin, initial treatment with RT is usually preferred because (1) the dose required to prevent recurrence of disease after a positive resection margin is similar to that required to control gross disease; (2) postoperative wound complications can delay the start of RT, providing an opportunity for disease progression; and (3) the side effects of combined surgery and high-dose radiation tend to be greater than those of radiation alone. In some cases, however, resection with a close margin followed by planned postoperative RT may be preferred over treatment with radiation alone if the surgeon believes negative margins can be achieved and if the estimated risk of postresection wound complications is low. The goal should always be to achieve the best chance of local control with the least morbidity (Chapter 3). Close cooperation and early consultation between the surgeon and radiation oncologist are key to achieving the best result.

Postoperative Radiation Therapy

Predictors of postvulvectomy local recurrence are discussed earlier in this chapter. The most common indications for postoperative vulvar radiation are a close or positive margin. However, other risk factors should be considered and, as will be discussed later in this chapter, the presence of lymph node metastases may influence the decision whether to treat the vulva.

For patients who have a close margin (closer than 8 to 10 mm), the recommended dose is influenced by several factors.

- *Confidence in the margin status.* The pathology report should include a clear description of the gross specimen, the size of the tumor-free margin (measured in mm), and the location of any close margin. Although discussion with the pathologist who handled the resection specimen may clarify the margin status, margins that are described as "negative" without a clear description of the relationship between the tumor and the surgical margins should always be regarded with suspicion.
- *Whether re excision had to be performed to "convert" an initially positive margin to negative.* Under such circumstances, the radiation oncologist should always speak directly with the surgeon to determine why the extent of the lesion was underestimated with the initial excision and to confirm that the surgeon is certain the re-excision removed tissue at the margin of the involved site. If a positive margin was obtained because of the tumor's proximity to critical structures, re-excision is unlikely to clear a positive margin. If there is doubt, the margin should be considered positive.
- *The time from surgery to the start of radiation therapy.* Postoperative RT should be initiated within 8 weeks and preferably within 4 to 6 weeks of excision. Although the effect of delay has not been closely studied in this specific setting, the time from surgery to the end of radiation has been proven to correlate with recurrence in other settings. We believe that delays in the initiation of postoperative RT (or breaks in the middle of treatment) justify an increase in the prescribed dose of radiation.

Viswanathan et al.[10] reported a high rate of local recurrence when close margins received ≤50 Gy and have recommended at least 56 Gy for any patient with a margin ≤10 mm. However, in our experience, vulvar recurrences are rare after 45 to 50 Gy given over 4 to 5 weeks if the tumor-free margin is 5 to 10 mm and if none of the above concerns pertain. For margins that are >1 to 2 mm but <5 mm, we recommend at least 50 Gy to the operative bed, and we usually give 54 to 56 Gy if the margin is <1 to 2 mm, particularly if there is extensive LVSI or if the tumor is an adenocarcinoma. When a patient is referred for treatment of a positive vulvar resection margin, a dose of at least 60 Gy to the operative bed (HRCTV–PTV) and a lower dose of 40 to 50 Gy to a surrounding vulvar CTV–PTV are recommended.

However, more detailed studies are needed to clarify the relationship between vulvar recurrence, radiation dose, and postoperative risk factors. The influence of concurrent chemotherapy on local control in this setting is uncertain. Also, as will be discussed later, it is critical that the technique used to administer RT delivers the desired dose to the entire operative bed with adequate margin.

Preoperative Radiation Therapy

In 1973, Boronow[22] introduced the concept of preoperative RT as an alternative to pelvic exenteration for treatment of locally advanced vulvar cancer; he cited a small personal experience and reviewed available case reports that suggested early encouraging results, particularly in view of the high perioperative mortality rates reported in that era for pelvic exenteration. Following Boronow's initial report, preoperative RT (usually administered with concurrent chemotherapy) became an increasingly accepted treatment option for vulvar cancers that were unresectable or that involved critical structures. These experiences are difficult to summarize because of the small numbers of patients treated, heterogeneous disease presentations, and methodological variations. However, several generalizations can be made from these studies:

- Clinical complete response rates 4 to 6 weeks after 40 to 50 Gy of preoperative chemoradiation generally ranged between 45% and 75%.[23–33]
- Patients whose postradiation vulvectomy specimen contained no histologic evidence of residual disease rarely had recurrence in the residual vulva.
- The outcome of patients who had even microscopic residual disease in the vulvectomy specimen was poor, with a high rate of locoregional recurrence.
- Comparison between the results of two Gynecologic Oncology Group phase II trials, GOG-101 (RT dose 40.9 to 47.8 Gy) and GOG 205 (RT target dose, 57.6 Gy), suggests that the tumor response rates are strongly correlated with radiation dose; for these two studies, the rates of clinical complete response in the vulva were 44% and 64%, respectively.[31,32] However, other factors including patient selection and differences in radiation treatment schedules, duration, and technique likely contributed to the broad range of reported response rates from smaller series. Also, in the era before 3-D planning, the prescribed doses at isocenter may not have accurately represented the actual doses delivered to the vulva, possibly clouding the tumor dose–response relationship.
- If unresectable or marginally resectable disease remains after the typical 4- to 6-week observation period used for evaluation of tumor response, the long break is likely to render any additional "boost" RT ineffective. This is a major weakness of the preoperative approach (Chapter 3).
- Most authors report frequent perioperative complications after preoperative RT, including high rates of wound breakdown and perioperative infection.[25,32] Of 50 patients who had post-RT vulvar resections in GOG-101, four died of complications in the immediate perioperative period.[32] Extensive groin dissection may contribute additional side effects of lymphedema and lymphocyst.

Although many patients have been cured with 40 to 50 Gy of preoperative RT followed by organ-sparing resection, the morbidity of combined treatment and the high recurrence rates observed in patients who have residual disease have increasingly led clinicians to explore treatment with definitive RT with or without concurrent chemotherapy.

For these reasons, for the past 20 years, our preference has been to treat most patients who are not candidates for initial organ-sparing surgery with definitive RT, usually with concurrent chemotherapy; vulvar resection is performed only if the tumor has not completely responded to high-dose radiation. This practice is reflected in recent reports of our experience[34] and in the case studies accompanying this chapter. However, the benefits of planned preoperative versus definitive RT for locally advanced vulvar cancers continue to be debated.

Radiation Therapy as Primary Treatment of the Vulva

Until recently, reports of definitive chemoradiation for vulvar cancer were largely confined to anecdotal reports of patients who did not undergo the intended resection after preoperative RT. In 2008, Landrum et al.[35] reported the outcome of 33 patients who had chemoradiation for stage III or IV vulvar cancers; these were large cancers (median diameter 6 cm), most involved critical structures or vagina, and 58% involved regional nodes. Eight patients had adjuvant surgical resection, but of the remaining 25 patients who were treated with chemoradiation alone, there were only three local recurrences, one of which was salvaged surgically.

Of 58 evaluable patients treated with chemoradiation in GOG 205, 29 had postradiation biopsies with negative results for residual disease and therefore did not undergo resection of the original tumor site; of these 29, 4 had recurrences in the vulva, 3 recurred outside the vulva, and 22 remained disease free at the time of the last evaluation. Of the 29 patients who had clinical or histologic evidence of persistent vulvar disease, only 6 were alive and disease free at the time of analysis. It appears that about 50% of the patients in this series had their vulvar cancers controlled with RT alone. However, the recommended dose of radiation used in this study was low (57.6 Gy), 20% of patients received less than 55 Gy, and median duration of radiation treatments was not specified.

In our experience, 60 Gy is the minimum dose required to achieve a high rate of vulvar disease control, and we prefer to treat large lesions with higher doses (66 to 68 Gy) if possible. In a recent report by Koay et al.,[34] the rate of vulvar disease control at 5 years was 83% for 74 patients who received >56 Gy. The median dose of RT to the vulva was 64 Gy, and the median duration of RT was 46 days; 85% of the patients in this series completed RT within 56 days or less.

Management of the Regional Nodes

As stated earlier, any vulvar cancer that has invaded more than 1 mm has a significant probability of lymph node metastasis. Because the prognosis of patients who have recurrence in the groin is much poorer than that of patients who have inguinal lymph node metastasis at diagnosis, the initial management of the groins is crucial to achieving a cure; diagnostic methods must be accurate and treatment definitive. However, the short- and long-term side effects of groin treatments can be substantial and, in some cases, can compromise an overall multidisciplinary treatment plan. The challenge for clinicians is to minimize these side effects without compromising locoregional disease control.

Physical examination is an inaccurate method of diagnosing or ruling out inguinal metastasis. Even a moderate subcutaneous fat layer obscures the contours of the medial femoral nodes and even very large nodes can be easily missed in obese patients (CS 12.8); for this reason, some form of tomographic imaging should be obtained to rule out the presence of enlarged lymph nodes in the groin.

Clinically Negative Groins—Surgical Management

For patients with early-stage vulvar cancer, the classic approach to the groin is a thorough inguinofemoral lymphadenectomy, unilateral for cancers that are more than 2 cm from midline and bilateral for midline tumors. If no metastases are found, most reports quote a groin recurrence rate of <2% to 5%.[21,36] With this procedure, however, wound complications (e.g., dehiscence, cellulitis, seroma) are frequent and the incidence of chronic leg edema, which can be debilitating in some cases, ranges between 25% and 50%. However, patients who have had less thorough groin dissections have had unacceptably high groin recurrence rates, particularly if they had poorly differentiated carcinomas.[37,38] For this reason, patients who have had only a superficial inguinal dissection or who have had fewer than 8 to 10 nodes in the lymphadenectomy specimen should, at a minimum, be followed closely with serial groin ultrasounds, particularly if no sentinel node ultrastaging has been performed.

A number of studies have explored the role of sentinel node biopsy in patients who have early-stage vulvar cancer.[2,36] These studies indicate that, for appropriately selected patients and in experienced hands, the finding of a negative sentinel node is sufficiently predictive to justify avoidance of lymphadenectomy. In one of the largest studies (GROINSS-V), the rate of groin recurrence after negative sentinel biopsy alone was 2.3%, comparable with the rates reported after lymphadenectomy; the rates of wound breakdown and infection were much less than with lymphadenectomy, and the rate of chronic lymphedema was reduced from 25% to ~2%. Patients who have multifocal disease or who have primary tumors >4 cm in diameter have an unacceptably high false-negative rate; these patients and any who fail to have a sentinel node identified require lymphadenectomy or RT. It is also important to note that a team of surgeons and pathologists experienced in sentinel node technique and ultrastaging is required to replicate the level of accuracy achieved in GROINSS-V.

Clinically Negative Groins—Treatment with Radiation Therapy Alone

In selected cases, particularly for patients who require RT for locally advanced disease in the vulva or known metastases in a contralateral groin, radiation may be considered as a primary treatment option for one or both groins (CS 12.3–12.6).

Although RT had clearly been proven effective as an adjuvant treatment after lymphadenectomy,[1] early experiences led many clinicians to question the effectiveness of RT alone to prevent recurrence. In GOG-88, a randomized trial conducted in the late 1980s, Stehman et al.[39] attempted to compare the effectiveness of RT versus lymphadenectomy in patients with early-stage disease and clinically negative groins (by physical examination). The study was closed early after five groin recurrences were noted in the first 25 patients treated with RT only. However, the RT used in this study was seriously flawed in several respects. CT, a relatively new study at the time, was not required for diagnosis or treatment planning. Hence, physical examination likely failed to detect the presence of gross disease requiring more than the specified dose of 50 Gy. In addition, patients were treated using a combination of appositional photon and electron beams prescribed to a depth of 3 cm. Electron beam irradiation was also a new technology at the time; Koh et al.[40] subsequently demonstrated that the techniques used would have underdosed the groin nodes by as much as 50%.

Other studies have suggested that radiation, when correctly applied, can be very effective. Katz et al.[37] reported an 11% rate of groin recurrence at 5 years in 30 patients who had locally advanced cancers and clinically negative groins treated with RT alone; in this series, the only two isolated groin recurrences occurred lateral to unusually narrow fields in patients treated in the early 1980s without CT planning.

In our experience, radiation alone rarely fails to prevent groin recurrence if the primary cancer is controlled and the following apply:

- Tomographic image guidance is used to generate a plan that provides adequate coverage of the inguinofemoral region, including the lateral circumflex nodes (Chapter 5).
- Imaging studies are carefully scrutinized for any suspicious nodes. Although in selected cases, ultrasound-guided biopsy may be used to evaluate small nodes, we tend to treat any node >8 to 10 mm in the high-risk region adjacent to the common femoral and saphenous vessels as positive. If they are not removed surgically, such nodes are typically boosted to a dose of 60 Gy.

Treatment of Clinically Positive Groins

As demonstrated in several of the case studies at the end of this chapter (CS 12.4–12.8), the treatment of patients who have grossly enlarged lymph nodes can be particularly challenging. The specific clinical situation and the resources available to the treating physicians dictate the optimal approach.

- *Radical lymphadenectomy followed by radiation therapy.* Although considered by some to be the standard approach to resectable groin disease, radical lymphadenectomy has a very high rate of perioperative and late morbidity, particularly when a very extensive dissection is required to clear N2 disease. Wound complications can delay adjuvant RT, potentially compromising its effectiveness. For patients who have nodal replacement by tumor or extracapsular extension, standard postoperative doses of 45 to 50 Gy are insufficient to achieve local control. In these cases, at least 60 Gy is probably required (Table 12.2).[5,16,17,41] When combined with a very extensive node dissection, high-dose RT is associated with a significant risk of late complications, including fibrosis and chronic lymphedema. For these reasons, we tend to favor a more limited operation or treatment with radiation alone.
- *Selective excision of enlarged nodes followed by radiation therapy.* In 2007, Hyde et al.[42] reported the combined experience of three centers, comparing outcome of patients who had either nodal debulking (17 patients) or full groin dissection (23 patients) for grossly positive nodes. All patients had postoperative RT. The patients who had a full dissection (all of whom were treated in a single center) had somewhat larger nodes but also received higher doses of postoperative RT. The groin recurrence rates were not significantly different for patients who had lymph node debulking or full lymphadenectomy before adjuvant RT, although the groin recurrence rates were high in both groups (~ 21% and 37%, respectively). We consider this approach for patients who have one or two enlarged nodes that are not fixed, particularly if the patient has a thin body habitus (CS 12.4).
- *Definitive radiation therapy.* For patients who have extensive inguinal lymphadenopathy, definitive RT (usually combined with concurrent chemotherapy) can be highly effective (CS 12.5–12.8). We generally recommend this approach for patients who have many enlarged nodes (that could be removed only with a very extensive dissection) or whose large body habitus would contribute to a high risk of wound complications. Between 1980 and 2010, 37 patients who had grossly enlarged inguinal lymph nodes received definitive groin RT at MD Anderson; although most of these patients had locally advanced vulvar cancers with extensive inguinal lymphadenopathy and (in many cases) pelvic node involvement,[20] only three had relapse in the groin (unpublished data); all three had fixed inguinal masses and two of these three had received only 55 to 60 Gy, less than would currently be recommended for bulky fixed nodes (Table 12.2). There were only three cases of posttreatment lymphedema, all of which were minor (grade 1).

TABLE 12.2 Recommended Radiation Doses for Lymph Node Metastases from Squamous Carcinomas of the Vulva[a]

Postoperative:	
Microscopic, no extracapsular extension (ECE), no suspicious nodes on postoperative imaging	45–50 Gy
Grossly enlarged nodes, no ECE, no suspicious nodes on postoperative imaging	50–56 Gy
ECE or total replacement of node by tumor	60–66 Gy
Gross residual disease	60–70 Gy
Definitive RT:	
Suspicious nodes <1 cm	56–60 Gy
Suspicious nodes 1–2 cm	60–66 Gy
Suspicious nodes >2 cm	64–70 Gy
Massive or fixed nodal disease	65–70 Gy

[a]*These are general recommendations that must be taken in the context of the patient's individual clinical situation. These doses also assume a fractional dose of 1.8–2 Gy per fraction.*

Surgical resection followed by RT has never been compared directly with definitive groin RT. However, we have found chemoradiation to be a highly effective and well-tolerated treatment for gross nodal disease. Definitive regional RT does require meticulous image-based planning to ensure that every potentially involved node receives an adequate dose of radiation, and dedicated on-treatment management to avoid treatment delays.

Although lymphadenectomy or selective nodal excision followed by RT is an accepted and effective approach for some patients, combined treatment also requires careful attention to detail. It is not unusual to find residual suspicious nodes after lymphadenectomy (CS 12.1 and 12.10); any residual node ≥8 to 10 mm that is in a site of primary or secondary nodal drainage should be treated as positive unless proven otherwise, usually with a radiation dose of at least 60 Gy.

Postoperative Radiation Therapy—The Evidence

It was GOG-37,[1,43] a prospective randomized trial conducted between 1977 and 1984, that firmly established the role of postoperative RT in the curative management of patients with vulvar cancer (Fig. 12.6). In that classic study, patients who were found to have lymph node metastases at the time of radical inguinal lymphadenectomy were randomly allocated to have an ipsilateral pelvic lymph node dissection (then considered standard treatment) or 45 to 50 Gy of adjuvant inguinal and pelvic RT. The trial was closed before reaching the planned accrual goal when an interim analysis demonstrated a significantly higher overall survival rate and a lower rate of inguinal recurrence for patients in the radiation treatment arm.

Impressive as they were, the results of GOG-37 probably underestimated the potential benefit of postoperative RT. The radiation dose was inadequate to reliably control disease in sites of extracapsular nodal extension, which would have been present in many of the cases.[16,41] Also, because CT was not commercially available when the trial was opened, residual

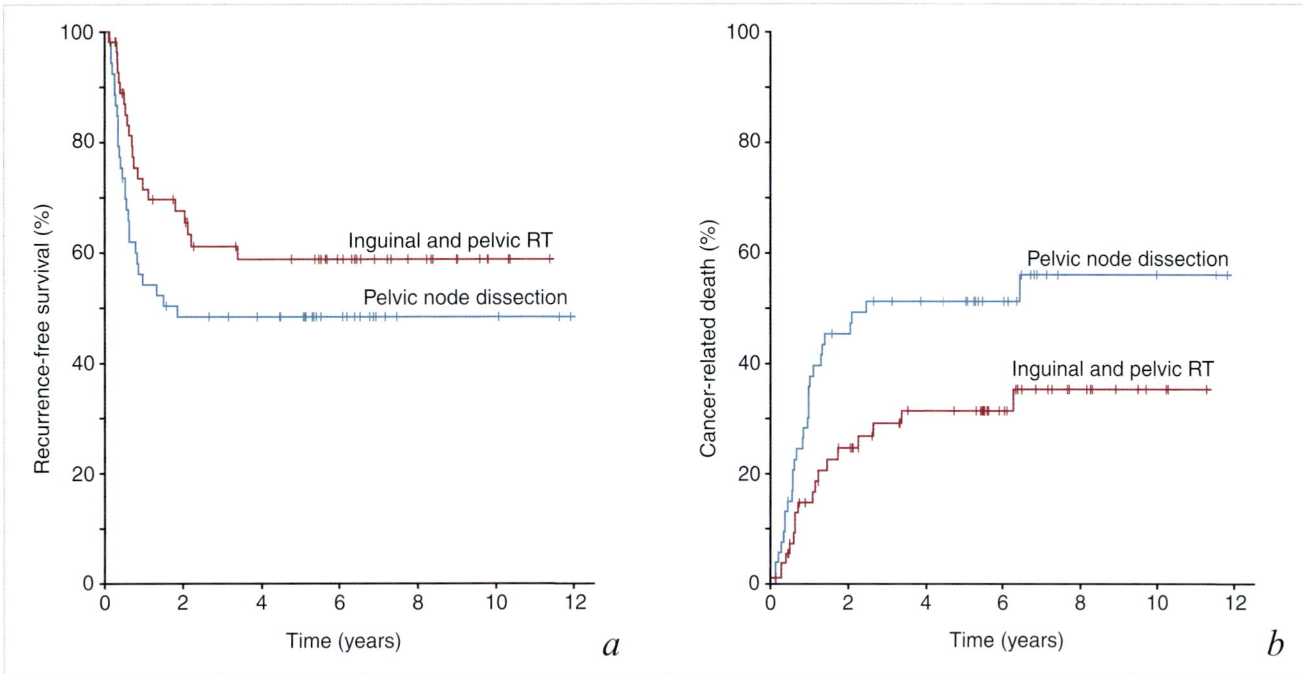

FIGURE 12.6 From GOG-88, the rates of recurrence-free survival (*a*) and the incidences of cancer-related death (*b*) for patients treated after vulvectomy and inguinal lymphadenectomy with either pelvic lymph node dissection or adjuvant inguinal and pelvic radiation. These curves were taken from the 2009 update of the trial first published in preliminary form by Homesley et al. in 1988. (Kunos C, Simpkins F, Gibbons H, et al. Radiation therapy compared with pelvic node resection for node-positive vulvar cancer: a randomized controlled trial. *Obstet Gynecol* 2009;114:537–546.)

gross disease in the pelvis or groins that would have required more than 50 Gy would not have been easily detected.

The low pelvic recurrence rate in GOG-37 has led some clinicians to doubt the need for pelvic treatment in node-positive patients and to limit their target to the inguinal operative bed(s).[18,39] However, patients with pelvic node involvement also tend to have advanced inguinal node disease[20] and are therefore at the highest risk for groin recurrence. In the absence of tomographic imaging, pelvic recurrences were unlikely to be detected in GOG-37; this is a likely explanation for the low pelvic recurrence rates, particularly in the surgical arm of the trial. MD Anderson data demonstrate that even clinically evident pelvic node involvement can be cured in up to 40% of cases.[20] In GOG-37, 28% of patients in the pelvic node dissection arm had histologic evidence of pelvic node involvement; for patients with clinically suspicious groin nodes, the rate was 45%. This is ample justification for treatment of at least the distal pelvic lymph nodes.

In 2015, Mahner et al.[18] published a large multi-institutional retrospective study of vulvar cancer patients treated in Germany between 1998 and 2008. Remarkably, only 41% of 447 patients with inguinal metastases received adjuvant RT to the ipsilateral groins and only 26% received inguinopelvic radiation. Although the patients who had groin irradiation tended to have more advanced groin disease, they had significantly better progression-free and overall survival rates than did patients who did not receive groin irradiation, confirming the results of GOG-37.

Postoperative Radiation Therapy—The Indications

Patients who have nodal metastases from vulvar cancer nearly always require postoperative RT. Retrospective series suggest that patients who have a thorough lymphadenectomy showing one or two nodes with microscopic intranodal metastases <5 mm may not require adjuvant radiation. However, *this is only in the context of a complete lymphadenectomy*, generally with >9 nodes removed, including the medial femoral nodes. Sentinel node biopsy alone is never sufficient treatment if even only a small focus of cancer is found in the ultrastaged specimen. In their review of GROINSS-V, Oonk et al.[44] reported an 11% rate of nonsentinel lymph node involvement, even when the focus of cancer in the sentinel node was ≤2 mm.

Any patient who has had a less than complete node dissection (particularly if no sentinel node has been examined) should have imaging of the groins with ultrasound-guided biopsy of any suspicious residual lymph nodes to determine the need for adjuvant RT (CS 12.10).

The dose of radiation depends on the extent of node involvement (Table 12.2).

The Role of Chemotherapy

Although there have been no randomized trials confirming the benefit of concurrent chemotherapy with RT, chemoradiation is an accepted standard for patients who can tolerate combined modality treatment. The justification for this is based on extrapolation from phase I evidence of benefit in other squamous carcinomas, particularly of the cervix and anus, and from reports of high response rates of locally advanced vulvar cancers to chemoradiation. Chemotherapy regimens typically are those favored for anal cancer (combinations of

5-fluorouracil and either mitomycin C or cisplatin) or treatments typically used for locally advanced cervical cancer (e.g., weekly cisplatin). We generally recommend concurrent chemoradiation with weekly cisplatin (40 mg/m^2) for patients who are receiving definitive RT for advanced primary tumors or positive margins and for patients who have regional metastases. However, radiation alone is also effective treatment if administered without treatment delays and is often the treatment of choice for patients who are frail or who have major contraindications to chemotherapy (**CS 12.3**).

Several phase II trials have explored the possible role of neoadjuvant chemotherapy followed by surgery with or without postoperative RT.[45–47] Complete response rates to chemotherapy ranged between 5% and 35%. In view of these modest complete response rates, patients require either postoperative radiation or thorough lymphadenectomy to ensure that regional metastases have been cleared; several patients in these series required pelvic exenteration to clear their local disease. However, there are some long-term survivors who had organ-sparing surgery without RT. The number of patients followed disease free for more than 3 to 5 years is still small, and this approach probably requires further study before routine use outside a protocol setting.

Chemotherapy is generally the treatment of choice for patients who have recurrent or metastatic disease that cannot be managed with surgery or radiation. However, response rates are low and usually of short duration; supportive care is an acceptable alternative, particularly for patients who are frail.[19]

Selecting among Options to Develop a Combined Approach to Treatment

The previous sections outlined the various treatment options for the primary site and groins of patients with carcinomas of the vulva. After multidisciplinary discussion, an overall treatment strategy must be established that integrates the treatment of the vulva and nodes to optimize the overall therapeutic ratio.

The following summarizes the factors that influence locoregional treatment strategy in specific clinical situations. Note that concurrent chemotherapy is recommended for most patients who are receiving radiation for treatment of gross disease as discussed in the previous section, "The Role of Chemotherapy."

Resectable Primary Tumor, Clinically Negative Groins

The treatment of choice is nearly always wide local excision of the primary site and either lymphadenectomy or sentinel node evaluation for the groin(s) as discussed earlier. Additional treatment is guided by the operative findings:

- *Negative margins, negative groins after adequate lymphadenectomy*: No further treatment is needed.
- *Positive or close vulvar margins, negative groins after adequate lymphadenectomy*: Re-excision of the vulva, if critical structures will not be compromised, or vulvar RT (**CS 12.2**), particularly if the margin was frankly positive or if a close margin abutted a critical structure.
- *Positive or close margins, with positive nodes*: RT to vulva and groins is recommended.
- *Positive or close margins, inadequate groin evaluation*: RT to vulva and groins is usually recommended.

Resectable Primary, Suspicious, or Positive Groin Nodes

Wide local excision is recommended for the primary site. The nodes should be managed according to the extent of disease, as discussed in the section "Management of the Regional Nodes." However, when adjuvant RT is indicated for nodal metastases, it can be difficult to decide whether to include the site of a completely excised vulvar cancer in the radiation fields. In general, when the inguinal nodes are positive, the threshold of risk for recommending postoperative vulvar treatment is low because lymph node involvement itself is a risk factor for vulvar recurrence and because it can be difficult and morbid to irradiate the primary site for recurrence after regional RT (**CS 12.10**). If the risk of local recurrence is >10% to 20%, we usually recommend vulvar treatment. (See the previous section, "Predictors of Vulvar Recurrence.") If the vulva is not included, an effort should be made to adequately treat the groin with as little exposure of the vulva as possible (**CS 12.9**).

Critically Situated Primary, Marginally Resectable

If the surgeon believes the primary tumor can be resected with a margin of at least a few millimeters and without compromising organ function, wide local excision is recommended for the primary tumor, usually followed by postoperative radiation. If the likelihood of positive margins is high, primary radiation is recommended for the primary tumor with nodal treatment as discussed above.

Unresectable Primary, Clinically Negative Groins

If the primary grossly involves critical structures or the surgeon indicates that the risk of a positive margin would be high after attempted resection, the vulva is usually treated with radiation. Our usual recommendation is treatment of the groins with radiation alone after thorough review of imaging to identify suspicious nodes that require a boost dose of radiation (**CS 12.6**).

Unresectable Primary, Suspicious Inguinal Nodes

Side effects of radical lymphadenectomy can delay necessary primary treatment and postoperative groin irradiation, potentially reducing treatment effectiveness. Fluctuating lymphocysts complicate treatment planning and can be a source of infection. We recommend definitive regional radiation (**Table 12.2**; **CS 12.5, 12.7, and 12.8**) or limited excision of gross nodes followed by RT (**CS 12.4**) to the groins and primary.

TECHNICAL CONSIDERATIONS

Many of the technical aspects of treatment are discussed in detail in Chapters 4 to 7 of this book. Several aspects deserve emphasis here.

- *The initial preparation for treatment is particularly critical* for vulvar cancer because diagnostic imaging rarely provides an adequate sense of the extent and orientation of vulvar disease. Examination at the time of simulation with placement of radio-opaque markers on tumor, scars, and critical structures is essential (Chapters 4 and 5).
- *Vulvar target volume definition is particularly challenging* because of the orientation of the vulva approximately tangential to the CT plane and because the normal and abnormal anatomy is extremely difficult to visualize on CT. In addition to radio-opaque markers, reference to MRI (ideally obtained in the treatment position) and surface reconstructions can assist in accurate contouring (Fig. 6.10).
- *The entire vulva should usually be treated to a dose of at least 40 Gy.* Any gross tumor or high-risk clinical target volumes (CTVs) should be covered with margin, and adequate planning target volume (PTV) margins should be used as discussed in Chapter 6. However, tolerance is directly related to the amount of irradiated skin and we do not believe, for example, that the entire mons needs to be treated in a patient who is receiving RT for a small perineal cancer. Today, intensity-modulated radiation therapy (IMRT) permits much greater tailoring of target volumes than was possible with anterior–posterior (AP)–posterior–anterior (PA) fields (Chapter 6). However, radiation oncologists are still learning how to use this tool effectively; clinicians who do not treat vulvar cancer regularly should consider using simpler techniques or referring patients to a center with subspecialty experience.
- *Attention to the dose at skin surface is particularly important.* If the patient is treated in a frog-leg position, bolus should be used to ensure adequate dose at the surface of exposed tumor and at least 2 cm of the surrounding skin. However, bolus that extends over skin that is not at risk for tumor involvement causes unnecessary acute and late skin damage. Bolus is usually not required on the groin areas unless there is skin involvement by tumor or the patient is very thin—if required, 3-mm bolus can be used over the inguinal target every other day. Due to the tangential beam orientation with IMRT, bolus is rarely needed over the groins; with 6 MV IMRT, bolus. May be used every other day on the vulva unless exposed skin is involved by tumor. However, the dose to exposed skin surfaces should always be confirmed with thermoluminescent dosimetry (TLDs).
- *Radiation fields should be large enough to extend at least 1 cm distal to the vulvar target.* To achieve this with some treatment planning systems, it may be necessary to create a false structure over the vulva in order to extend the PTV beyond the vulvar skin during IMRT optimization (Figure 6.9).
- *Appositional perineal electron beam treatment may be useful in selected cases if the target volume is superficial.* We occasionally use an appositional electron field for a final boost treatment **(CS 12.9)**. However, this is a specialized technique that requires stirrups fitted to the treatment table. The depth of the target, influence of irregular surface contours, and the effects of electron beam constriction at depth must be carefully considered. We do not recommend the use of appositional perineal photon fields because of the unnecessary dose delivered to deeper pelvic structures. Perineal ports should never be used in the same treatment session as anterior or posterior inguinopelvic fields. The change in patient position makes it impossible to rule out overlaps between fields that would cause tissues to receive twice the prescribed fractional radiation dose.
- *In most cases, treatment in daily fractions of 1.8 to 2 Gy is recommended to reduce the severity of acute and late effects.* Mild hypofractionation (2 to 3 Gy per fraction) may be considered to treat regions of gross disease if the target can be treated with adequate PTV margin without exceeding normal tissue tolerance limits.
- *The importance of infection control during treatment cannot be overemphasized.* Early skin reactions that cause clinicians to halt treatment are nearly always related to bacterial or fungal infection (Chapter 7).

References

1. Homesley HD, Bundy BN, Sedlis A, et al. Radiation therapy versus pelvic node resection for carcinoma of the vulva with positive groin nodes. *Obstet Gynecol.* 1986;68:733–740.
2. Oonk MH, Hollema H, de Hullu JA, et al. Prediction of lymph node metastases in vulvar cancer: a review. *Int J Gynecol Cancer.* 2006;16:963–971.
3. Moskovic EC, Shepherd JH, Barton DP, et al. The role of high resolution ultrasound with guided cytology of groin lymph nodes in the management of squamous cell carcinoma of the vulva: a pilot study. *Br J Obstet Gynaecol.* 1999;106:863–867.
4. Stehman FB, Bundy BN, Ball H, et al. Sites of failure and times to failure in carcinoma of the vulva treated conservatively: a Gynecologic Oncology Group study. *Am J Obstet Gynecol.* 1996; 174:1128–1132; discussion 1132–1123.
5. Bogani G, Cromi A, Serati M, et al. Predictors and patterns of local, regional, and distant failure in squamous cell carcinoma of the vulva. *Am J Clin Oncol.* 2014.
6. Heaps JM, Fu YS, Montz FJ, et al. Surgical-pathologic variables predictive of local recurrence in squamous cell carcinoma of the vulva. *Gynecol Oncol.* 1990;38:309–314.
7. Rouzier R, Haddad B, Plantier F, et al. Local relapse in patients treated for squamous cell vulvar carcinoma: incidence and prognostic value. *Obstet Gynecol.* 2002;100:1159–1167.
8. Woolderink JM, de Bock GH, de Hullu JA, et al. Patterns and frequency of recurrences of squamous cell carcinoma of the vulva. *Gynecol Oncol.* 2006;103:293–299.
9. Chan JK, Sugiyama V, Pham H, et al. Margin distance and other clinico-pathologic prognostic factors in vulvar carcinoma: a multivariate analysis. *Gynecol Oncol.* 2007;104:636–641.
10. Viswanathan AN, Pinto AP, Schultz D, et al. Relationship of margin status and radiation dose to recurrence in post-operative vulvar carcinoma. *Gynecol Oncol.* 2013;130:545–549.
11. Tantipalakorn C, Robertson G, Marsden DE, et al. Outcome and patterns of recurrence for International Federation of Gynecology and Obstetrics (FIGO) stages I and II squamous cell vulvar cancer. *Obstet Gynecol.* 2009;113:895–901.

12. Faul CM, Mirmow D, Huang Q, et al. Adjuvant radiation for vulvar carcinoma: improved local control. *Int J Radiat Oncol Biol Phys.* 1997;38:381–389.
13. Faul CM, Miramow D, Gerzten K, et al. Isolated local recurrence in carcinoma of the vulva: prognosis and implications for treatment. *Int J Gynecol Cancer.* 1998;8:409–414.
14. Homesley HD, Bundy BN, Sedlis A, et al. Prognostic factors for groin node metastasis in squamous cell carcinoma of the vulva (a Gynecologic Oncology Group study). *Gynecol Oncol.* 1993;49:279–283.
15. Aragona AM, Cuneo NA, Soderini AH, et al. An analysis of reported independent prognostic factors for survival in squamous cell carcinoma of the vulva: is tumor size significance being underrated? *Gynecol Oncol.* 2014;132:643–648.
16. Origoni M, Sideri M, Garsia S, et al. Prognostic value of pathological patterns of lymph node positivity in squamous cell carcinoma of the vulva stage III and IVA FIGO. *Gynecol Oncol.* 1992;45:313–316.
17. Raspagliesi F, Hanozet F, Ditto A, et al. Clinical and pathological prognostic factors in squamous cell carcinoma of the vulva. *Gynecol Oncol.* 2006;102:333–337.
18. Mahner S, Jueckstock J, Hilpert F, et al. Adjuvant therapy in lymph node–positive vulvar cancer: the AGO-CaRE-1 study. *J Natl Cancer Inst.* 2015;107.
19. Hacker NF, Eifel PJ. Vulvar cancer. In: Berek JS, Hacker NF, eds. *Gynecologic Oncology*. Philadelphia, PA: Wolters Kluwer; 2015:560–607.
20. Thaker NG, Klopp AH, Jhingran A, et al. Survival outcomes for patients with stage IVB vulvar cancer with grossly positive pelvic lymph nodes: time to reconsider the FIGO staging system? *Gynecol Oncol.* 2015;136:269–273.
21. Homesley HD, Bundy BN, Sedlis A, et al. Assessment of current International Federation of Gynecology and Obstetrics staging of vulvar carcinoma relative to prognostic factors for survival (a Gynecologic Oncology Group study). *Am J Obstet Gynecol.* 1991;164:997–1003; discussion 1003–1004.
22. Boronow RC. Therapeutic alternative to primary exenteration for advanced vulvovaginal cancer. *Gynecol Oncol.* 1973;1:233–255.
23. Boronow RC, Hickman BT, Reagan MT, et al. Combined therapy as an alternative to exenteration for locally advanced vulvovaginal cancer. II. Results, complications, and dosimetric and surgical considerations. *Am J Clin Oncol.* 1987;10:171–181.
24. Akl A, Akl M, Boike G, et al. Preliminary results of chemoradiation as a primary treatment for vulvar carcinoma. *Int J Radiat Oncol Biol Phys.* 2000;48:415–420.
25. Landoni F, Maneo A, Zanetta G, et al. Concurrent preoperative chemotherapy with 5-fluorouracil and mitomycin C and radiotherapy (FUMIR) followed by limited surgery in locally advanced and recurrent vulvar carcinoma. *Gynecol Oncol.* 1996;61:321–327.
26. Berek JS, Heaps JM, Fu YS, et al. Concurrent cisplatin and 5-fluorouracil chemotherapy and radiation therapy for advanced-stage squamous carcinoma of the vulva. *Gynecol Oncol.* 1991;42:197–201.
27. Beriwal S, Shukla G, Shinde A, et al. Preoperative intensity modulated radiation therapy and chemotherapy for locally advanced vulvar carcinoma: analysis of pattern of relapse. *Int J Radiat Oncol Biol Phys.* 2013;85:1269–1274.
28. Eifel PJ, Morris M, Burke TW, et al. Prolonged continuous infusion cisplatin and 5-fluorouracil with radiation for locally advanced carcinoma of the vulva. *Gynecol Oncol.* 1995;59:51–56.
29. Gerszten K, Selvaraj RN, Kelley J, et al. Preoperative chemoradiation for locally advanced carcinoma of the vulva. *Gynecol Oncol.* 2005;99:640–644.
30. Hacker NF, Berek JS, Juillard GJ, et al. Preoperative radiation therapy for locally advanced vulvar cancer. *Cancer.* 1984;54:2056–2061.
31. Moore DH, Ali S, Koh WJ, et al. A phase II trial of radiation therapy and weekly cisplatin chemotherapy for the treatment of locally-advanced squamous cell carcinoma of the vulva: a gynecologic oncology group study. *Gynecol Oncol.* 2012;124:529–533.
32. Moore DH, Thomas GM, Montana GS, et al. Preoperative chemoradiation for advanced vulvar cancer: a phase II study of the Gynecologic Oncology Group. *Int J Radiat Oncol Biol Phys.* 1998;42:79–85.
33. Russell AH, Mesic JB, Scudder SA, et al. Synchronous radiation and cytotoxic chemotherapy for locally advanced or recurrent squamous cancer of the vulva. *Gynecol Oncol.* 1992;47:14–20.
34. Koay EJ, Jhingran A, Klopp AH, et al. Factors associated with long-term survival in locally-advanced squamous cell carcinoma of the vulva treated with definitive radiation therapy. *Int J Radiat Oncol Biol Phys.* 2013;87:S129.
35. Landrum LM, Skaggs V, Gould N, et al. Comparison of outcome measures in patients with advanced squamous cell carcinoma of the vulva treated with surgery or primary chemoradiation. *Gynecol Oncol.* 2008;108:584–590.
36. Van der Zee AG, Oonk MH, De Hullu JA, et al. Sentinel node dissection is safe in the treatment of early-stage vulvar cancer. *J Clin Oncol.* 2008;26:884–889.
37. Katz A, Eifel PJ, Jhingran A, et al. The role of radiation therapy in preventing regional recurrences of invasive squamous cell carcinoma of the vulva. *Int J Radiat Oncol Biol Phys.* 2003;57:409–418.
38. van Beekhuizen HJ, Auzin M, van den Einden LC, et al. Lymph node count at inguinofemoral lymphadenectomy and groin recurrences in vulvar cancer. *Int J Gynecol Cancer.* 2014;24:773–778.
39. Stehman FB, Bundy BN, Thomas G, et al. Groin dissection versus groin radiation in carcinoma of the vulva: a Gynecologic Oncology Group study. *Int J Radiat Oncol Biol Phys.* 1992;24:389–396.
40. Koh WJ, Chiu M, Stelzer KJ, et al. Femoral vessel depth and the implications for groin node radiation. *Int J Radiat Oncol Biol Phys.* 1993;27:969–974.
41. van der Velden J, van Lindert AC, Lammes FB, et al. Extracapsular growth of lymph node metastases in squamous cell carcinoma of the vulva. The impact on recurrence and survival. *Cancer.* 1995;75:2885–2890.
42. Hyde SE, Valmadre S, Hacker NF, et al. Squamous cell carcinoma of the vulva with bulky positive groin nodes-nodal debulking versus full groin dissection prior to radiation therapy. *Int J Gynecol Cancer.* 2007;17:154–158.
43. Kunos C, Simpkins F, Gibbons H, et al. Radiation therapy compared with pelvic node resection for node-positive vulvar cancer: a randomized controlled trial. *Obstet Gynecol.* 2009;114:537–546.
44. Oonk MH, van Hemel BM, Hollema H, et al. Size of sentinel-node metastasis and chances of non-sentinel-node involvement and survival in early stage vulvar cancer: results from GROINSS-V, a multicentre observational study. *Lancet Oncol.* 2010;11:646–652.
45. Aragona AM, Cuneo N, Soderini AH, et al. Tailoring the treatment of locally advanced squamous cell carcinoma of the vulva: neoadjuvant chemotherapy followed by radical surgery: results from a multicenter study. *Int J Gynecol Cancer.* 2012;22:1258–1263.
46. Domingues AP, Mota F, Durao M, et al. Neoadjuvant chemotherapy in advanced vulvar cancer. *Int J Gynecol Cancer.* 2010;20:294–298.
47. Geisler JP, Manahan KJ, Buller RE. Neoadjuvant chemotherapy in vulvar cancer: avoiding primary exenteration. *Gynecol Oncol.* 2006;100:53–57.

Case Studies

The case studies for this chapter were selected to demonstrate various disease presentations that can be managed by radiation therapy. The reasons for the final treatment strategy alternative approaches are discussed, as are the methods used to prepare patients for treatment and the management of treatment-related side effects. It should be noted that none of the patients described in these case studies required treatment breaks and all had completed treatment in 5 to 7 weeks, depending on the prescribed radiation dose. IMRT is now used to treat most vulvar cancers in our department and the following cases reflect that practice. However, two cases that were treated using 3-D conformal techniques are also included as examples **(CS 12.6 and 12.9)**.

List of Case Studies for Chapter 12:

Abbreviations Used in the Case Studies:

AP	Anterior–Posterior
BMI	Body mass index
CTV	Clinical target volume
CT	Computed tomography
EBRT	External beam radiotherapy
ECE	Extracapsular extension
EI	External iliac
EUA	Examination under anesthesia
FIGO	International Federation of Gynecology and Obstetrics
FDG	Fluorodeoxyglucose
GTV	Gross tumor volume
HPV	Human papilloma virus
HRCTV	High-risk clinical target volume
IMRT	Intensity-modulated radiation therapy
ITV	Internal target volume
KPS	Karnofsky performance status
LVSI	Lymph-vascular space invasion
MRI	Magnetic resonance imaging
NED	No evidence of disease
PET	Positron emission tomography
PA	Posterior–anterior
PTV	Planning target volume
SUV	Standard uptake value
TLD	Thermo-luminescent dosimeter
WBC	White blood cell
VIN	Vulvar intraepithelial neoplasia

CS 12.1 • Vulvar Cancer Following Local Excision with High-Risk Features, Positive Nodes, and Infectious Complications

History: A 56-year-old woman with a 2.5-cm ulcerated mass in the left posterior vestibule of the vagina had wide local excision, left sentinel node biopsy, and left groin dissection. Postoperatively, the patient developed a vulvar cellulitis that responded to 7 days of intravenous vancomycin.

Pathology: Poorly differentiated squamous carcinoma invading 8 mm with perineural invasion and LVSI. The initial margin was focally positive; re-excision of the urethral margin was negative but the surgeon remained concerned about the proximity of the deep margin near the rectum. One of two left sentinel nodes was positive; no other nodes in the specimen.

Evaluation at Diagnosis: *CT*: prominent nodes in the left groin (***a***, ***b***).

Evaluation 5 Weeks after Surgery: *Exam*: 75 kg; NED; incisions healing well with no erythema. *KPS*: 90.

Treatment Plan: Chemo-RT. With one of two nodes involved and a paramedian primary, both groins were at risk for residual disease. Planning CT revealed a lymphocyst in the left groin (***c***) as well as bilateral 1–1.5 cm nodes that had increased in size (*arrows*, ***b***, ***d***). These may have been inflammatory but because 48 Gy would be insufficient if the nodes were involved, a boost was planned. Findings of high grade, LVSI, perineural invasion, and uncertain margins indicated a high risk of vulvar recurrence. The role of chemotherapy is unproven but is supported by retrospective studies and level 1 evidence from other sites.

EBRT** (completed in 39 days):**

Set up: Frog-leg in a cradle; 3-mm bolus on the posterior vulva. The vulvar scar was marked with wire and BBs (*red arrows*, ***f***).

IMRT was used to reduce the dose of RT to critical structures and skin. The vulva, groins, and external and internal iliac nodes (CTV) were treated to 43.2 Gy in 24 fractions; an integrated boost to the groins, distal pelvic nodes, and vulvar operative bed (HRCTV) brought the dose to these regions to 48 Gy (***e***, ***f***). Following this, electrons were used to boost suspicious nodes in the groins (***g***, *arrows*) to a total dose of 60 Gy.

Chemotherapy: Weekly cisplatin ×3

Outcome: Severe diarrhea began in the first week of RT. The early onset and history of intravenous vancomycin suggested *Clostridium difficile* infection, which was eventually confirmed. Metronidazole was begun and the patient improved although she had two relapses treated with oral vancomycin. Skin erythema in the 3rd week responded to fluconazole. By the 5th week, she had patchy moist desquamation but with sitz baths, infection control, and pain management, she completed RT without a break. Persistent *C. difficile* infection was eventually treated successfully with a fecal transplant. At 2 years, the patient had NED with no vulvar, bladder, or bowel complaints but with 1+ left leg edema.

Comment: Postoperative imaging should always be scrutinized for possible residual disease. Bacterial and candidal infections are common in patients receiving vulvar RT but are often misinterpreted as direct effects of treatment. With infection management, local care, and pain management, treatment delays are rarely necessary.

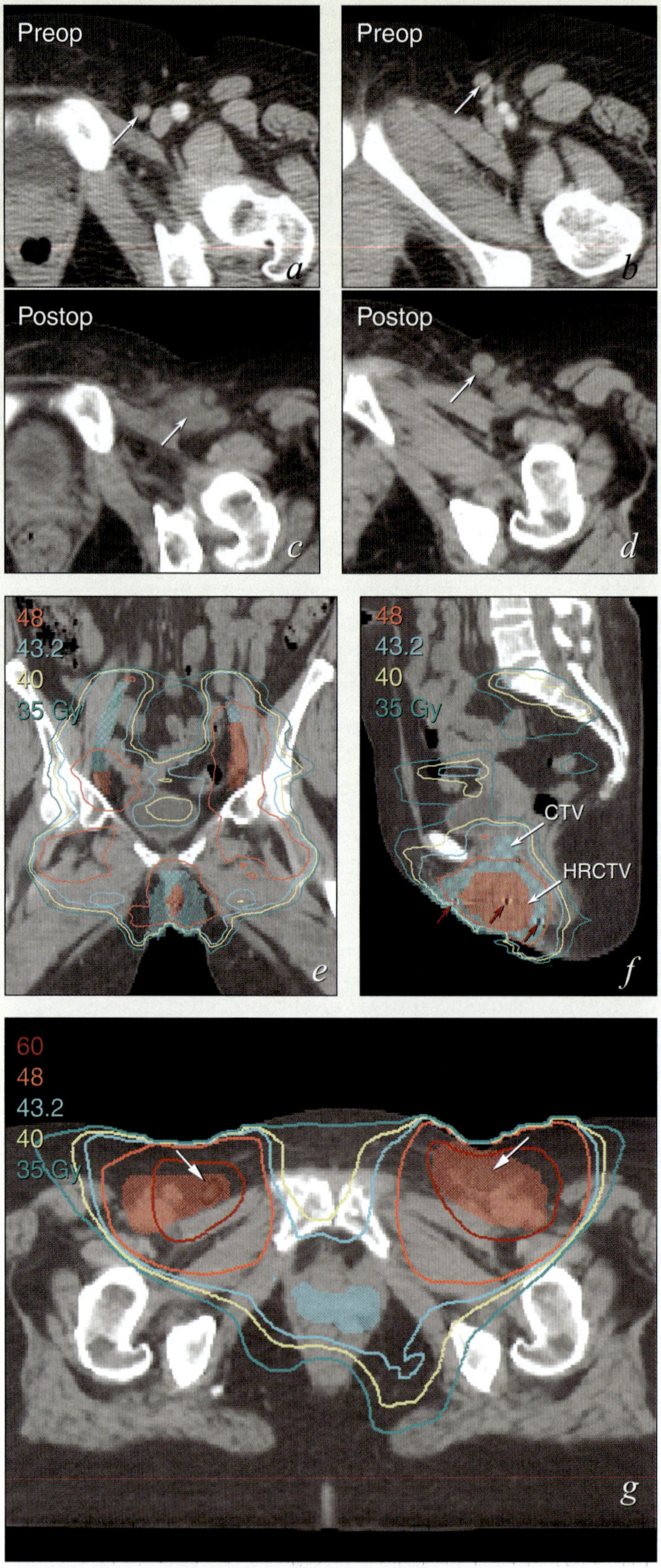

CS 12.2 • Multifocal Squamous Carcinoma of the Vulva Treated with Resection with Close Margins and Negative Nodes

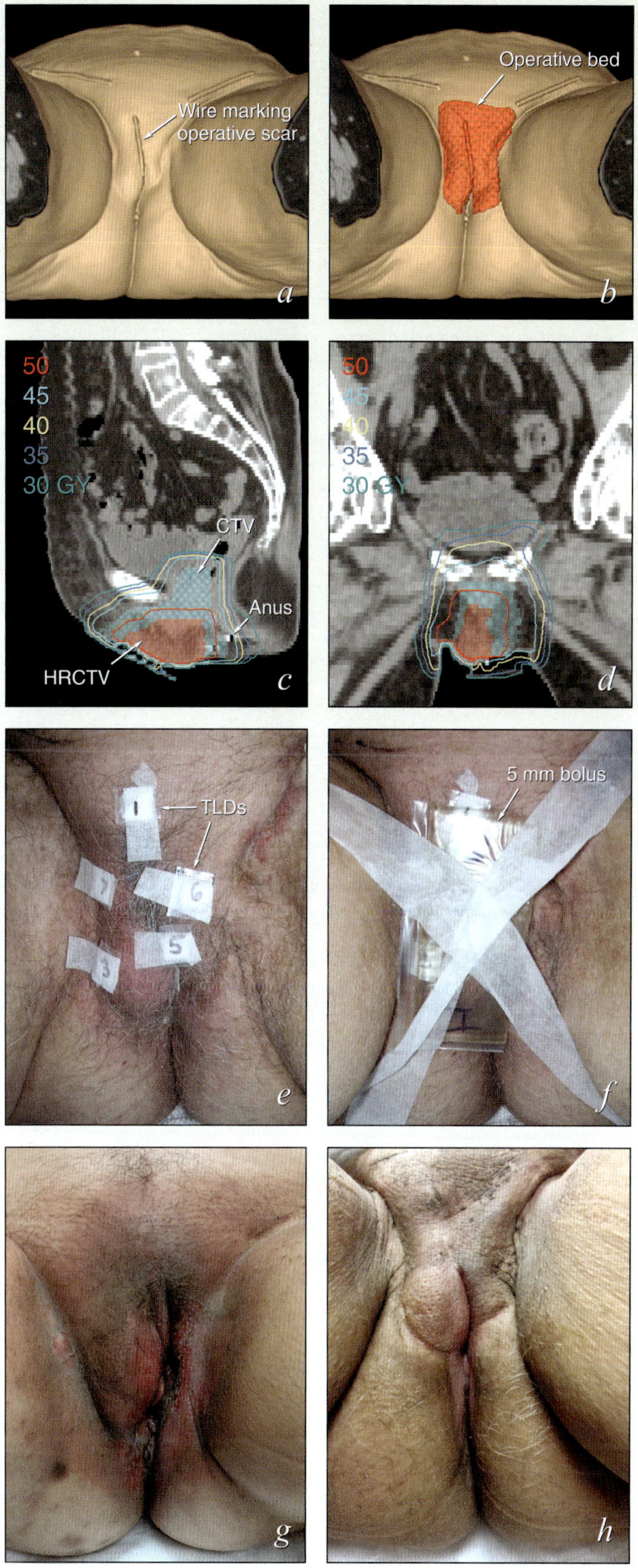

History: A 75-year-old woman with a long history of lichen sclerosis had two abnormal lesions noted on the vulva. After biopsies showed invasive squamous carcinoma, the patient was referred for evaluation and treatment.

Evaluation at Diagnosis: *Exam*: A 1 × 1.5 cm ulcerated, thickened right periclitoral lesion and a separate 2 × 1.5 cm ulcerated, raised lesion on the left labium minus at 3 o'clock; no palpable nodes. *KPS*: 100. *Chest x-ray*: NED.

Surgery: Wide radical excision of the two vulvar lesions in a single specimen. Bilateral sentinel lymph node mapping and biopsy; bilateral inguinal lymphadenectomy.

Pathology: Multifocal moderate to poorly differentiated squamous carcinoma invading 4.5 mm with focal LVSI in a background of severe dysplasia; close (1.5 mm) deep lateral margin on the right; three right and seven left inguinal nodes negative, including bilateral sentinel nodes.

Treatment Plan: The resection had been extended to the deep fascia and the surgeon was not confident that re-resection could improve the margin status. Features other than the deep margin (high grade, LVSI, and multifocality) already placed the patient at higher than usual risk for local recurrence. However, the risk of recurrence in the groins was low. There is no evidence to support the use of chemotherapy in this setting. The plan was to use vulvar RT to reduce the risk of local recurrence.

EBRT *(completed in 32 days)*:
Set up: Frog-leg in a custom cradle. To assist target definition, wires were placed at simulation to mark the operative incision (***a***, ***b***), and BBs were placed on the urethra and anal verge; 5-mm bolus was placed over the central vulva (***f***). On the first day of treatment, TLDs were placed to verify the adequacy of the skin dose (***e***, ***f***). The target volume included the entire vulva just up to the anal verge posteriorly and the distal half of the vagina. IMRT was used rather than appositional electrons to enable coverage of the vestibule and distal vagina. An integrated boost was used to increase the dose to the region of the close margin in the right vulva.

IMRT (VMAT) (***c***, ***d***):
In 25 fractions:

Vulvar CTV (+7 mm): 45 Gy (180 cGy/fraction)

HRCTV (+7 mm): 50 Gy (200 cGy/fraction)

Chemotherapy: None.

Outcome: Vulvar pruritus and erythema at day 13 (26 Gy) improved with fluconazole and sitz baths. At 42 Gy (***g***), there was brisk erythema of the vulva, with patches of moist desquamation in the bolused region. At 3 months (***h***), NED with occasional diarrhea requiring loperamide; no vulvar or urinary complaints. At 2 years, followed at home with NED.

Comment: Had the margin been frankly positive, a higher dose (usually 60 Gy) would have been given to the HRCTV.

CS 12.3 • Locally Recurrent Vulvar Cancer in a Patient with Morbid Obesity and Chronic Venous Stasis

History: A 79-year-old woman with vulvar pruritus had a cluster of warty perineal lesions. The largest, a 2-cm exophytic lesion excised from the posterior fourchette, contained well-differentiated squamous carcinoma, with >1 mm invasion; three smaller lesions were cauterized without biopsy. The patient was observed without further treatment for 9 months until she developed two new lesions in the same region and was referred for evaluation. The patient was obese with severe arthritis, urinary incontinence, and lower extremity venous stasis with a chronic leg ulcer receiving wound care. She required a walker or scooter for ambulation.

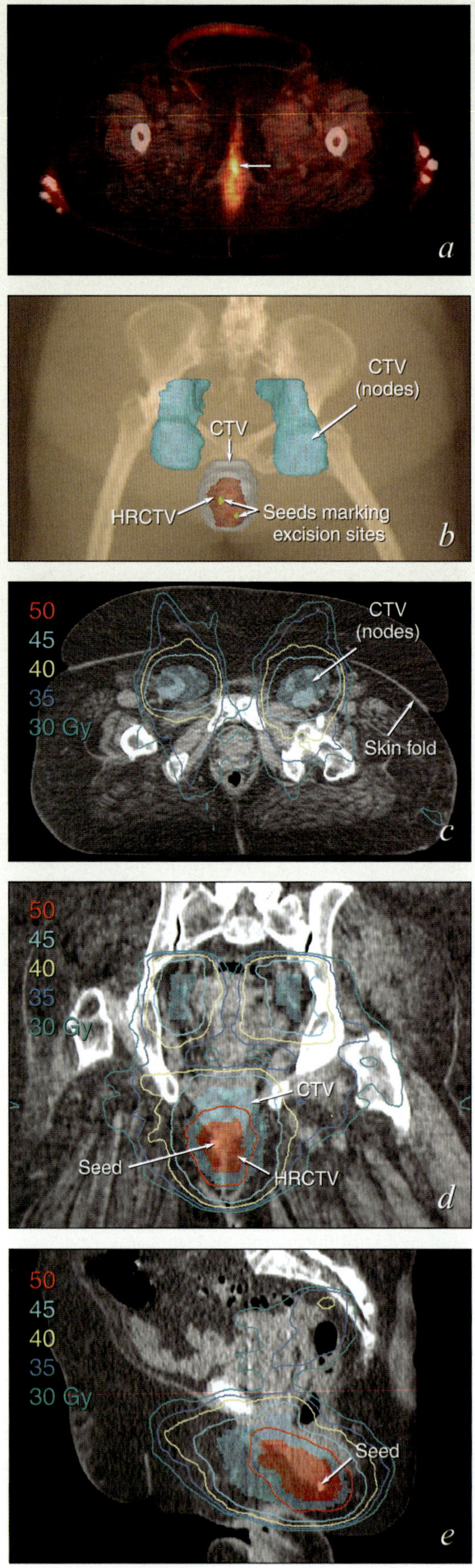

Evaluation: Alert, oriented. Weight: 140 kg (BMI, 65); *Exam (EUA)*: two raised lesions in the posterior vulva measuring 1.5 × 1.2 cm and 2.5 × 1.2 cm, respectively. *PET–CT*: NED except for a focal area of FDG uptake in the vulva (***a***). KPS 70.

Treatment Plan: The goal was to prevent recurrence with as little short- and long-term morbidity as possible. It was felt that a lymph node dissection would attend an unacceptable risk of wound complications and lymphedema, which could have severe consequences in the context of the patient's chronic stasis. Because of the location and presence of two lesions about 2–3 cm apart, a wide resection of the vulva would have been difficult to close primarily. However, the gynecologic oncologist felt that simple excisions could be accomplished with close but negative margins, reducing the dose of radiation required to achieve local control.

Plan: Simple excision of vulvar lesions followed by radiotherapy to the primary site and bilateral groins. The radiation oncologist, who was present at EUA, inserted fiducial markers adjacent to each excision site.

Pathology: Both lesions showed invasive squamous carcinoma. Depths of invasion were 3 and 3.5 mm, respectively, with 3-mm tumor-free margins; no LVSI.

Radiation Therapy *(completed in 32 days)***:**

Setup: Supine, custom cradles with legs apposed. Any effort to separate the legs would have increased the lateral diameter without reducing the skin dose in this obese patient. The subpannicular and intergluteal skin folds were contoured and, wherever possible, the dose to these folds was kept below 20–30 Gy. Fiducial markers placed at EUA and the PET assisted vulvar target definition (***b***). IMRT was used to enable adequate coverage of the groin and protection of femoral heads, skin folds, and other critical structures. Because of the large skin-to-target distances, 18-MV beams were used for several of the beams. Treatment began 3 weeks after excisional biopsies.

IMRT (***c–e***): The vulva, bilateral groins, and distal pelvic node CTVs (+1 cm) were treated to 45 Gy in 25 fractions. Using an integrated boost, the region surrounding the resection beds (HRCTV) +1 cm was treated to 50 Gy.

Chemotherapy: None.

Outcome: At treatment end, there were 3–4 cm patches of moist desquamation in the groins and posterior vulva. With sitz baths, skin barrier, and antifungal treatments, the skin had healed with only mild erythema at 3.5 weeks. At 2.5 years, NED with mild radiation changes in the posterior vulva.

Comments: Because the depth from the surface to the femoral vessels was 14–15 cm, electrons could not be used to treat the groins. Conformal 3-D techniques would have delivered a significantly higher dose to the femoral heads and skin folds than IMRT.

CS 12.4 • Stage III Vulvar Cancer with a Small, Posterior Vulvar Lesion and Inguinal Lymphadenopathy

History: A 43-year-old woman with a history of three laser ablations for VIN noted a mass in the right groin. Biopsy of an asymptomatic vulvar lesion showed squamous carcinoma. After her physician recommended radical excision with the possibility of colostomy, the patient sought another opinion.

Evaluation at Diagnosis: *Exam*: 4 × 3 cm right groin node; 2-cm ulcerated lesion on the posterior fourchette, inseparable from the anal sphincter; *MRI*: 3-cm superficial right groin node (***a***) and a deeper 1-cm node in the inguinal canal (***b***); also, a 2-cm enhancing, nodular area in the perineum (***c***); *CT*: Inguinal lymphadenopathy; otherwise NED; *KPS*: 100. Chest x-ray NED.

Treatment Plan: The dominant site of disease was the large groin node, which would have required 65–70 Gy to achieve a high probability of control with RT alone. The patient's thin body habitus would have limited skin sparing with RT but reduced the risk of wound complications after surgical excision. Because the primary site was felt to be too close to the anus and rectum to achieve negative surgical margins without compromising anal function, definitive RT was recommended for the primary. *Plan*: excision of right inguinal lymphadenopathy followed by chemo-RT.

Surgery: A 3 × 4 cm node was adherent but able to be dissected away from the saphenous vein. On pathology review, the node was completely replaced by squamous carcinoma; additional groin tissue was removed but contained no lymph nodes. Postoperative imaging showed that the smaller node seen on preoperative CT was still present.

EBRT *(completed in 39 days)*:

Set up: Frog-leg, custom cradle. BBs were placed on the vulvar tumor (*red arrow*) and other key structures (***d***).

Because there was ECE, the inguinal scar was treated and the nodal bed was treated to 60 Gy. An initial integrated boost included only the vulvar GTV–PTV, which was defined using fused MRI images and clinical exam. A final sequential boost was more generous, including a surrounding HRCTV margin, as well as the GTV. A 5-mm bolus was applied to the right groin and vulva for 20 treatments and was then removed. Doses were confirmed using TLDs.

IMRT:

Fractions 1–25 (***d–f***):

CTV vulva, pelvic nodes, left groin (+6 mm): 45 Gy (180 cGy/fraction)

GTV vulva and HRCTV right groin (+6 mm): 50 Gy (200 cGy/fraction)

Fractions 26–30:

HRCTV R groin: 10 Gy (***g***); HRCTV and GTV vulva (+6 mm): 10 Gy (***h***); based on composite plans (not shown), all areas of gross disease and the HRCTV groin received at least 60 Gy; the HRCTV vulva received 55 Gy.

Chemotherapy: Weekly cisplatin ×6.

Outcome: At 4 months, NED by PET and exam; minimal skin changes with mild atrophy and scarring of the posterior fourchette (***i, j***). At 2.5 years, NED and fully active, with intermittent constipation.

Comment: Because the primary lesion was small and confined to the perineum and the rest of the vulva was completely normal, the anterior vulva and mons were not targeted.

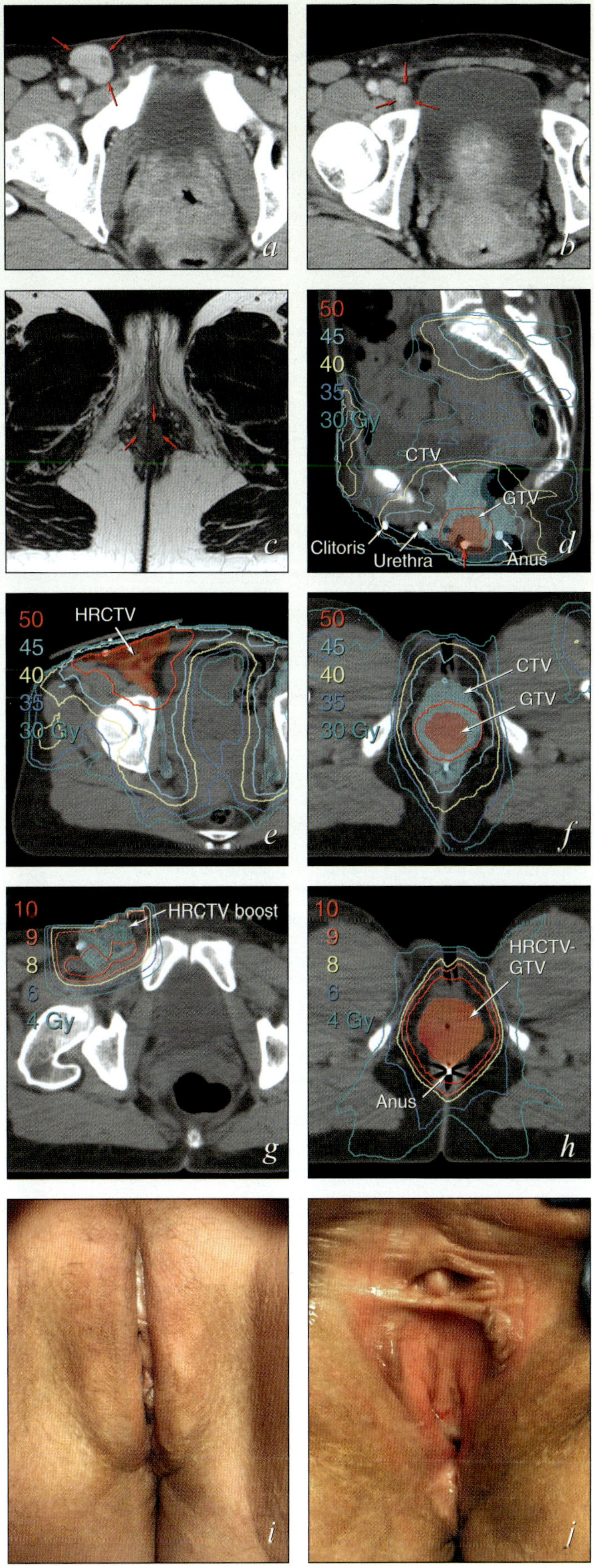

CS 12.5 • Extensive Vulvar Cancer Involving Perineum, Vagina, and Nodes

History: A 64-year-old woman who had an enlarging vulvar mass and purulent discharge was referred after her physician biopsied the mass and incised a separate lesion on the adjacent buttock. The patient had diabetes mellitus and a history of hemorrhoidectomy.

Evaluation: *Exam*: A 5-cm mass involving the right vulva and perineum extended to the anal verge and posterior distal vagina; a separate 2-cm lesion involved the skin of the buttock. *KPS*: 80–90. *MRI, CT pelvis*: 6 × 3.5 × 5 cm mass in the right and posterior vulva, involving the vagina, abutting the anus, and extending to the right medial thigh (***a***); 5.6 ×3.7 right inguinal mass (***b***); prominent right EI nodes; *CT abdomen, chest*: NED; *biopsies* (*vulva, buttock*): moderately differentiated squamous carcinoma.

Treatment Plan: Radical vulvar resection would have required sacrifice of the rectum. Although an argument could have been made to excise the largest groin node, the patient's habitus facilitated sparing of the inguinal skin, permitting high-dose RT. Equivocal distal EI nodes were treated as positive because of their location just proximal to the large groin node. Final plan: Definitive chemo-RT.

Radiation Therapy (*completed in 46 days*)**:**
Set up: Frog-leg in a custom cradle.

Treatment was delivered using an initial IMRT plan with integrated boosts to the vulva and to the involved nodes; this was followed by a sequential boost to the primary GTV and to the largest inguinal node. On the first day of treatment, TLD measurements verified that adequate dose was delivered to all the regions of skin involvement (***f***). Presumably because of the tangential incidence of beams, even the relatively exposed buttock lesion received >90% of the dose so no bolus was used in this case. Because of the patient's body habitus, all other regions of gross disease were more than 1 cm deep to the surface and therefore received approximately 100% of the prescribed dose.

The final boost targets were modified to reflect some reduction in tumor mass effect but included all initial areas of infiltration, particularly in the left buttock.

Fractions 1–30 (***c–e***):

HRCTV (including GTV-vulva) (+10 mm): 60 Gy (200 cGy/fraction)

GTV-inguinal and EI nodes (+10 mm): 62 Gy (207 cGy/fraction)

CTV nodes and ITV vulva (+7 mm): 51 Gy (170 cGy/fraction)

Fractions 31–34 (***g, h***):

GTV-vulva (+9 mm): 8 Gy (total dose 68 Gy)

GTV-largest groin node (+9 mm): 8 Gy (total dose, 70 Gy)

Chemotherapy: Weekly cisplatin ×4.

Outcome: During RT, antibiotics were required for a UTI and for a boil on the left labium that grew out methicillin-resistant *Staphylococcus aureus*. Erythema and patchy moist desquamation were treated with fluconazole and local care.

At 3.5 months, NED in the vulva by exam and MRI and marked reduction in the right groin node. At 7 months, NED by PET. At 1 year, underwent fistulotomy for a left transsphincteric perianal fistula; this healed over 2 months without sequelae. At 4 years, NED by exam; moderate prepubic and left leg edema; normal bowel function.

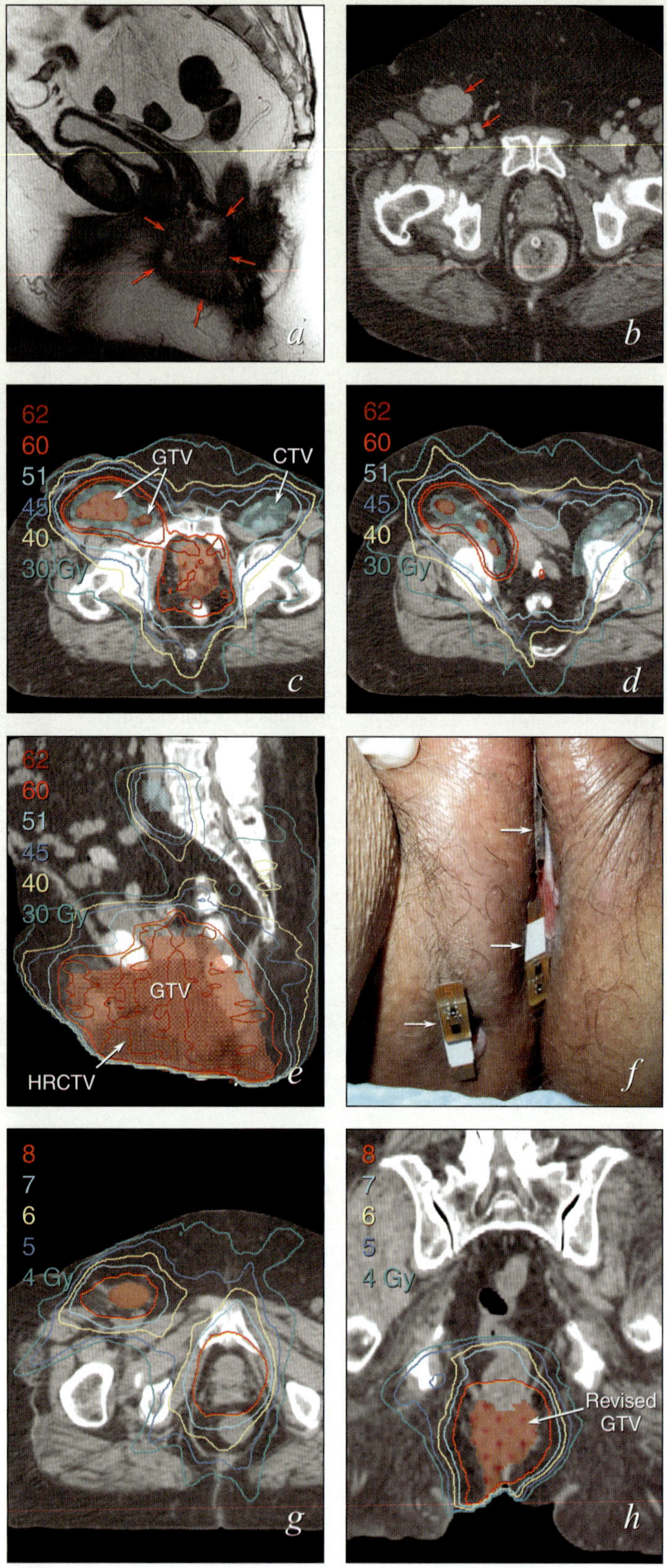

CS 12.6 • Squamous Carcinoma of Bartholin's Region with Groin Metastases

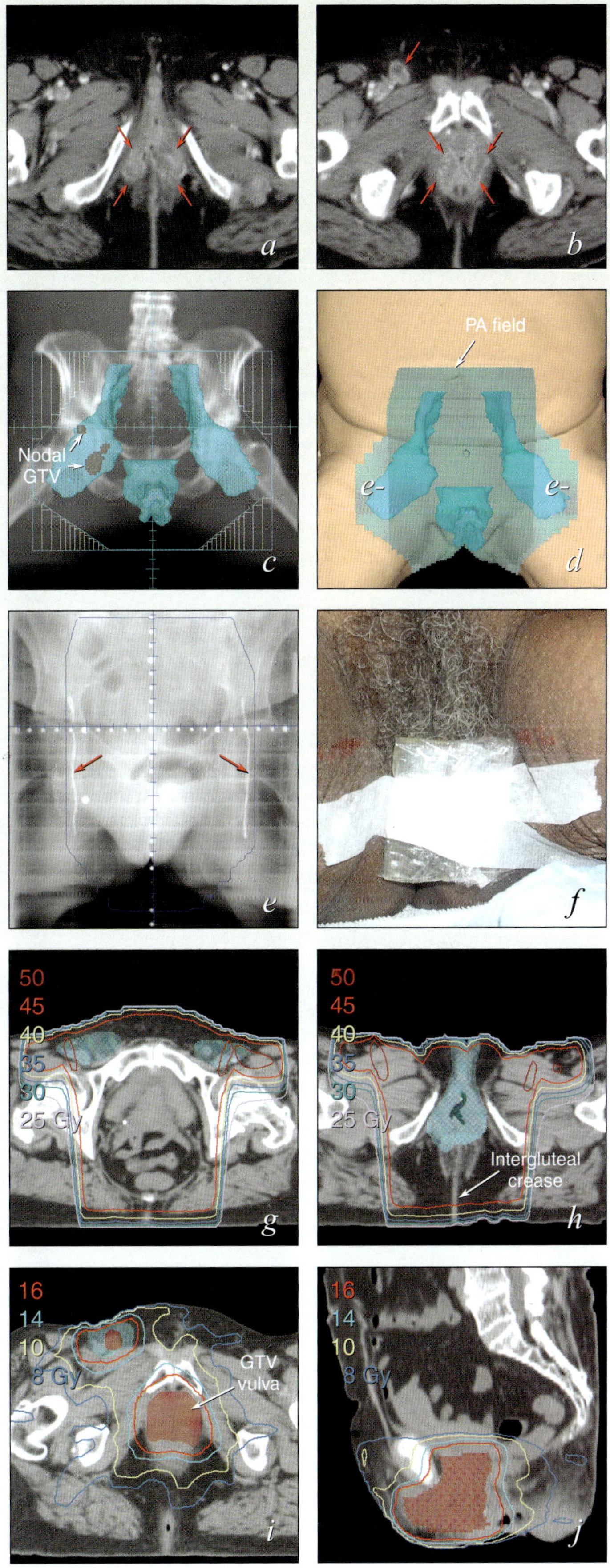

History: A 65-year-old woman had a 2-year history of a "lump" in the left vulva. This was presumptively diagnosed as a Bartholin gland cyst, but despite several courses of antibiotics, the mass continued to grow. The patient eventually had EUA for planned incision and drainage; however, when the mass was entered, the physician encountered solid tumor. The patient was referred for further evaluation and treatment.

Evaluation: *Exam*: A large defect with thickened, friable tissue in the posterior vestibule and vaginal wall; the left portion was submucosal, suggesting possible origin in the Bartholin gland but the lesion also extended across midline posteriorly; tumor approximated but did not grossly involve the anus or rectal mucosa; a 2-cm node was palpated in the right groin; *KPS*: 90; *CT pelvis, abdomen, chest*: peripherally enhancing hypodense mass in the left vulva and distal vagina (***a***, ***b***); 1.7-cm right inguinal node (***b***); otherwise NED; *biopsies* (*vulva*): Poorly differentiated squamous carcinoma; *FNA* (*right inguinal node*): squamous carcinoma.

Treatment Plan: Radical vulvar resection would have required at least a posterior exenteration and might not have achieved negative margins because of tumor abutting the pelvic floor musculature. Final plan: Definitive chemo-RT to the vulva and regional nodes.

Radiation Therapy (*completed in 51 days*)**:**
Setup: Frog-leg in a custom cradle. Bolus (5 mm) on the posterior vulva (***f***).

Using a 3-D technique, a wide anterior 6-MV photon field encompassed the entire target volume with margin (***c***); a narrow 18-MV posterior field included the vulva, distal iliac, and medial inguinal nodes, and 12-MeV electrons were used to supplement the lateral groins (***d***). These fields were weighted to achieve a homogeneous dose of 45 Gy in 25 fractions (***g***, ***h***). During treatment, setup accuracy was verified with portal films; wires were placed on the medial borders of the electron fields to confirm accurate alignment with the borders of the posterior field (***e***).

The vulva, involved groin node, and two adjacent 7–10 mm lymph nodes were then treated using IMRT to bring the total doses to these regions to 61 Gy (***i***, ***j***)

Chemotherapy: Weekly cisplatin ×4.

Outcome: In week 5 of RT, sudden onset of confluent moist desquamation primarily involving the intergluteal region responded to antibiotics and fluconazole; the patient continued with her boost, which excluded much of the affected area. At 2 weeks, there was marked improvement but the site of the tumor was still healing. At 5 years, followed with NED at an outside facility.

Comments: We do not favor extensive lymphadenectomy in this situation because wound complications tend to delay definitive management of the primary; however, excision of the node followed by RT would have been an alternative approach.

Compared with IMRT, AP–PA treatment reduces the risk of geometric misses of the target but invariably exposes more skin to full dose, particularly in the intergluteal crease (***h***). IMRT would have facilitated delivery of a somewhat higher dose of 64–66 Gy, which we prefer for such a large tumor.

CS 12.7 • Massive T4 Vulvar Cancer Involving Anus and Satellite Lesions

History: A 38-year-old woman with a large vulvar lesion, severe pain, leg edema, anorexia, and a 40-lb weight loss sought a second opinion after pelvic exenteration was recommended.

Evaluation: *Exam* (***a***): A 20-cm fungating mass bilaterally involved the entire vulva with two satellite lesions on the buttocks (*arrows*); bilateral enlarged groin nodes; *weight*: 44 kg; *KPS*: 70; *WBC* 15,000; *Hgb*: 7.0; *albumin*: 1.8; *PET* (***b***): Large, intensely hypermetabolic vulvar lesion and multiple enlarged mildly hypermetabolic inguinal nodes (SUV 3–4); *MRI* (***c, d***): Extensive perineal tumor infiltrating skin and subcutaneous tissues of the vulva, perineum, urethra, and gluteal folds with circumferential involvement of anus extending cephalad to the levator ani; *biopsy* (*vulva*): squamous carcinoma.

Treatment Plan: The patient was admitted for transfusion, infection control, and pain management with improvement. It was decided to attempt cure because the patient had no apparent distant metastases. However, she was a poor candidate for surgery because of her performance status and disease extent. With extensive skin and organ involvement, even ultraradical surgery would have had difficulty clearing her primary disease. It was decided not to attempt to resect the nodes. The low SUV of lateral inguinal lymph nodes and regression following initial antibiotic therapy suggested that much of the lymphadenopathy was due to inflammation. Only a very extensive bilateral LAD could rule out metastasis, and the associated risk of wound complications and postoperative delays was felt to outweigh any benefit. The greatest challenge would be control of the vulvar lesion. The plan was to treat with definitive chemo-RT.

Radiation Therapy (*completed in 46 days*):
Setup: Frog-leg with 1-cm bolus on the vulva. A large tumor cavity was packed with wet gauze. Initial treatment included an integrated hypofractionated boost to the center of the tumor to promote rapid regression. Enlarged inguinal nodes were treated to 55–60 Gy, with the most suspicious medial nodes treated to 60 Gy. The plan was adapted twice to accommodate to regression. Doses were confirmed with TLD measurements.

IMRT Plan:
Fractions 1–20 (***e, f***): CTV (+7 mm): 36 Gy; vulva GTV (+10 mm): 40 Gy; nested internal GTV: 44 Gy

Fractions 21–28: CTV 12.5 Gy; GTV nodes and vulva: 16 Gy

Fractions 29–33: GTV vulva and PET+ nodes: 8 Gy

Total doses (***g–i***):

CTVs: 48.5 Gy in 28 fractions; vulva GTV: 63–68 Gy in 32 fractions (based on composite of varying contours); enlarged nodes: 55–60 Gy in 28–32 fractions

The patient received intensive local care and dietary and pain management throughout the treatment.

Chemotherapy: Because of initial performance status and compliance issues, she completed only 40 mg/m^2 cisplatin ×2.

Outcome: Rapid tumor response. At 2 months, NED with a healing defect at the former site of vulvar skin involvement (***j***), good bowel and bladder function, and 9 kg weight gain. At 4 years, NED with follow-up at an outside facility.

Comments: This complex treatment required many steps and committed multidisciplinary management. This good outcome cannot be routinely expected but justified the decision to treat with curative intent.

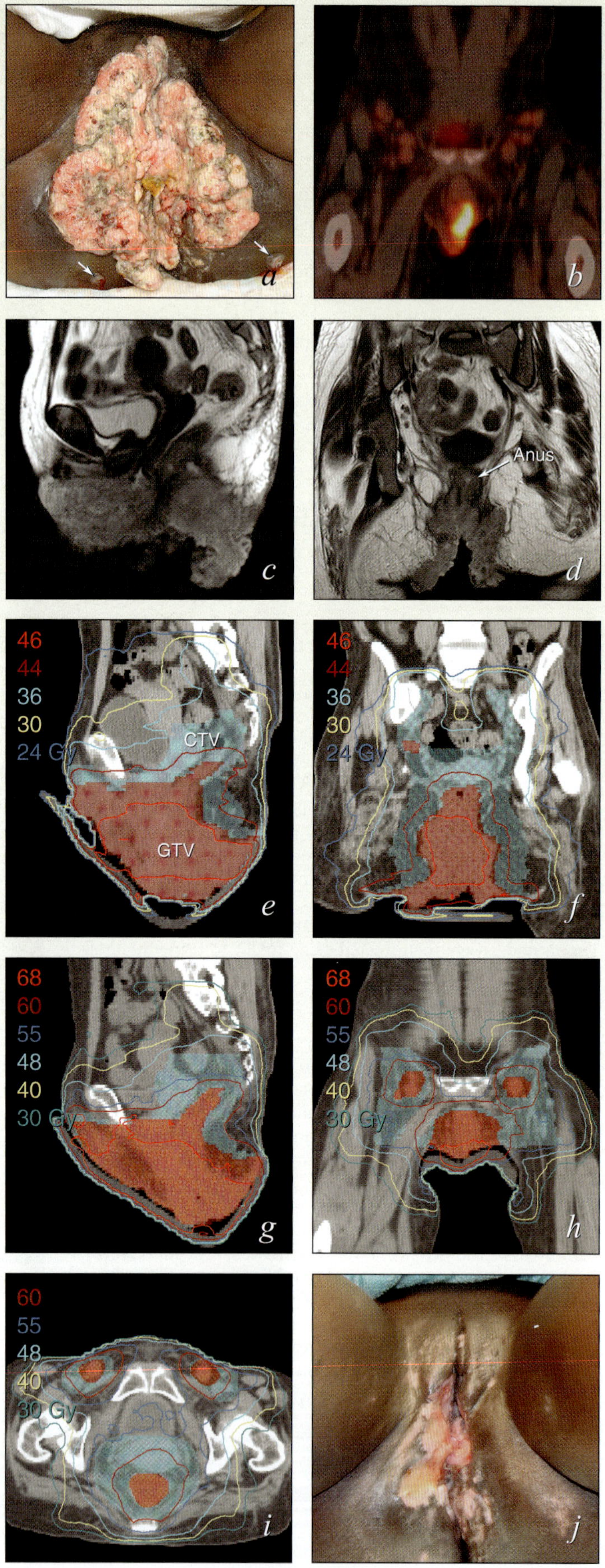

CS 12.8 • Stage IVB Periclitoral Cancer with Extensive Groin and Pelvic Lymphadenopathy

History: A 62-year-old woman had a 1-year history of an enlarging groin node that progressed after initial response to antibiotics. A 5-cm left groin mass was excised, showing squamous carcinoma; a subsequent wound infection responded to antibiotics. No primary site was identified, and she was referred for evaluation and treatment.

Evaluation: *Exam* (*EUA*): A 3×2 cm nodular periclitoral tumor and a separate 2-cm perihymenal suburethral lesion that extended superficially to the junction of the middle and distal vagina; no lymphadenopathy was appreciated; the left inguinal incision was well healed; *KPS*: 90. *MRI, CT*: multiple enlarged nodes up to 2 cm in diameter (***a***); a 4-cm left external iliac node (***a, b***); the primary tumor was not seen, and chest and abdomen CTs showed NED; *biopsy* (*left groin node*): squamous carcinoma, HPV-16 positive.

Treatment Plan: The primary lesion could not be resected without sacrificing bladder function. Resection of the large pelvic node was considered but her disease had already progressed during treatment of postsurgical infection, and resection of all nodal disease would have required very extensive additional surgery. *Plan*: Definitive chemoradiation.

Radiation Therapy (*completed in 41 days*):*
Setup (***c, d***): Frog-leg; bolus on the vulva and inguinal incision was removed after 15 treatments to moderate the dose to uninvolved skin.

IMRT was delivered to multiple targets using a single plan with integrated boosts (***e–g***).

Total doses (in 28 fractions):

Vulvar GTV (+10 mm), inguinal and left pelvic node GTVs (+10 mm): 64.4 Gy (230 cGy/fraction)

Small, equivocal right pelvic node GTV (+10 mm): 60.2 Gy (215 cGy/fraction)

HRCTV left groin (+7 mm): 57.4 Gy (205 cGy/fraction)

Vulvar and vaginal CTV (+7 mm): 54.6 Gy (195 cGy/fraction)

Iliac node CTVs (+7 to 10 mm): 44.8 Gy (160 cGy/fraction)

Chemotherapy: Weekly cisplatin ×5.

Outcome: During treatment, yeast infection was treated with fluconazole and sitz baths. By the conclusion, there was brisk erythema of the skin with patchy moist desquamation in the inguinal creases and on the labia minora. At 4 months, NED by exam and CT. At 10 years, NED with mild skin changes except for epilation and telangiectasia localized to the highest dose region (***h, i***); mild left leg and prepubic edema; normal bowel and bladder function.

Comments: Imaging and physical examination were both needed to define the target volumes. Lymphadenopathy was apparent only on imaging but a fairly extensive vulvar primary was appreciated only on physical examination.

IMRT allowed treatment of gross disease to high dose without major long-term sequelae. Although treatment was remarkably well tolerated, today we are more likely to use a combination of integrated and sequential boosts to reduce the range of daily fraction sizes and would use a 5- to 7-mm PTV margin for integrated boosts. We would also likely give a slightly higher effective dose (60 Gy) to the site of ECE in the left groin.

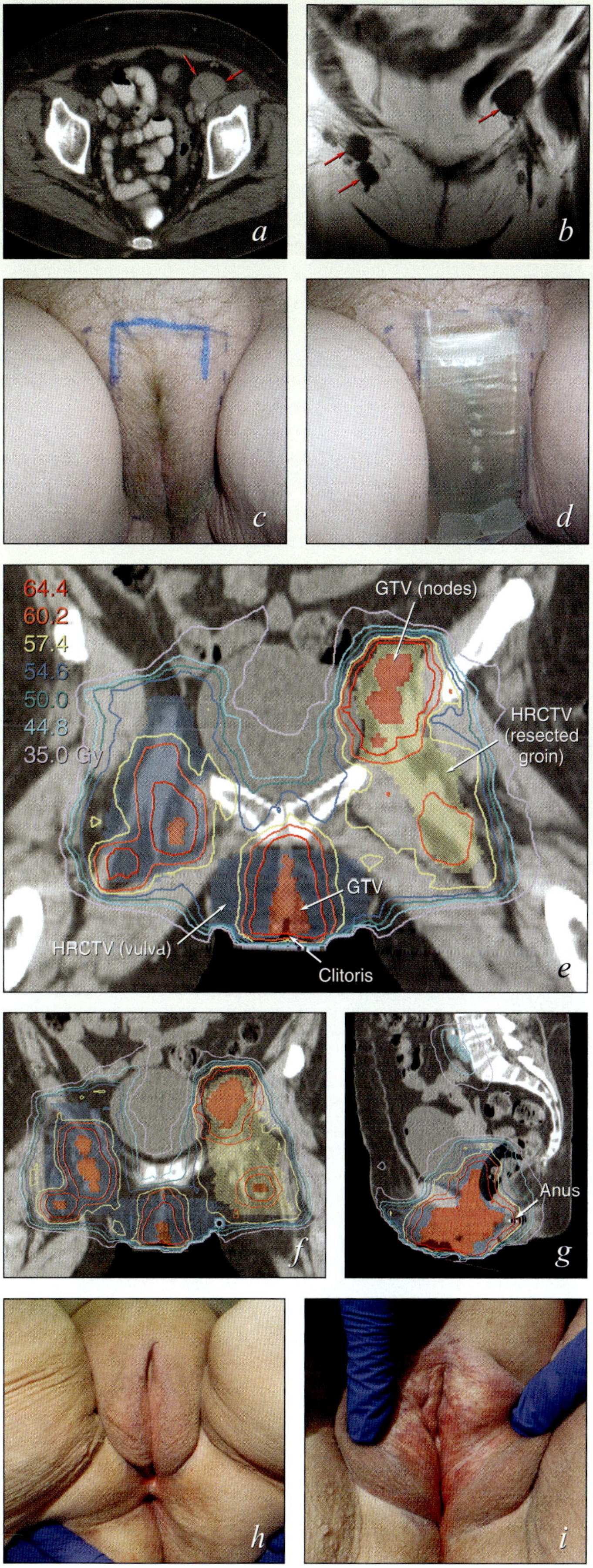

*For illustration purposes, this early IMRT plan was reoptimized using the original doses and target volumes. Figure 5.11 shows additional images of this patient's right groin contours.

CS 12.9 • Radiation Therapy for Vulvar Cancer after Previous Groin Irradiation

History: A 76-year-old woman had left inguinal lymphadenectomy with excision of a 4-cm node containing poorly differentiated squamous carcinoma. After no primary source was found, she had adjuvant RT to the left groin using AP–PA photon fields for 45 Gy and then 12-MeV electrons to bring the total dose to 60 Gy. The vulva was not targeted, but the margins of the AP–PA fields included a portion of the lateral vulva (***a***).

Six months later, a 2-cm ulcerative lesion was noted in the left labium, and CT revealed a new 3-cm right inguinal lymph node. Wide excision of the vulvar lesion demonstrated poorly differentiated squamous carcinoma; a positive lateral margin was re-excised but the lateral margin of the second specimen was also positive. Lymphadenectomy revealed metastasis in one of two right groin nodes with ECE. The patient sought a second opinion for treatment recommendations.

Postoperative Evaluation: *Exam*: Hyperpigmentation and telangiectasia of skin overlying the left groin; a 5 × 6 cm lesion on the left labium was consistent with granulation tissue and residual cancer; induration extended to the border of the irradiated skin; no lymphadenopathy. *KPS*: 90–100. *CT*: review confirmed no evidence of distant disease.

Treatment Plan: Although retreatment required some overlap with the previous field, the only chance of cure in this case was with definitive RT. Chemotherapy response rates for vulvar cancer are poor, and the consequences of locoregional progression would be severe, exceeding the risks of retreatment. The plan was definitive chemoradiation.

Radiation Therapy (*completed in 42 days*):
Setup: Supine with legs apposed in a cradle. The vulva, right groin, and distal iliac nodes were treated using a combination of 6- and 18-MV photons and 12-MeV electrons (***b***, ***c***). These fields were weighted to deliver 50 Gy in 25 fractions to the groin and anterior vulva and 45 Gy to deeper structures. A slight field reduction after 20 fractions reduced the dose to the overlap region.

The left groin and vulvar HRCTV (***d***) were then boosted to a total dose of 60 Gy using appositional electron beams.

Chemotherapy: Concurrent low-dose continuous infusion of cisplatin and 5-fluorouracil.

Outcome: At 5 weeks, an exudative erythematous skin reaction was treated with antibiotics and fluconazole with improvement. At 1 year, arthroplasty for left femoral neck fracture; at 2 years, arthroplasty for right femoral neck fracture. At 10 years, she was treated for breast cancer and had the onset of recurrent episodes of cellulitis in the left leg that compromised her quality of life. However, at 14 years (age 90), she remains NED, independent, and quite active with good bowel and bladder function but with chronic skin changes in the perineum and intergluteal folds (***e***), moderate left leg edema, and generalized osteoporosis.

Comments: Vulvar cancer was undoubtedly the source of the initial left groin node. This case demonstrates some of the challenges of delivering vulvar RT to a patient who has had previous groin irradiation.

Treatment in a frog-leg position would have reduced the reaction in the medial thighs. IMRT might have improved posterior tissue sparing but would have been hampered by the need to minimize the use of lateral field angles. Proton beam therapy, although technically challenging in this location, might have held some advantages had it been available.

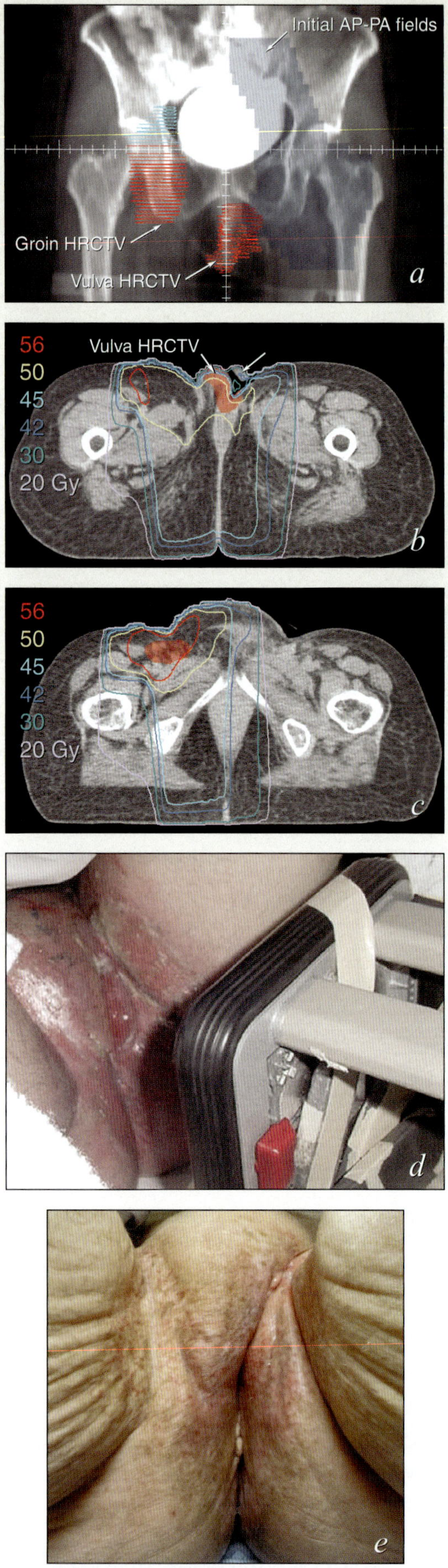

CS 12.10 • Inguinal Node Recurrence after Partial Radical Vulvectomy and Negative Sentinel Node Biopsies

History: A 70-year-old woman noted a thickened area on her vulva. Her physician performed a biopsy and referred her for treatment.

Evaluation at Diagnosis: *Exam*: A 2 × 4 cm left periclitoral lesion, 5 mm from the urethra; no lymphadenopathy; *CT, chest x-ray*: NED; *KPS*: 100; *biopsy* (*vulva*): moderately differentiated squamous carcinoma.

Surgery: The patient opted for primary surgical treatment after counseling that the clitoris might need to be sacrificed. A radical partial vulvectomy and distal urethrectomy were performed, demonstrating a 2 × 3 cm squamous carcinoma, invading 6 mm with no LVSI; right and left sentinel nodes and three additional groin nodes had NED.

Interval Evaluations: The patient was followed with serial groin ultrasounds. At 5 months, a left inguinal node with a hypoechoic nodule (*arrows*, ***c***) and increased vascularity was considered suspicious. *Biopsy* (*FNA*): Squamous carcinoma; *CT*: Left groin node increased from 1.5 × 0.8 cm preoperatively (***a***) to 1.5 × 1.2 cm (***b***); otherwise NED. *Exam*: Extensive granulation tissue in the healing operative bed was negative for recurrence on biopsy.

Surgery: A left inguinal lymphadenectomy showing a 5-mm focus of squamous carcinoma (***d***) with no ECE in one of five nodes.

Treatment Plan: EBRT to the left inguinal operative bed and distal left pelvic lymph nodes (***e***). It was decided not to treat the vulva, which initially had widely negative margins. There was some concern that the extensive granulation tissue in the periurethral region might harbor recurrent disease despite negative biopsies. If it did, 45 Gy would have been inadequate to achieve local control, but without proof, the morbidity of high-dose radiation (e.g., ≥60 Gy) could not be justified. For these reasons, fairly strict avoidance limits were set for the central vulva to enable subsequent treatment, if required. The right groin, which had a negative sentinel node at first surgery and no suspicious nodes 6 months later, was also considered low risk and was not treated, although this was a more controversial choice.

At the time of planning CT, an enlarged node was noted near the lateral circumflex vein, just superolateral to the operative bed (*arrows*, ***f***, ***g***). Although this node (which was <5 mm on preoperative CT) was probably inflammatory, it was decided to boost the region because a second recurrence in this site would almost certainly have been fatal.

EBRT** (completed in 32 days):**

Setup: Frog-leg, custom cradle (***e***).

Using IMRT, the inguinal CTV (+7 mm) was treated to 50 Gy, and the distal iliac CTV (+7 mm) was treated to 45 Gy in 25 fractions (***f***, ***g***). Following this, the suspicious groin node was boosted, initially with 20 MeV e− and then with 12 MeV e−, to bring the total dose to 62 Gy (***h***, ***i***).

Chemotherapy: The patient declined chemotherapy.

Outcome: At treatment end, erythema and dry desquamation in the inguinal fold. At 4.5 years (5 years after initial diagnosis), NED with mild hyperpigmentation in the inguinal fold and no lymphedema.

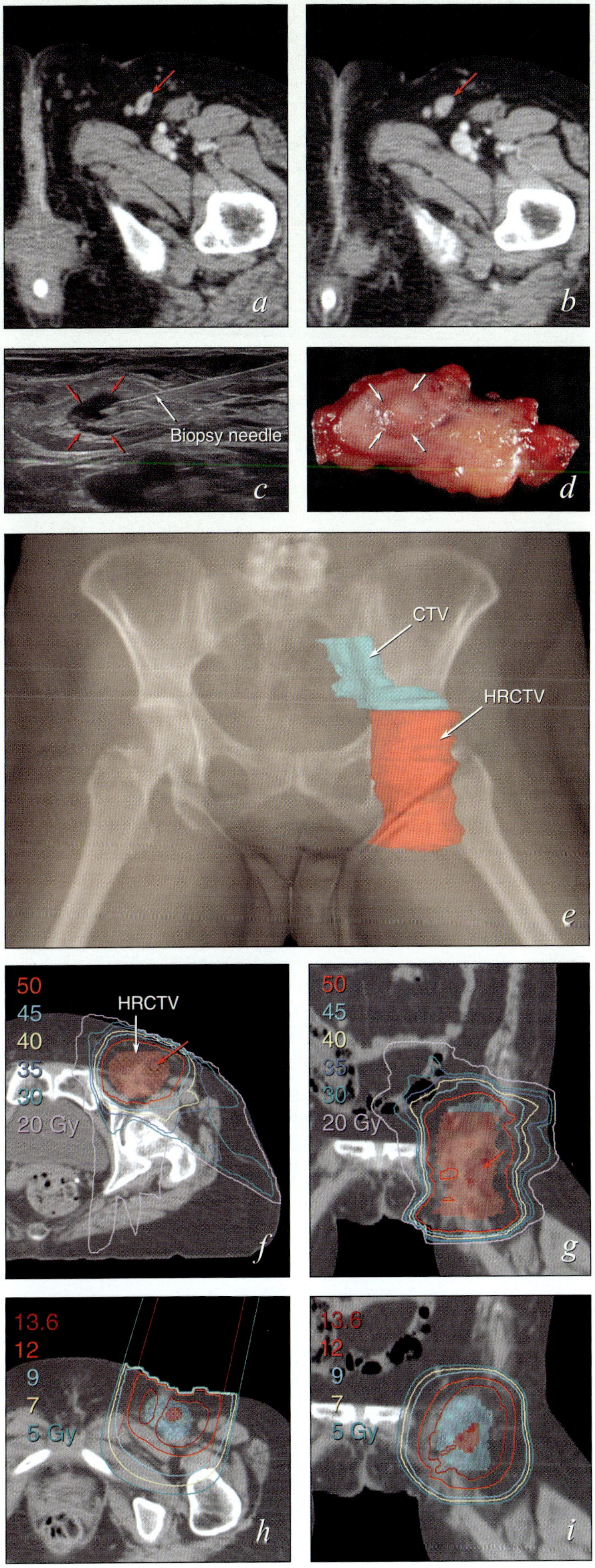

CHAPTER 13

Uterine Cancer

INTRODUCTION

Most endometrial cancers are cured by simple removal of the uterus. For this reason, investigators have tended to focus their attention on improving methods of identifying the minority subset of patients who are at risk for recurrence after hysterectomy alone and on the selection of effective adjuvant treatments for patients with known or suspected extrauterine disease. Over the past 30 years, many studies have attempted to define the roles of surgical staging, adjuvant radiation therapy, and adjuvant chemotherapy. However, despite years of study, many long-standing questions remain about the roles of these adjuvant treatments. Several factors have contributed to this:

- *Although endometrial cancer is the most common gynecologic malignancy diagnosed in developed countries, locally advanced and high-risk endometrial cancers are relatively uncommon.* For example, the estimated number of uterine cancers diagnosed in the United States in 2015 is 55,000, but the estimated number of disease-related deaths is only about 10,000.[1] This low rate of disease-specific mortality reflects the fact that most endometrial cancers are low-grade tumors diagnosed at an early stage.
- *Most of the recurrence risk resides in a small subset of patients who have multiple risk factors.* When studies mix patients who have more favorable cancers with the relatively small number of higher-risk patients, the benefits of adjuvant treatments are difficult to detect (Chapter 2).
- *The staging and histologic classification systems have changed several times during the past 30 years.* These changes complicate efforts to generalize results from early studies to current practice.
- *Large discrepancies exist among pathologists in the assessment of histologic risk factors and even in the diagnosis of cancer versus hyperplasia.* Review of histologic material by expert gynecologic pathologists leads to significant reinterpretation of results in up to 40% of cases,[2–5] making it difficult to generalize results from trials and large single-institutional experiences to different practice settings.

To understand and to be able to articulate the potential benefits and risks of adjuvant treatments, clinicians must navigate a complex and often flawed set of trials and retrospective studies. Because the ability to understand and explain the rationale behind treatment decisions is so critical to the effective management of endometrial cancers, a primary goal of this chapter will be to summarize available data, to suggest how those data can be applied to individual clinical situations, and to explain the sources of continued controversy.

Because the aforementioned issues tend to dominate the discourse, technical aspects of radiation therapy for endometrial cancer are often taken for granted. However, a recent survey of practice at MD Anderson Cancer Center indicated that fewer than 20% of the patients receiving external beam therapy with curative intent had stage I disease; another 20% had stage II, while the majority had stage III disease or locoregional recurrences. Although the nature of our practice undoubtedly contributes to this distribution, the past decade has seen a general decrease in the use of external beam therapy for early-stage cases and an increasing appreciation of the role of radiation therapy for locoregionally advanced cancers that may require extended radiation fields, boosts to regions of high-risk or gross disease, or combined modality treatment. As a result, endometrial cancers now represent some of our most technically challenging cases. The case studies associated with this chapter will focus on some of these more complex problems.

PRETREATMENT EVALUATION

At Initial Diagnosis

The initial treatment of most patients with newly diagnosed endometrial cancer is surgery, and the results of surgery are used to assign a FIGO stage (**Table 13.1**) and determine the need for additional treatment. For most patients, the yield from preoperative tomographic imaging is very low, and hence, most guidelines recommend only a chest x-ray in addition to a history and physical examination and laboratory studies. However, additional preoperative imaging studies may be helpful in some cases:

- *Patients who have high-risk histologic subtypes.* Because patients who have serous carcinomas or carcinosarcomas have relatively high rates of extrauterine spread, CT or PET–CT may be indicated to rule out metastases, particularly if the patient has symptoms. Some clinicians also recommend a baseline CA-125 for patients with high-risk subtypes.
- *Preoperative evaluation of disease extent within the uterus.* MRI can provide information about the depth of myometrial invasion that can be used to guide the extent of surgical staging. However, the accuracy of MRI is heavily dependent on the methods of image acquisition.[6]

TABLE 13.1 Evolution of the FIGO Staging System for Carcinomas of the Endometrium

Stage[a]	1971–1987 (Based on clinical findings)	1988–2008 (Based on operative findings)	2009– (Based on operative findings)
I	Carcinoma is confined to the uterine body		
IA	The length of the uterine cavity is 8 cm or less[a,b]	Tumor limited to the endometrium	Tumor confined to the uterus, no or <1/2 myometrial invasion[c]
IB	The length of the uterine cavity is more than 8 cm[a,b]	Invasion to less than one-half the endometrium	Tumor confined to the uterus, >1/2 myometrial invasion[c]
IC		Invasion to more than one-half the endometrium	
II	Carcinoma has involved the corpus and the cervix but has not extended outside the uterus[a]		Carcinoma involves the cervical stroma but is not beyond the uterus[c]
IIA		Endocervical glandular involvement only	
IIB		Cervical stromal invasion	
III	Carcinoma has extended outside the uterus but not outside the true pelvis		
IIIA		Tumor involves serosa or adnexa or positive peritoneal cytology[d]	Tumor invades serosa or adnexa[d]
IIIB		Vaginal metastases	Vaginal or parametrial involvement
IIIC		Metastases to pelvic or paraaortic nodes	IIIC1 pelvic node involvement IIIC2 paraaortic involvement
IVA	Spread to adjacent organs	Invasion of bladder and/or bowel mucosa	
IVB	Spread to distant organs	Distant metastases including abdominal metastases and or inguinal lymph nodes	

[a]*After 1988, FIGO mandated that the histologic grade of the tumor should be specified with the stage for all stages. According to the 1971–1987 staging system, only the stage I category was subdivided by grade using a system that was based strictly on the architectural pattern of the tumor. The grades were designated as "grade 1, highly differentiated; grade 2, moderately differentiated with partly solid areas; grade 3, predominantly solid or entirely undifferentiated carcinoma." After 1988, a more detailed grading system was adopted that recognized the importance of special histologic variants and nuclear atypia* (**Table 13.2**).

[b]*Prior to 1988, the presence of cervical involvement was determined by fractional dilatation and curettage.*

[c]*In 2009, tumors confined to the endometrium were grouped with other tumors that invaded <½ the myometrium, and the number of stage I subcategories was reduced from 3 to 1. Tumors that involved endocervical glands without stromal invasion were moved from the stage II to the stage I category.*

[d]*In 1988, positive peritoneal cytology was made a criterion for inclusion in stage IIIA. In 2008, after data suggested that peritoneal cytology was a weak independent predictor of prognosis, it was removed from consideration in the FIGO system.*

TABLE 13.2 FIGO Histologic Grading System (1988–)

Grade 1	5% or less of a nonsquamous or nonmorular solid growth pattern
Grade 2	6%–50% of a nonsquamous or nonmorular solid growth pattern
Grade 3	More than 50% of a nonsquamous or nonmorular solid growth pattern

Notes on pathologic grading:
- Notable nuclear atypia, inappropriate for the architectural grade, raises the grade of a grade 1 or a grade 2 tumor by 1.
- In serous adenocarcinomas, clear cell adenocarcinomas, and squamous cell carcinomas, nuclear grading takes precedence.
- Adenocarcinomas with squamous differentiation are graded according to the nuclear grade of the glandular component.

- *Patients who have gross cervical or vaginal involvement.* In these cases, MRI can help to clarify the site of origin (cervix or uterus) and the extent of disease in the fundus, cervix, and vagina; this in turn helps guide the initial approach to treatment with surgery or radiation therapy (**CS 13.2 and 13.3**).

Genetic counseling and testing to rule out Lynch syndrome should be considered for women who are <50 years old or who have a strong family history of colorectal and uterine cancers (Chapter 1).

After Hysterectomy, Prior to Initiation of Adjuvant Therapy

Any patient who is being considered for postoperative adjuvant external beam irradiation or chemotherapy should have high-quality tomographic imaging. Such imaging serves several purposes:

- *To rule out extrapelvic nodes that might indicate a need for extended radiation fields.* As discussed in Chapter 5, cancers involving the uterine fundus can metastasize directly to the infrarenal paraaortic nodes. For patients with high-risk endometrial cancer, it is recommended that the simulation CT extend to include the renal vessels to permit reexamination of this region, particularly if there is no recent diagnostic imaging.
- *To document areas of gross disease prior to the delivery of chemotherapy for stage III disease.* If the patient is subsequently referred for consolidation treatment or for disease progression, it is important to have documentation of the initial extent of disease, because more than 45 Gy is recommended to all sites of initial gross disease, even if there has been a response to chemotherapy.
- *To rule out suspicious nodes within the radiation therapy fields.* Even modestly enlarged nodes should be considered for an integrated or sequential boost (**CS 13.5 and 13.6**).
- *To rule out distant disease.* CT of the chest is recommended for most patients who have advanced-stage disease or high-risk subtypes.

Tomographic imaging should be obtained even if the patient has had an apparently complete pelvic and paraaortic lymphadenectomy. It is not unusual for residual nodes to be detected after lymphadenectomy. In our experience, the most frequent sites of residual disease after lymphadenectomy are as follows:

- Posterior to and just distal to the left renal vessels
- Deep to the vessels in the aortocaval space
- Deep to the vessels at the point of bifurcation of the common iliac vessels (particularly on the left)
- In the distal obturator region

If results for preoperative imaging obtained within 6 to 8 weeks of adjuvant treatment are negative, postoperative contrast-enhanced imaging may not be needed, although all images should be carefully scrutinized by the treating radiation oncologist and compared with the postoperative treatment planning CT to confirm that all abnormal nodes have been removed. In some cases, a contrast-enhanced CT is needed to obtain good views of the nodal regions. For patients who have very extensive nodal disease, PET can be very helpful in defining radiation target volumes, although false positives due to postoperative inflammation reduce the value of PET in the immediate postoperative setting.

Before Definitive Treatment (Medically or Surgically Inoperable Cancer)

If possible, pelvic MRI should be obtained to clarify the distribution of gross disease within the uterine cavity and to assist in external beam and brachytherapy treatment planning (**CS 13.2 and 13.10**). For patients with high-risk histologic types, CT of the chest, abdomen, and pelvis or PET–CT should be obtained to rule out metastatic disease.

RISK ASSESSMENT

To determine the need for adjuvant therapy and to select the treatment most likely to maximize therapeutic gain, a careful assessment of risks should be undertaken to estimate:

- The risk of vaginal recurrence
- The risk of extravaginal pelvic recurrence
- The risk of paraaortic nodal recurrence
- The risk of distant recurrence

This section reviews factors that have been correlated with overall outcome and describes how these factors can be used to predict possible patterns of recurrence. Subsequent sections of this chapter address evidence that various treatments can alter these recurrence patterns and possibly contribute to cure. Ultimately, the potential gains must then be weighed against the risks of treatment-related side effects (Chapter 9).

Primary Tumor Characteristics

Several primary tumor characteristics have been commonly correlated with the outcome of patients with endometrial cancer:

- Histologic subtype
- Histologic grade
- Presence and depth of myometrial invasion
- Presence and depth of cervical stromal invasion
- Lymph vascular space invasion
- Tumor size

These features have all been associated with the presence of lymph node metastasis, which is in turn a strong predictor of outcome. Other extrauterine features that correlate with prognosis include vaginal, adnexal, bladder, and rectal involvement, although these are relatively rare findings. Peritoneal cytology, lower uterine segment (LUS) involvement, and cervical glandular involvement do not have a clear independent influence on outcome. Older age and African American ethnicity have been associated with poorer outcomes, although these correlations reflect, at least in part, the tendency for patients in these groups to have higher-risk tumor characteristics. Combinations of risk factors can provide much stronger predictive value than any individual feature. The current FIGO staging system (**Tables 13.1 and 13.2**) incorporates many but not all of the known risk factors.

Adjuvant treatment decisions are based primarily on a pathologist's report of the operative findings. Because diagnostic errors can easily lead to inappropriate treatments, it is critical that clinicians be aware of the expertise of the pathologists interpreting their patients' specimens (Chapter 3) and of any potential sources of error or misinterpretation. The pathologist should be consulted directly to resolve any ambiguities. Whenever possible, *endometrial cancer specimens should be reviewed by a specialized gynecologic pathologist before adjuvant treatment is initiated.*

The following sections discuss some of the most important predictors of outcome, with emphasis on potential sources of misdiagnosis or misinterpretation.

Histologic Variants

The five major subtypes of endometrial cancer have been categorized as type I or type II cancers according to their overall behavior:

Type I cancers tend to have a relatively favorable prognosis:

- *Endometrioid* (75% to 80%). The differentiated features of endometrioid cancers resemble normal endometrial epithelium. Various patterns have been described, including papillary and villoglandular forms; these must not be confused with serous cancers, which also tend to have a papillary architecture but are much more aggressive. Endometrioid cancers often contain a squamous component, the grade of which typically follows that of the glandular component. Adenosquamous carcinomas are high-grade endometrioid cancers with a malignant squamous component. When low-grade cancers contain squamous elements, the squamous regions usually have a benign appearance; such cancers, which are sometimes referred to as adenoacanthomas, have a prognosis similar to that for pure adenocarcinomas of similar grade. The risk of developing endometrioid cancer is increased in patients who have been exposed to excess exogenous or endogenous estrogens, and many such cancers are to some degree hormone responsive (Chapter 1).
- *Mucinous* (1% to 5%). The differentiated features of mucinous cancers often recapitulate cervical glandular epithelium. They typically have prominent intracytoplasmic mucin and can be difficult to differentiate from primary cervical cancers although, unlike cervical cancers, uterine cancers are usually HPV negative. Their prognosis is similar to that of endometrioid cancers.[7]

Type II cancers tend to be hormone independent and have a relatively aggressive behavior, even when initially confined to the uterus:

- *Serous* (8% to 10%). The differentiated features of serous carcinomas recapitulate normal fallopian tube epithelium. Referred to in the past as "uterine papillary serous carcinoma (UPSC)," this variant is more appropriately called "uterine serous carcinoma (USC)" to accommodate cancers that have the immunohistochemical characteristics of a serous carcinoma without a distinct papillary architecture (Chapter 1).[8] Virtually, all USCs are high grade, with frequent recurrence and metastasis to nodes, peritoneal cavity, and elsewhere; in this, their behavior tends to mirror that of high-grade serous cancers originating in other sites. Although USC represents only 8% to 10% of endometrial cancers, it is responsible for 40% to 50% of recurrences. Because the clinical significance of USC was not widely recognized until the mid-1980s,[9,10] studies including patients treated before then should be assumed to include undetected cases of serous carcinoma. Also, because the pre-1988 grading system was strictly based on architectural appearance, USCs were often given a grade 1 or 2 assignment, further compromising the generalizability of early trials to current management. Serous carcinoma is often admixed with other subtypes. Although some authors have argued that the prognosis is somewhat better for mixed tumors than for pure serous cancers, the presence of USC tends to dominate the prognosis even when its proportion is as little as 10%.[11] Underdiagnosis and overdiagnosis of serous carcinoma can lead to serious errors in treatment selection, so expert review is particularly critical.
- *Clear cell carcinomas* (1% to 5%): Clear cell carcinoma is a rare subtype characterized by glands and papillae composed of hobnail cells having abundant clear cytoplasm. Although

they have been classified as type II, clear cell carcinomas that have no serous elements are usually grade 2 and have a better prognosis than other type II cancers, with 5-year survival rates for stage I disease ranging between 75% and 95%.[12] It is important to recognize that most cancers with "clear cell features" are not clear cell carcinoma. In particular, endometrioid cancers frequently have clear cytoplasm due to accumulation of glycogen, lipid, mucin, or other substances.[13] Again, expert review is recommended to avoid errors in diagnosis.

- *Carcinosarcoma* (1% to 2%): Carcinosarcomas (previously called malignant mixed müllerian tumors) are high-grade neoplasms that contain admixed malignant epithelial and mesenchymal elements. They usually occur in postmenopausal women (median age, 65) and in some cases may follow a history of pelvic radiation therapy[14] or treatment with tamoxifen. Carcinosarcomas typically present as bulky, polypoid tumors that protrude through the cervical os. Deep myometrial invasion, lymph vascular space invasion (LVSI), and lymph node metastases are frequent, and pelvic and distant recurrences are common; intraperitoneal metastases are more frequent than with type I cancers, but the rate is uncertain because most authors do not distinguish between intraperitoneal and retroperitoneal abdominal metastases. In most cases, the metastases from carcinosarcomas are purely epithelial but the prognosis appears to be poorer than that for other type II cancers.

Although carcinosarcomas were previously classified as a type of uterine sarcoma or a true mixture of carcinoma and sarcoma, molecular analyses have demonstrated that most are monoclonal, with carcinomatous and sarcomatoid elements thought to represent divergent differentiation or metaplastic evolution from a common epithelial precursor.[15] Carcinosarcomas are frequently subclassified as homologous (having mesenchymal elements native to the uterus) or heterologous (having foreign mesenchymal elements with features of, e.g., cartilage, bone, striated muscle, or fat), and the epithelial components can be endometrioid, serous, or clear cell. However, neither the presence of heterologous elements nor the epithelial pattern has been clearly demonstrated to be correlated with outcome.[16]

Histologic Grade

The current FIGO grading system is summarized in **Table 13.2**. Although histologic grade is one of the strongest predictors of outcome, evolving definitions and variations in the application of the current system are frequent sources of confusion:

- With the 1988 system, vague definitions were made more specific and, for the first time, pathologists were advised to increase the grade if the degree of nuclear atypia was inconsistent with the architectural grade (**Table 13.2**). This led to a major shift in grade assignments, with a greater tendency for tumors to be diagnosed as grade 1 and with a few tumors (e.g., clear cell and serous carcinomas) assigned a higher grade than had been possible under the previous system. Because of these changes, histologic grade assignments should be viewed with skepticism for any study that included patients with tumors diagnosed before the late 1980s.
- Over time, pathologists also shifted their criteria for diagnosing cancer, reclassifying some of the most well-differentiated lesions as atypical hyperplasia.[17] It is likely that many patients entered in studies prior to the mid-1980s would not be diagnosed as having cancer by current criteria; even today, the distinction between low-grade cancer and benign abnormalities can sometimes be difficult.[18]
- Even in the modern era, studies have demonstrated major inconsistencies in the way grade is assigned.[2,5] In a notable example, central pathology review of the postoperative radiation therapy in endometrial cancer (PORTEC) trials led to reassignment of ~40% of cancers to a lower grade.[19–21] Studies from the United States suggest a similar rate of reassignment when tumors initially diagnosed by general pathologists are subjected to expert review.[2,5]

Myometrial Invasion

Lymph node metastasis, recurrence, and death from endometrial cancer are all strongly correlated with the depth of myometrial invasion by tumor. Although lymph node involvement is extremely rare in patients whose cancers are confined to the endometrium, as tumor invades the underlying muscle it has access to a rich network of lymphatics that can carry metastases to the regional nodes (Chapter 5). Many methods have been used to describe the extent of myometrial infiltration. The FIGO staging system uses a threshold of 50% invasion for distinguishing stages IA and IB. Although this simple dichotomization produces two groups with different outcomes, it also diminishes the predictive power of this important variable. Strong arguments have been made for describing the degree of invasiveness in thirds,[22] as a continuous variable[23] or as an absolute rather than a fractional measurement.[24] Although measurement of the depth of invasion is usually straightforward, significant errors can occur. Ali et al.[25] reported reassignment of FIGO (1988) stage in 12% of referred cases after review by an expert pathologist. Tumors that are exophytic or involve adenomyosis can pose particular challenges. Endometrioid cancers frequently involve foci of adenomyosis that can exist deep within the uterine wall. When cancer arising in adenomyosis extends to invade adjacent myometrium, the tumor is staged according to the location of the invasive focus; however, some authors have suggested that measurement from the endomyometrial junction of the adenomyosis would more accurately predict the prognosis of such tumors.[26,27]

Lymph Vascular Space Invasion

LVSI has consistently been correlated with the probabilities of lymph node metastasis and locoregional recurrence[23,28]; these risks are increased if the LVSI is extensive.[26] However, there is considerable interobserver variability in the assessment of LVSI, due in part to artifacts of processing that can mimic LVSI. Several investigators have noted that LVSI is more likely to be diagnosed and is less likely to be correlated with lymph node involvement if the uterine specimen was removed laparoscopically.[29] It has been hypothesized that the balloon tip intrauterine manipulators used during laparoscopic hysterectomy can displace tumor cells into vascular spaces, causing so-called "vascular pseudoinvasion." In some cases, this may be indistinguishable from true LVSI. More study will be needed to determine how this potential source of error should influence the use of LVSI as a prognostic factor in endometrial cancers.

Tumor Size

Several authors have found significant correlations between the diameter of the primary tumor (≤2 cm vs. >2 cm) and the presence of lymph node metastasis[23,30]; the tumor diameter has been variously defined as the average[30] or the maximum diameter as measured on fresh tissue.[23] The significance of tumor size seems to be independent of invasion depth or tumor grade.

Cervical Involvement

The presence of cervical involvement has classically been considered to be an independent risk factor for recurrence, although robust evidence supporting this can be difficult to find. Most studies of stage II disease have included patients who were classified using the inaccurate pre-1988 clinical staging system (**Table 13.1**) or who had FIGO 1988 stage IIA disease. Also, nearly all studies are confounded by treatment selection bias. That said, several investigators have cited cervical stromal involvement as an independent predictor of lymph node involvement.[23,31] Investigators from the Mayo Clinic also reported that cervical stromal involvement was associated with poorer overall survival for patients with grade 3 or type II carcinomas but that it was not correlated with survival of patients with lower-grade cancers.[32] It seems likely that the depth of cervical stromal invasion is important; however, the only studies that have examined this are small and confounded by treatment selection bias.[33,34] It should be recognized that the indistinct junction between the LUS and endocervix can be a cause of significant intraobserver variability in the designation of cervical stromal involvement. Early stromal involvement can also be difficult to distinguish from involvement of invaginating endocervical glands.[35]

LUS Involvement

The most notable feature of tumors originating in the LUS is the high incidence (about 30%) of associated Lynch syndrome.[36] Although tumors *arising* in the LUS are, due to their proximity to the cervix, more likely to be stage II disease, they do not seem to have an increased incidence of lymph node involvement. On the other hand, fundal carcinomas that extend to involve the LUS are likely to be large tumors with other high-risk features associated with advanced disease. The mixture of these two presentations has led to inconsistent conclusions about the prognostic significance of LUS involvement. There is, however, little evidence that LUS involvement *per se* is an independent predictor of prognosis when tumor size, depth of invasion, and other risk factors are taken into account.

Lymph Node Involvement and Its Influence on Prognosis

All of the adverse risk factors discussed above have been associated with an increased rate of lymph node metastases and most are independent predictors of metastasis. In 2013, AlHilli et al.[23] proposed a nomogram for predicting the likelihood of lymphatic dissemination. This tool, based on findings in 883 patients from the Mayo Clinic who had lymphadenectomy or who were observed without adjuvant treatment (**Fig. 13.1**), demonstrates the complex relationship between intrauterine risk factors and lymph node metastasis. A reconfiguration of the Mayo Clinic data (**Fig. 13.2**) clearly illustrates why a simple combination of grade and depth of invasion is insufficient to predict the risk of metastasis. Although the quantitative accuracy of the Mayo Clinic nomogram needs to be validated with another dataset, it is one of the more useful tools currently available for predicting the relative risk of lymph node involvement and the need for adjuvant treatment, particularly for patients who have not had lymphadenectomy.

As discussed in Chapter 5, cancers involving the uterine fundus can spread directly to the paraaortic lymph nodes, in some cases even without evidence of pelvic node metastasis. In a prospective study of intermediate- to high-risk local features, Mariani et al.[37] reported that, of 57 patients who had formal pelvic and paraaortic lymphadenectomy, 51% had involvement of both the pelvic and paraaortic nodes, 33% had pelvic node involvement only, and 16% had only paraaortic node involvement. Of 26 patients who had detailed information about the location of paraaortic nodes, 77% had metastases superior to the inferior mesenteric artery. This pattern of nodal dissemination is very different from that of cervical cancer and has important implications for radiation therapy planning.

Lymph node involvement is undoubtedly a predictor of poorer prognosis. However, several factors may influence the survival rates reported in clinical series:

- Adjuvant external beam therapy reduces the rate of regional recurrence and, as will be discussed later, adjuvant treatment probably improves survival.
- Variations in the extent of surgical evaluation and in the methods of histologic processing of lymph nodes are sources of significant stage migration in patients with endometrial cancer. In particular, recent interest in lymphatic mapping with sentinel node evaluation is likely to increase the proportion of patients found to have very early micrometastases or isolated tumor cells in sentinel nodes[38]; this may lead to an appearance of improved survival rates for patients with stage IIIC disease.

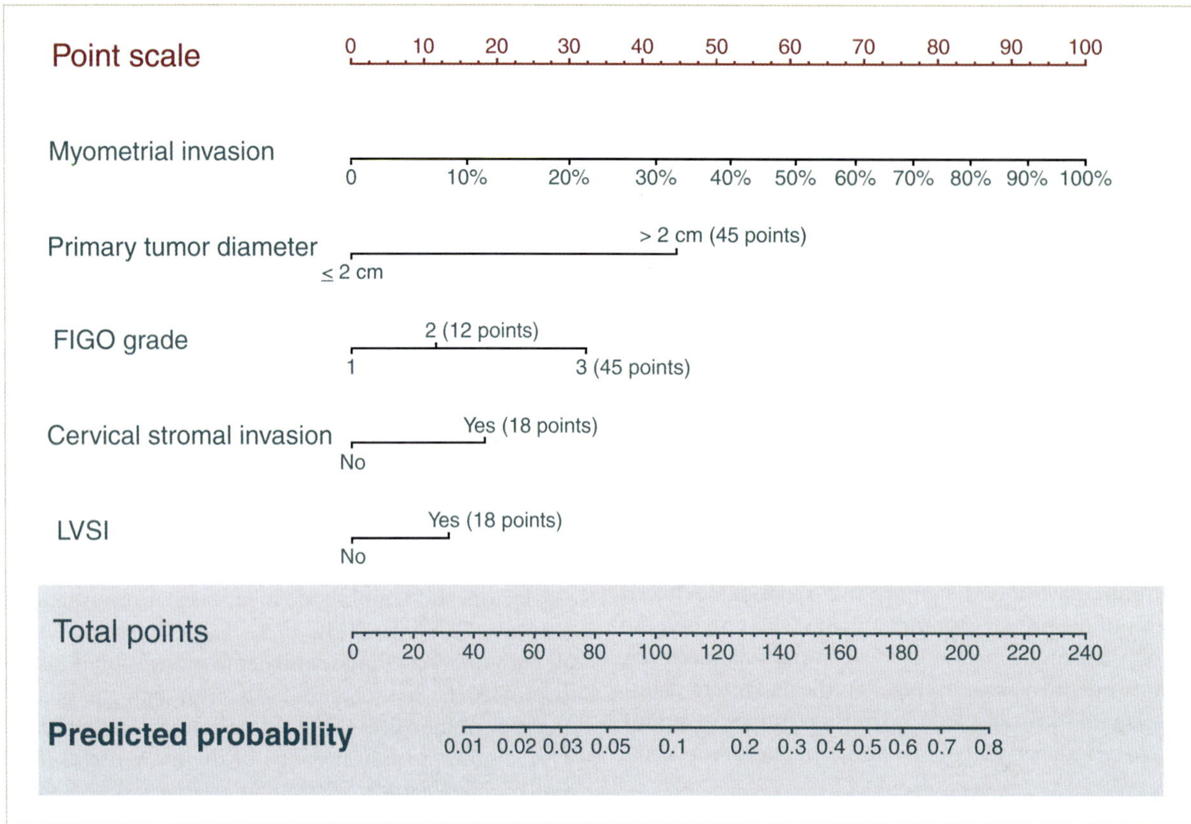

FIGURE 13.1 Mayo Clinic nomogram for the prediction of lymph node metastases, as proposed by AlHilli et al.[23] The study was based on 883 patients with type I cancers who had pelvic and paraaortic lymph node dissection or who were followed without adjuvant treatment. (LVSI, lymph vascular space invasion.)

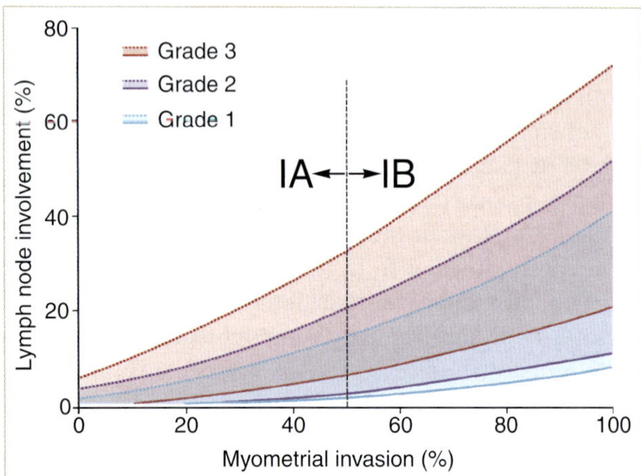

FIGURE 13.2 In this figure, the predicted lymph node rates specified in the Mayo Clinic nomogram shown in Figure 13.1[23] **have been reconfigured to illustrate why the risks of node involvement cannot be accurately predicted using grade and depth of invasion alone.** The lower (*solid*) lines of each color represent the predicted rate of lymph node metastases for patients with grade 1, 2, or 3 disease who have tumors <2 cm without lymph vascular space invasion (LVSI). The upper (*dotted*) lines represent the predicted rates for each grade if patients have larger tumors with LVSI. Note the marked overlap in risk depending on the presence or absence of risk factors other than grade and depth of invasion.

Evidence suggests that with appropriate volume-directed treatment, the prognosis of stage IIIC2 disease is not markedly different from that of stage IIIC1 tumors of similar grade.[39] The influence of other nodal factors including the number of nodes, nodal ratio, and presence of gross disease has been studied to a very limited degree, with various conclusions.[39–42]

Other Factors

Peritoneal Cytology

Although peritoneal cytology was for many years included as a criterion for FIGO staging (Table 13.1), most evidence suggests that it is not a useful independent predictor of prognosis. For this reason, it was removed from the FIGO staging of endometrial cancer in 2009. Peritoneal cytology may have served as a surrogate for undetected serous cancers in early reviews. However, serous cancers tend to recur intraperitoneally despite negative cytology results, and endometrioid cancers rarely recur intraperitoneally even in the context of positive washings. The excellent outcome of patients who have positive results for peritoneal cytology without other risk factors suggests that the development of intraperitoneal metastasis has more to do with cancer biology than with the presence of free-floating intraperitoneal tumor cells. Some authors have reported an increased incidence of tumor cells in the peritoneal cytology of patients undergoing laparoscopic (as opposed to open abdominal) hysterectomy for low-grade cancers[43]; although there is no evidence that this alters prognosis, some clinicians have advocated tying the fallopian tubes to prevent tumor egress during uterine manipulation.

Molecular Markers

Investigators are currently studying a host of molecular markers that promise to refine our predictive capabilities, although none are in routine use today. See Chapter 1 for discussion of this topic.

Patient Factors

Most authors have found a correlation between increasing age and poor prognosis. This reflects, in part, the fact that older patients are more likely to have serous and other high-grade tumor types, whereas young women with endometrial cancer tend to have low-grade endometrioid cancers. However, age is often reported to be an independent predictor of prognosis even after adjustment for other known prognostic factors.[37] For this reason, age is included in several definitions of "high intermediate-risk" stage I disease.[19,22] Other patient factors that may be correlated with the rate of relapse are race, obesity, and diabetes mellitus.[44] Overall survival is also heavily influenced by the comorbid illnesses that are often present in this group of patients[32]; intercurrent death is another factor that can reduce the influence of adjuvant treatments.

FIGO Stage

The FIGO staging system was converted from a clinical to a pathologic staging system in 1988 and was further modified in the most recent (2009) version (Tables 13.1 and 13.2). The current system incorporates some of the most important predictors of prognosis and is correlated with outcome, although there are few large series that have prospectively employed the 2009 version. The FIGO system is unusual for staging systems in that it requires an assessment of tumor grade and specifies criteria for assigning grade. However, as discussed above, the outcomes and proportions of patients falling into various subgroups are dependent on the experience of pathologists assigning grade, the rigor of surgical staging, and possibly on the methods of adjuvant treatment used to treat high-risk disease.

Mechanisms and Risk Factors for Vaginal Recurrence

An understanding of the mechanism of vaginal recurrences has important implications for the development of an effective preventive strategy. Dissemination through the vaginal lymphatics has been suggested as a potential route for vaginal metastasis leading to recurrence. However, several features of vaginal recurrence suggest that posthysterectomy implantation of tumor cells in surgically disturbed vaginal tissues, possibly encouraged by growth factors produced by the healing process (Chapter 3), may provide a more likely explanation.

- More than 80% of recurrences are isolated and localized to the vaginal apex, usually in the region of the vaginal incision. Regional lymphatic anatomy does not readily explain such a selective route for metastasis from the uterine fundus.
- Most vaginal recurrences can be prevented by treating only the vaginal apical mucosa, indicating that vaginal recurrence is not part of a broader pattern of lymphatic dissemination.
- It is not uncommon to see vaginal recurrences after removal of high-grade tumors that had little or no invasion of myometrium or lymphatic spaces.[45,46] In fact, multivariate analyses suggest that LVSI, which is a strong predictor of regional recurrence and disease-related death, is not a major predictor of vaginal recurrence.[26,45]
- The fact that vaginal metastases are far less common as a site of initial involvement (<1% of cases) than as a site of recurrence speaks against lymphatic dissemination as an important mechanism.
- Adenocarcinomas have the well-known capacity to implant in other operative sites, including abdominal incisions, port sites (CS 13.9), and even episiotomy sites.

Histologic grade is probably the most powerful predictor of vaginal recurrence.[46,47] The rates of locoregional recurrence (most of which are vaginal) have been reported to be 20% or more even for superficially invasive grade 3 carcinomas[48] (Fig. 13.3). Fewer data are available for patients with deeply

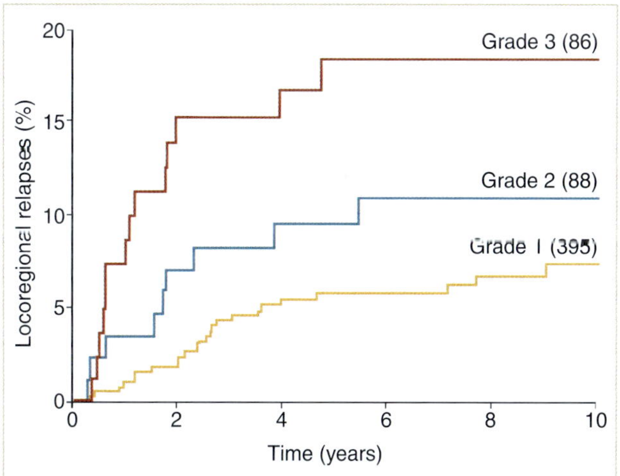

FIGURE 13.3 From PORTEC-1, the probability of locoregional (vaginal or pelvic) relapse according to revised histologic grade (following central pathology review); ~75% of the locoregional recurrences in this trial were confined to the vagina. These curves underestimate the risk of local recurrence for untreated patients because half of the patients contributing to these curves received pelvic radiation therapy, which reduced the overall rate of locoregional recurrence by about 75%. Locoregional recurrence rates by grade were not given for the two arms, but from these data, one can estimate a local recurrence rate of more than 25% in untreated patients with grade 3 disease. Because deeply invasive grade 3 tumors were excluded from the trial, this high recurrence rate was for patients who had stage IA, grade 3 disease. (From Creutzberg CL, van Putten WL, Koper PC, et al. Survival after relapse in patients with endometrial cancer: results from a randomized trial. *Gynecol Oncol.* 2003;89:201–209.)

invasive grade 3 disease because they usually receive some form of adjuvant treatment. However, in PORTEC trials, local recurrences were three times as frequent for stage IB, grade 2 cancers than for stage IA, grade 2 cancers, suggesting that the depth of myometrial invasion is also a risk factor for vaginal recurrence.[48]

DEVELOPING A MULTIDISCIPLINARY TREATMENT STRATEGY

Surgical Management

Although the initial surgical management of uterine cancer was traditionally performed via laparotomy, today the operation is increasingly being performed using a laparoscopic or robot-assisted laparoscopic technique. Randomized trials have demonstrated that laparoscopic surgery is associated with longer operating times but shorter hospital stays, fewer serious postoperative complications, and less postoperative pain.[49,50] Long-term follow-up suggests that survival rates are similar. Late complication rates have not yet been analyzed for patients treated with adjuvant radiation in large randomized trials. However, a retrospective study of patients who had postoperative pelvic radiation after hysterectomy suggested that the rate of nonrectal bowel injury was significantly lower for patients whose surgery was performed laparoscopically rather than via laparotomy.[51] Laparoscopic port-site recurrences are uncommon (0.24% in the LAP2 randomized trial[52]) but are important to recognize because they can often be cured with local treatment **(CS 13.9)**.[53]

Hysterectomy for Endometrial Cancer

In most cases, the surgical treatment of endometrial cancer includes a total (type I) hysterectomy (Chapter 3) and bilateral salpingo-oophorectomy. The adnexa are removed because they are a potential site of metastasis or, occasionally, second primary ovarian cancers (Chapter 1). For patients with cervical stromal involvement, a radical or modified radical hysterectomy may be indicated, particularly if there is extensive cervical invasion or a wish to avoid postoperative pelvic radiation therapy.[54]

Lymph Node Evaluation

Although pathologic nodal evaluation has been incorporated in the FIGO staging system since 1988 (**Table 13.1**), questions persist about the value of universal surgical staging. Pelvic and paraaortic lymphadenectomies markedly increase the rates of perioperative and long-term complications[55] (Chapter 3). These side effects may be difficult to justify for patients with minimally invasive, low-grade cancers that have a negligible probability of lymph node metastases and perhaps even for those who have a sufficiently high risk that adjuvant treatment would be recommended even in the face of a negative dissection.

Two randomized trials that evaluated the benefit of surgical staging each failed to demonstrate any improvement in survival for the patients who had lymphadenectomy.[56,57] Although most patients in these trials did not have high-risk intrauterine features, these studies clearly argued against the routine use of pelvic lymphadenectomy for low-risk endometrial cancers. Retrospective cohort studies suggest that there may be some benefit for higher-risk patients if a much more extensive pelvic and paraaortic lymphadenectomy is performed[58]; however, this question has not yet been explored in a controlled prospective trial.

Although there is little evidence that lymphadenectomy is actually therapeutic, knowledge about lymph node involvement can be very useful for triaging patients to receive adjuvant treatments. The ideal strategy would be a method that would obtain this information without subjecting all patients to the side effects of extensive lymphadenectomy. Two approaches to a more selective form of lymph node evaluation have been studied:

- *Intraoperative evaluation.* The Mayo Clinic group has recommended intraoperative evaluation of the uterus with frozen section analysis to determine the grade, depth of invasion, and primary tumor diameter. In their experience, the rate of lymph node metastases is very low if the tumor is grade 1–2, invades <50%, and measures <2 cm in diameter or if it is grade 3 and <2 cm with no myometrial invasion; lymphadenectomy is not recommended for such cases.[59] These authors reported a discordance rate between intraoperative and final assessments of only 1.3%; other authors have reported higher discordance rates but most have not incorporated tumor diameter in their intraoperative assessments.[59]
- *Sentinel node evaluation.* Several investigators have explored the potential role of lymphatic mapping with sentinel node evaluation in patients with uterine cancer.[38,60,61] This intriguing though still investigational approach may provide important diagnostic information without the morbidity of a full lymphadenectomy. Although several investigators have used intrauterine injections to map the sentinel nodes, a more practical approach may be to inject the cervix, which shares its pelvic lymphatic drainage with the uterus; in experienced hands, low false-negative rates can be achieved, although there is a steep learning curve.[61] Ultrastructural staging of sentinel nodes detects some small micrometastases including isolated tumor cells that would otherwise go undetected; the significance of these very small metastases remains uncertain. One disadvantage of the cervical injection method is that it does not identify possible paraaortic sentinel nodes,[38] although the probability of paraaortic metastases seems to be low if the pelvic sentinel nodes are negative.

Staging of Type II Cancers

Because of their predilection to intraperitoneal spread, serous tumors and carcinosarcomas should be staged like an ovarian cancer (Chapter 14) with omentectomy and peritoneal biopsies.

The Role of Chemotherapy

Although chemotherapy has come to have a widely accepted role in the adjuvant treatment of advanced-stage endometrial cancer, the evidence of benefit, particularly as a single modality, is actually very weak, resting almost entirely on the interpretation of a single trial (GOG-122) that, at least in retrospect, had serious flaws.

GOG 122—Chemotherapy versus Whole-Abdominal Radiation Therapy

In 2006, the Gynecologic Oncology Group published results of GOG-122, a randomized trial conceived in the early 1990s, that compared adjuvant chemotherapy with whole abdominal radiation therapy (WART) for patients who had stage III or IV endometrial cancers limited to the abdomen and pelvis.[62] The results of GOG-122 were interpreted as showing significantly better relapse free and overall survival for patients who had chemotherapy. Its publication led to a marked increase in the use of adjuvant chemotherapy, and the trial continues to be the primary source cited as evidence of the superiority of chemotherapy over radiation therapy in treatment of high-risk disease. However, close examination of the trial reveals flaws that may call into question the validity of the authors' conclusions.

- The acute side effects of WART undoubtedly contributed to many incomplete or protracted treatments. These large fields, now known to be unnecessary for many of the subgroups included in this trial, compromised the intensity and probably the effectiveness of radiation.
- At least 16% of patients were known to have gross residual disease remaining after surgery. However, because no preoperative or postoperative tomographic imaging was required for patients in GOG-122, it is likely that the extent of residual disease was often underestimated. The specified dose of radiation given in this study was probably not adequate to control gross disease. Furthermore, many of the patients in the trial had stage IV disease with peritoneal involvement.
- Subset analysis of GOG-122 revealed a higher survival rate for patients with endometrioid cancers treated with chemotherapy but failed to demonstrate any benefit for patients with serous cancers.
- The actual relapse-free survival rates for the two treatment arms were similar (**Fig. 13.4**). It was only after correction for an imbalance in the stage distribution between the two arms that the chemotherapy arm was found to have superior outcome. Because patients did not have consistent nodal staging, the validity of this correction can be questioned.
- Although the uncorrected overall survival rates seem to favor chemotherapy, the difference between the overall and relapse-free survival rates of patients treated with chemotherapy (**Fig. 13.4**) suggests that many chemotherapy failures were salvaged; the authors state that many patients received radiation therapy salvage treatment. This leads to the question of whether more patients were cured with chemotherapy or whether salvage was simply more likely to be feasible for patients who had not already received an incomplete or inadequate course of radiation. Subsequent trials have not confirmed the value of chemotherapy alone as an adjuvant.

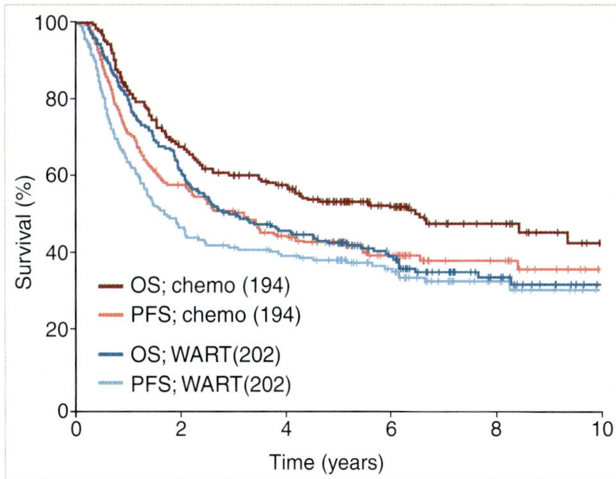

FIGURE 13.4 Progression-free survival (PFS) and overall survival (OS) for patients treated with either whole-abdominal radiation therapy (WART) or chemotherapy (doxorubicin and cisplatin) in the Gynecologic Oncology Group (GOG)-122 Trial. The curves have been superimposed to highlight the relationships between PFS and OS rates for the two arms. Without the statistical adjustment made in the final analysis, the difference in PFS between the two treatment arms was small. For patients treated with WART, the OS meets the PFS curve, suggesting that patients on average survived 1 to 2 years after recurrence with few salvages. In contrast, the OS curve for patients treated with chemotherapy remains well above the PFS curve even at 10 years, suggesting that the higher OS of patients treated with chemotherapy resulted from successful salvage of chemotherapy failures. (Figure adapted from Randall ME, Filiaci VL, Muss H, et al. Randomized phase III trial of whole-abdominal irradiation versus doxorubicin and cisplatin chemotherapy in advanced endometrial carcinoma: a Gynecologic Oncology Group Study. *J Clin Oncol.* 2006;24:36–44.)

Other Randomized Trials

Two trials have compared adjuvant pelvic radiation versus chemotherapy, but neither has demonstrated a difference in survival between the two treatments.[63,64] A third trial, GOG-249,[65] randomized patients to receive either adjuvant chemotherapy (carboplatin and paclitaxel) plus vaginal brachytherapy or pelvic radiation; this as-yet unpublished trial was reported at the 2014 annual meeting of the Society of Gynecologic Oncologists to show no difference in survival between the two arms, but patients treated with chemotherapy had higher rates of pelvic recurrence and acute toxicity.

Probably, the most compelling evidence that adjuvant chemotherapy can contribute to the curative treatment of endometrial cancer comes from the 2010 report by Hogberg et al.[66] of the combined results of two randomized trials of radiation alone versus radiation plus chemotherapy. The study is difficult to summarize because the eligibility criteria and treatments differed between the two trials and because the contributing trials allowed a variety of chemotherapy regimens and sequences. However, the combined results did demonstrate a significantly better relapse-free survival and a trend toward improved overall survival ($p = 0.07$) for patients who received chemotherapy in addition to radiation therapy.

Retrospective Studies

Retrospective data suggest that radiation therapy alone or combined with chemotherapy may be more effective than chemotherapy alone, at least for patients with stage III disease[39,67] (discussed further below).

Schedules of Combined Chemotherapy and Radiation

A variety of schedules and sequences have been used to combine chemotherapy with radiation. A sandwich technique of radiation inserted in the middle of a six-cycle course of chemotherapy gained popularity after an encouraging report published by Secord et al.[68] in 2009; however, subsequent analysis from this group failed to confirm the advantage of this approach over other sequential schedules.[67] We tend to prefer a schedule of concurrent chemoradiation followed by adjuvant chemotherapy, because this approach does not delay the start of radiation and avoids a break in the course of chemotherapy (Chapter 3) **(CS 13.3, 13.6, and 13.7)**. However, more comparative studies are needed to determine when combined therapy is indicated and the most effective schedule of administration.

Most of the randomized studies of adjuvant chemotherapy have used combinations of cyclophosphamide, doxorubicin, and cisplatin (CAP).[62–64,66] However, today clinicians are increasingly favoring the use of carboplatin and paclitaxel, a regimen that seems in nonrandomized studies to have a response rate at least similar to that for CAP. GOG-249[65] and several ongoing trials are evaluating the efficacy of carboplatin and paclitaxel in a randomized setting.

Cisplatin is most commonly used in concurrent chemoradiation schedules. We have found that most patients can tolerate at least four courses of subsequent carboplatin and paclitaxel, even after extended field irradiation.[69]

In summary, there is currently no evidence that chemotherapy alone is superior to radiation as adjuvant therapy for locoregionally confined disease. However, there is evidence that chemotherapy may be beneficial when added to radiation in selected situations. Specific examples are discussed below and in case studies at the end of this chapter.

MANAGEMENT CONSIDERATIONS ACCORDING TO DISEASE EXTENT

Stage I, Type I Cancers

The value of adjuvant radiation therapy for early-stage disease has been evaluated in six prospective randomized trials comparing pelvic radiation with either observation or vaginal brachytherapy (**Table 13.3**).[19,21,22,70–72] None of these trials has demonstrated a significant difference in overall survival. However, all of these trials were hampered by the inclusion of a large number of patients with very favorable cancers; this is evidenced by the small number of endometrial cancer-related deaths in the control arms of the trials (**Table 13.3**). For example, in GOG-99,[22] 40% of patients had grade 1 tumors and 59% had less than 50% invasion. The PORTEC trials excluded patients with deeply invasive grade 3 disease; however, postentry expert pathology review also indicated that community pathologists had repeatedly overinterpreted the grade of endometrial lesions—in the final analysis, 59% of patients entered in PORTEC-1 and 78% of patients in PORTEC-2 had grade 1 cancers. This probably explains why only about 6% of patients in either trial died of endometrial cancer-related causes. PORTEC-2, which randomized patients between vaginal cuff brachytherapy and pelvic radiation, seems to have included very few patients having multiple risk factors but does indicate that vaginal treatment is sufficient to prevent recurrence for most patients with intermediate-risk disease.

In a *post hoc* analysis of GOG-99, the authors identified a subgroup of patients with "high intermediate-risk disease" (**Table 13.4**) who represented one-third of the study population but had two-thirds of the disease-related events; survival analysis suggested that pelvic radiation was beneficial in this group of patients (**Fig. 13.5**). However, patients with these high intermediate-risk factors are relatively uncommon, and it can be difficult to design trials with these restrictive entry criteria. In their subsequent trial, GOG-249,[65] the Gynecologic Oncology Group used a looser definition of high intermediate risk, undoubtedly lessening the margin for improvement with adjuvant treatments. The PORTEC group also tried to define a high intermediate-risk group from the results of PORTEC-1; however, the more restrictive criteria and disproportionate entry of grade 1 tumors in PORTEC-2 still resulted in a cohort of patients with relatively low-risk disease. Ultimately, none of the trials listed in **Table 13.3** included patients with sufficient risk to have any chance of detecting a benefit from external beam therapy.

When considering whether to recommend adjuvant treatment, it is important to consider:

- Risk factors for vaginal or lymph node recurrence (see section "Risk Assessment")
- The status of lymph nodes and extent of lymph node dissection
- Risk factors for radiation-related complications

TABLE 13.3 Randomized Trials Evaluating the Role of Pelvic Radiation Therapy in Patients with Early-Stage Endometrial Cancer

Trial	Eligibility	Randomization	Number of patients	Endometrial cancer deaths (percent of total)	Outcome
Norwegian Radium Hospital[72]	Clinical stage I (FIGO 1971)	VBT VBT + pelvic RT	277 260	25 (9%) 28 (11%)	OS: no significant difference
GOG-99[22]	IB, IC, II (occult) (FIGO 1988)	Observation Pelvic RT	202 190	19 (9%) 15 (8%)	LRR: decreased with pelvic RT (14% vs. 4%) OS: no significant difference
PORTEC-1[19]	ICG1 or G2 or IAG3 or IB G3 (FIGO 1988)	Observation Pelvic RT	361 354	18 (5%) 23 (6%)	LRR: decreased with pelvic RT (7% vs. 2%) OS: no significant difference
ASTEC/EN.5 Study Group[71]	I or IIA with >50% MI or G3 (FIGO 1988)	Observation or VBT Pelvic RT	453 452	41 (9%) 37 (8%)	OS: no significant difference
PORTEC-2[21]	FIGO 1988	VBT Pelvic RT	213 214	15 (7%) 10 (5%)	LRR: no significant difference DFS, OS: no significant difference
Swedish cooperative group[70]	Stage I, nuclear G1–G2 and G3 or >50% MI or DNA aneuploidy	VBT VBT + pelvic RT	223 224	27 (12%) 15 (7%)	LRR: no significant difference OS: no significant difference

VBT, vaginal brachytherapy; RT, radiation therapy; OS, overall survival; LRR, locoregional recurrence rate; GOG, Gynecologic Oncology Group; PORTEC, postoperative radiation therapy in endometrial cancer; MI, myometrial invasion; G, grade.

On the basis of randomized trials and other available data, pelvic radiation generally should not be recommended for stage I disease unless the patient has either (1) GOG-99 high intermediate-risk disease (if lymphadenectomy has been performed) or (2) multiple risk factors of deep invasion, LVSI, grade, and tumor size that predict a significant risk of lymph node involvement (if adequate lymphadenectomy has not been performed) (Fig. 13.1). In general, if the estimated risk of nodal metastasis is >15% to 20%, we tend to recommend pelvic radiation therapy if there are no major contraindications.

In most cases, patients who have intermediate-risk factors that do not meet these criteria should be observed or treated with vaginal brachytherapy only. Using trial data (particularly

TABLE 13.4 Definitions of "High Intermediate-Risk Disease" in GOG and PORTEC Trials

Trial	Definition	Comments
GOG-99[22]	Risk factors: G2 or G3; LVSI; outer 1/3 myometrial invasion <50 years old: 3 risk factors ≥50, <70 years old: 2 risk factors ≥70 years old: 1 risk factors	"Selective bilateral pelvic and paraaortic lymphadenectomy" required Stage I or stage II "occult" (FIGO 1988)
GOG-249[65]	Risk factors: G2 or G3; LVSI; outer 1/2 myometrial invasion <50 years old: 3 risk factors ≥50, <70 years old: 2 risk factors ≥70 years old: 1 risk factors	Lymphadenectomy performed in 89% of patients Stage I, IIA, or IIB disease (FIGO 1988)
PORTEC-2[21]	>60 years old plus stage ICG1 or ICG2 or stage IIA plus G1–G2 or G3 with <50% myometrial invasion	Most patients did not have lymphadenectomy; deeply invasive grade 3 tumors were excluded from this definition

LVSI, lymph vascular space invasion; G, grade.

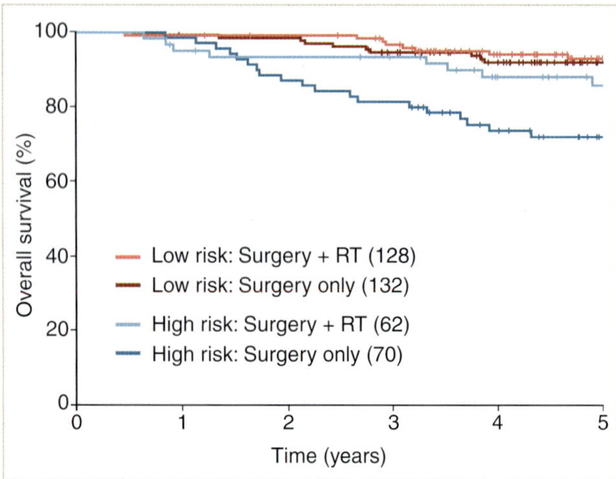

FIGURE 13.5 Overall survival of patients with low- or high intermediate-risk endometrial cancer treated in the Gynecologic Oncology Group (GOG)-99 trial. For patients with low intermediate-risk disease (two-thirds of the patients entered), the overall survival was high for patients who received no adjuvant treatment and was not improved with pelvic radiation. However, in this unplanned subset analysis, patients with high intermediate-risk disease seemed to have a better survival rate if they received adjuvant radiation therapy (RT). (Figure reprinted from Keys HM, Roberts JA, Brunetto VL, et al. A phase III trial of surgery with or without adjunctive external pelvic radiation therapy in intermediate risk endometrial adenocarcinoma: A Gynecologic Oncology Group study. *Gynecol Oncol.* 2004;92:744-751.)

GOG-99 risk criteria) and risk factor analyses summarized in the section "Risk Assessment," recommendations can be made for the use of adjuvant vaginal brachytherapy or pelvic radiation therapy (Table 13.5). However, no table can fully summarize the complex combinations of patient and tumor risk factors in all their gradations.

The Role of Vaginal Brachytherapy

As discussed in the section "Mechanisms and Risk Factors for Vaginal Recurrence," the vagina is one of the most common sites of recurrence after hysterectomy. These recurrences can usually be prevented with intracavitary vaginal brachytherapy. Although vaginal recurrences can often be cured, the morbidity of salvage treatment is considerably higher than that of prophylactic treatment. Because the recurrence rate is particularly high for patients with type II or grade 3 cancers, and because the salvage rate of high-grade recurrences is <50%, we recommend treatment with at least vaginal brachytherapy for nearly all high-grade cancers as well as for patients who do not receive pelvic radiation therapy for high intermediate-risk disease (Table 13.5).

Because ~80% of vaginal recurrences are localized to the apex, we usually recommend treatment of only the proximal one-third of the vagina. Recurrences that occur distal to the apical vagina tend most often to be suburethral; prevention of such recurrences requires treatment of the entire vagina, which would be expected to significantly increase vaginal shortening and narrowing. However, many clinicians

TABLE 13.5 Suggested Adjuvant Treatment for Patients with Stage I, Type I Endometrial Cancers

	Lymph nodes evaluated[a]		Lymph nodes not evaluated[a]	
	No added risk factors	With risk factors[b]	No added risk factors	With risk factors[b]
Grade 1, inner 1/3	Observe	Observe	Observe	Observe
Grade 1, middle 1/3	Observe	±VBT	Observe	±VBT
Grade 1, outer 1/3	±VBT	VBT or pelvic RT[c]	±VBT	Pelvic RT or VBT[c]
Grade 2, inner 1/3	Observe	±VBT	Observe	Observe or VBT
Grade 2, middle 1/3	±VBT	VBT or pelvic RT[c]	±VBT	VBT or pelvic RT[c]
Grade 2, outer 1/3	VBT	Pelvic RT	VBT or pelvic RT[d]	Pelvic RT
Grade 3, inner 1/3	VBT	VBT	VBT	VBT or pelvic RT[c]
Grade 3, middle 1/3	VBT	VBT or pelvic RT[c]	VBT or pelvic RT[d]	Pelvic RT
Grade 3, outer 1/3	VBT or pelvic RT[d]	Pelvic RT	Pelvic RT	Pelvic RT

[a]*Patients who have a random sampling with fewer than two or three nodes are not usually considered to have an adequate node dissection, although stricter criteria have been used. In experienced hands, negative sentinel node evaluation may contribute to the level of confidence in a negative evaluation.*

[b]*Risk factors to be considered include LVSI, tumor diameter, and age >70 years as well as the depth of invasion within these categories.*

[c]*Choice based on the number of risk factors present as well as risk factors for side effects.*

[d]*Choice based on the depth of invasion within this category and risk factors for side effects.*

[e]*Choice based on the depth of invasion within this category, extent of lymph node dissection, and risk factors for side effects.*

VBT, vaginal brachytherapy; RT, radiation therapy.

recommend treatment of the upper two-thirds of the vagina, and the two approaches have never been directly compared.

Various brachytherapy schedules have been used for patients who require only vaginal treatment. One of the most popular is a schedule of three fractions of 7.5 Gy each, prescribed to a depth of 0.5 cm beneath the vaginal surface. Depending on the applicator diameter, the vaginal surface dose with this schedule is 11 to 12 Gy per fraction, equating to a BED_{3Gy} of about 160 and an equivalent vaginal surface dose at 2 Gy per fraction (EqD2) of ~95 Gy. This BED is nearly identical to that of the higher-dose regimen given in a Swedish randomized trial that compared six fractions of either 5 Gy or 2.5 Gy prescribed at 0.5 cm (Fig. 8.14).[73] In that trial, there was no difference in vaginal recurrence rates (which were <1% for patients in both arms), but the amount of vaginal shortening at 5 years was markedly greater for patients who received the high-dose regimen. We recommend a regimen that falls between the two Swedish schedules: five fractions of 6 Gy each, delivered to the surface of the proximal one-third of the vagina over 1.5 weeks. In our experience, this schedule is highly effective and causes little late vaginal toxicity. See Chapter 8 for more discussion of brachytherapy technique.

The value of a brachytherapy boost after pelvic radiation therapy is uncertain. Although retrospective and prospective studies have generally reported low vaginal recurrence rates after pelvic radiation therapy alone, the baseline risk in most of these studies was low. We currently add a modest dose of vaginal brachytherapy (usually 10-Gy vaginal surface dose in 2 fractions) after 45 Gy of external beam irradiation when we are treating patients who have high-risk disease.

Cervical Stromal Involvement

The treatment of stage II endometrial cancer must take into account the extent of disease in the cervix and the distribution of disease in the uterine body. Whenever possible, cancer involving the uterine fundus should be treated with hysterectomy, because the geometry and physics of intracavitary brachytherapy make it difficult to achieve adequate radiation doses to sterilize disease in the apical and lateral fundus. On the other hand, extensive cervical involvement can sometimes be difficult to clear surgically with adequate margins.

The literature on this topic is particularly difficult to interpret because the definition of stage II has shifted over time, most studies are small, and treatment selection factors (particularly measures of the extent of cervical involvement) are poorly characterized. Until recently, even cervical glandular involvement was routinely considered an indication for pelvic radiation. However, there is a small but growing body of data that can be used to guide management of stage II disease. It is also useful to consider cervical cancer management principles (Chapter 10) when deciding how to approach patients who have gross cervical involvement, and in the postoperative setting, the so-called "Sedlis criteria"[74] for postoperative treatment of node-negative cervical cancer (GOG-92) can be helpful in determining the need for adjuvant treatment of stage II endometrial cancers. Notably, in subset analysis of GOG-92, it was the adenocarcinomas of the cervix that appeared to derive the greatest benefit from postoperative pelvic radiation therapy, a finding that undoubtedly has some relevance for the treatment of müllerian adenocarcinomas that secondarily involve the cervix.

Microscopic Cervical Stromal Invasion

Early cervical stromal involvement is often discovered as an incidental finding after simple hysterectomy. On the basis of available data correlating prognosis with depth of stromal invasion,[23,31] small series of patients treated without pelvic radiation therapy,[75,76] and studies of postoperative treatment of cervical cancer,[74] we suggest the following guidelines:

- If there is <3 mm of cervical stromal invasion, no LVSI, no evidence of nodal metastasis after adequate surgical assessment, and no intrauterine findings suggesting the need for additional treatment, patients can probably be safely treated with vaginal brachytherapy only, even after simple hysterectomy.
- If there is invasion of the outer one-third of the cervical stroma or invasion of the middle one-third with LVSI, we usually recommend treatment with adjuvant pelvic radiation therapy.
- If these criteria are not met and there are no intrauterine risk factors suggesting a need for pelvic radiation, radical hysterectomy (or if simple hysterectomy was performed, parametrectomy) followed by vaginal cuff brachytherapy is probably sufficient.
- If the patient has not had an adequate surgical evaluation of the pelvic lymph nodes, pelvic radiation therapy is recommended for most patients who have more than 2 to 3 mm of cervical stromal invasion, particularly if the tumor is high grade.

Gross Involvement of the Cervix

If there is gross involvement of the cervix, the extent and distribution of disease should, if possible, be assessed preoperatively with MRI. If the results suggest that the disease can be resected with negative margins, radical hysterectomy with appropriate surgical staging is usually indicated. Depending on the operative findings, this is usually followed by external beam irradiation followed, particularly in cases of gross cervical involvement, by a brachytherapy boost to the vaginal apex.

If imaging suggests that there is near full-thickness invasion of the cervix (particularly in the region of the cervicovesical junction) or if there is suspicion of parametrial or proximal vaginal extension, initial treatment with radiation therapy may be indicated to avoid a surgical procedure that leaves positive margins (Chapter 3).

If there is both extensive uterine and cervical involvement, radiation may be initiated with tentative preoperative intent. In such a case, several things must be considered:

- Abdominopelvic CT or PET/CT should always be obtained before radiation to evaluate for possible extrauterine disease. Disease that would dictate a palliative treatment intent should be biopsied. Any suspicious nodes should be treated with a definitive dose of at least 60 Gy before surgery.
- In some cases, particularly for type II cancers, pretreatment laparoscopic staging to rule out intra-abdominal metastases may be indicated.
- *To avoid an unacceptable risk of postoperative fistula, the dose of brachytherapy to critical structures should be limited to no more than 70% to 75% of usual threshold doses* (after 45 Gy of pelvic radiation).
- In most cases, only a type I extrafascial hysterectomy should be performed; although a modified radical hysterectomy can be performed if there is no alternative, the risk of major complications is high.
- If the risk of an unsuccessful operation is greater than the 8% to 10% risk of intrauterine recurrence after definitive radiation therapy, hysterectomy may not be appropriate.
- For patients who have massive uterine disease and very extensive cervical or paracervical involvement, initial chemotherapy may be considered to attempt to reduce the disease volume. However, this neoadjuvant approach has its own set of challenges (Chapter 3).

In some cases, particularly if MRI indicates that the uterine fundus is spared or only superficially involved, the preferred local treatment may be definitive radiation therapy **(CS 13.2)**.

Fortunately, these cases are rare. Because of their complexity, they are best treated in a setting of close multidisciplinary cooperation.

Stage IIIC Disease

Many adjuvant approaches have been recommended for patients who have regional lymph node involvement:

- Radiation therapy only
- Concurrent chemoradiation plus adjuvant chemotherapy
- Sequential chemotherapy and radiation therapy with either radiation followed by chemotherapy or chemotherapy followed by radiation therapy
- Sandwich therapy, usually three courses of chemotherapy followed by radiation and then additional chemotherapy
- Chemotherapy alone

No prospective randomized trials have been dedicated to comparing these options for patients with stage IIIC disease. Subset analysis of the 190 patients with stage IIIC disease entered in GOG-122 found no significant difference in progression-free survival of patients treated with chemotherapy or WART. The MaNGO ILIADE-III study included only 63 patients with stage IIIC disease, an insufficient number to draw conclusions about the relative benefits of pelvic radiation versus combined radiation and chemotherapy.

Evidence of Radiation Therapy Benefit

Retrospective studies of stage IIIC disease do provide strong evidence of the benefit of radiation therapy in these cases.

The largest retrospective study of stage IIIC disease was reported by Secord et al.[67] (**Fig. 13.6**) in 2013. They reported the combined experiences of several institutions, comparing the outcome of 265 patients who received various adjuvant treatments for optimally cytoreduced (i.e., <1 cm) residual disease. Several conclusions could be drawn from this experience:

- Patients treated with chemotherapy alone had a significantly poorer survival rate than those treated with radiation even though patients treated with chemotherapy only were, on average, younger and had lower-grade cancers.
- The outcome of 45 patients treated with radiation therapy alone did not differ from the outcome for 161 patients treated with sequential chemotherapy and radiation.
- This update differed from an earlier report,[68] in that it found no advantage of sandwich treatment over other sequential regimens.

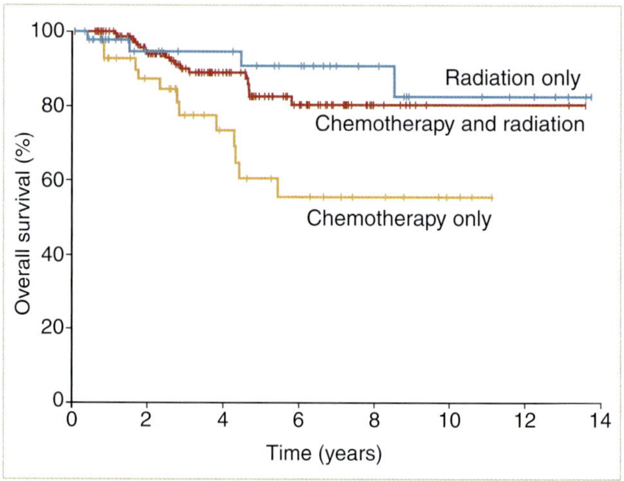

FIGURE 13.6 Overall survival of 265 patients with optimally resected stage IIIC endometrial cancer. In this retrospective review, Secord et al. reported a significantly higher pelvic recurrence rate and poorer overall survival rate for patients who did not receive external beam radiation therapy ($p = 0.005$). There was no significant difference between patients who had radiation therapy with or without chemotherapy. (Figure adapted from Secord AA, Geller MA, Broadwater G, et al. A multicenter evaluation of adjuvant therapy in women with optimally resected stage IIIC endometrial cancer. *Gynecol Oncol.* 2013;128:65-70.)

A second, smaller experience reported by Klopp et al.[39] yielded similar results, with significantly improved regional control and overall survival for patients who received radiation therapy.

When Is Combined Modality Adjuvant Treatment Indicated?

Five-year survival rates for patients with stage IIIC, grade 1 or 2 disease are 70% to 80%, even after treatment with radiation therapy alone. However, survival rates are poorer for patients with grade 3 or type II cancers and for patients with adnexal or cervical involvement.[39,77] Although the evidence of benefit is limited, we do recommend combined treatment for patients with grade 3 disease, serous cancers, or carcinosarcomas and for patients with gross residual disease. Combined modality options are discussed in detail in Chapter 3 and earlier in this chapter in the section titled "The Role of Chemotherapy."

For patients who have completely resected grade 1 or 2 cancers, the margin for improvement over radiation alone is narrower and should be balanced against the side effects of combined modality treatment **(CS 13.4)**. For reasons discussed in Chapter 3, we prefer the use of concurrent chemoradiation followed by adjuvant chemotherapy over regimens that delay radiation or cause breaks in chemotherapy delivery.

For patients with stage IIIC1 disease, the decision of whether to treat the paraaortic nodes can be a difficult one. Lymphadenectomy data show that 50% to 70% of patients who have pelvic node involvement also have involvement of the paraaortic nodes.[37] In all cases, imaging of the aortic region should be carefully scrutinized before pelvic radiation is initiated. Patients who have multiple or grossly enlarged pelvic nodes and whose tumors are located in the uterine fundus have a particularly high probability of paraaortic involvement; in such cases, an argument can be made to treat the paraaortic region prophylactically. Alternatively, the patient can be closely watched using CT after pelvic radiation; if detected early, paraaortic recurrence can often be cured with additional radiation.[78]

Other Rare Presentations

Adnexal Involvement

Expert pathology review is often needed to distinguish metastasis to the adnexa from simultaneous primary cancers. Simultaneous primary cancers are usually low-grade, endometrioid cancers of early stage in each respective site. Optimal treatments for each site should be integrated after multidisciplinary discussion. Patients who have true metastasis to the ovary have a poor prognosis. Chemotherapy plays a major role, although radiation therapy is often indicated to prevent local failure. The decision of whether to treat the vaginal cuff or pelvis is based on intrauterine risk factors.

Vaginal Involvement

The vagina is involved in <1% of cases at diagnosis. The approach to treatment of such patients must be individualized with a strategy developed in close cooperation between radiation oncologists and gynecologic oncologists. For patients who have apical vaginal involvement that can be cleared surgically, initial surgery is usually indicated. If there is isolated metastasis in the distal vagina, hysterectomy may be followed by radiation therapy with appropriate external or brachytherapy boost. If the hysterectomy cannot be performed without cutting through gross vaginal disease, preoperative radiation may be indicated after careful staging **(CS 13.3)**.

Medically Inoperable Endometrial Cancer

With improvements in minimally invasive surgical techniques, many patients who would previously have been referred for definitive radiation therapy can be safely treated surgically. Today, patients who are referred for definitive radiation therapy on the basis of medical inoperability generally have very severe medical conditions or extreme obesity.

In many cases, body habitus or medical conditions limit the diagnostic options. However, if possible, either MRI or PET should be obtained to provide information about the distribution of disease within the uterus and to assess for possible lymph node involvement. CT may be helpful but has limited utility in assessment of intrauterine tumor extent.

Pretreatment evaluation should always include a thorough medical assessment with specific attention to the risks of definitive surgery and of possible sedation methods for brachytherapy. Even in experienced hands, the risk of intrauterine recurrence after definitive radiation therapy including brachytherapy is usually 8% to 10%[79,80]; this risk must be carefully weighed against the risks of major morbidity or mortality from surgery.

Today, patients who are referred to radiation therapy specifically because of obesity typically have a body mass index (BMI) of 50 or more. Definitive treatment of patients of this size poses special technical challenges, for both external beam irradiation and brachytherapy, that are discussed in Chapters 6 and 8, respectively, and in **CS 13.1 and 13.10**.

The treatment strategy for patients who are deemed to have inoperable disease due to severe medical comorbidity must take into consideration the nature and severity of the patient's medical conditions and risk factors related to their endometrial cancer. Grade 1 tumors are sometimes treated with hormonal approaches; if this fails or is not deemed appropriate and the uterus is small, patients may be treated effectively with brachytherapy alone. For higher grade or larger lesions, a combination of external beam and brachytherapy is usually recommended. Brachytherapy techniques and schedules should take into consideration the risk of many procedures versus the risk and practicality of a hospital stay for low-dose rate or twice-daily fractionated HDR brachytherapy. Brachytherapy technique is important, and applicators that can be adjusted to reach the full length of the uterine cavity are preferred. For patients who have very short life expectancy or who cannot tolerate conventional external beam or brachytherapy, a hypofractionated course of external irradiation may be indicated to control symptoms (Chapter 16).

Recurrent Disease

Locoregional recurrences of endometrial cancer can frequently be cured with aggressive multimodality treatment. The prognosis is best for patients who have low-grade cancers, but even high-grade, type II cancers can sometimes be cured with locoregional treatment (CS 13.8). Long follow-up may be required to determine the effect of recurrence on survival rates. Although most vaginal recurrences occur within 3 years of endometrial cancer diagnosis, recurrences can be seen more than 5 years after hysterectomy (Fig. 13.3), and even distant metastatic disease can have an indolent course, particularly for patients who have low-grade cancers (CS 13.9).

Vaginal Recurrence

The vagina, particularly the vaginal apex, is a frequent site of recurrence. Most recurrences are detected on routine physical examination or after the patient notices vaginal bleeding. Most isolated recurrences can be cured, but the prognosis is correlated with the size and grade of the recurrence and whether there is associated extravaginal disease.[48,81] Overall, 5-year survival rates of 60% to 70% can be expected for patients treated definitively for low-grade recurrences; recurrences of high-grade cancers are less likely to be salvaged, with cure rates of 40% or less.

The techniques used to treat vaginal recurrences of endometrial cancer are essentially identical to those used to treat primary vaginal cancers (Chapter 11). The value of concurrent and adjuvant chemotherapy is currently being studied in a prospective Gynecologic Oncology Group trial. In the meantime, we usually recommend concurrent chemotherapy for recurrences that are high-grade, large, or associated with regional involvement. Small, low-grade recurrences are usually curable with radiation therapy alone. Vaginal recurrences occurring after previous radiation therapy pose special challenges to achieve local control without exceeding normal tissue tolerance (CS 13.8 and 13.9).

Isolated Nodal Recurrence

Although the prognosis for patients with regionally recurrent disease is poorer than that for patients presenting with initial stage IIIC disease, isolated nodal recurrences are often curable and should be treated with definitive intent. If the patient has not had any previous adjuvant therapy, radiation therapy is recommended, using techniques, target volumes, and doses similar to those used for stage IIIC disease. Any regions of gross disease should receive at least 60 Gy. If the disease has recurred after chemotherapy, sites of pre-chemotherapy gross disease should be given a boost dose of radiation (usually to a total of 55–60 Gy), even if they are not enlarged at the time of recurrence. In most cases, the clinical target volume (CTV) should include the iliac nodes bilaterally; if there is evidence of paraaortic involvement, extended fields are treated similar to those used for stage IIIC2 disease. IMRT is recommended, particularly if there is extensive gross disease. Concurrent and adjuvant chemotherapy is usually recommended unless recurrence has occurred less than 6 months after chemotherapy.

The decision of whether to include uninvolved vagina in the target volume depends on the time interval since hysterectomy and previous treatment (CS 13.6).

Isolated paraaortic recurrences that occur after pelvic radiation are often curable.[78] Because they are often located above the inferior mesenteric artery, there is frequently a gap between the recurrent paraaortic disease and the proximal border of the previous radiation field. However, the CTV should be extended distally to the upper limit of the previous field to prevent recurrences between the radiation fields; the proximal paraaortic field border should extend at least 1 to 2 cm above the renal vessels, as described for stage IIIC2 disease.

Except in cases of massive nodal disease, isolated infield recurrences are rare if patients have received an optimal dose with their initial radiation therapy. Although definitive treatment of infield recurrences may not be possible without causing unacceptable morbidity, in selected cases stereotactic body radiation therapy (SBRT), hypofractionated IMRT, or proton therapy may be used to achieve palliation of symptoms and even prolonged disease-free intervals (CS 13.5).

Uterine Sarcomas

Primary uterine sarcomas are rare but fall into three major groups, leiomyosarcomas, endometrial stromal sarcomas, and adenosarcomas. In 2008, FIGO recommended that these cancers be staged using a separate staging system that borrows from sarcoma staging systems used for other sites.[82] Because the roles for radiation therapy are very limited in uterine sarcomas, they will be discussed only briefly.

Leiomyosarcomas

Leiomyosarcomas usually arise from uterine smooth muscle, although they may rarely arise from within benign leiomyomas. The focus of management is similar to that for sarcomas arising in other sites, with surgical resection being the cornerstone of curative management. Lymph node metastases are rare and generally found only in patients who have advanced cancers with other sites of extrauterine disease, so lymphadenectomy is not generally indicated. No evidence suggests that adjuvant radiation therapy improves the survival rate of patients with leiomyosarcoma. Although retrospective studies have hinted that radiation may improve local control, a 2008 randomized trial[83] demonstrated no significant difference in the rates of local control or overall survival between 50 patients who were observed and 49 patients treated with pelvic radiation therapy after hysterectomy for leiomyosarcoma. Most recurrences include distant metastases to lung, abdomen, or other sites. Although adjuvant chemotherapy is sometimes given to patients who have large cancers, the benefit remains uncertain.[84]

Endometrial Stromal Sarcomas

These are rare tumors that typically occur in women in their 1940s and 1950s. Five-year survival rates are 75% to 80%.[85] Endometrial stromal sarcomas usually contain estrogen and progesterone receptors and typically respond well to progestins or aromatase inhibitors, which are the most effective treatments for advanced or recurrent disease.[86] These tumors do respond to radiation therapy, and several studies have suggested that local recurrences can be reduced with adjuvant radiation therapy[87]; however, hormone therapy is generally the treatment of choice for advanced or recurrent disease, and radiation is rarely recommended except for rare cases of hormone refractory disease. Undifferentiated uterine sarcomas were at one time called high-grade endometrial stromal sarcomas. However, because they lack features of endometrial stroma and have a very different behavior with a poor prognosis, they are no longer referred to as endometrial stromal sarcomas.

Adenosarcomas

Adenosarcomas are very rare tumors composed of benign epithelium with a malignant mesenchymal component. They should not be confused with carcinosarcomas, which have a malignant epithelial component and a much poorer prognosis than adenosarcomas. More than 80% of adenosarcomas are diagnosed as stage I or II disease; lymph node involvement is rare (<5%), and the 5-year survival rate is ~80%.[88] Hysterectomy alone is sufficient treatment in most cases. A small proportion of cases that exhibit sarcomatous overgrowth have a poorer prognosis, but these cases are so rare that there are virtually no data available regarding the effectiveness of radiation therapy or chemotherapy.[89]

References

1. Siegel RL, Miller KD, Jemal A. Cancer statistics, 2015. *CA Cancer J Clin.* 2015;65:5–29.
2. Scholten AN, Smit VT, Beerman H, et al. Prognostic significance and interobserver variability of histologic grading systems for endometrial carcinoma. *Cancer.* 2004;100:764–772.
3. Cunha TM, Felix A, Cabral I. Preoperative assessment of deep myometrial and cervical invasion in endometrial carcinoma: comparison of magnetic resonance imaging and gross visual inspection. *Int J Gynecol Cancer.* 2001;11:130–136.
4. Zaino RJ. FIGO staging of endometrial adenocarcinoma: a critical review and proposal. *Int J Gynecol Pathol.* 2009; 28:1–9.
5. Kwon JS, Francis JA, Qiu F, et al. When is a pathology review indicated in endometrial cancer? *Obstet Gynecol.* 2007;110:1224–1230.
6. Rauch GM, Kaur H, Choi H, et al. Optimization of MR imaging for pretreatment evaluation of patients with endometrial and cervical cancer. *Radiographics.* 2014;34:1082–1098.
7. Ross JC, Eifel PJ, Cox RS, et al. Primary mucinous adenocarcinoma of the endometrium. A clinicopathologic and histochemical study. *Am J Surg Pathol.* 1983;7:715–729.
8. Cancer Genome Atlas Research Network; Kandoth C, Schultz N, et al. Integrated genomic characterization of endometrial carcinoma. *Nature.* 2013;497:67–73.
9. Hendrickson M, Ross J, Eifel P, et al. Uterine papillary serous carcinoma: a highly malignant form of endometrial adenocarcinoma. *Am J Surg Pathol.* 1982;6:93–108.
10. Hendrickson M, Ross J, Eifel PJ, et al. Adenocarcinoma of the endometrium: analysis of 256 cases with carcinoma limited to the uterine corpus. Pathology review and analysis of prognostic variables. *Gynecol Oncol.* 1982;13:373–392.
11. Boruta DM II, Gehrig PA, Fader AN, et al. Management of women with uterine papillary serous cancer: a Society of Gynecologic Oncology (SGO) review. *Gynecol Oncol.* 2009;115:142–153.
12. Fadare O, Zheng W, Crispens MA, et al. Morphologic and other clinicopathologic features of endometrial clear cell carcinoma: a comprehensive analysis of 50 rigorously classified cases. *Am J Cancer Res.* 2013;3:70–95.
13. Fadare O, Parkash V, Dupont WD, et al. The diagnosis of endometrial carcinomas with clear cells by gynecologic pathologists: an assessment of interobserver variability and associated morphologic features. *Am J Surg Pathol.* 2012;36:1107–1118.
14. Pothuri B, Ramondetta L, Eifel P, et al. Radiation-associated endometrial cancers are prognostically unfavorable tumors: a clinicopathologic comparison with 527 sporadic endometrial cancers. *Gynecol Oncol.* 2006;103:948–951.
15. Samarnthai N, Hall K, Yeh IT. Molecular profiling of endometrial malignancies. *Obstet Gynecol Int.* 2010;2010:162363.
16. Zhang C, Hu W, Jia N, et al. Uterine carcinosarcoma and high-risk endometrial carcinomas: a clinicopathological comparison. *Int J Gynecol Cancer.* 2015;25:629–636.
17. Eifel PJ, Hendrickson M. Stage I endometrial carcinoma: the importance of pathologic review in retrospective analyses. *Int J Radiat Oncol Biol Phys.* 1990;18:1271–1273.
18. McKenney JK, Longacre TA. Low-grade endometrial adenocarcinoma: a diagnostic algorithm for distinguishing atypical endometrial hyperplasia and other benign (and malignant) mimics. *Adv Anat Pathol.* 2009;16:1–22.
19. Creutzberg CL, Nout RA, Lybeert ML, et al. Fifteen-year radiotherapy outcomes of the randomized PORTEC-1 trial for endometrial carcinoma. *Int J Radiat Oncol Biol Phys.* 2011;81:e631–e638.
20. Creutzberg CL, van Putten WL, Koper PC, et al. Surgery and postoperative radiotherapy versus surgery alone for patients with stage-1 endometrial carcinoma: multicentre randomised trial. PORTEC Study Group. Post Operative Radiation Therapy in Endometrial Carcinoma. *Lancet.* 2000;355:1404–1411.
21. Nout RA, Smit VT, Putter H, et al. Vaginal brachytherapy versus pelvic external beam radiotherapy for patients with endometrial cancer of high-intermediate risk (PORTEC-2): an open-label, non-inferiority, randomised trial. *Lancet.* 2010;375:816–823.
22. Keys HM, Roberts JA, Brunetto VL, et al. A phase III trial of surgery with or without adjunctive external pelvic radiation therapy in intermediate risk endometrial adenocarcinoma: a Gynecologic Oncology Group study. *Gynecol Oncol.* 2004;92:744–751.
23. AlHilli MM, Podratz KC, Dowdy SC, et al. Risk-scoring system for the individualized prediction of lymphatic dissemination in patients with endometrioid endometrial cancer. *Gynecol Oncol.* 2013;131:103–108.
24. Geels YP, Pijnenborg JM, van den Berg-van Erp SH, et al. Absolute depth of myometrial invasion in endometrial cancer is superior to the currently used cut-off value of 50%. *Gynecol Oncol.* 2013;129:285–291.

25. Ali A, Black D, Soslow RA. Difficulties in assessing the depth of myometrial invasion in endometrial carcinoma. *Int J Gynecol Pathol.* 2007;26:115–123.
26. Bosse T, Peters EE, Creutzberg CL, et al. Substantial lymph-vascular space invasion (LVSI) is a significant risk factor for recurrence in endometrial cancer—a pooled analysis of PORTEC 1 and 2 trials. *Eur J Cancer.* 2015;51:1742–1750.
27. Hanley KZ, Dustin SM, Stoler MH, et al. The significance of tumor involved adenomyosis in otherwise low-stage endometrioid adenocarcinoma. *Int J Gynecol Pathol.* 2010;29:445–451.
28. Morrow CP, Bundy BN, Kurman RJ, et al. Relationship between surgical-pathological risk factors and outcome in clinical stage I and II carcinoma of the endometrium: a Gynecologic Oncology Group study. *Gynecol Oncol.* 1991;40:55–65.
29. Folkins AK, Nevadunsky NS, Saleemuddin A, et al. Evaluation of vascular space involvement in endometrial adenocarcinomas: laparoscopic vs abdominal hysterectomies. *Mod Pathol.* 2010;23:1073–1079.
30. Schink JC, Rademaker AW, Miller DS, et al. Tumor size in endometrial cancer. *Cancer.* 1991;67:2791–2794.
31. Euscher E, Fox P, Bassett R, et al. The pattern of myometrial invasion as a predictor of lymph node metastasis or extrauterine disease in low-grade endometrial carcinoma. *Am J Surg Pathol.* 2013;37:1728–1736.
32. AlHilli MM, Mariani A, Bakkum-Gamez JN, et al. Risk-scoring models for individualized prediction of overall survival in low-grade and high-grade endometrial cancer. *Gynecol Oncol.* 2014;133:485–493.
33. Ferriss JS, Brix W, Tambouret R, et al. Cervical stromal invasion predicting survival in endometrial cancer. *Obstet Gynecol.* 2010;116:1035–1041.
34. Orezzoli JP, Sioletic S, Olawaiye A, et al. Stage II endometrioid adenocarcinoma of the endometrium: clinical implications of cervical stromal invasion. *Gynecol Oncol.* 2009;113:316–323.
35. McCluggage WG, Hirschowitz L, Wilson GE, et al. Significant variation in the assessment of cervical involvement in endometrial carcinoma: an interobserver variation study. *Am J Surg Pathol.* 2011;35:289–294.
36. Westin SN, Lacour RA, Urbauer DL, et al. Carcinoma of the lower uterine segment: a newly described association with Lynch syndrome. *J Clin Oncol.* 2008;26:5965–5971.
37. Mariani A, Dowdy SC, Cliby WA, et al. Prospective assessment of lymphatic dissemination in endometrial cancer: a paradigm shift in surgical staging. *Gynecol Oncol.* 2008;109:11–18.
38. Touboul C, Bentivegna E, Uzan C, et al. Sentinel lymph node in endometrial cancer: a review. *Curr Oncol Rep.* 2013;15:559–565.
39. Klopp AH, Jhingran A, Ramondetta L, et al. Node-positive adenocarcinoma of the endometrium: outcome and patterns of recurrence with and without external beam irradiation. *Gynecol Oncol.* 2009;115:6–11.
40. Toptas T, Simsek T. Stage IIIC endometrial cancer: the need for novel subgrouping according to the ratio of metastatic lymph nodes. *Arch Gynecol Obstet.* 2015;291:391–398.
41. Polterauer S, Khalil S, Zivanovic O, et al. Prognostic value of lymph node ratio and clinicopathologic parameters in patients diagnosed with stage IIIC endometrial cancer. *Obstet Gynecol.* 2012;119:1210–1218.
42. Bristow RE, Zahurak ML, Alexander CJ, et al. FIGO stage IIIC endometrial carcinoma: resection of macroscopic nodal disease and other determinants of survival. *Int J Gynecol Cancer.* 2003;13: 664–672.
43. Sonoda Y, Zerbe M, Smith A, et al. High incidence of positive peritoneal cytology in low-risk endometrial cancer treated by laparoscopically assisted vaginal hysterectomy. *Gynecol Oncol.* 2001;80:378–382.
44. Ko EM, Walter P, Clark L, et al. The complex triad of obesity, diabetes and race in Type I and II endometrial cancers: prevalence and prognostic significance. *Gynecol Oncol.* 2014;133:28–32.
45. Desrosiers L, Fadare O, Xiao ZF, et al. Lymphovascular space invasion does not predict vaginal relapses in stage I endometrioid adenocarcinoma of the endometrium. *Ann Diagn Pathol.* 2008;12:112–117.
46. Scholten AN, van Putten WL, Beerman H, et al. Postoperative radiotherapy for Stage 1 endometrial carcinoma: long-term outcome of the randomized PORTEC trial with central pathology review. *Int J Radiat Oncol Biol Phys.* 2005;63:834–838.
47. Mariani A, Dowdy SC, Keeney GL, et al. Predictors of vaginal relapse in stage I endometrial cancer. *Gynecol Oncol.* 2005;97:820–827.
48. Creutzberg CL, van Putten WL, Koper PC, et al. Survival after relapse in patients with endometrial cancer: results from a randomized trial. *Gynecol Oncol.* 2003;89:201–209.
49. Janda M, Gebski V, Brand A, et al. Quality of life after total laparoscopic hysterectomy versus total abdominal hysterectomy for stage I endometrial cancer (LACE): a randomised trial. *Lancet Oncol.* 2010;11:772–780.
50. Walker JL, Piedmonte MR, Spirtos NM, et al. Laparoscopy compared with laparotomy for comprehensive surgical staging of uterine cancer: Gynecologic Oncology Group Study LAP2. *J Clin Oncol.* 2009;27:5331–5336.
51. Ghezzi F, Cromi A, Serati M, et al. Radiation-induced bowel complications: laparoscopic versus open staging of gynecologic malignancy. *Ann Surg Oncol.* 2011;18:782–791.
52. Walker JL, Piedmonte MR, Spirtos NM, et al. Recurrence and survival after random assignment to laparoscopy versus laparotomy for comprehensive surgical staging of uterine cancer: Gynecologic Oncology Group LAP2 Study. *J Clin Oncol.* 2012;30:695–700.
53. Grant JD, Garg AK, Gopal R, et al. Isolated port-site metastases after minimally invasive hysterectomy for endometrial cancer: outcomes of patients treated with radiotherapy. *Int J Gynecol Cancer.* 2015;25:869–874.
54. Wright JD, Fiorelli J, Kansler AL, et al. Optimizing the management of stage II endometrial cancer: the role of radical hysterectomy and radiation. *Am J Obstet Gynecol.* 2009;200:419.e1–419.e7.
55. Dowdy SC, Borah BJ, Bakkum-Gamez JN, et al. Prospective assessment of survival, morbidity, and cost associated with lymphadenectomy in low-risk endometrial cancer. *Gynecol Oncol.* 2012;127:5–10.
56. Benedetti Panici P, Basile S, Maneschi F, et al. Systematic pelvic lymphadenectomy vs. no lymphadenectomy in early-stage endometrial carcinoma: randomized clinical trial. *J Natl Cancer Inst.* 2008;100:1707–1716.
57. Kitchener H, Swart AM, Qian Q, et al. Efficacy of systematic pelvic lymphadenectomy in endometrial cancer (MRC ASTEC trial): a randomised study. *Lancet.* 2009;373:125–136.
58. Todo Y, Kato H, Kaneuchi M, et al. Survival effect of para-aortic lymphadenectomy in endometrial cancer (SEPAL study): a retrospective cohort analysis. *Lancet.* 2010;375:1165–1172.
59. Kumar S, Medeiros F, Dowdy SC, et al. A prospective assessment of the reliability of frozen section to direct intraoperative decision making in endometrial cancer. *Gynecol Oncol.* 2012;127:525–531.

60. Touhami O, Trinh XB, Gregoire J, et al. Predictors of non-sentinel lymph node (non-SLN) metastasis in patients with sentinel lymph node (SLN) metastasis in endometrial cancer. *Gynecol Oncol.* 2015;138:41–45.
61. Abu-Rustum NR. Sentinel lymph node mapping for endometrial cancer: a modern approach to surgical staging. *J Natl Compr Canc Netw.* 2014;12:288–297.
62. Randall ME, Filiaci VL, Muss H, et al. Randomized phase III trial of whole-abdominal irradiation versus doxorubicin and cisplatin chemotherapy in advanced endometrial carcinoma: a Gynecologic Oncology Group Study. *J Clin Oncol.* 2006;24:36–44.
63. Maggi R, Lissoni A, Spina F, et al. Adjuvant chemotherapy vs radiotherapy in high-risk endometrial carcinoma: results of a randomised trial. *Br J Cancer.* 2006;95:266–271.
64. Susumu N, Sagae S, Udagawa Y, et al. Randomized phase III trial of pelvic radiotherapy versus cisplatin-based combined chemotherapy in patients with intermediate- and high-risk endometrial cancer: a Japanese Gynecologic Oncology Group study. *Gynecol Oncol.* 2008;108:226–233.
65. McMeekin DS, Filiaci VL, Aghajanian C, et al. A randomized phase III trial of pelvic radiation therapy versus vaginal cuff brachytherapy followed by paclitaxel/carboplatin chemotherapy in patients with high risk, early stage endometrial cancer: a Gynecologic Oncology Group trial. *Gynecol Oncol.* 2014;134:438.
66. Hogberg T, Signorelli M, de Oliveira CF, et al. Sequential adjuvant chemotherapy and radiotherapy in endometrial cancer—results from two randomised studies. *Eur J Cancer.* 2010;46:2422–2431.
67. Secord AA, Geller MA, Broadwater G, et al. A multicenter evaluation of adjuvant therapy in women with optimally resected stage IIIC endometrial cancer. *Gynecol Oncol.* 2013;128:65–70.
68. Secord AA, Havrilesky LJ, O'Malley DM, et al. A multicenter evaluation of sequential multimodality therapy and clinical outcome for the treatment of advanced endometrial cancer. *Gynecol Oncol.* 2009;114:442–447.
69. Klopp A, Jhingran A, Pardeshi V, et al. Chemoradiation followed by adjuvant chemothrapy for management of stage IIIC2 endometrial cancer. *Int J Radiat Oncol Biol Phys.* 2011;81:S191.
70. Sorbe B, Horvath G, Andersson H, et al. External pelvic and vaginal irradiation versus vaginal irradiation alone as postoperative therapy in medium-risk endometrial carcinoma—a prospective randomized study. *Int J Radiat Oncol Biol Phys.* 2012;82:1249–1255.
71. Blake P, Swart AM, Orton J, et al. Adjuvant external beam radiotherapy in the treatment of endometrial cancer (MRC ASTEC and NCIC CTG EN.5 randomised trials): pooled trial results, systematic review, and meta-analysis. *Lancet.* 2009;373:137–146.
72. Aalders J, Abeler V, Kolstad P, et al. Postoperative external irradiation and prognostic parameters in stage I endometrial carcinoma: clinical and histopathologic study of 540 patients. *Obstet Gynecol.* 1980;56:419–427.
73. Sorbe B, Straumits A, Karlsson L. Intravaginal high-dose-rate brachytherapy for stage I endometrial cancer: a randomized study of two dose-per-fraction levels. *Int J Radiat Oncol Biol Phys.* 2005;62:1385–1389.
74. Rotman M, Sedlis A, Piedmonte MR, et al. A phase III randomized trial of postoperative pelvic irradiation in stage IB cervical carcinoma with poor prognostic features: follow-up of a gynecologic oncology group study. *Int J Radiat Oncol Biol Phys.* 2006;65:169–176.
75. Paydar I, DeWees T, Powell M, et al. Adjuvant radiotherapy in Stage II endometrial carcinoma: is brachytherapy alone sufficient for local control? *Brachytherapy.* 2015;14:427–432.
76. Rittenberg PV, Lotocki RJ, Heywood MS, et al. Stage II endometrial carcinoma: limiting post-operative radiotherapy to the vaginal vault in node-negative tumors. *Gynecol Oncol.* 2005;98:434–438.
77. Mariani A, Webb MJ, Keeney GL, et al. Stage IIIC endometrioid corpus cancer includes distinct subgroups. *Gynecol Oncol.* 2002;87:112–117.
78. Shirvani SM, Klopp AH, Likhacheva A, et al. Intensity modulated radiation therapy for definitive treatment of paraortic relapse in patients with endometrial cancer. *Pract Radiat Oncol.* 2013;3:e21–e28.
79. Kupelian PA, Eifel PJ, Tornos C, et al. Treatment of endometrial carcinoma with radiation therapy alone. *Int J Radiat Oncol Biol Phys.* 1993;27:817–824.
80. Podzielinski I, Randall ME, Breheny PJ, et al. Primary radiation therapy for medically inoperable patients with clinical stage I and II endometrial carcinoma. *Gynecol Oncol.* 2012;124:36–41.
81. Jhingran A, Burke TW, Eifel PJ. Definitive radiotherapy for patients with isolated vaginal recurrence of endometrial carcinoma after hysterectomy. *Int J Radiat Oncol Biol Phys.* 2003;56:1366–1372.
82. Prat J FIGO staging for uterine sarcomas. *Int J Gynaecol Obstet.* 2009;104:177–178.
83. Reed NS, Mangioni C, Malmstrom H, et al. Phase III randomised study to evaluate the role of adjuvant pelvic radiotherapy in the treatment of uterine sarcomas stages I and II: an European Organisation for Research and Treatment of Cancer Gynaecological Cancer Group Study (protocol 55874). *Eur J Cancer.* 2008;44:808–818.
84. Dinh TA, Oliva EA, Fuller AF Jr, et al. The treatment of uterine leiomyosarcoma. Results from a 10-year experience (1990–1999) at the Massachusetts General Hospital. *Gynecol Oncol.* 2004;92:648–652.
85. Brooks SE, Zhan M, Cote T, et al. Surveillance, epidemiology, and end results analysis of 2677 cases of uterine sarcoma 1989–1999. *Gynecol Oncol.* 2004;93:204–208.
86. Rauh-Hain JA, del Carmen MG. Endometrial stromal sarcoma: a systematic review. *Obstet Gynecol.* 2013;122:676–683.
87. Schick U, Bolukbasi Y, Thariat J, et al. Outcome and prognostic factors in endometrial stromal tumors: a Rare Cancer Network study. *Int J Radiat Oncol Biol Phys.* 2012;82:e757–e763.
88. Arend R, Bagaria M, Lewin SN, et al. Long-term outcome and natural history of uterine adenosarcomas. *Gynecol Oncol.* 2010;119:305–308.
89. Friedlander ML, Covens A, Glasspool RM, et al. Gynecologic Cancer InterGroup (GCIG) consensus review for mullerian adenosarcoma of the female genital tract. *Int J Gynecol Cancer.* 2014;24:S78–S82.

Case Studies

The case studies for this chapter focus on some of the more complex technical challenges with patients requiring radiation for endometrial cancer, particularly patients who had extrauterine involvement at the time of hysterectomy or who were treated for recurrent disease. Many of these patients were treated using IMRT partly because they had regions of unresected gross disease within the target volume. However, **CS 13.2–13.4** were treated using relatively simple three-dimensional conformal techniques. **CS 13.1, 13.5, 13.9, and 13.10** address some special considerations associated with treatment of very obese patients with endometrial cancer. Technical aspects of external beam and brachytherapy treatment are also discussed in Chapters 4 to 8.

List of Case Studies for Chapter 13

CS 13.1. Stage IB, grade 2 endometrioid cancer with high intermediate-risk features

CS 13.2. Stage II, grade 2 endometrioid cancer with high intermediate-risk features

CS 13.3. Uterine serous carcinoma involving the midvagina (Stage IIIB)

CS 13.4. Stage IIIC2, grade 2 endometrial cancer

CS 13.5. Simultaneous uterine and ovarian adenocarcinomas with nodal recurrence after pelvic RT

CS 13.6. Stage IIIC2 uterine carcinosarcoma recurrent in iliac nodes after chemotherapy

CS 13.7. Stage IIIC1 endometrioid cancer recurrent after chemotherapy in PANs

CS 13.8. Vaginal recurrence after adjuvant vaginal brachytherapy for stage II disease

CS 13.9. Stage IA, grade 2 with multiple recurrences including the distal vagina and abdominal wall

CS 13.10. Endometrial cancer inoperable due to severe obesity

Abbreviations Used in the Case Studies

AP	Anterior–posterior
BMI	Body mass index
BSO	Bilateral salpingo-oophorectomy
CT	Computed tomography
CTV	Clinical target volume
D&C	Dilatation and curettage
DM	Distant metastasis
EBRT	External beam radiotherapy
FDG	Fluorodeoxyglucose
FIGO	International Federation of Gynecology and Obstetrics
FNA	Fine needle aspirate
GOG	Gynecologic Oncology Group
GTV	Gross tumor volume
HDR	High-dose rate
HRCTV	High-risk clinical target volume
IMRT	Intensity-modulated radiation therapy
ITV	Internal target volume
KPS	Karnofsky performance status
LND	Lymph node dissection
LVSI	Lymph vascular space invasion
MRI	Magnetic resonance imaging
NED	No evidence of disease
PA	Posterior–anterior
PAN	Paraaortic node
PET	Positron emission tomography
PDR	Pulsed-dose rate
RT	Radiation therapy
SBRT	Stereotactic body radiation therapy
TAH	Total abdominal hysterectomy

CS 13.1 • Stage IB, Grade 2 Endometrioid Cancer with High Intermediate-Risk Features

History: A 63-year-old woman had postmenopausal bleeding after anticoagulation for knee replacement surgery; she was treated several times with antibiotics with temporary improvement but after about 1 year of intermittent symptoms, a transvaginal ultrasound was performed showing a thickened endometrial stripe. Endometrial biopsy was called grade 1 adenocarcinoma. The patient underwent robot-assisted laparoscopic hysterectomy, BSO, and lymph node dissection. On the basis of the findings, treatment with vaginal brachytherapy alone was recommended, but the patient sought a second opinion.

Pathology: A 4 × 2 × 2 cm endometrioid carcinoma invading 13 of 15 mm with multiple foci of LVSI; on review, the tumor was categorized as grade 2. Five pelvic lymph nodes were examined, and all were negative.

Evaluation: *Exam*: NED. *Weight*: 159 kg; *BMI*: 63; *KPS*: 100; *CT chest abdomen and pelvis*: NED.

Treatment Plan: The patient's age (≥60) and hysterectomy findings (including three high-risk features) placed her squarely in the GOG-99 high intermediate-risk group. The risk of vaginal involvement was probably at least 15%–20%, but the risk of undetected node involvement was also substantial. According to the Mayo Clinic nomogram, the estimated risk of lymph node involvement in a patient with her intrauterine findings is 40%–50% (***a***). Although her lymph nodes were negative, with only five nodes examined the likelihood of undetected metastases remained high. For these reasons, pelvic radiation therapy was recommended.

Although treatment was initiated 5 days after initial consultation, the patient was by then more than 8 weeks beyond the date of her hysterectomy. For this reason, a slightly higher than usual dose of radiation was prescribed.

Radiation Therapy (*completed in 42 days*):
Setup: Supine in a custom cradle. Full (***b***) and empty (***c***) bladder scans were used to designate a vaginal ITV. The patient's right to left diameter exceeded the maximum field of view set by the treatment planning system, this limited the angles available for IMRT (*arrows*, ***d***, ***e***).

***EBRT*:** The nodal CTV (+7 mm) and vaginal ITV (+7 mm) were treated to a total dose of 46.8 Gy in 26 fractions.

***Brachytherapy*:** Using a Delclos dome cylinder, the proximal one-third of the vagina was treated using HDR brachytherapy to a surface dose of 10 Gy in 2 fractions.

Outcome: At 1 year NED in active follow-up.

Comments: Although this patient could have been treated using a three-dimensional conformal external beam technique, her body habitus would have required an arrangement using oblique fields (Fig. 6.11). Because this would have significantly increased the volume of bowel treated to high dose, it was decided to use IMRT.
The proximal border of this patient's external treatment was about 2 or 3 cm higher than usual to encompass some small common iliac nodes of uncertain significance.

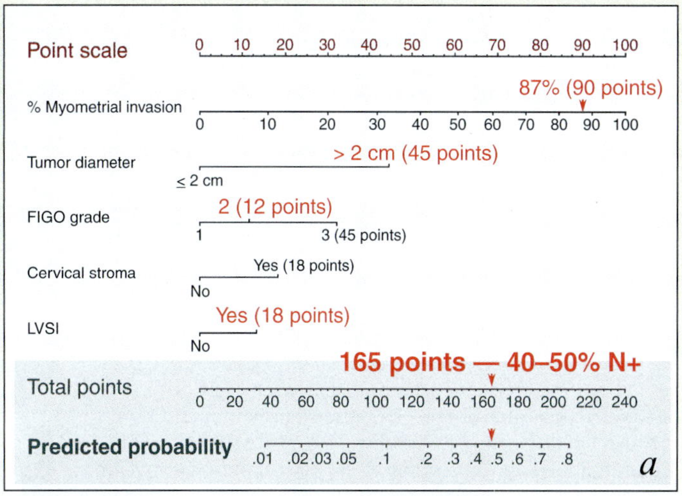

a

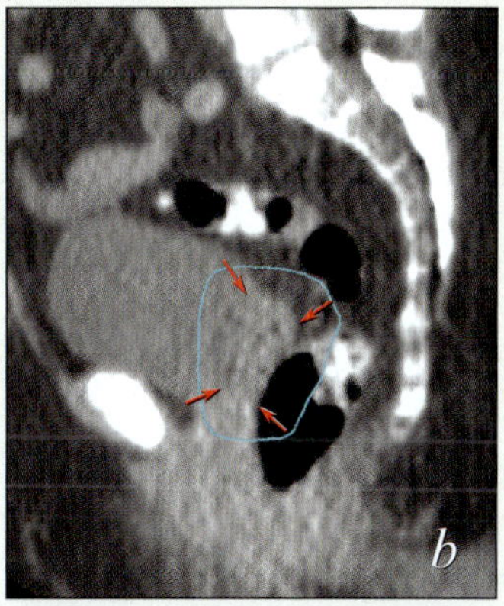

b

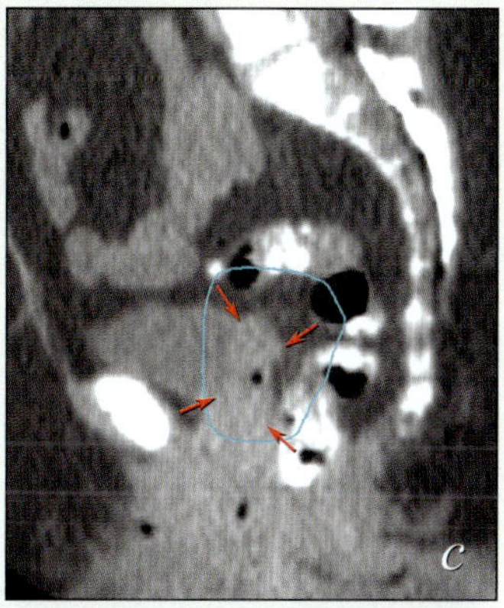

c

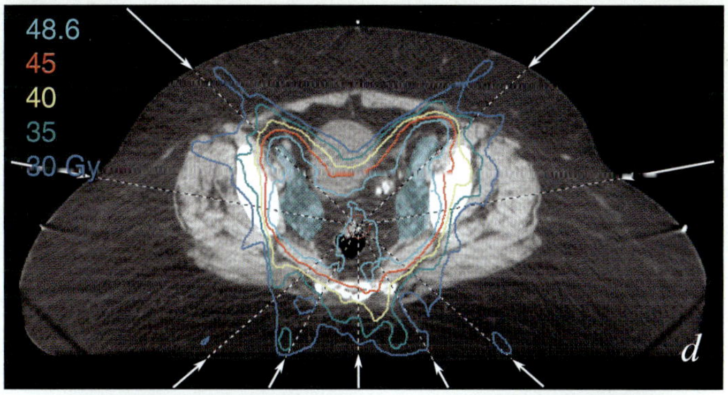

d

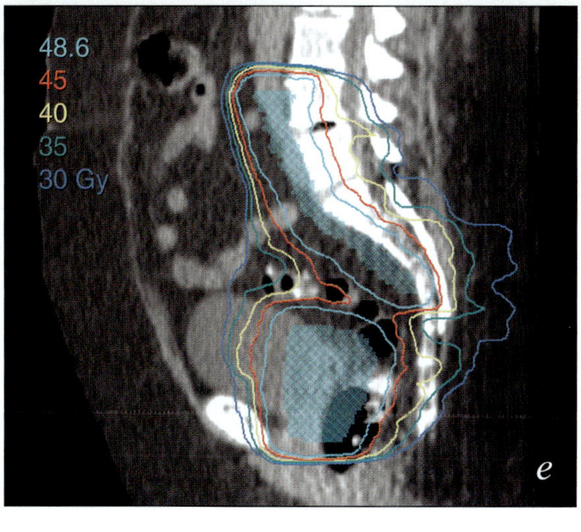

e

CS 13.2 • Stage II, Grade 2 Endometrioid Cancer with High Intermediate-Risk Features

History: A 73-year-old woman with postmenopausal bleeding had an endometrial biopsy showing adenocarcinoma. She had multiple medical problems including poorly controlled diabetes mellitus, hypertension, and obesity.

Evaluation: *Exam*: 2- to 3-cm cervix with a small tongue of tissue protruding through the os. *Weight*: 83 kg; *BMI*: 38; *KPS*: 90; *MRI (**a, b**) and CT*: A large tumor involved the lower uterine segment and cervix with near full-thickness involvement anteriorly (*arrows, **a***); no lymphadenopathy. Medical assessment was that she could tolerate surgery with minimally increased risk. *Endometrial biopsy*: Grade 2 endometrioid adenocarcinoma.

Treatment Plan: Deep anterior cervical infiltration raised concern about the ability to achieve a negative margin with hysterectomy (***a**, white arrow*). Despite extensive lower uterine segment involvement, the fundus was spared and the deepest stromal invasion was in the distal uterus and cervix. With a sufficiently long tandem, brachytherapy should be able to encompass this tumor volume, particularly if there was a good response to initial external beam irradiation. It was decided to begin pelvic radiation and reevaluate with MRI before brachytherapy to give a definitive dose or a reduced dose of brachytherapy followed by hysterectomy. Although there is limited evidence supporting the use of chemotherapy, concurrent weekly cisplatin was recommended to maximize the chance of an excellent tumor response.

Radiation Therapy:
Setup: Supine in a custom cradle.

EBRT*:** The nodal CTV (+7 mm) and vaginal ITV (+7 mm) were treated to a total dose of 45 Gy in 25 fractions using a four-field technique with 18-MV photons (c–f***).

Interim Evaluation: MRI showed an excellent response (***b***); however, there was still deep cervical stromal infiltration near the bladder *(white arrow)*. The uterine fundus was free of tumor. It was decided to proceed with a definitive brachytherapy dose.

***Brachytherapy* (*g, h*):** An intrauterine tandem was placed in the uterus with the length adjusted to reach the fundus; 3-cm cylinders were placed in the vagina. In two PDR treatments of 44 hours each, a total dose of 30 Gy was delivered to Point A. The HRCTV D90 received ~40 Gy (total dose 85 Gy). Because there was no initial gross disease at the fundus, the loading at the tandem tip was decreased for the second placement.

Chemotherapy: Concurrent weekly cisplatin ×4.

All treatment was completed in 47 days.

Outcome: At 4 months, NED by PET (***i***) and MRI (***j***). At 4 years, NED in active follow-up and with normal bowel and bladder function.

Comments: Although the primary treatment for most endometrial cancers is hysterectomy, definitive RT may be preferred in selected cases. Cancers limited to the fundus are nearly always better treated surgically because it is difficult to deliver an adequate radiation dose to the fundus of the uterus with brachytherapy and because surgical evaluation permits staging of the cancer. However, because of the unusual distribution of tumor in this case, the risk of a positive surgical margin was felt to be greater than the risk of local failure with radiation therapy.

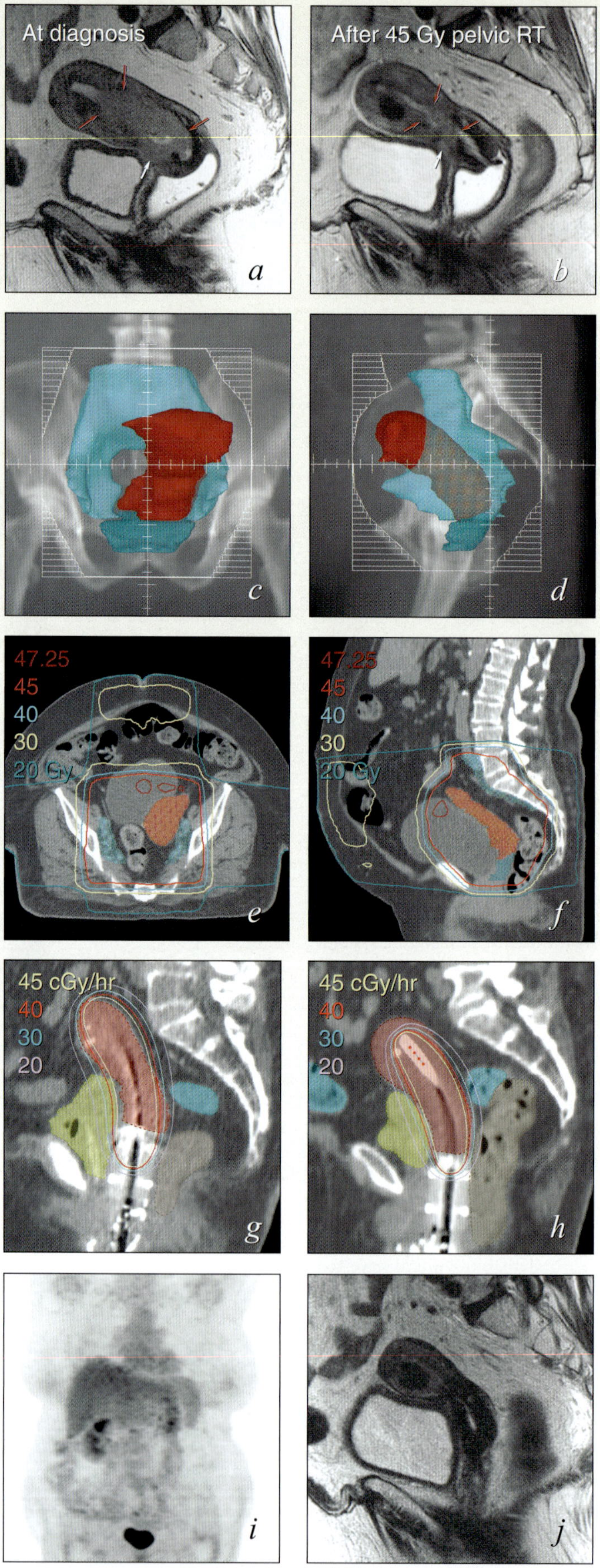

CS 13.3 • Uterine Serous Carcinoma Involving the Midvagina (Stage IIIB)

History: A 76-year-old woman in good health had postmenopausal bleeding.

Evaluation: *Exam*: Enlarged, retroverted uterus; 3-cm cervix; 2-cm papular lesion in the upper vagina up to the middle third; *KPS*: 80; *MRI* (***a***, ***b***): Severely retroflexed uterus; 7.5 × 6.5 cm tumor in the uterine fundus, tumor replacing the cervix, tumor plaque on right vaginal wall (*arrows*, ***b***); *CT chest, abdomen, pelvis*: no lymphadenopathy or DM; *Uterine D&C*: mixed serous and grade 2 endometrioid adenocarcinoma; *Vaginal biopsy*: grade 2 endometrioid carcinoma.

Treatment Plan: The large intrauterine tumor required hysterectomy to achieve the best chance of local control. However, the surgeon felt that hysterectomy could not be achieved without a high risk of positive margin at the bladder or vagina. The aggressive histology and stage suggested that chemotherapy also should play a role.

Combined modality treatment was recommended beginning with concurrent chemo-RT followed by brachytherapy, completion hysterectomy, and adjuvant carboplatin and paclitaxel.

The overall goal was to sterilize the vaginal disease and decrease the volume of disease in the cervix and uterus with preoperative RT. The dose to the vaginal surface in the region of the future vaginal incision would be limited to no more than 80 Gy to minimize the risk of surgical complications.

***EBRT (c–f)*:** In 25 fractions: 45 Gy to the pelvis using a four-field technique. The target volume included the presacral nodes (because of the cervix involvement), and the distal field border was lower than usual because of the vaginal involvement and aggressive histologic type.

***Brachytherapy (g)*:** *Findings*: The vaginal lesion was no longer visible or palpable. The cervix was 3 cm; the uterus was slightly enlarged.

Applicator selection: The primary goal was to boost the dose to the cervix and vagina. Because of this and the severe retroflexion, it was decided not to attempt to treat the uterine fundus. A 4.5-cm tandem was inserted with three 3-cm vaginal cylinders. A 5-mm diameter tandem was used to minimize risk of perforation. PDR brachytherapy was delivered in 70 hourly pulses.

Total RT doses (completed in 40 days):

Point A: 64 Gy; cervix GTV and HRCTV >70 Gy

Vaginal surface (upper 1/3): 70–80 Gy (total dose)

Vaginal surface (middle 1/3): 65–70 Gy

Pelvic CTV: 45 Gy (in 34 days)

Chemotherapy: Concurrent weekly cisplatin; adjuvant carboplatin and paclitaxel ×3.

Hysterectomy (4 weeks after RT completion): mixed serous and endometrioid adenocarcinoma with treatment effect; 2-cm intrauterine tumor (4.5/11 mm invasion); small superficial residual in cervix. All surgical margins were negative.

Outcome: The patient had a 1-cm area of vaginal apex necrosis noted after her third cycle of adjuvant chemotherapy. This was treated with antibiotics and healed after 2–3 months. Because of this, the planned fourth cycle of adjuvant chemotherapy was not given. At 5 years, NED with stable chemotherapy-related peripheral neuropathy.

Comments: These uncommon cases require close multidisciplinary collaboration. Had there been less cervical involvement and the vaginal lesion a bit more proximal, initial hysterectomy would have been preferred.

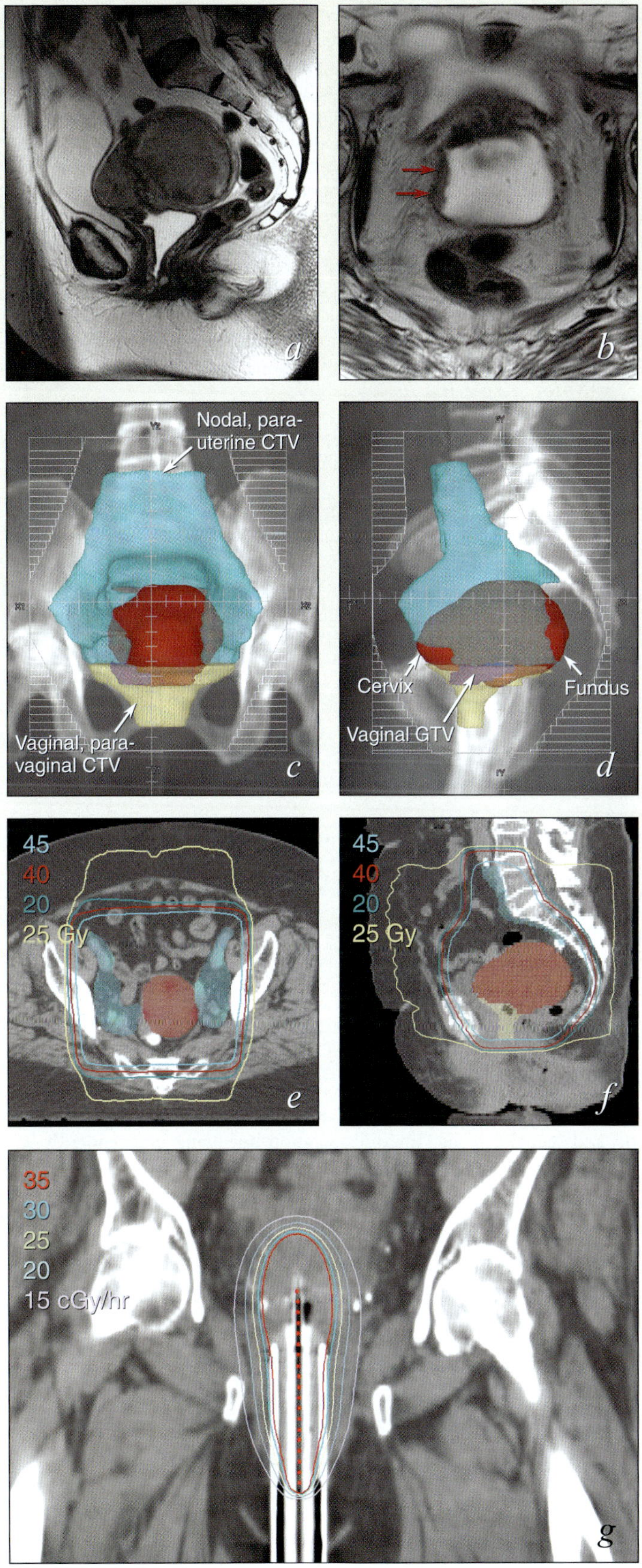

CS 13.4 • Stage IIIC2, Grade 2 Endometrial Cancer

History: An 80-year-old woman who was being followed for thyroid cancer developed postmenopausal bleeding. Endometrial curettage was diagnosed as grade 1 adenocarcinoma in a background of hyperplasia. The patient underwent laparoscopic hysterectomy and BSO; because intraoperative evaluation and frozen section demonstrated a grade 2 tumor invading at least one-third of the myometrial thickness, it was decided to perform a pelvic and paraaortic LND. Postoperatively, the patient had a minor hypotensive episode and required transfusion for a hemoglobin of 8 but was discharged on the fourth postoperative day. Her postoperative course was otherwise unremarkable.

Pathology: A 4 × 1.1 cm, grade 2 endometrioid carcinoma with a minor component of papillary endometrioid carcinoma; the cancer invaded 9 of 24 mm (38%), and there were multiple foci of LVSI including one in the cervix, which was otherwise negative for tumor involvement. Of 18 PANs examined, 5 contained isolated tumor cells in subcapsular spaces. Three pelvic nodes were negative for metastasis.

Evaluation: *Exam*: NED. *Weight*: 59 kg; *BMI*: 63; *KPS*: 100; *Chest x-ray*: NED; *CT abdomen and pelvis*: no lymphadenopathy or DM.

Treatment Plan: Although the volume of disease was small, the finding of tumor cells in multiple PANs was felt to be sufficient to justify adjuvant radiation therapy. However, in view of the small volume of nodal disease and the relatively low grade of her tumor, it was decided that the theoretical benefit of chemotherapy was insufficient to justify combined modality treatment in this relatively healthy but elderly woman. The plan was for extended field radiation therapy alone.

Radiation therapy (*completed in 42 days*):
Setup: Supine in upper and lower custom cradles with arms up. The bladder was empty for simulation, but the patient was encouraged to fill her bladder during treatment.

EBRT*:** The pelvic and PANs were treated to a total dose of 45 Gy in 25 fractions using a four-field technique of 18-MV photons (a–d***). To protect the kidneys (***b***), the fields were weighted to give more radiation dose through AP and PA fields rather than lateral fields.

***Brachytherapy*:** Using a 2-cm Delclos dome cylinder, the proximal one-third of the vagina was treated using HDR brachytherapy to a vaginal surface dose of 15 Gy in 3 fractions.

***Chemotherapy*:** None.

Outcome: At 10 years, NED; followed for cardiovascular disease, mild arthritis, and sequelae of her thyroid operation but living independently without genitourinary, gastrointestinal, or other complaints referable to her endometrial cancer or RT.

Comments: With sentinel node ultrastaging, the diagnosis of isolated tumor cells in nodes is becoming more frequent. The significance of this finding is still being studied, but in this case with five involved nodes, there was little doubt that the patient was at high risk for recurrence. Today, we would probably treat this patient using IMRT, which would give somewhat greater sparing of pelvic small bowel and sacral bone; however, the four-field technique used here also provided a very acceptable dose distribution for delivery of the 45-Gy dose required to achieve regional control. Although we add a modest dose of vaginal brachytherapy to boost the vaginal apex in high-risk patients, the benefit of this is unproven.

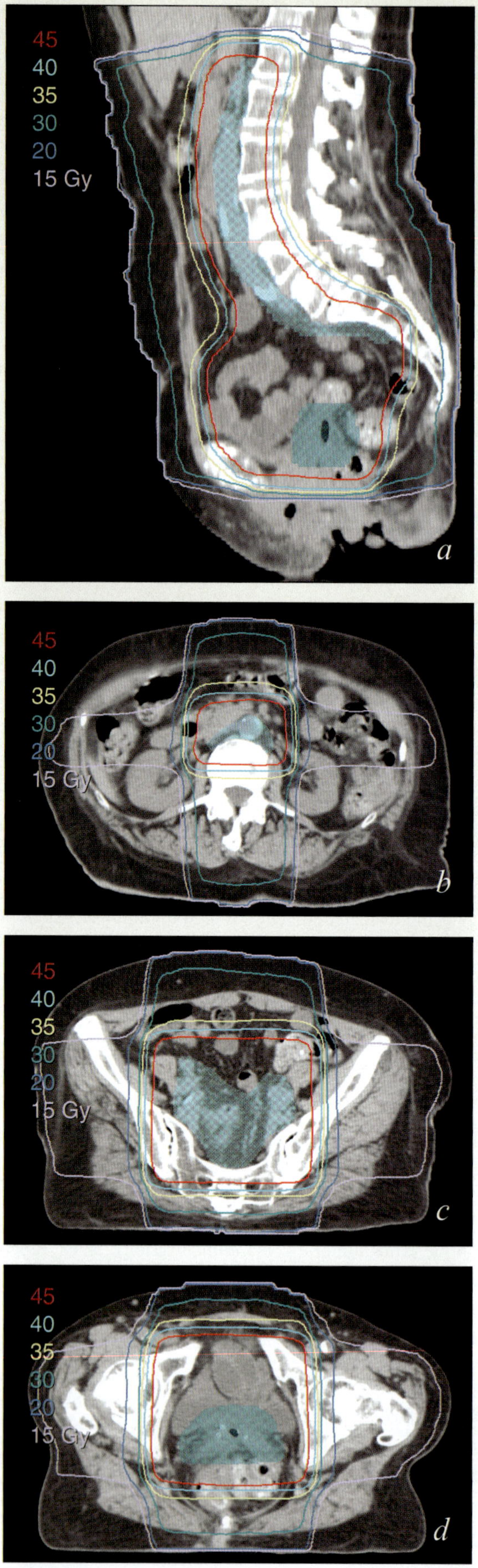

History: A 33-year-old nulliparous woman had emergency TAH-BSO for an acute vaginal hemorrhage.

Histologic examination revealed a deeply invasive grade 1 endometrioid carcinoma of the endometrium and bilateral grade 2 endometrioid carcinomas of the ovary, measuring 9 × 7 cm and 4 × 3 cm, respectively. No nodes were sampled. CT (***a***) showed no lymphadenopathy but was of poor quality. The patient received adjuvant pelvic RT with concurrent carboplatin followed by four courses of carboplatin and paclitaxel. She was followed with NED until 9 years later when she had onset of fatigue, bloating, and abdominal pain. When CT revealed lymphadenopathy, she was referred for evaluation and treatment.

Evaluation: *Exam*: *Weight*: 172 kg; *BMI*: 62; *Pelvic exam*: NED; *KPS*: 90; *PET–CT* (***b***, ***c***): FDG-avid lymphadenopathy including a 4-cm distal common iliac mass with associated ureteral obstruction and a 3.5-cm aortocaval mass, otherwise NED; *Biopsy (FNA, left iliac node)*: adenocarcinoma.

Treatment Plan: After multidisciplinary discussion, initial chemotherapy was recommended to be followed by RT. After six courses of carboplatin and paclitaxel with a partial response, the residual pelvic and paraaortic masses measured about 2.8 cm and 2.3 cm, respectively.

Although the pelvic mass was completely contained within the previous RT fields (***d***), several factors made it reasonable to consider retreatment in this case. The long interval since pelvic RT permitted some recovery of irradiated tissues. Also, the patient's morbid obesity reduced the amount of bowel in close proximity to tumor, although it also degraded the accuracy of diagnostic setup verification methods.

Radiation Therapy:

Setup: Supine with upper and lower cradles; arms above the head. A single isocenter was placed between the two nodal masses near the iliac mass to maximize setup accuracy in this region. Separate beam arrangements and fractionation were used above and below the isocenter. For the pelvic mass, a hypofractionated schedule was used to deliver a dose equivalent to 60 Gy to the GTV and <40 Gy to adjacent critical structures, including bowel, bone, and sacral plexus. The PAN recurrence, which was well outside the previous radiation fields (***d***), was treated with more conventional fractionation (***e***, ***h***).

IMRT:

Pelvic mass (in 20 fractions, ***e–g****)*:

GTV (+4 mm): 55 Gy (270 cGy/fraction)

GTV (+7 mm): 40 Gy (200 cGy/fraction)

PANs (in 30 fractions, ***e***, ***h****)*:

GTV (+7 mm): 60 Gy

CTV (+10 mm): 50 Gy

Chemotherapy: Weekly paclitaxel ×6.

Outcome: Treatment tolerated well with only mild diarrhea. At 3 years, NED by PET.

Comments: Although SBRT was considered for the pelvic mass, tight margins were impractical because of the uncertainties caused by the patient's obesity; we preferred to use a fractionated schedule that would permit somewhat larger targets without exposing critical structures to large fractional doses.

This patient exhibited several features classically associated with multiple müllerian primaries: nulliparity, young age, bilateral ovarian tumors, and low-grade endometrioid histology. It is, of course, impossible to know which primary led to the nodal recurrence.

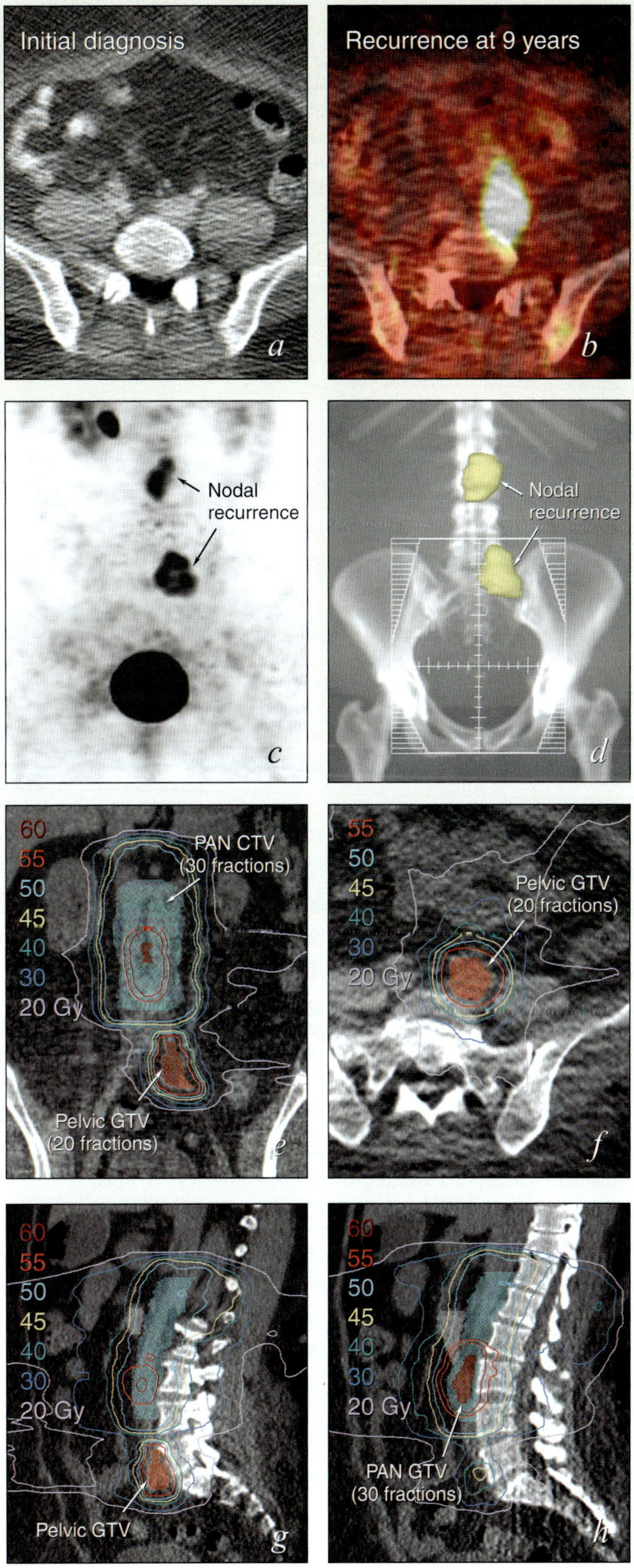

CS 13.6 • Stage IIIC2 Uterine Carcinosarcoma Recurrent in Iliac Nodes after Chemotherapy

History: A 65-year-old woman with bleeding and an enlarged uterus had an endometrial biopsy showing carcinosarcoma. TAH-BSO, LND, and omentectomy revealed carcinosarcoma invading the myometrium 4 of 11 mm; 5 of 22 pelvic and 1 of 6 PA nodes were microscopically positive; omentum and peritoneal biopsies were negative. She had vaginal cuff brachytherapy followed by six courses of carboplatin and paclitaxel. One year later, a rising CA-125 prompted further evaluation.

Evaluation: *CT* (***a***, ***b***): enlarged iliac nodes (*arrows*) up to the aortic bifurcation; PET (***g***): FDG-avid iliac and PA nodes; no DM. *Node biopsy*: high-grade adenocarcinoma. *Exam*: NED. *KPS*: 100.

Treatment Plan: Carcinosarcomas tend to spread hematogenously and intraperitoneally. However, patients who have isolated regional metastasis are sometimes curable with regional treatment. The large nodes, high grade, and 1-year interval since chemotherapy were felt to support the use of concurrent and adjuvant chemotherapy to achieve the greatest chance of cure.

Studies suggest that treatment with chemo-RT followed by carboplatin/paclitaxel is well tolerated and may be superior to chemotherapy alone for stage IIIC G3 disease.

EBRT (*completed in 43 days*): Because of the common iliac and prior PAN involvement, the CTV margin included the PANs up to 3 cm proximal to the renal veins (***c–f***). Paravaginal tissues (but not the previously treated vagina) were included in the CTV (***c***). The isocenter was placed in the center of the GTV to optimize setup accuracy in this region.

The CTV (+7 mm) was treated to 45 Gy in 25 fractions with a 5-Gy integrated boost to the GTV (+5 mm) (***c***, ***d***); the largest node received a 7.5-Gy integrated boost (***c***). This treatment was followed by a 14-Gy boost (in 7 fractions) to all PET+ nodes (+5 mm) (***e***, ***f***), bringing the total GTV dose to 64–66.5 Gy. In part because visceral fat distanced bowel somewhat from the GTV targets, the dose to critical structures was kept well within tolerance limits.

Chemotherapy: Concurrent weekly cisplatin ×2, discontinued because of pancytopenia. Adjuvant carboplatin and paclitaxel ×3.

Outcome: PET at the end of chemotherapy showed complete resolution of all prior regions of increased FDG uptake (***h***). Note: hyperactive marrow outside the RT field in this PET obtained shortly after completion of chemotherapy (***h***). Two years after RT and 3.5 years after initial diagnosis, the patient has no evidence of carcinosarcoma and a normal CA-125. However, she was treated for early-stage breast cancer in the interim.

Comments: Further studies are needed to determine the optimal treatment of stage IIIC carcinosarcoma. However, in most cases, chemotherapy alone is not curative. RT significantly reduces the rate of local recurrence and should be considered as part of the initial treatment plan.

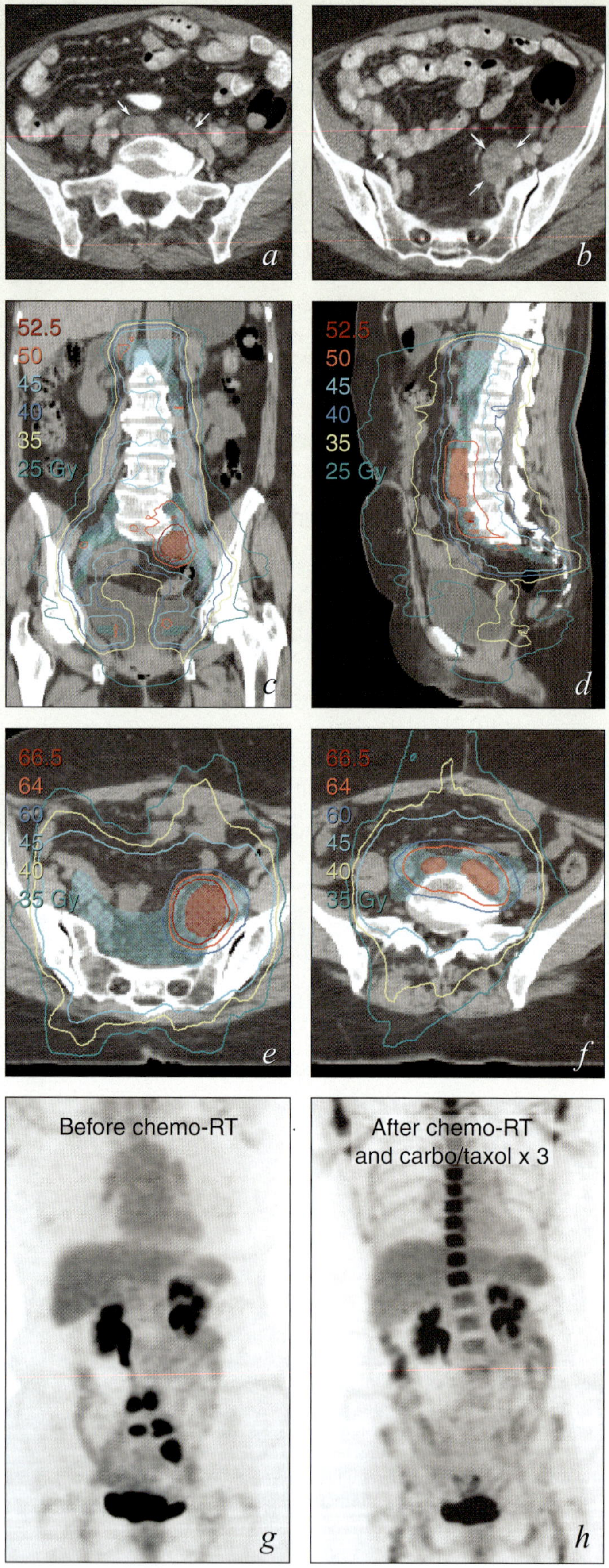

CS 13.7 • Stage IIIC1 Endometrioid Cancer Recurrent after Chemotherapy in PANs

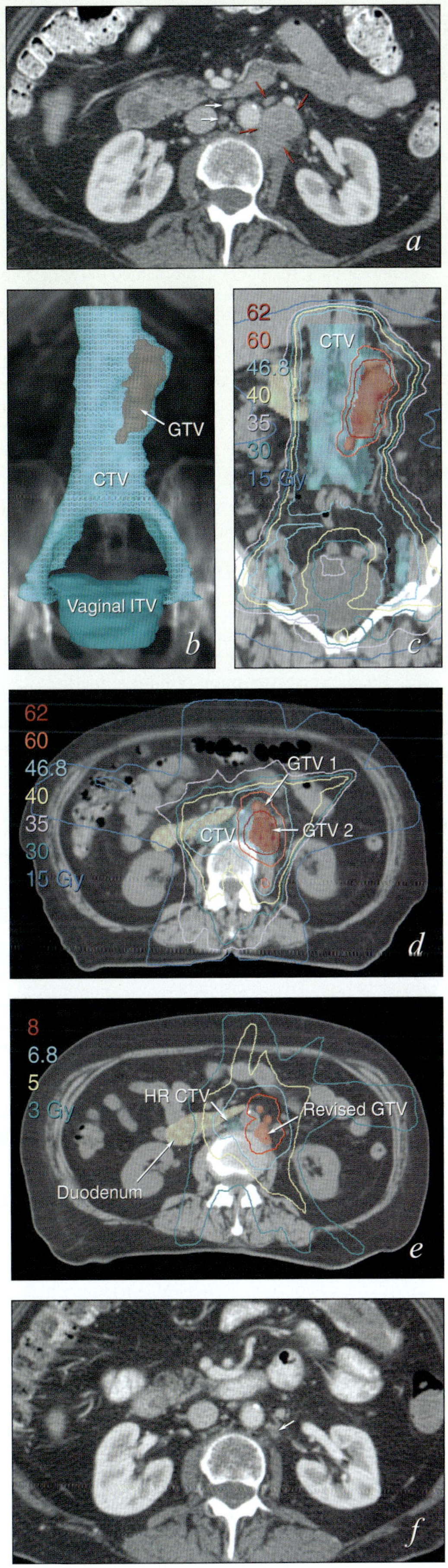

History: A 72-year-old woman with postmenopausal bleeding had an endometrial biopsy showing adenocarcinoma. TAH-BSO and pelvic LND revealed grade 2 endometrioid carcinoma invading the myometrium 2 of 18 mm; there was superficial cervical stromal invasion but no LVSI. Cancer involved 1 of 9 right and 0 of 8 left pelvic nodes; no PANs were sampled. After five courses of carboplatin and paclitaxel, there was NED by CT.

Six months later, CT revealed a 1 × 2 cm PAN. FNA showed "rare atypical cells suspicious for malignancy." PET demonstrated FDG-avidity in the node but otherwise NED. The patient was told that surgery would not be helpful and was offered a choice of palliative chemotherapy or observation; RT was not suggested. After 3 months of observation, the node had increased in size and she sought a second opinion.

Evaluation: *Exam*: NED; *KPS*: 100; *CT*: a confluent mass of enlarged nodes measuring up to 3 cm in axial diameter occupied the left paraaortic space (***a***, *red arrows*) and extended from the renal vein to the aortic bifurcation (***b***); several small aortocaval nodes (***a***, *white arrows*) were of uncertain significance. *Biopsy (FNA, left PAN)*: adenocarcinoma.

Treatment Plan: Surgical resection was not recommended because of the very extensive disease infiltrating posterior to the renal vein. With a 6-month interval to recurrence, it was felt that the tumor might still be platinum sensitive. After some debate, it was decided to recommend concurrent chemo-RT in an effort to maximize the chance of local control.

Radiation Therapy (*completed in 42 days*): The pelvic lymph nodes and vagina (***b***) were included because of the relatively short time interval since her initial treatment and because there had been initial evidence of pelvic node metastasis. The PANs were treated to the top of T12. The small aortocaval nodes were designated a HRCTV and treated to a higher dose than the rest of the CTV. A repeat CT at 3 weeks did not show enough tumor regression to justify modification of the initial plan, but the GTV was revised for the final boost (***e***).

Setup: Supine with upper and lower cradles; arms above the head.

IMRT was delivered to multiple targets using integrated and sequential boosts (***c–e***).

Fractions 1–26 (***c, d***):

Nodal CTV and vaginal ITV (+7 mm): 46.8 Gy (1.8 Gy/fraction)

PAN GTV (+7 mm; included several small nodes proximal to the main mass): 52 Gy (2 Gy/fraction)

Bulky PANs (+3 mm): 55.9 Gy (2.15 Gy/fraction)

Fractions 27–31 (***e***):

Residual GTV (+7 mm): 8 Gy (2 Gy/fraction); total dose, 63.9 Gy.

Aortocaval HRCTV (+7 mm): 6.8 Gy (1.7 Gy/fraction); total dose, 53.6 Gy.

Chemotherapy: Weekly cisplatin ×4, discontinued because of neutropenia; adjuvant carboplatin and paclitaxel.

Outcome: Rapid response during treatment (***e***) with only a tiny indistinct node remaining at 4 months (***f***, *arrow*). At 5 years (6.5 years after initial diagnosis), NED. Her only symptoms were arthritis pain and continued tingling and numbness of the lower extremities.

Comments: At diagnosis, we would have recommended postoperative RT after obtaining an abdominal CT (which was not performed at that time) to rule out the presence of paraaortic disease. The value of adjuvant chemotherapy in this setting is uncertain and probably was responsible for her neurologic symptoms.

CS 13.8 • Vaginal Recurrence after Adjuvant Vaginal Brachytherapy for Stage II Disease

History: A 67-year-old woman with postmenopausal bleeding was found to have a large uterine mass (***a***, *arrows*); biopsy showed adenocarcinoma. A total laparoscopic hysterectomy, BSO, and pelvic LND was performed, revealing a 4-cm grade 2 endometrioid carcinoma of the lower uterine segment invading 12 mm of a 16-mm thick myometrium. There was deep cervical stromal invasion and LVSI. Six pelvic nodes were negative for metastasis.

The patient was referred to a radiation oncologist who recommended intracavitary vaginal brachytherapy only; the proximal half of the vagina received three treatments of 7 Gy each prescribed at 0.5 cm depth. Applicator position was verified with orthogonal films but without fiducial markers in the vagina. Estimated bladder and rectal doses were 7–7.5 Gy per fraction.

One year later, the patient complained of dysuria and pelvic pressure. MRI and PET showed a 2 cm mass in the left vaginal apex with no other evidence of disease.

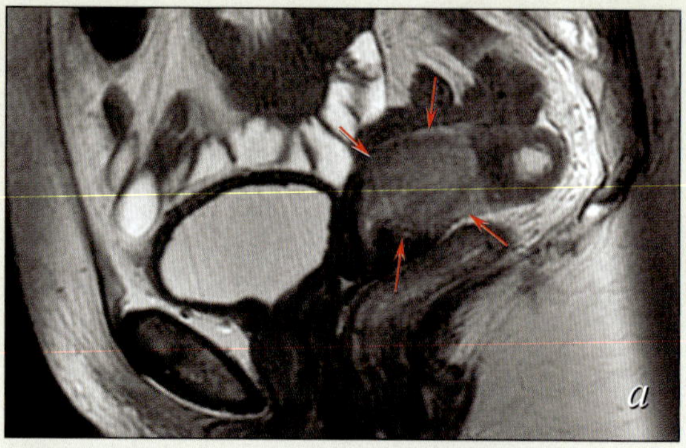

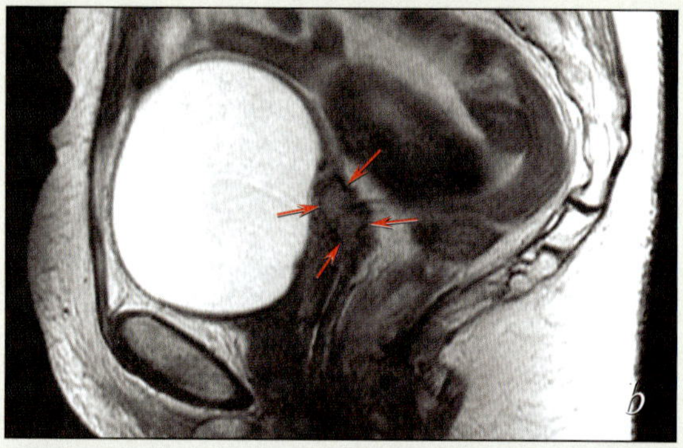

Evaluation: *Exam (EUA)*: Narrowed upper vagina with a 1 × 2 cm mass above the left vaginal apex and eroding through the mucosa (***b***, *arrows*). *KPS*: 90. *Cystoscopy and proctoscopy*: No visible radiation changes or tumor involvement. Fiducial markers were inserted in the apex to assist in treatment planning and monitoring. *Biopsy (vagina)*: adenocarcinoma.

Treatment Plan: Definitive chemo-RT. Although the risk of complications was higher than usual, surgical treatment would have required pelvic exenteration, and chemotherapy alone would not have been curative.

Radiation Therapy (*completed in 43 days*): The pelvic lymph nodes and vagina were treated using IMRT with integrated and sequential boosts. To minimize internal motion, initial treatment was delivered with 250–300 mL in the bladder, confirmed daily with ultrasound. For the final boost, a bladder catheter was inserted daily and the bladder filled with a fixed volume of 250 mL. Also, the correct position of fiducial markers was verified daily with KV imaging.

Setup: Supine in a custom cradle.

Fractions 1–25 (***c, d***):

GTV-ITV (+5 mm): 50 Gy (200 cGy per fraction)

Upper vaginal ITV (+7 mm): 47.5 Gy (190 cGy per fraction)

Vaginal ITV (+7 mm): 45 Gy (180 cGy per fraction)

Fractions 26–32 (***e***):

GTV-ITV (+5 mm): 14 Gy (200 cGy per fraction)

GTV-ITV (+7 mm): 12.25 Gy (175 cGy per fraction)

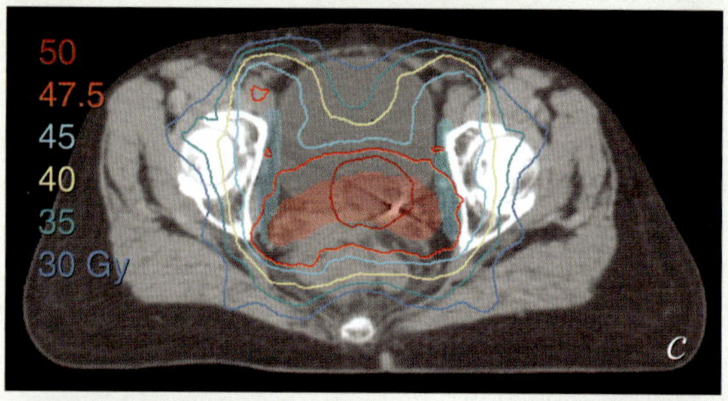

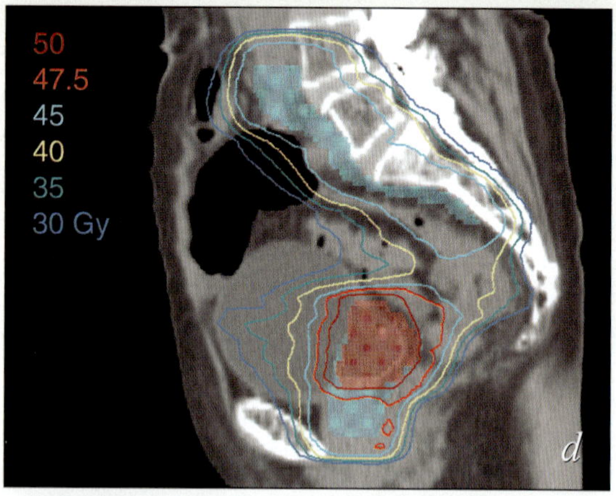

Chemotherapy: Weekly cisplatin ×5.

Outcome: At 4 months, NED by exam and MRI. At 18 months, onset of intermittent rectal bleeding; colonoscopy showed only hemorrhoids. At 2 years, increased bleeding with a hemoglobin of 6. Proctoscopy showed neovascularization of the anterior rectal wall. After transfusion and treatment with Rowasa enemas, the bleeding improved. At 5 years, NED with continued mild intermittent hematochezia but stable hemoglobin levels of 11–11.5.

Comments: In cases of stage II disease with very extensive cervical stromal involvement, adjuvant pelvic RT is usually recommended, particularly if only a simple hysterectomy has been performed.

One disadvantage of the three-fraction adjuvant brachytherapy regimen used in this case is the relatively high effective dose to the bladder and rectum, which increases the risk of complications after retreatment (Chapter 8).

An alternative approach for treatment of the recurrence would have been to boost the vaginal GTV with interstitial brachytherapy; this would have required laparoscopic guidance or, possibly, real-time MRI guidance and image-based planning to control the dose to previously treated bladder and rectum.

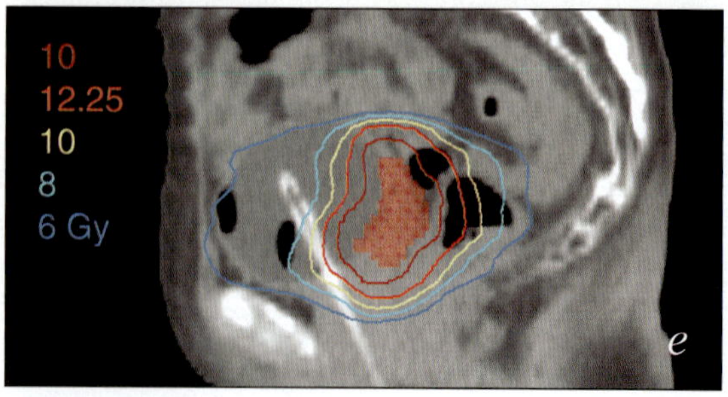

CS 13.9 • Stage IA, Grade 2 with Multiple Recurrences Including the Distal Vagina and Abdominal Wall

History: A 47-year-old woman with menometrorrhagia had a laparoscopic hysterectomy and BSO after uterine biopsy showed grade 1 adenocarcinoma. Final pathology showed a 2.5 cm, grade 2 endometrioid carcinoma invading 5 of 33 mm with LVSI; no nodes were sampled. She received vaginal cuff brachytherapy consisting of 5 doses of 6 Gy each prescribed to the surface of the apical vagina. Six months later, a distal vaginal nodule was noted on exam.

Evaluation: *Exam*: 3-cm eroded lesion in the posterior distal vagina, about 2 cm from the introitus; *Weight*: 150 kg; *BMI*: 53.4; *CT chest, abdomen and pelvis*: NED. *Node biopsy*: Grade 2 endometrioid carcinoma.

Treatment Plan: Definitive RT including EBRT and brachytherapy. The previous vaginal brachytherapy delivered less than 20 Gy to the bladder or rectum and did not overlap with the new GTV so it was not felt to add significantly to the risks of retreatment. The medial inguinal nodes were included in the nodal CTV because of the distal location of the tumor.

EBRT (*completed in 39 days*): The nodal CTV and the entire vagina and paravaginal tissues were treated to a total dose of 45 Gy in 25 fractions using a four-field technique of 18-MV photons. At the conclusion of EBRT, a residual 2-cm diameter plaque extended cephalad from the hymenal ring.

Brachytherapy (*e, f*): The perineum was deemed sufficiently thick to accommodate an interstitial implant. Under direct palpation, six interstitial needles were inserted transperineally and secured around a 3-cm domed cylinder. Using PDR, a total dose of 30 Gy was delivered to the GTV with 1-cm margin over 67 hours at 45 cGy per hour.

Chemotherapy: None.

Outcome: At 8 months, NED by exam and CT with no treatment-related complaints.

At 3.5 years, a 9 × 6.5 cm abdominal wall mass (*arrows*, ***g***) was biopsied, showing recurrent adenocarcinoma. After evaluation otherwise showed NED, an en bloc resection with abdominal wall reconstruction was performed. Because the lateral resection margins were <0.5 mm, postoperative IMRT was recommended (***h***). The HRCTV (including the close margin) received 60 Gy and a wider CTV received 52.5 Gy. Wherever possible, the previous high-dose (45 Gy) region was avoided, although there was some overlap inferolaterally.

At 5 years, a solitary lung nodule (*arrow*, ***i***) was resected.

At 6 years, the patient had a seizure; MRI showed a solitary left parietal brain metastasis, which was also resected; at 8 years, the patient had NED but medical problems related to her obesity and treatment, including poorly controlled diabetes, cardiopulmonary disease, chronic renal insufficiency, and a persistent seizure disorder.

Comments: The natural history of low-grade endometrial cancer can be protracted, and long follow-up is required to fully determine the impact of disease recurrence. The abdominal wall recurrence probably originated in a laparoscopy port site; these recurrences are frequently curable and should be treated aggressively if no other disease is found. This patient never received chemotherapy, probably because her complicating medical problems increased the risk of unproven adjuvant treatment.

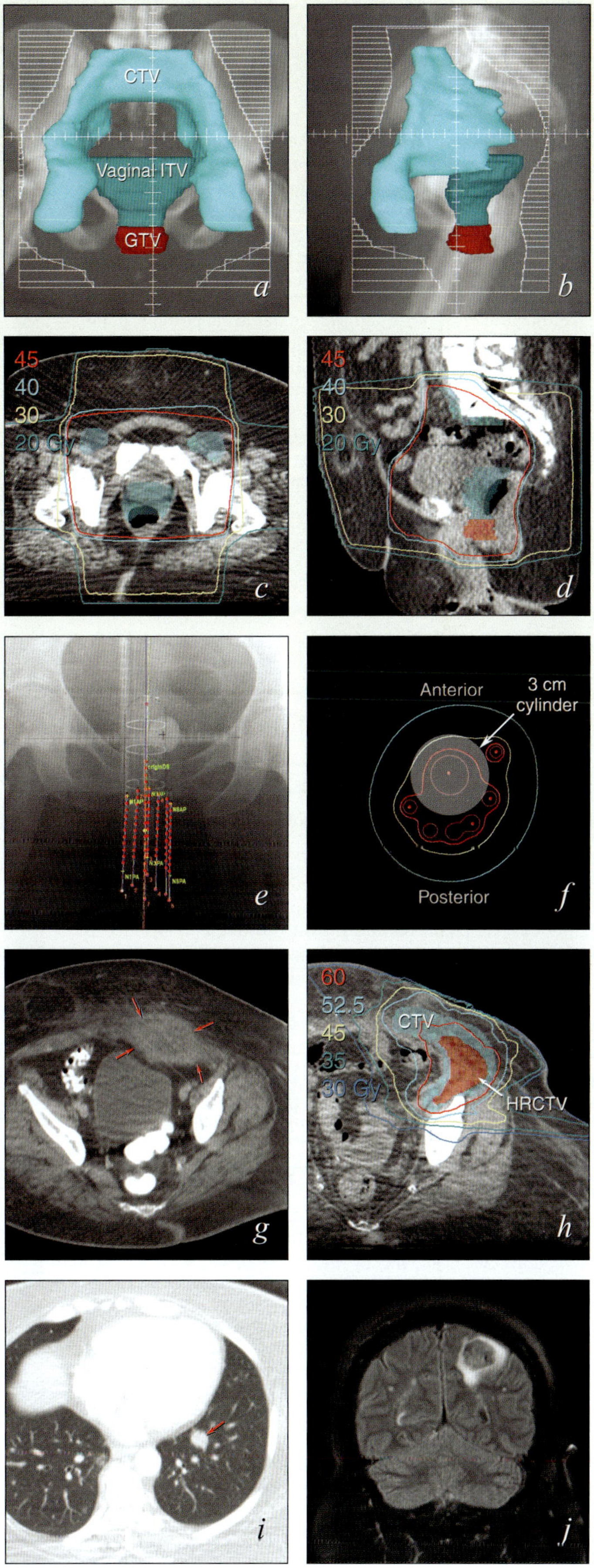

CS 13.10 • Endometrial Cancer Inoperable Due to Severe Obesity

History: A 54-year-old woman with vaginal bleeding and a thickened endometrial stripe on ultrasound had a biopsy showing endometrial adenocarcinoma. The patient, who weighed 210 kg, was placed on a weight loss program and referred for treatment recommendations.

Evaluation: *Exam*: NED. *Weight*: 195 kg; *BMI*: 76; *KPS*: 90; *MRI (**a**, **b**) and PET–CT (**c**, **d**)*: 3 × 3 × 2 cm FDG-avid lesion invading the myometrium of the right cornu (***a***, ***c***, *arrows*); bilateral FDG-avid (SUV, 4–6) pelvic, left paraaortic, axillary, and inguinal lymph nodes. *Pathology*: grade 1 endometrioid adenocarcinoma; *Biopsy (FNA) axillary and inguinal nodes*: no carcinoma, although low-grade lymphoma could not be ruled out; the pelvic and PANs could not be biopsied because of the patient's habitus.

Treatment Plan: The risk of operation was felt to be too high for surgical management and the uterine disease too extensive for hormonal treatment. After multidisciplinary discussion, it was decided to treat with definitive RT. Because metastatic involvement of the pelvic nodes could not be ruled out, they were prescribed a dose intended to sterilize gross disease. It was decided to observe the paraaortic node and attempt to obtain more tissue from extrapelvic lymph nodes if they did not resolve on follow-up scans.

Radiation Therapy:

EBRT (IMRT): The available beams were limited because the patient's width exceeded the limits of the treatment planning system; 18-MV photons were needed to achieve a homogeneous dose.

In 25 fractions (***e***, ***f***):

Nodal CTV (+7 mm); uterine and vaginal ITVs (+7 mm): 45 Gy (1.8 Gy/fraction)

Nodal GTV (+7 mm): 50 Gy (2.0 Gy/fraction)

Brachytherapy (g, h): The uterus accommodated a single tandem; 3-cm cylinders were added in the vagina. Although the goal was to deliver 35 Gy to the uterine GTV and HRCTV, brachytherapy coverage of the right cornu was poor (*arrows*, ***g***, ***h***), and it was estimate that the dose to this region could not exceed 20–25 Gy without exceeding sigmoid tolerance.

For this reason, IMRT was used to boost the uterine fundus and nodal GTV; this boost was treated with empty bladder to minimize uncertainties. The second brachytherapy dose was adjusted to avoid exceeding normal tissue tolerances, bringing the minimum dose to the GTV to ~80 Gy. The apical vagina received a total surface dose of 75 Gy.

EBRT boost:

In 5 fractions:

Nodal and uterine GTV (+7 mm): 10 Gy (2.0 Gy/fraction)

Chemotherapy: Concurrent weekly cisplatin ×4

Treatment was completed in 54 days.

Outcome: At 5 months, NED by PET–CT. No treatment-related symptoms. At 1 year, NED by MRI.

Comments: Treatment of very obese patients frequently requires difficult compromises. In this case, the disease was in a particularly challenging location for definitive RT because the uterine horn is the most difficult part of the uterus to treat with intracavitary brachytherapy. Also, had surgery been possible, management of the pelvic and PANs would likely have been different.

An alternative three-dimensional technique would have been to use four oblique fields (Chapter 6), but this would have increased the bowel dose and would have precluded an integrated nodal boost.

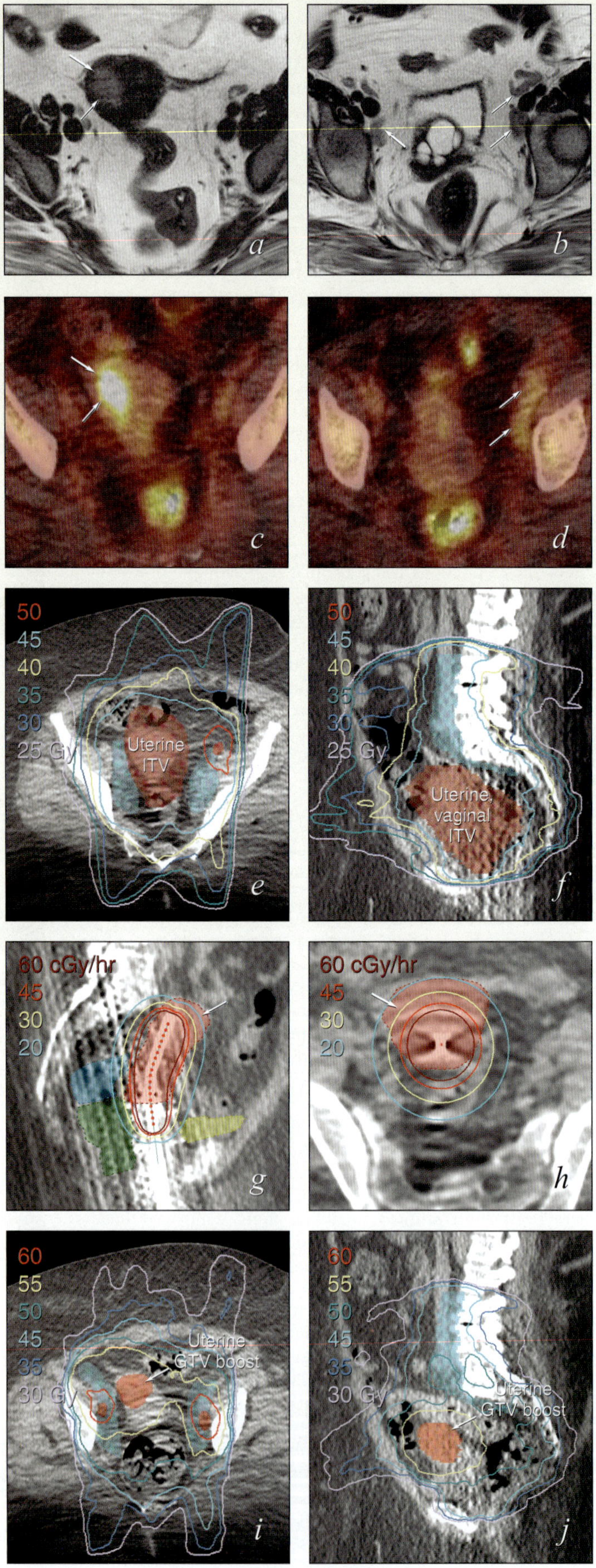

CHAPTER 14

Ovarian Cancer

INTRODUCTION

As will be shown later in this chapter, there is strong evidence that radiation therapy (RT) can play an important role in the curative treatment of selected patients with ovarian cancer. However, the decision to use RT, particularly with curative intent, should be made only after very careful consideration of the risks and benefits of all treatment options. Unfortunately, it has been difficult to achieve a cohesive strategy for the use of RT for ovarian cancer, for a number of reasons:

- Most patients with ovarian cancer either have or are at high risk for developing intra-abdominal carcinomatosis and are therefore not good candidates for definitive local treatment.
- Although RT was once strongly considered in the initial treatment of patients with minimal or no gross disease, the development of more effective chemotherapy and the adverse effects of early RT methods led to a decline in the use of RT for this indication. Eventually, many gynecologic oncologists entirely abandoned the use of RT for definitive treatment.
- RT is often considered only as a treatment of last resort, offered after the patient has already undergone several operations and many courses of chemotherapy. These previous treatments increase the risk of major radiation-related complications, narrowing the therapeutic window for complication-free definitive treatment.
- More than 20 years have passed since the role of RT for ovarian cancer was last investigated in a large prospective trial. Although retrospective studies suggest that RT may have a role in selected patients, radiation treatment methods have been inconsistent, making it difficult to formulate definitive recommendations.

The case studies at the end of this chapter demonstrate that some patients enjoy long disease-free intervals and may even be cured after receiving RT for localized recurrence of ovarian cancer. Furthermore, population-based studies suggest that certain subsets of patients with ovarian cancer might benefit sufficiently from adjuvant RT to justify its use in the initial management of their disease. However, RT for ovarian cancer remains highly controversial. To understand how RT can contribute to the management of ovarian cancer, radiation oncologists must understand the natural history of this disease and be familiar with surgery and chemotherapy options and their expected outcomes.

PRESENTATION AND PATTERNS OF SPREAD

The typical presenting symptoms of ovarian cancer are pain, dysuria, bloating, and early satiety. These symptoms are often vague and may not occur until the cancer is already advanced. At diagnosis, about 70% of patients have disease that has extended or metastasized beyond the ovary.

Disease is bilateral at diagnosis in 25% to 30% of cases. Ovarian cancer may extend directly from the ovary to the rectosigmoid, ureters, pelvic sidewall, or other adjacent tissues. The most common form of metastasis from ovarian cancer is transcoelomic metastasis, in which detached malignant cells following the pattern of flow of peritoneal fluid implant on peritoneal surfaces and form metastatic growths. Common sites of involvement resulting from this type of metastasis are the pelvic cul-de-sac (rectouterine pouch), omentum, paracolic gutters, and undersurface of the right hemidiaphragm. However, not all patients with malignant cells found in peritoneal fluid have or develop peritoneal tumor involvement, suggesting that not all cancers have the capacity to implant and grow on serosal surfaces.

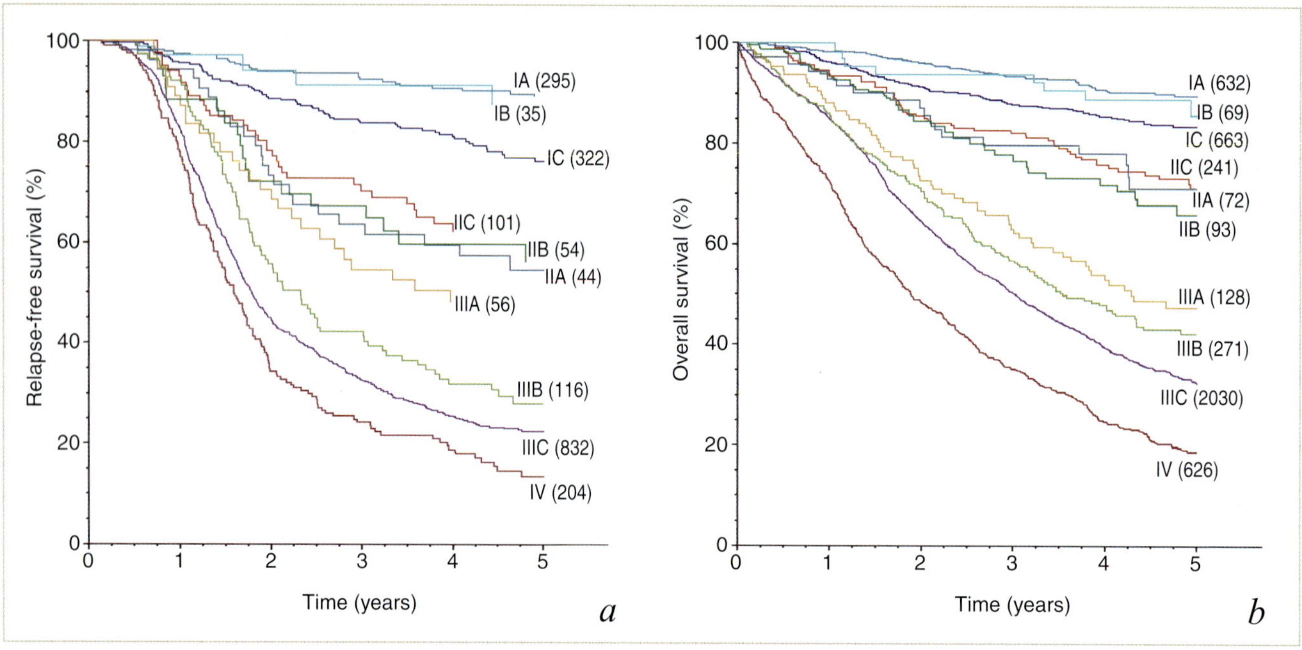

FIGURE 14.1 Relapse-free survival (*a*) and overall survival (*b*) of patients with epithelial ovarian cancer by FIGO substage. Stage categories in this figure refer to the 2006 FIGO stage categories. (From Heintz AP, Quinn MA, Benedet JL, et al. Carcinoma of the ovary. FIGO 26th Annual Report on the Results of Treatment in Gynecological Cancer. *Int J Gynaecol Obstet.* 2006;95(suppl 1):S161–S192.)

Ovarian cancer can spread directly to pelvic, paraaortic, or occasionally, inguinal lymph nodes (Chapter 5). Lymphadenectomy series indicate that 50% to 80% of patients with stage III or IV disease and at least 20% of patients who would otherwise be classified as having stage I or II disease have pelvic or paraaortic lymph node metastases.[1]

Hematogenous metastases are present in only 2% to 3% of patients at diagnosis. About one-third of patients with stage III or IV disease at diagnosis eventually develop metastases in the lung, liver, brain, bone, subcutaneous tissues, or other sites.

PROGNOSTIC FACTORS

FIGO Stage

The FIGO staging system is based on clinical findings and on the results of intra-abdominal surgical exploration. Both recurrence-free survival (**Fig. 14.1**) and overall survival are strongly correlated with FIGO stage.[2] However, about half of all patients have stage III disease, and most of those have stage IIIC disease (**Fig. 14.2**).

In 2014, FIGO published a revised staging system for ovarian cancer (**Table 14.1**).[3] In this new version, ovarian, fallopian tube, and primary peritoneal cancers were for the first time covered by a single staging system, reflecting the similar natural histories and approaches to treatment for carcinomas arising in these sites. Also, the stage IC category was subdivided to reflect findings concerning the relationships between tumor spill and outcome.

However, the most significant changes in the 2014 FIGO staging system involved the classification of ovarian cancer with nodal metastases. In the 2006 FIGO staging system, all cases with lymph node metastases were classified as at least stage IIIC. Since then, retrospective studies demonstrated that patients who had pelvic or aortic lymph node metastases without peritoneal carcinomatosis had a better prognosis than other patients with stage IIIC disease.[1,4] For this reason, in the 2014 system, FIGO designated a separate category (stage IIIA1) for pelvic or aortic nodal metastases without

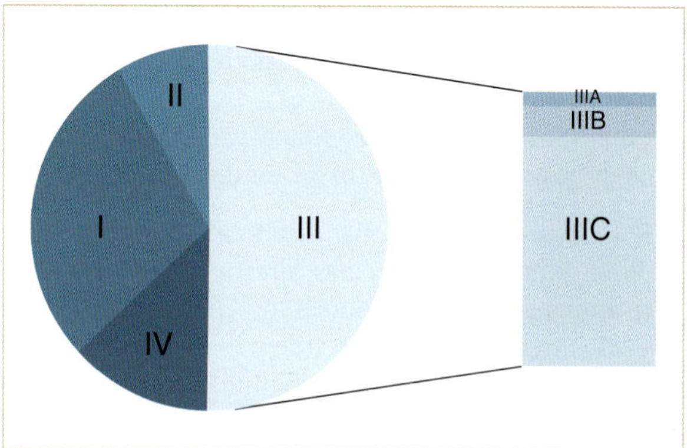

FIGURE 14.2 Distribution of patients with newly diagnosed epithelial ovarian cancer by FIGO stage. Stage categories in this figure refer to the 2006 FIGO stage categories. (Data from Heintz AP, Quinn MA, Benedet JL, et al. Carcinoma of the ovary. FIGO 26th Annual Report on the Results of Treatment in Gynecological Cancer. *Int J Gynaecol Obstet.* 2006;95(suppl 1):S161–S192.)

TABLE 14.1 FIGO Staging for Primary Cancers of the Ovary, Fallopian Tube, and Peritoneum (Effective January 1, 2014)

Stage I	**Tumor confined to ovaries or fallopian tubes**
IA	Tumor limited to one ovary (capsule intact) or fallopian tube; no tumor on ovarian or fallopian tube surface; no malignant cells in ascites or peritoneal washings
IB	Tumor limited to both ovaries (capsule intact) or fallopian tubes; no tumor on ovarian or fallopian tube surface; no malignant cells in ascites or peritoneal washings
IC	Tumor limited to one or both ovaries or fallopian tubes, with any of the following:
IC1	Surgical spill intraoperatively
IC2	Capsule ruptured before surgery or tumor on ovarian or fallopian tube surface
IC3	Malignant cells in ascites or peritoneal washings
Stage II	**Tumor involves one or both ovaries or fallopian tubes with pelvic extension (below the pelvic brim) or primary peritoneal cancer**
IIA	Extension and/or implants on the uterus, fallopian tubes, or ovaries
IIB	Extension to other pelvic intraperitoneal tissues
Stage III	**Tumor involves one or both ovaries or fallopian tubes or peritoneal cancer, with cytologically or histologically confirmed spread to the peritoneum outside the pelvis or metastasis to the retroperitoneal lymph nodes**
IIIA	Metastasis to the retroperitoneal lymph nodes with or without microscopic peritoneal involvement beyond the pelvis
IIIA1	Positive retroperitoneal lymph nodes only (histologically proven), either ≤10 mm in greatest dimension (IIIA1i) or >10 mm (IIIA1ii)
IIIA2	Microscopic extrapelvic (above the pelvic brim) peritoneal involvement with or without positive retroperitoneal lymph nodes
IIIB	Macroscopic peritoneal metastases beyond the pelvic brim ≤2 cm in greatest dimension with or without metastases to retroperitoneal nodes
IIIC	Macroscopic peritoneal metastases beyond the pelvic brim >2 cm in greatest dimension, with or without metastases to retroperitoneal nodes
Stage IV	**Distant metastasis excluding peritoneal metastases**
IVA	Pleural effusion with positive cytology
IVB	Metastases to extra-abdominal organs (including inguinal lymph nodes and lymph nodes outside of the abdominal cavity)

peritoneal carcinomatosis. For radiation oncologists, this separate designation for apparently locoregionally confined disease will help to clarify the initial distribution of disease when patients are referred for treatment of subsequent recurrences.

In the 2014 staging system, FIGO also shifted isolated inguinal node metastases from stage IIIC to stage IVB. There are few data documenting the outcomes of patients with this rare presentation; however, the groin is a primary echelon site of lymphatic drainage from the ovaries (Chapter 5), and anecdotal reports of prolonged survival after local treatment for isolated groin recurrences (CS 14.8)[5] suggest that the prognosis may not be as grave as the stage IVB designation suggests.

Histologic Subtype

The stage of ovarian cancer at presentation is strongly correlated with the histologic subtype (Fig. 14.3).[2] Differences in the behaviors of these subtypes provide important insights for clinicians interested in defining the role of local treatment in the management of ovarian cancer.

Because about two-thirds of ovarian cancers are serous, undifferentiated, or of mixed histologic subtype with a serous component, the behavior of these cancers dominates clinical impressions of the disease. Serous carcinomas, whether they originate in the ovary, fallopian tube, uterus, or peritoneum, have a strong predilection for transcoelomic spread. Although a small subset of ovarian serous cancers may lack the ability to implant on peritoneal surfaces (CS 14.3, 14.4, and 14.7), approximately 80% of patients with ovarian serous cancer present with advanced disease, usually with abdominal carcinomatosis. Undifferentiated cancers and carcinosarcomas exhibit similarly aggressive behaviors.

Mucinous, clear cell, and endometrioid cancers are much less likely to spread intraperitoneally; about two-thirds of these cancers are confined to the pelvis at diagnosis

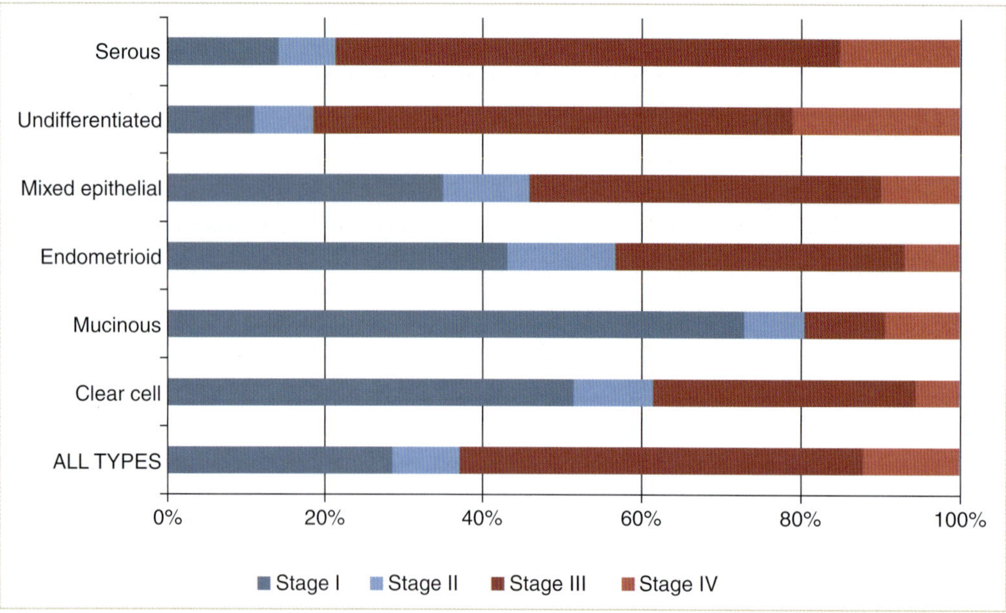

FIGURE 14.3 Relationship between histologic subtype and FIGO stage in patients with epithelial ovarian cancer. Stage categories in this figure refer to the 2006 FIGO stage categories. (Data from Heintz AP, Quinn MA, Benedet JL, et al. Carcinoma of the ovary. FIGO 26th Annual Report on the Results of Treatment in Gynecological Cancer. *Int J Gynaecol Obstet.* 2006;95(suppl 1):S161–S192.)

(**Fig. 14.3**). Several authors have reported that locoregionally confined ovarian cancers of these subtypes have a relatively good prognosis after treatment with involved-field RT.[5–7] As data accumulate, it will also be interesting to note whether patients with these subtypes are more likely to present with isolated pelvic or aortic lymph node metastases (i.e., stage IIIA1 disease).

Patients with early-stage (FIGO stage I or II) serous, mucinous, and clear cell carcinomas have similar prognoses. However, mucinous and clear cell carcinomas tend to respond more poorly to chemotherapy than other histologic subtypes, and therefore, patients with advanced mucinous or clear cell carcinomas have a relatively poor prognosis.[2] Because mucinous and clear cell cancers have a greater tendency to remain localized and have relatively poor chemoresponsiveness, patients with these cancers are relatively good candidates for RT under appropriate circumstances.

Grade

In general, patients with ovarian cancer with grade 1 tumors tend to survive longer than patients with grade 2 or 3 tumors of similar stage,[2] although studies have demonstrated significant inter- and intraobserver variation in the assignment of tumor grade.

ROLES OF SURGERY AND CHEMOTHERAPY

Surgery and chemotherapy are the cornerstones of treatment for epithelial ovarian cancer. While RT can play an important role in individual cases, it can only be recommended after careful consideration of the risks and potential benefits of all available treatments. For this reason, the roles of surgery and chemotherapy in patients with early-stage, advanced, and recurrent ovarian cancer are reviewed here.

Surgery

Early-Stage Disease

In a patient with an adnexal mass, the first step in management is to assess the risk of malignancy using pelvic ultrasonography and measurement of the serum CA-125 level. If the findings are suggestive of malignancy, the patient should be referred to a gynecologic oncologist for surgical evaluation. If intraoperative frozen section is positive for invasive ovarian cancer, full surgical staging should be performed.[8]

The standard surgical treatment and evaluation for early-stage ovarian cancer includes total abdominal hysterectomy with bilateral salpingo-oophorectomy (TAH-BSO) (ideally with intact removal of the ovarian tumor), omentectomy, and pelvic and paraaortic lymph node dissection. Peritoneal surfaces should be explored, and suspicious lesions should be biopsied. In addition, random biopsies of the cul-de-sac, paracolic gutters, intestinal mesenteries, and diaphragm should be performed, and ascitic fluid or pelvic washings should be collected.

A horizontal suprapubic (Pfannenstiel) incision does not provide adequate access for the evaluation of the upper abdomen; studies of patients who have had re-exploration through a more appropriate midline incision reveal that the stage is increased as a result in at least 30% of those initially thought to have stage I or II disease.[9]

Advanced Disease

Patients with more advanced disease who are medically fit and who do not have metastases in organ parenchyma usually undergo initial cytoreductive surgery, including TAH-BSO, omentectomy, lymph node dissection, and resection of as much metastatic disease as possible; the goal of surgery is to achieve an *optimal cytoreduction* leaving no more than microscopic residual disease.[8]

Cytoreductive surgery typically provides immediate benefit by relieving gastrointestinal symptoms caused by intestinal compression or obstruction, thereby improving the patient's overall nutritional status. A number of more theoretical benefits of cytoreductive surgery include removal of poorly vascularized regions that might not receive adequate concentrations of chemotherapy; reduction in the proportion of nonproliferating, relatively chemoresistant cells; reduction in the proportion of hypoxic cells; and reduction (potentially by several logs) in the overall number of cancer cells that must be killed by chemotherapy. However, the prognosis of patients with bulky (>10 cm) metastatic deposits or extensive carcinomatosis remains poor even after an optimal cytoreduction.[8]

Patients with advanced disease who, for medical or other reasons, are unable to undergo primary cytoreductive surgery typically have a diagnosis made by biopsy and then receive 3 or more cycles of neoadjuvant chemotherapy. If repeat evaluation after neoadjuvant chemotherapy demonstrates a satisfactory initial response, the patient usually undergoes an interval debulking surgery with the goal of achieving an optimal cytoreduction before administration of additional chemotherapy.

There is fairly strong evidence that achievement of optimal primary cytoreduction, which requires effort and skill, is associated with improved survival rates; however, the poorer survival rates of patients with suboptimal cytoreduction may, in part, reflect confounding adverse prognostic factors.[2,10]

Recurrent Disease

Surgery performed to achieve optimal cytoreduction of disease that has recurred after chemotherapy is termed *secondary cytoreduction*. Patients whose cancer progresses or recurs within 6 months of the completion of platinum-based chemotherapy (i.e., platinum-resistant cancer) do not appear to benefit from secondary cytoreduction. However, retrospective studies indicate that secondary cytoreduction may benefit selected patients with relatively late, localized recurrences that can be completely resected.

Additional notes about surgery for ovarian cancer.

- Although lymph node dissections are increasingly being included in routine surgical staging, these are often limited nodal samplings; a thorough lymphadenectomy, which adds significantly to the length and potential adverse effects of surgery, is frequently not performed.
- There has been a move toward increasingly thorough surgical staging, which has improved the quality of information used to select treatments but has also resulted in stage migration toward more advanced stages, causing improvements in survival to appear more encouraging when viewed stage by stage than when examined for the overall population.[2]
- A 2012 SEER analysis found that 48% of patients undergoing surgical staging for ovarian cancer have at least one perioperative complication. The ~16% of patients who had multiple complications were more likely to have delayed initiation of chemotherapy and a poor outcome.[11]
- Cytoreductive surgeries are often long, open operations that involve bowel resections, ureterolysis, extensive lymph node dissections, and other procedures that traumatize critical structures. These surgical manipulations undoubtedly contribute to the risk of adverse effects from subsequent RT.

Chemotherapy

The current standard chemotherapy for most patients with newly diagnosed epithelial ovarian cancer is combination chemotherapy including a platinum compound (usually carboplatin) and a taxane (usually paclitaxel). Patients who have early-stage disease may be treated with combination chemotherapy or with carboplatin only. The only patients for whom chemotherapy is not recommended are those with FIGO (2014) stage IA or IB, grade 1 disease.[8] A brief review of the studies leading to this standard will help to put the evolving role of RT for ovarian cancer in context.

Early-Stage Disease

Adjuvant chemotherapy is usually recommended for patients who have stage IC or II disease or grade 2 or 3 disease of any stage.[8,12] Although there is no definitive evidence that chemotherapy improves survival in patients with early-stage disease who have had thorough surgical staging, recent studies suggest that some patients with early-stage disease may derive greater benefit from adjuvant chemotherapy than others.

In the late 1980s, three trials that compared combination chemotherapy (cisplatin and cyclophosphamide) with either observation or intraperitoneal instillation of phosphorus 32 demonstrated lower recurrence rates for patients who received adjuvant chemotherapy but no differences in overall survival rates.[13,14]

In the 1990s, two large European randomized trials compared platinum-based chemotherapy with observation in patients with early-stage disease.[15] Although both trials demonstrated significant improvements in survival for patients who received chemotherapy, many of the patients in these trials did not have optimal surgical staging. When a subset analysis was performed that was limited to patients who had optimal surgical staging, no significant survival improvement was seen with chemotherapy.[11,15]

In a subsequent Gynecologic Oncology Group (GOG) trial (GOG-157),[16] there was no difference in outcome for 3 versus

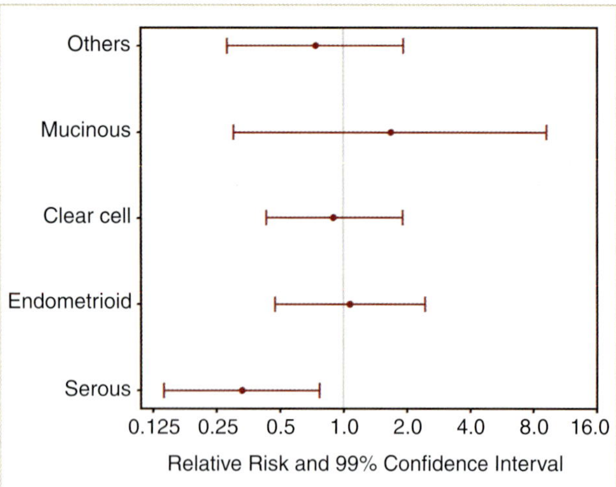

FIGURE 14.4 Relative risk of recurrence for 427 patients with ovarian cancer who received 6 versus 3 cycles of carboplatin and paclitaxel in GOG-157 by histologic subtype. (From Chan JK,Tian C, Fleming GF, et al. The potential benefit of 6 vs. 3 cycles of chemotherapy in subsets of women with early-stage high-risk epithelial ovarian cancer: an exploratory analysis of a Gynecologic Oncology Group study. *Gynecol Oncol.* 2010;116(3):301-306, doi:10.1016/j.ygyno.2009.10.073.)

6 cycles of carboplatin and paclitaxel in patients with early-stage, high-risk (stage IA, grade 3; stage IB, grade 3; clear cell; or any stage IC or II) epithelial ovarian cancer. Interestingly, an exploratory subset analysis showed that for 97 patients with serous carcinomas, the recurrence rate was significantly less for patients randomized to receive 6 cycles,[17] whereas for 266 patients with endometrioid, clear cell, or mucinous cancers, the number of cycles had no influence on the recurrence rate, providing additional evidence of the different behavior of these subtypes (Fig. 14.4).

Advanced Disease

Dozens of prospective randomized trials conducted over more than 40 years have led to the current standard treatments for advanced ovarian cancer. Although these studies have led to some incremental improvements, most patients with advanced disease eventually die of causes related to ovarian cancer (Fig. 14.1).[2]

In the 1970s, the standard treatment for ovarian cancer was single-agent chemotherapy with alkylating agents such as melphalan, cyclophosphamide, or chlorambucil. Investigators sought to improve outcomes by combining these agents with other available cytotoxic drugs, but more than a dozen trials failed to improve on the results achieved with single agents.[18] At the time, patients who had minimal residual disease after surgery often had pelvic RT added to alkylating agent therapy. Two trials that compared this standard with whole abdominal RT are discussed in the section "Historical Evidence of Benefit from RT" later in this chapter.

After cisplatin was made available for clinical use in the late 1970s, it was soon demonstrated to be superior to cyclophosphamide as a single agent, increasing the median survival of patients with advanced disease from 12 to 19 months.[19] A meta-analysis of trials that tested combinations that did or did not include cisplatin also suggested a benefit from cisplatin treatment.[20] However, randomized trials comparing cisplatin alone or in combination with other agents yielded inconclusive results.[20]

In the late 1980s, two drugs were introduced that would eventually form the backbone of ovarian cancer treatment: carboplatin and paclitaxel. Carboplatin, introduced in 1989, was found to be as effective as cisplatin but with less nephrotoxicity and fewer gastrointestinal toxic effects[20]; it soon replaced cisplatin in the treatment of ovarian cancer. In the early 1990s, two large prospective trials compared a combination of carboplatin and paclitaxel with the then-standard regimen of carboplatin and cyclophosphamide; both trials demonstrated significantly improved response rates, progression-free survival, and eventually, overall survival for the paclitaxel-containing combination.[21] Combinations of carboplatin and paclitaxel have continued to form the standard primary treatment for ovarian cancer for 20 years.

Several studies have tried to improve on the results seen with carboplatin and paclitaxel by adding new agents.

- *Addition of other cytotoxic agents.* A massive 5-arm multinational trial added topotecan, liposomal doxorubicin, or gemcitabine to the carboplatin–paclitaxel backbone in various combinations. None of these combinations improved upon the 2-drug control treatment.[22]
- *Addition of bevacizumab.* Two large randomized trials failed to demonstrate improved survival with addition of concurrent or maintenance bevacizumab to the combination of carboplatin and paclitaxel.[23,24] One study showed a 2-month delay in time to progression, but the progression-free survival curves converged a few months after maintenance bevacizumab was discontinued.[24] This minimal gain, coupled with the cost and toxic effects of bevacizumab, has prevented the drug from becoming standard for initial treatment of ovarian cancer, although it is sometimes used to treat recurrence.

Perhaps more successful have been efforts to improve outcome by increasing treatment intensity. Recent studies have focused on two methods of dose intensification: intraperitoneal chemotherapy and dose-dense chemotherapy.

- *Intraperitoneal chemotherapy.* Several randomized trials have demonstrated significantly improved survival rates with the combination of intraperitoneal and intravenous administration of chemotherapy.[25] The benefits of this approach appear to be greater for patients who have had optimal cytoreduction and less for patients with mucinous, clear cell, and low-grade tumors. Intraperitoneal chemotherapy is associated with increased toxic effects, including bowel adhesions, and may be associated with an increase in the rate of adhesion-related bowel obstruction.[26] There are very few data available on the risks of RT after intraperitoneal chemotherapy, but this form of chemotherapy should be considered a possible risk factor for post-RT bowel complications.

- *Dose-dense chemotherapy.* In 2009, the Japanese Gynecologic Oncology Group published results of a trial that compared standard every 3 weeks carboplatin and paclitaxel with an intensified regimen that combined standard-dose carboplatin with weekly paclitaxel[27]; the total paclitaxel dose was increased by 30% in the dose-dense regimen. Both progression-free survival and median survival were significantly better for patients in the dose-dense arm. Patients who had residual disease measuring at least 1 cm in diameter appeared to derive the greatest benefit. This result has not yet been independently confirmed, but several trials of dose-dense chemotherapy are ongoing.

Several studies have evaluated the possible role of maintenance chemotherapy for advanced ovarian cancer. A 2013 meta-analysis of eight trials concluded that there was no evidence that adding maintenance therapy with platinum, doxorubicin, or paclitaxel to standard primary chemotherapy was more effective than observation alone.[28]

Recurrent Disease

Recurrent ovarian cancer is rarely curable with chemotherapy. However, the times to recurrence and death in patients treated for ovarian cancer are variable. Although most recurrences occur within 2 years of an initial complete response, first recurrences may occur 5 or more years after treatment (**Fig. 14.1**; **CS 14.1**). In some cases, a poor response to first-line chemotherapy and rapid disease progression lead to the patient's death in weeks or months. In other cases, ovarian cancer becomes a chronic disease with a course spanning many years and many therapeutic interventions **(CS 14.1, 14.3, and 14.7)**; in these cases, clinicians are challenged to balance the adverse effects of tumor and treatment in a way that maximizes the duration and the quality of the patient's life.

Patients who experience progression or recurrence within 6 months of completing an initial course of platinum-based chemotherapy are considered to have platinum-resistant disease; their rates of response to second-line cytotoxic chemotherapy are generally <10%, and their median overall survival is usually reported to be about 12 months.[8]

Patients who experience recurrence more than 6 months after completing primary chemotherapy are considered to have platinum-sensitive disease. These patients are much more likely than patients with platinum-resistant disease to respond to retreatment with a platinum agent, usually given in combination with paclitaxel, doxorubicin, or gemcitabine. However, the duration of response tends to be short: the most effective combinations yield median progression-free survival times of 10 to 12 months. At least 75% of patients who begin second-line chemotherapy can be expected to have active disease 1 year later, and more than 90% will have experienced progression by 2 years.

After second recurrence, some patients will continue to respond to chemotherapy but typically with progressively shorter response durations and increasing treatment-related toxic effects.

Toxic Effects of Chemotherapy

Although combinations of carboplatin and paclitaxel are usually relatively well tolerated, they cause a number of toxic effects, including alopecia, nausea, anorexia, fatigue, myelosuppression, and neurotoxic effects. Paclitaxel-associated peripheral neuropathy can be dose limiting and may compromise the patient's quality of life. See Chapter 3 for a more detailed review of the toxic effects of these and other drugs used in the treatment of ovarian cancer.

ROLE OF RT

Historical Evidence of Benefit from RT

A brief review of historical experiences will help to explain geographic differences in attitudes toward the use of RT in the treatment of ovarian cancer.

In the 1960s and early 1970s, several retrospective studies suggested that adjuvant pelvic RT resulted in better than expected outcome for patients with early-stage, particularly stage II, ovarian cancer.[29] However, it was clear that abdominal recurrences prevented local RT from having a major curative role.

In 1963, Delclos et al.[30] described the first practical method of delivering whole abdominal RT (WART) using a cobalt-moving-strip technique. This advance led to a series of randomized trials comparing WART with alkylating agent chemotherapy. In the first, the MD Anderson Cancer Center group compared WART with single-agent melphalan in patients with stage I or II disease; they reported similar survival with the two approaches but less severe gastrointestinal toxic effects in the patients treated with chemotherapy. The trial was later criticized because of flaws in the WART technique.[31] However, on the basis of the results of this trial and the introduction of cisplatin a few years later, WART was largely abandoned as an initial treatment for ovarian cancer in the United States.

A second trial, published a few years later by the Princess Margaret Hospital in Toronto, yielded different results. In that study, Dembo et al. compared cobalt-moving-strip WART with a combination of pelvic RT and chlorambucil in patients with stage IB–III disease. After excluding patients who had incomplete pelvic operations, the authors found that the recurrence-free survival rate was significantly higher for patients who had WART than for those treated with chemotherapy (64% vs. 40%).[32] The same group later demonstrated that WART administered using a single large "belly bath" field appeared to be as effective as WART delivered with the cobalt-moving-strip technique.[33] A subsequent multi-institutional Canadian trial[34] and other smaller trials failed to confirm the superiority of WART over alkylating agent chemotherapy. However, the

Princess Margaret Hospital study demonstrated that some patients could be cured with RT. It also led Canadian physicians to retain interest in RT as a treatment for ovarian cancer.

During the 1980s, a number of investigators evaluated the use of WART as salvage therapy for patients in whom multiagent chemotherapy failed to control disease. Although there were anecdotal successes, most of the patients in these series had chemotherapy-resistant, high-grade neoplasms and compromised bone marrow reserve, which limited the deliverability and effectiveness of WART.[35,36]

Predictors of Benefit from RT

Although historical experiences indicated that some patients with ovarian cancer benefitted from RT, the results have been difficult to apply to modern practice. A major weakness of early studies was the inclusion of many patients who were later identified as poor candidates for RT. Subsequent retrospective analyses of these experiences began to define prognostic factors that predicted relatively good outcome with RT.

In 1993, the Princess Margaret group sought to validate and refine previous prognostic classification systems for ovarian cancer.[37] They analyzed outcomes of 472 patients with stage I–III ovarian carcinoma who had "optimal" (defined as <2 cm) residual disease; all patients received equivalent doses of ~27.5 Gy to the whole abdomen and 50 Gy to the pelvis. Their study confirmed earlier impressions that recurrence-free survival was strongly correlated with stage, histologic subtype, and grade. In particular, patients with grade I cancers and with stage I–II mucinous or endometrioid cancers tended to have a favorable outcome. There were few patients with clear cell carcinoma in this series.

A 2011 population-based study by Swenerton et al. from Vancouver, Canada, refined understanding of the relationship between histologic subtype and the effectiveness of RT.[7] In 1985, the British Columbia Cancer Agency developed guidelines for treatment of women with optimally cytoreduced intermediate- to high-risk ovarian cancer. The guidelines recommended 3 cycles of platinum-based chemotherapy followed by either WART or 3 additional cycles of chemotherapy, according to physician preference. From the British Columbia Cancer Agency tumor registry database, Swenerton et al. identified 703 eligible patients who had received either chemotherapy only (351 patients) or chemotherapy followed by WART (352 patients). For the 281 women with serous carcinomas, there were no differences in survival or disease-specific survival between the two treatments. However, for the 399 women with endometrioid, mucinous, or clear cell carcinomas, RT was associated with a 40% reduction in mortality and a 43% reduction in disease-specific mortality compared to chemotherapy only (**Fig. 14.5**). A second analysis that focused on women with clear cell carcinoma of the ovary demonstrated that those with stage II or stage IC disease due to capsular involvement had significantly better relapse-free survival if they had RT (usually WART) in combination with carboplatin and paclitaxel rather than chemotherapy alone (relative risk of relapse, 0.54; $p = 0.02$).[6] It is interesting that GOG-157 demonstrated no difference between 3 versus 6 cycles of chemotherapy for patients with endometrioid, mucinous, or clear cell carcinoma (**Fig. 14.4**).

These studies leave a number of questions unanswered. First and perhaps most important, does the whole abdomen

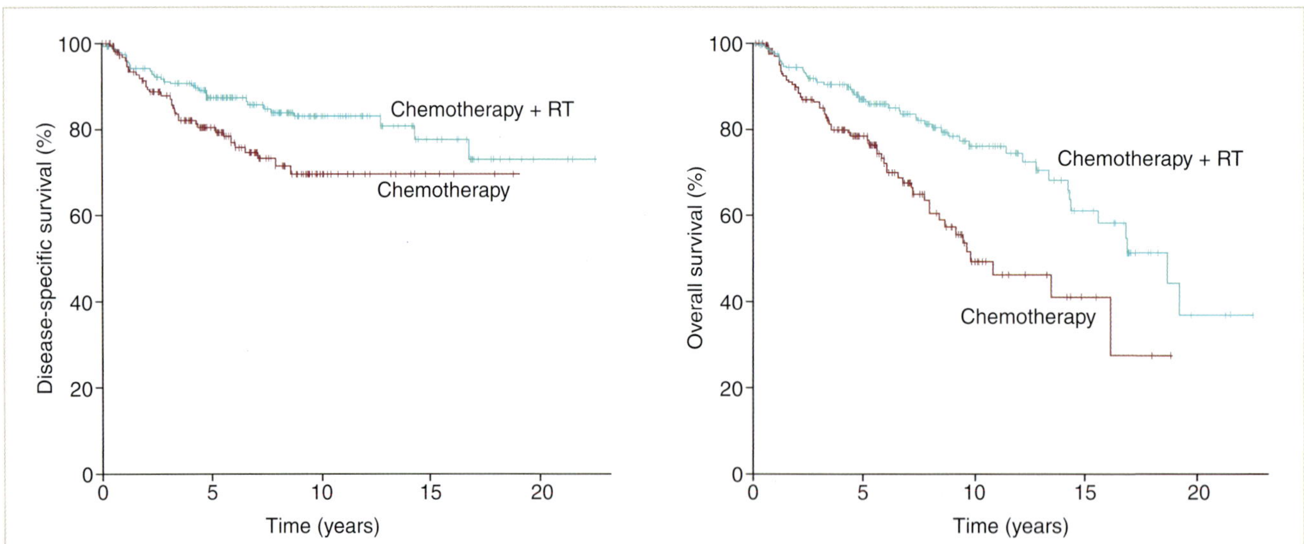

FIGURE 14.5 Disease-specific survival (*a*) and overall survival (*b*) for patients with stage I and II clear cell, endometrioid, and mucinous ovarian cancers treated with 6 cycles of carboplatin and paclitaxel or with 3 cycles of carboplatin and paclitaxel followed by WART. (Swenerton KD, Santos JL, Gilks CB, et al. Histotype predicts the curative potential of radiotherapy: the example of ovarian cancers. *Ann Oncol.* 2011;22(2):341–347, doi:10.1093/annonc/mdq383.)

need to be treated in order for RT to provide a benefit? Second, is the relatively low dose of radiation delivered to peritoneal surfaces with WART sufficiently effective to justify the added morbidity of large-field treatment, or is it the pelvic treatment that is most important? The patients who benefitted most from WART were those with stage I and II disease of histologic subtypes that are less likely than serous cancer to involve peritoneal surfaces early in the course of the disease. Third, how important is the treatment of the paraaortic region, a primary echelon site of nodal involvement? Given the compelling evidence from the Canadian studies and given the reluctance to use WART outside of Canada, it may be time to explore the value of local, volume-directed RT in selected women with ovarian cancer. In the meantime, because there have been no major studies of adjuvant local RT, the best clues to answer these questions may come from retrospective studies of RT for postchemotherapy recurrence.

RT for Recurrent Disease

Retrospective studies of women treated for postchemotherapy recurrence of ovarian cancer provide evidence of the potential curative role of involved-field RT in this disease.[5,38] In 2013, Brown et al.[5] reported the outcomes of 102 patients treated with definitive involved-field RT for localized postchemotherapy recurrence. Most of the patients were heavily pretreated: patients in the series had received a median of three courses of chemotherapy and had undergone a median of two resections before being referred for RT. Typically, patients were referred because their tumors were not responding to chemotherapy or because toxic effects no longer permitted patients to receive systemic therapy. Despite these unfavorable features, the 5-year progression-free and overall survival rates were 24% and 40%, respectively (**Fig. 14.6**). Several patients with recurrence at a second site

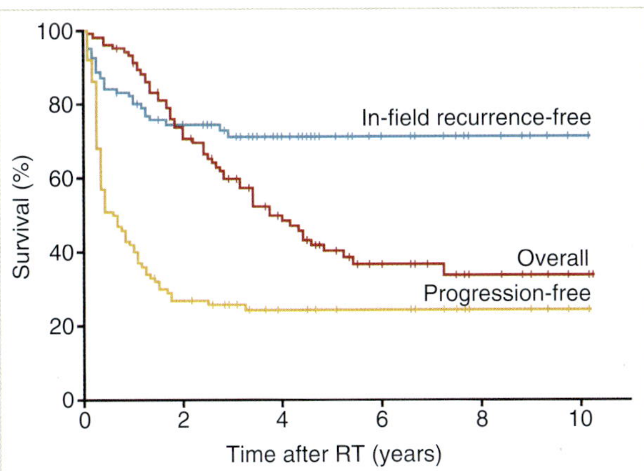

FIGURE 14.6 Outcome from the time of RT for 102 women treated with curative intent for recurrent epithelial ovarian cancer at MD Anderson Cancer Center from 1999 to 2009. (From Brown AP, Jhingran A, Klopp AH, et al. Involved-field radiation therapy for locoregionally recurrent ovarian cancer. *Gynecol Oncol.* 2013;130(2): 300–305, doi:10.1016/j.ygyno.2013.04.469.)

after RT had successful salvage treatment, and other patients had prolonged treatment breaks before requiring additional treatment. The eight patients with recurrent clear cell carcinoma had a particularly favorable prognosis compared to other patients (5-year relapse-free survival rate, 75% vs. 20%, $p = 0.01$). Other predictors of a good outcome were initial platinum sensitivity and a tumor diameter <3 cm at the time of RT. However, the long-term survivors also included a number of patients with platinum-resistant, high-grade serous, or bulky unresectable cancers. Several of the case studies at the end of this chapter describe cases reported in this series.

Palliative RT

RT can be very effective for palliation of symptoms from a dominant lesion. The most common indications for palliative RT are vaginal bleeding, pain, and rectosigmoid compression from a pelvic mass. Painful paraaortic disease may also be an indication for palliative RT. Hematogenous metastases from ovarian cancer are relatively uncommon, but some patients do develop painful bone metastases or brain metastases that require symptom relief. Palliative strategies and treatments are discussed in more detail in Chapter 16.

DEVELOPING A RADIATION TREATMENT STRATEGY

This section and the case studies at the end of this chapter will focus mainly on the selection, evaluation, and treatment of patients with recurrence of ovarian cancer after chemotherapy because that has been the context of most of our experience. However, the data presented in this chapter strongly suggest that there may also be a role for adjuvant RT, so we will begin with a discussion of RT as adjuvant treatment.

RT as Adjuvant Treatment

Clear cell, mucinous, and endometrioid cancers tend to be localized at presentation and have repeatedly been demonstrated to have favorable outcomes after RT. The fact that these subtypes, particularly clear cell and mucinous cancers, also respond relatively poorly to chemotherapy suggests an opportunity for RT, probably in combination with chemotherapy, to improve outcome. Stage IIB and IIIA1 cancers of favorable subtype would be the most obvious candidates for such an up-front combined modality approach. However, in the United States, RT is rarely considered as an initial treatment; in current National Comprehensive Cancer Network guidelines, RT is not mentioned as a treatment option for ovarian cancer of any stage.[39]

RT for Recurrent Disease

Patient Selection

The ideal candidate for definitive salvage treatment is probably one who has a tumor of favorable histologic subtype that has recurred in a single nodal site (paraaortic, pelvic, or inguinal) (**CS 14.6 and 14.8**) or in the initial pelvic operative bed (e.g., at the vaginal apex or in the cul-de-sac) (**CS 14.2**). That said, even patients with high-grade serous tumors can be good candidates for definitive RT in the rare cases in which the tumor never colonizes the peritoneal cavity despite repeated local or nodal recurrences (**CS 14.3 and 14.7**).

Patients who have never had peritoneal disease are probably better candidates for RT than patients who have had peritoneal disease. However, sometimes patients with platinum-sensitive cancer that initially involved the peritoneum will subsequently develop stubbornly recurrent disease in a single site (**CS 14.4**). These patients will occasionally do well after local treatment of the recurrence; however, before definitive treatment is initiated, every effort should be made to rule out peritoneal or distant involvement, particularly if there are still some viable options for systemic treatment.

Before RT is recommended, there should always be a detailed multidisciplinary discussion to determine whether surgical resection would improve the likelihood of local control sufficiently to justify the risks of surgery (Chapter 3). In many cases, RT will be recommended to prevent postsurgical recurrence. The decision whether to recommend combined modality treatment or RT alone is based on the following factors:

1. The size of the tumor. Tumors >3 cm in diameter can often be controlled with RT alone but have a higher likelihood of post-RT recurrence than smaller tumors.
2. The likelihood that complete resection can be achieved without sacrifice of organ function.
3. The proximity of tumor to adjacent critical structures that could be injured by administration of definitive RT (**CS 14.2**).
4. The probability that surgery will increase the likelihood of radiation-related adverse effects.
5. The possible benefit of restaging to rule out microscopic peritoneal disease.

Pre-RT Evaluation

When a patient is being considered for definitive RT, a thorough evaluation should be performed to (1) rule out the presence of distant metastases or peritoneal involvement that would shift the treatment goal from curative to palliative; (2) accurately define the extent of gross disease; and (3) define any other regions that might be at relatively high risk for recurrence.

In some cases, PET–CT can be very valuable both for ruling out distant disease and for defining the extent of gross disease in the potential treatment region. For patients with recurrent pelvic disease, computed tomography with a contrast agent helps to differentiate gross disease from adjacent bowel loops and to define the extent of possible regional nodal involvement. Pelvic examination is important to define the presence and extent of vaginal involvement (Chapter 4).

The pretreatment evaluation should always include a detailed review of all previous imaging, operative, and pathology reports. This review may suggest a region adjacent to the recurrence site that is at sufficiently high risk to justify expansion of the clinical target volume (CTV) or designation of a high-risk CTV.

RT Doses

Although the data from studies of WART seem to suggest that low radiation doses are sometimes effective in the treatment of ovarian cancer, our experiences with RT for gross disease suggest that the doses required to control ovarian carcinomas are similar to those for müllerian carcinomas arising in other sites. In most cases, we recommend delivering the equivalent of 60 to 66 Gy at 2 Gy per fraction to regions of gross disease, with the cumulative dose depending on the size of the metastatic deposit and the proximity of critical structures. CTVs are usually treated to 45 to 50 Gy. However, a higher dose may be given if the risk of disease is considered higher than usual because of any of the following:

1. The finding of equivocal nodes close to the gross tumor volume
2. Extracapsular nodal extension
3. Close or positive surgical margins
4. Prechemotherapy sites of involvement that are adjacent to the primary target volume

Although forward-planned three-dimensional conformal RT with curative intent can be delivered successfully, intensity-modulated RT is particularly valuable for the treatment of ovarian cancer recurrent after chemotherapy because of the frequent presence of gross disease requiring relatively high doses; the greater than usual risk of radiation-related complications because of prior treatments; and the frequent close proximity of recurrent tumor to sensitive critical structures.

However, because there is a significant risk of microscopic disease adjacent to known gross tumor, tightly conforming fields that include only the gross tumor apparent on imaging are not recommended. In most cases, the target volume should be expanded to include a CTV encompassing regions of possible soft tissue infiltration and immediately adjacent regional nodes. However, the extent of regional coverage may be less than for other gynecologic RT treatments because the extensive preradiation treatments received by most ovarian cancer patients may contribute to a higher than usual risk of side effects. As for all radiation treatments, a realistic PTV margin should always be added to the primary target volumes (Chapter 6).

Site-Specific Treatment Recommendations

Treatment of Pelvic Recurrences

Frequent sites of recurrence are in the presacral space (**CS 14.1**), perirectal space (**CS 14.2**), cul-de-sac (often with extension to the apical vagina) (**CS 14.3**), and iliac nodes. These are often sites of extensive prior surgery, and the risk to adjacent critical structures (particularly bowel anastomoses) must be carefully considered in the decision whether to treat and what to include in the CTV. However, concerns about the risk of treatment-related side effects must be balanced against the risk of marginal recurrence **(CS 14.3)**. It is always wise to include a margin of adjacent soft tissue and proximate lymph nodes in a CTV. Although the extent of the CTV may vary according to the factors discussed above, some general principles should guide treatment planning. For infiltrating soft tissue lesions, we generally include any soft tissue that was involved before chemotherapy response or resection; in most cases, an additional CTV margin of at least 1.5 cm (excluding uninvolved bone, muscle, and bowel) is added to the gross tumor volume (GTV). For lesions involving the cul-de-sac, the CTV usually includes the entire cul-de-sac, apical vagina, and adjacent perirectal space **(CS 14.2)**. For paravaginal lesions, potential internal organ motion should be carefully considered, and a realistic internal target volume (ITV) should be designated (Chapter 5). For patients with isolated pelvic nodal recurrences, we typically extend the nodal CTV at least 3 to 4 cm proximal and 1 to 2 cm distal to the site of known lymph node involvement.

Treatment of Paraaortic Nodes

The paraaortic nodes are one of the most common sites of isolated recurrence **(CS 14.4–14.7)**. The paraaortic nodes most frequently involved are the nodes posterior and just distal to the left renal vessels and the paracaval nodes near the insertion of the gonadal vessels (Chapter 5). For definitive treatment, the recommended CTV usually covers the paracaval and paraaortic nodal compartments, extending distally at least 2 to 3 cm beyond the most distal positive node and proximally at least 2 to 3 cm above the renal vessels. See Chapter 5 for more detailed descriptions of paraaortic nodal target volumes. If many nodes are involved, we usually extend the field distally at least to the bifurcation of the aorta. The paracaval nodes most frequently involved are those lying just posterior to the duodenum; particular care must be taken not to exceed the tolerance limits for this structure (Chapter 6).

Treatment of the Inguinal Nodes

The groin is a possible primary echelon site of nodal spread from the ovary (Chapter 5), and inguinal node recurrences can sometimes be cured with regional RT alone or after groin dissection. The target should include the entire inguinofemoral compartment (Fig. 5.6) and operative bed, if applicable. Inclusion of the distal external and internal iliac nodes in the CTV is usually recommended **(CS 14.8)**.

Treatment of Oligometastases in Extra-abdominal Sites

Although patients who develop extra-abdominal disease (other than in the groin) probably are rarely curable with local therapy, long-term disease-free intervals are occasionally observed after treatment of localized extra-abdominal, particularly nodal, metastases **(CS 14.5)**. That said, Brown et al.[5] were unable to identify a method for predicting these rare, but notable, successes. In patients with localized extra-abdominal metastases, several factors should be carefully considered before a definitive treatment course is recommended, including the pace of disease, likelihood of achieving local control with RT, potential morbidity of high-dose RT, and presence or absence of systemic treatment options.

RT FOR NONEPITHELIAL OVARIAN CANCERS

Nonepithelial ovarian cancers are very rare, and the role of RT in the treatment of these cancers is minor. However, a few specifics deserve mention here.

Dysgerminoma

Dysgerminoma, the most common germ cell tumor in females, is nearly identical to seminoma in males in terms of histologic appearance, behavior, and treatment response profile. Like seminomas, dysgerminomas are very sensitive to RT: after 25 to 35 Gy, local control rates are nearly 100%. However, unlike seminomas, which peak in incidence during the third decade of life, dysgerminomas tend to occur in young, often perimenarchal girls. The primary treatment after removal of the involved ovary is chemotherapy, which is nearly always curative. Because RT at young ages is associated with the added risks of second malignancy, growth delay, premature menopause, and other adverse effects, RT for dysgerminoma is indicated only in very rare instances of recurrent disease.

Granulosa Cell Tumors

Granulosa cell tumors derive from ovarian sex cords and mesenchyme. They are low-grade tumors that are usually confined to the ovary at presentation but can recur many years later. The primary treatment is surgical. Because of the long natural history and rarity of granulosa cell tumors, it has been difficult to study the effects of adjuvant treatments. Although granulosa cell tumors sometimes respond to chemotherapy and RT, there is no proof that any adjuvant treatment improves survival. RT may be considered if there is localized residual disease after surgery and can provide effective palliation of symptoms for patients with localized recurrences. In a review of 34 patients with granulosa cell tumors treated with RT at MD Anderson Cancer Center over a 40-year period,[40] 6 of 14 patients with gross disease had objective responses to RT, and 3 of those patients remained free of disease 10 to 21 years after treatment.

References

1. Berek JS. Lymph node-positive stage IIIC ovarian cancer: a separate entity? *Int J Gynecol Cancer.* 2009;19(suppl 2):S18–S20, doi:10.1111/IGC.0b013e3181bf8111.
2. Heintz AP, Quinn MA, Benedet JL, et al. Carcinoma of the ovary. FIGO 26th Annual Report on the Results of Treatment in Gynecological Cancer. *Int J Gynaecol Obstet.* 2006;95(suppl 1):S161–S192.

3. Prat J; Oncology FCoG, Belhadj H, et al. Staging classification for cancer of the ovary, fallopian tube, and peritoneum. *Int J Gynaecol Obstet.* 2014;124(1):1–5, doi:10.1016/j.ijgo.2013.10.001.
4. Kleppe M, Slangen BF, Kruse AJ, et al. Lymph node metastasis in stages I and II ovarian cancer: a review. *Gynecol Oncol.* 2011;123(3):610–614, doi:10.1016/j.ygyno.2011.09.013.
5. Brown AP, Jhingran A, Klopp AH, et al. Involved-field radiation therapy for locoregionally recurrent ovarian cancer. *Gynecol Oncol.* 2013;130(2):300–305, doi:10.1016/j.ygyno.2013.04.469.
6. Hoskins PJ, Le N, Gilks B, et al. Low-stage ovarian clear cell carcinoma: population-based outcomes in British Columbia, Canada, with evidence for a survival benefit as a result of irradiation. *J Clin Oncol.* 2012;30(14):1656–1662, doi:10.1200/JCO.2011.40.1646.
7. Swenerton KD, Santos JL, Gilks CB, et al. Histotype predicts the curative potential of radiotherapy: the example of ovarian cancers. *Ann Oncol.* 2011;22(2):341–347, doi:10.1093/annonc/mdq383.
8. Berek JS, Friedlander ML, Hacker NF. Epithelial ovarian, fallopian tube, and peritoneal cancer. In: Berek JS, Hacker NF, eds. *Gynecol Oncol.* Philadelphia, PA: Wolters Kluwer; 2014:464–529.
9. Young RC, Decker DG, Wharton JT, et al. Staging laparotomy in early ovarian cancer. *JAMA.* 1983;250(22):3072–3076, doi:10.1001/jama.1983.03340220040030.
10. Hacker NF, Berek JS, Lagasse LD, et al. Primary cytoreductive surgery for epithelial ovarian cancer. *Obstet Gynecol.* 1983;61(4):413–420.
11. Wright JD, Herzog TJ, Neugut AI, et al. Effect of radical cytoreductive surgery on omission and delay of chemotherapy for advanced-stage ovarian cancer. *Obstet Gynecol.* 2012;120(4):871–881, doi:10.1097/AOG.0b013e31826981de.
12. Winter-Roach BA, Kitchener HC, Lawrie TA. Adjuvant (post-surgery) chemotherapy for early stage epithelial ovarian cancer. *Cochrane Database Syst Rev.* 2012;3:CD004706.
13. Bolis G, Colombo N, Pecorelli S, et al. Adjuvant treatment for early epithelial ovarian cancer: results of two randomised clinical trials comparing cisplatin to no further treatment or chromic phosphate (32P). G.I.C.O.G.: Gruppo Interregionale Collaborativo in Ginecologia Oncologica. *Ann Oncol.* 1995;6(9):887–893.
14. Young RC, Brady MF, Nieberg RK, et al. Adjuvant treatment for early ovarian cancer: a randomized phase III trial of intraperitoneal 32P or intravenous cyclophosphamide and cisplatin—a gynecologic oncology group study. *J Clin Oncol.* 2003;21(23):4350–4355, doi:10.1200/JCO.2003.02.154.
15. Trimbos JB, Parmar M, Vergote I, et al. International Collaborative Ovarian Neoplasm trial 1 and Adjuvant ChemoTherapy in Ovarian Neoplasm trial: two parallel randomized phase III trials of adjuvant chemotherapy in patients with early-stage ovarian carcinoma. *J Natl Cancer Inst.* 2003;95(2):105–112, doi:10.1093/jnci/95.2.113.
16. Bell J, Brady MF, Young RC, et al. Randomized phase III trial of three versus six cycles of adjuvant carboplatin and paclitaxel in early stage epithelial ovarian carcinoma: a Gynecologic Oncology Group study. *Gynecol Oncol.* 2006;102(3):432–439, doi:10.1016/j.ygyno.2006.06.013.
17. Chan JK, Tian C, Fleming GF, et al. The potential benefit of 6 vs. 3 cycles of chemotherapy in subsets of women with early-stage high-risk epithelial ovarian cancer: an exploratory analysis of a Gynecologic Oncology Group study. *Gynecol Oncol.* 2010;116(3):301–306, doi:10.1016/j.ygyno.2009.10.073.
18. Advanced Ovarian Cancer Trialists Group. Chemotherapy in advanced ovarian cancer: an overview of randomised clinical trials. *Br Med J. 1991*;303(6807):884–893.
19. Lambert HE, Berry RJ. High dose cisplatin compared with high dose cyclophosphamide in the management of advanced epithelial ovarian cancer (FIGO stages III and IV): report from the North Thames Cooperative Group. *Br Med J.* 1985;290(6472):889–893, doi:10.1136/bmj.290.6472.889.
20. Aabo K, Adams M, Adnitt P, et al. Chemotherapy in advanced ovarian cancer: four systematic meta-analyses of individual patient data from 37 randomized trials. Advanced Ovarian Cancer Trialists' Group. *Br J Cancer.* 1998;78(11):1479–1487, doi:10.1038/bjc.1998.710.
21. Piccart MJ, Bertelsen K, Stuart G, et al. Long-term follow-up confirms a survival advantage of the paclitaxel–cisplatin regimen over the cyclophosphamide–cisplatin combination in advanced ovarian cancer. *Int J Gynecol Cancer.* 2003;13(suppl 2):144–148, doi:10.1111/j.1525-1438.2003.13357.x.
22. Bookman MA, Brady MF, McGuire WP, et al. Evaluation of new platinum-based treatment regimens in advanced-stage ovarian cancer: a Phase III Trial of the Gynecologic Cancer Intergroup. *J Clin Oncol.* 2009;27(9):1419–1425, doi:10.1200/JCO.2008.19.1684.
23. Burger RA, Brady MF, Bookman MA, et al. Incorporation of bevacizumab in the primary treatment of ovarian cancer. *N Engl J Med.* 2011;365(26):2473–2483, doi:10.1056/NEJMoa1104390.
24. Perren TJ, Swart AM, Pfisterer J, et al. A phase 3 trial of bevacizumab in ovarian cancer. *N Engl J Med.* 2011;365(26):2484–2496, doi:10.1056/NEJMoa1103799.
25. Hess LM, Benham-Hutchins M, Herzog TJ, et al. A meta-analysis of the efficacy of intraperitoneal cisplatin for the front-line treatment of ovarian cancer. *Int J Gynecol Cancer.* 2007;17(3):561–570, doi:10.1111/j.1525-1438.2006.00846.x.
26. Armstrong DK, Bundy B, Wenzel L, et al. Intraperitoneal cisplatin and paclitaxel in ovarian cancer. *N Engl J Med.* 2006;354(1):34–43, doi:10.1056/NEJMoa052985.
27. Katsumata N, Yasuda M, Isonishi S, et al. Long-term results of dose-dense paclitaxel and carboplatin versus conventional paclitaxel and carboplatin for treatment of advanced epithelial ovarian, fallopian tube, or primary peritoneal cancer (JGOG 3016): a randomised, controlled, open-label trial. *Lancet Oncol.* 2013;14(10):1020–1026, doi:10.1016/S1470-2045(13)70363-2.
28. Mei L, Chen H, Wei DM, et al. Maintenance chemotherapy for ovarian cancer. *Cochrane Database Syst Rev.* 2013;(6):CD007414.
29. Fuks F. External radiotherapy of ovarian cancer: standard approaches and new frontiers. *Semin Oncol.* 1975;2:253–266.
30. Delclos L, Braun EJ, Herrera JR, Jr., et al. Whole abdominal irradiation by cobalt-60 moving-strip technic. *Radiology.* 1963;81:632–641, doi:10.1148/81.4.632.
31. Dembo AJ. Epithelial ovarian cancer: the role of radiotherapy. *Int J Radiat Oncol Biol Phys.* 1992;22:835–845, doi:10.1016/0360-3016(92)90777-F.
32. Dembo AJ, Bush RS, Beale FA, et al. The Princess Margaret Hospital study of ovarian cancer: stages I, II, and asymptomatic III presentations. *Cancer Treat Rep.* 1979;63:249–254.
33. Fyles AW, Thomas GM, Pintilie M, et al. A randomized study of two doses of abdominopelvic radiation therapy for patients with optimally debulked Stage I, II, and III ovarian cancer. *Int*

J Radiat Oncol Biol Phys. 1998;41(3):543–549, doi:10.1016/S0360-3016(98)00066-2.

34. Klaassen D, Shelley W, Starreveld A, et al. Early stage ovarian cancer: a randomized clinical trial comparing whole abdominal radiotherapy, melphalan, and intraperitoneal chromic phosphate: a National Cancer Institute of Canada Clinical Trials Group report. *J Clin Oncol.* 1988;6(8):1254–1263.
35. Eifel PJ, Gershenson DM, Delclos L, et al. Twice-daily, split-course abdominopelvic radiation therapy after chemotherapy and positive second-look laparotomy for epithelial ovarian carcinoma. *Int J Radiat Oncol Biol Phys.* 1991;21(4):1013–1018, doi:10.1016/0360-3016(91)90743-N.
36. Thomas GM. Is there a role for consolidation or salvage radiotherapy after chemotherapy in advanced epithelial ovarian cancer? *Gynecol Oncol.* 1993;51(1):97–103, doi:10.1006/gyno.1993.1253.
37. Carey MS, et al. Testing the validity of a prognostic classification in patients with surgically optimal ovarian carcinoma: a 15-year review. *Int J Gynecol Cancer.* 1993;3(1):24–35, doi:10.1046/j.1525-1438.1993.03010024.x.
38. Lee LJ, Dembo AJ, Simm JE, et al. Nonserous histology and platinum-sensitivity are prognostic in localized recurrent ovarian cancer treated with radiation therapy. *Int J Radiat Oncol Biol Phys.* 2012;84(3):S96.
39. National Cancer Center Network. Ovarian cancer including fallopian tube cancer and primary peritoneal cancer. Version 3.2014: National Comprehensive Cancer Network; 2014 [updated 5/9/2014; cited 2015 2/22/2015]. Available from: http://www.nccn.org/professionals/physician_gls/pdf/ovarian.pdf
40. Wolf JK, Mullen J, Eifel PJ, et al. Radiation treatment of advanced or recurrent granulosa cell tumor of the ovary. *Gynecol Oncol.* 1999;73(1):35–41, doi:10.1006/gyno.1998.5287.

Case Studies

The eight case studies appended to this chapter demonstrate that some patients enjoy long disease-free intervals and may even be cured after receiving RT for localized recurrence of epithelial ovarian cancer. Several of these cases were selected from the study by Brown et al.,[5] which provides additional information about the selection criteria and patient outcomes. Approximately 25% to 30% of the patients in that study had a particularly favorable outcome after receiving RT with curative intent. Other patients in that study, not described here, experienced only palliation of symptoms or were treated with hope of cure only to have disease progress shortly after completion of treatment. Unfortunately, although we have been able to define some subgroups of patients who have a particularly good chance of long-term disease-free survival after RT,[5] review of our experience has not helped us to further refine our patient selection criteria. However, in view of the limited options remaining to most of these patients when they were referred, the reported outcomes support the use of definitive RT in selected cases.

List of Case Studies for Chapter 14

CS 14.1. Stage IIB ovarian cancer multiply recurrent in the presacral space

CS 14.2. Perirectal recurrence treated with resection and postoperative RT

CS 14.3. Ovarian cancer with sigmoid involvement multiply recurrent after chemotherapy and RT

CS 14.4. Stage IIIC serous carcinoma of the ovary with paraaortic node recurrence

CS 14.5. Ovarian carcinosarcoma with sequential recurrences in the paraaortic nodes and left neck

CS 14.6. Clear cell carcinoma of the ovary with isolated paraaortic node recurrence

CS 14.7. High-grade serous ovarian cancer multiply recurrent in paraaortic nodes

CS 14.8. Isolated inguinal recurrence of endometrioid carcinoma of the ovary

Abbreviations Used in the Case Studies

BSO	Bilateral salpingo-oophorectomy
CA-125	Cancer antigen 125
CT	Computed tomography
CTV	Clinical target volume
CXR	Chest x-ray
EBRT	External beam radiotherapy
FDG	Fluorodeoxyglucose
FNA	Fine needle aspirate
GTV	Gross tumor volume
HRCTV	High-risk clinical target volume
IMRT	Intensity-modulated radiation therapy
ITV	Internal target volume
IVC	Inferior vena cava
KPS	Karnofsky performance status
MRI	Magnetic resonance imaging
NED	No evidence of disease
PAN	Paraaortic node
PET	Positron emission tomography
PTV	Planning target volume
TAH	Total abdominal hysterectomy

CS 14.1 • Stage IIB Ovarian Cancer Multiply Recurrent in the Presacral Space

History: A 66-year-old woman was referred for consideration of RT. Eighteen years earlier, she had been diagnosed with stage IIB high-grade mixed carcinoma involving the ovary and fallopian tube with direct extension to the cul-de-sac. She was treated at that time with 6 cycles of carboplatin and cyclophosphamide and followed until 3 years later, when she had a first pelvic recurrence. She was retreated with 9 cycles of carboplatin and then followed for the next 15 years without definite evidence of disease, although she was periodically noted to have a small nodule in the sigmoid mesocolon. Sixteen years after the initial diagnosis of ovarian cancer, the nodule was noted to have increased to 1.5 cm in diameter. Two years later, CT revealed that the nodule measured 3.2 × 3.5 cm (***a***). Fine needle aspiration revealed high-grade adenocarcinoma consistent with ovarian cancer. The patient was treated with 6 cycles of carboplatin and paclitaxel, at the end of which the mass measured 1.5 × 2 cm (***b***). After returning home for holidays, the patient returned, having been referred for consideration of RT. CA-125 levels had always been normal.

Evaluation: *Exam*: Normal posthysterectomy findings. *KPS*: 90. *PET–CT*: Three months after the previous, postchemotherapy CT scan, the mass in the sigmoid mesocolon had regrown to about 3 cm in diameter (***c***). There was no other evidence of disease.

Treatment Plan: Definitive RT. In several respects, this patient was an ideal candidate for definitive local therapy. She had never had extrapelvic disease, and her recurrences were confined to a single site. Her local disease had been platinum sensitive, but the most recent progression suggested that the disease was becoming chemoresistant. For a tumor 3 cm in diameter, the probability of local control with RT alone is about 80%.[5]

EBRT (IMRT): Supine position, custom cradle. The target volume included the residual mass (GTV) as well as the surrounding vascular compartment (HRCTV) (***d***, ***e***). Because of the short field length and fixed target, accurate setup was anticipated with daily KV imaging. For this reason, and to minimize exposure to adjacent bowel, a tight PTV margin was used for the 60-Gy target volume. A nested internal volume excluding all normal tissue was treated to 63 Gy.

Total RT doses (in 30 fractions):

GTV and HRCTV (+7 mm): 51 Gy (170 cGy/fraction)

GTV and HRCTV (+3 mm): 60 Gy (200 cGy/fraction)

GTV and HRCTV (no margin): 63 Gy (210 cGy/fraction)

Outcome: Treatment was well tolerated; the only complaint was mild fatigue. At 7 years, NED by imaging and exam. Four years after treatment, the patient was treated for *BRCA1*–mutation-positive breast cancer.

Comments: Surgical resection could have been considered in this case. Because of the multiply recurrent disease, we would probably have recommended postoperative RT even after a gross total resection, but the dose might have been less. On the other hand, each operation probably increases the risk of RT-related complications, particularly if gross residual disease or a positive margin necessitates high-dose RT.

For this posterior lesion, prone treatment with a belly board might have reduced bowel exposure if the intestines shifted away from the target. Because of the persistent disease in a single location over many years, relatively small proximal and distal margins were used.

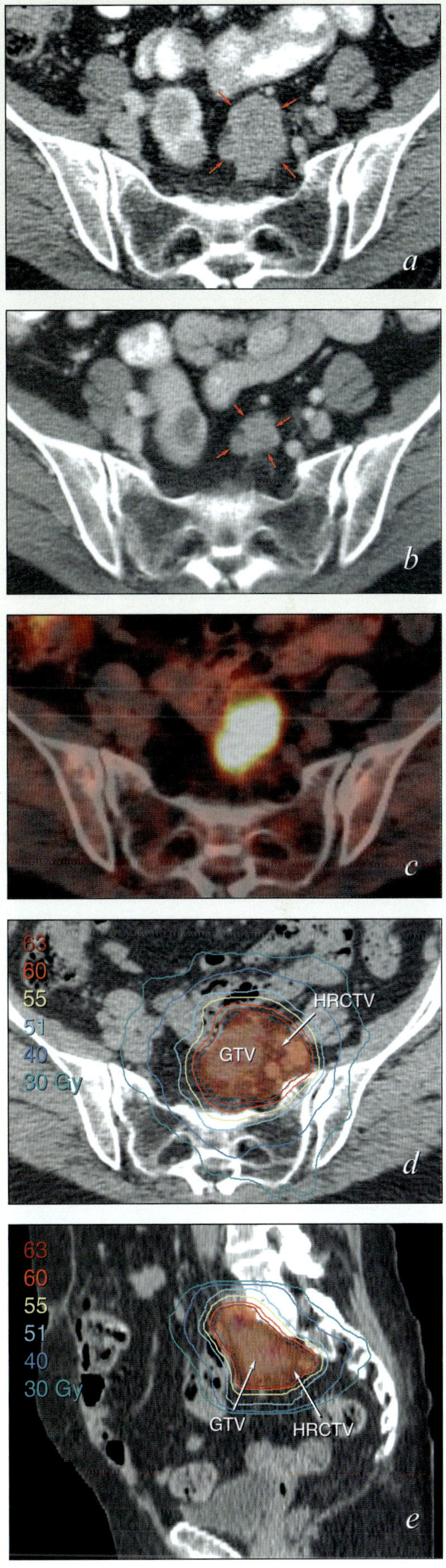

CS 14.2 • Perirectal Recurrence Treated with Resection and Postoperative RT

History: A 45-year-old woman with unexplained anemia was found to have a large pelvic mass. A TAH-BSO was performed with removal of a 15 × 9 × 7.5-cm right ovarian tumor that was adherent in the rectouterine space. An apparently separate mass that wrapped around the rectum was not removed. No additional staging was performed. The patient was referred for evaluation and treatment.

Initial Evaluation: *Exam*: A large, fixed mass was palpable on the right between the vagina and rectum. *KPS*: 90–100. *CT (abdomen, pelvis)*: An irregular mass extended posteriorly from the vaginal cuff and was inseparable from the rectosigmoid; findings for small external iliac lymph nodes were equivocal (***a***). *CA-125*: <7 U/mL. *CXR*: NED. *Pathology review (ovary and biopsy from cul-de-sac)*: High-grade carcinoma with transitional and endometrioid features.

Initial Treatment: To improve the chances of achieving optimal resection without colostomy, the patient initially was treated with 3 cycles of carboplatin and paclitaxel. CT showed an excellent response with only minimal residual thickening extending from the right vaginal cuff to the mesorectum (***b***). The patient then had an exploratory laparotomy with right parametrectomy, omentectomy, and biopsies. No tumor was found in any of the surgical specimens. The patient then had 4 additional cycles of carboplatin and paclitaxel followed by 1 year of paclitaxel maintenance therapy.

Recurrence: One year after chemotherapy was completed, a new, 2-cm perirectal nodule was noted on CT and pelvic exam (***c***, *arrow*). CT was otherwise negative for disease. Biopsy revealed recurrent adenocarcinoma.

Surgery: A 2-cm nodule abutting the rectal mucosa was completely resected without injury to the rectum. Surgical clips were placed to mark the operative bed. The nodule contained high-grade adenocarcinoma. Numerous biopsy specimens from the pelvic and abdominal peritoneum were negative for disease. Because of the localized recurrence and close surgical margin, the patient was referred for RT.

EBRT (*d, e*): After review of the initial distribution of the patient's disease, it was decided to include the entire cul-de-sac, perirectal spaces, and distal iliac nodes in the CTV. A HRCTV, including the resection bed with margin, was defined using preoperative imaging and surgical clips. IMRT was delivered in 28 fractions over 38 days. The CTV-ITV (+7 mm) was treated to 50 Gy (178 cGy/fraction). Using an integrated boost, the HRCTV (+5 mm) was treated to 56 Gy (200 cGy/fraction).

Chemotherapy: Carboplatin and paclitaxel were administered after RT but discontinued after 2 cycles because of myelosuppression.

Outcome: At 4.5 years after completion of RT (7 years after initial diagnosis), NED by PET and exam; the patient had occasional postcoital spotting but no dyspareunia and no bowel or bladder complaints.

Comments: For a 2-cm nodule, the probability of control with 60–65 Gy of RT alone is high. However, preoperative imaging suggested that the recurrent nodule could be resected without compromising the rectum. Surgery permitted restaging of the abdomen, and resection allowed delivery of a somewhat lower radiation dose. An argument could have been made to treat only the operative bed with a margin. However, after review of the patient's initial disease extent, it was felt that the entire cul-de-sac and perirectal spaces were at risk. A marginal recurrence would probably not have been curable without major organ compromise, so more inclusive treatment was chosen.

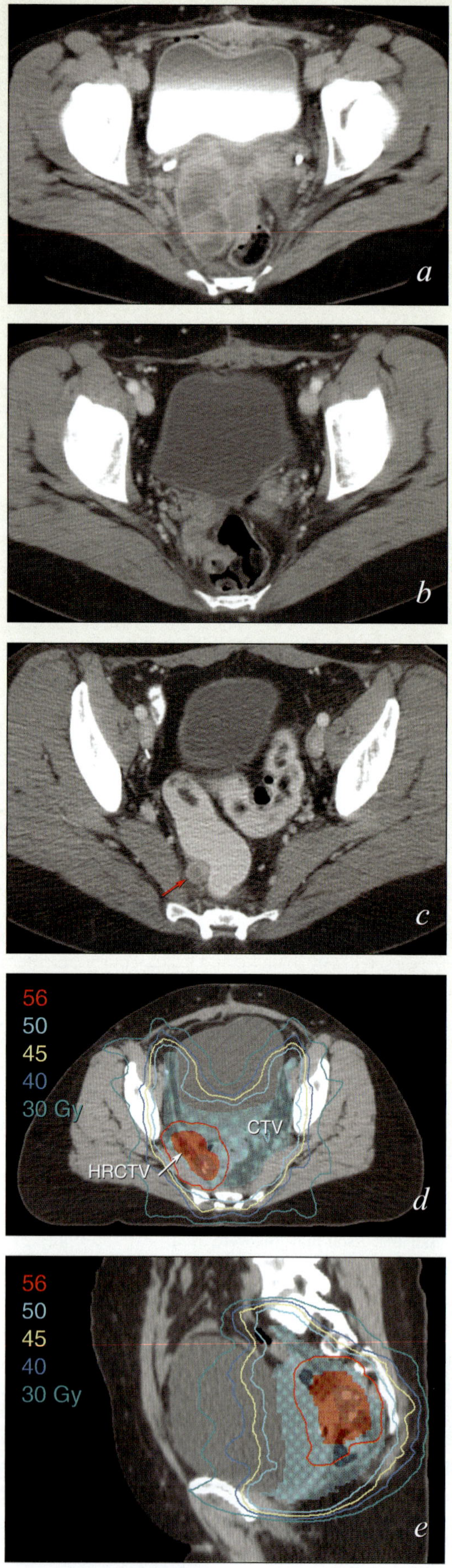

CS 14.3 • Ovarian Cancer with Sigmoid Involvement Multiply Recurrent after Chemotherapy and RT

History: A 52-year-old woman with bilateral ovarian cancer had TAH-BSO and optimal cytoreduction, including excision of a metastatic deposit on the sigmoid. Although the cancer had been categorized as stage IVB, it was confined to the pelvis and was probably actually stage IIB. After 6 cycles of carboplatin and paclitaxel, the serum CA-125 level fell to <10 U/mL from a preoperative high of >5,000 U/mL. However, the CA-125 level soon began to rise again, and 6 months after completion of chemotherapy, a paravaginal mass was noted on CT. The patient was referred for treatment recommendations.

Evaluation: *Exam*: 5- to 6-cm mass at the vaginal apex. *Colonoscopy*: Localized infiltration of sigmoid mucosa by probable tumor. *KPS*: 90. *CT* (***a**, arrows*): 4.5-cm solid vaginal-apex mass with an adjacent 4-cm cystic component situated between the bladder and rectum just below the sigmoid. *Biopsies* (*vagina, sigmoid*): Adenocarcinoma.

Initial Treatment of Recurrence: Investigational treatment with carboplatin and interferon. Although the tumor responded, the regimen was poorly tolerated because of drug-related hepatitis and diabetes aggravated by corticosteroid administration for carboplatin hypersensitivity. After 9 cycles of chemotherapy, RT was recommended to achieve local control.

Pre-RT Evaluation: *Exam*: 2-cm raised, mobile mass at the vaginal apex. *CT*: Small, spiculated residual soft tissue density beneath the sigmoid at the apex of the vagina.

EBRT (*b–d*): Supine position, custom cradle.

Fractions 1–25 (4-field, 18-MV photons):

Distal pelvis: 45 Gy

Fractions 26–34 (IMRT):

GTV, vaginal ITV (+7 mm): 15 Gy; GTV, vaginal ITV (+5 mm): 17 Gy

Brachytherapy: 4 Gy to the surface of the proximal third of the vagina using a domed cylinder.

Treatment was completed in 45 days.

Outcome: NED until 15 months after RT, when examinations revealed a rising CA-125 level and an ulcerated rectosigmoid mass (***e**, arrows*) that was biopsy positive for adenocarcinoma. The patient responded to cisplatin and gemcitabine with normalization of CA-125 level (***f***). However, when chemotherapy was discontinued after 9 cycles, the tumor rapidly progressed. For the following 5 years, the patient was treated with a variety of cytotoxic and biologic agents with progressively severe symptoms related to tumor and chemotherapy. She eventually required colostomy for sigmoid perforation and nephrostomies for ureteral obstruction. She died of complications of progressive pelvic cancer 6.5 years after RT and 10 years after initial diagnosis.

Comments: Although this patient was not cured, RT provided her only prolonged chemotherapy-free interval (***f***). The location of the recurrence near the proximal border of the radiation fields (***c**, arrow*) suggests that more generous coverage of the cul-de-sac and sigmoid might have improved the effectiveness of treatment. Today, a patient like this would also be treated using daily image guidance with close monitoring of the vaginal position.

This case demonstrates the variable natural history of ovarian cancer. Although most serous neoplasms disseminate rapidly to peritoneum or distant sites, this cancer remained confined to the pelvis for more than 10 years.

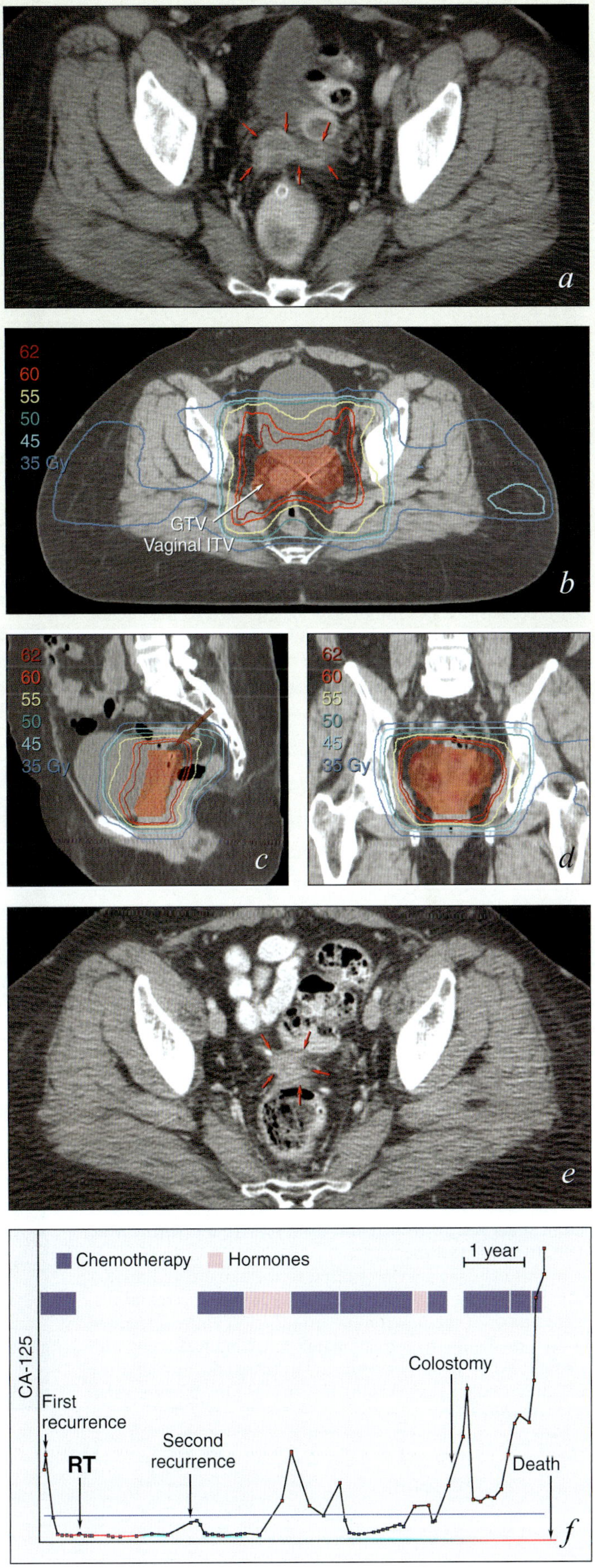

CS 14.4 • Stage IIIC Serous Carcinoma of the Ovary with Paraaortic Node Recurrence

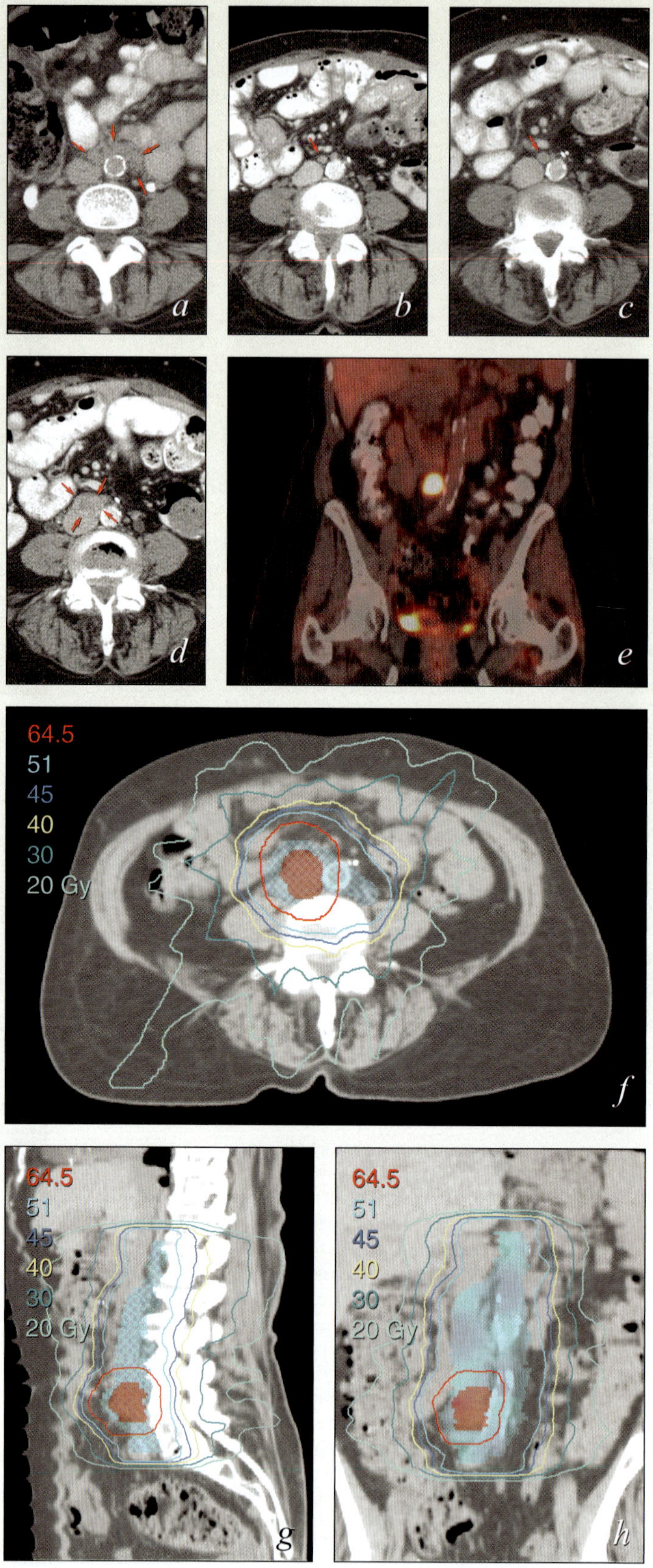

History: A 73-year-old woman with fatigue, anorexia, and early satiety had CT, which showed a large pelvic mass and paraaortic lymphadenopathy (*arrows*, ***a***). The patient underwent optimal cytoreduction of a high-grade serous carcinoma of the left ovary. The omentum and one omental node were involved, and there was transmural sigmoid involvement necessitating sigmoid resection. None of the 22 pelvic and paraaortic nodes sampled contained cancer. The patient was treated with 6 cycles of carboplatin and paclitaxel. The CA-125 level fell to 8.5 U/mL from a prechemotherapy value of 22 U/mL. However, over the next year, the CA-125 level rose to 20 U/mL, and a distal aortocaval node enlarged from 5 mm (*arrow*, ***b***) to 8 mm (***c***). The patient initially declined intervention, but 6 months later (2 years after initial diagnosis), when the node had enlarged to 2.5 × 2 cm (*arrows*, ***d***), she was reevaluated for treatment.

Evaluation: Exam: NED. *KPS*: 90–100. *PET–CT* (***e***): 2.5-cm hypermetabolic paraaortic node; no other evidence of disease. *Biopsy* (*paraaortic node*): High-grade müllerian carcinoma.

Treatment Plan: The patient was offered several options, including chemotherapy, resection, and RT. She was extremely reluctant to have more chemotherapy and ultimately chose RT. IMRT was used to minimize the dose to bowel and other adjacent structures. The entire paraaortic nodal region was included in the CTV. Although most of the enlarged PANs sampled at her initial surgery were negative, the patient's recurrence proved that her tumor had metastasized to this region; secondary spread to proximal aortocaval nodes was possible and several small, <5 mm nodes in this region, though within normal limits, were considered at risk because of their proximity to the involved site.

EBRT (IMRT) (*f–h*): Supine position, arms above head in upper and lower custom cradles.

Total RT doses (in 30 fractions):

GTV (+7 mm): 64.5 Gy (215 Gy/fraction)

CTV (+7 mm): 51 Gy (170 Gy/fraction)

Outcome: Treatment was well tolerated with minimal adverse effects. Repeat CT at 4 weeks did not demonstrate sufficient regression of the GTV to require modification of the IMRT plan. At 4 months, NED by PET with normal CA-125. At 7 years (9 years after initial diagnosis), NED without pain or complications of treatment. The patient required no additional treatment after RT.

Comments: Patients with serous cancer involving peritoneum or omentum usually have widespread disease recurrences; however, as demonstrated by this case, there are exceptions to this rule. In particular, patients who have platinum-sensitive disease (i.e., NED for at least 6 months after chemotherapy) and a single site of recurrent disease sometimes benefit from definitive local treatment.

In this case, the GTV was distal to the kidneys and duodenum, facilitating treatment planning. Because visceral fat displaced most of the bowel away from the GTV, the integrated boost was slightly hypofractionated to enable treatment with a single IMRT plan. However, today we would probably use a slightly smaller (e.g., 5 mm) PTV margin for the integrated GTV (Chapter 6).

CS 14.5 • Ovarian Carcinosarcoma with Sequential Recurrences in the Paraaortic Nodes and Left Neck

History: A 57-year-old woman with bloating, abdominal pain, and DVT was found to have a large pelvic mass.

Initial Treatment: After placement of an IVC filter, the patient had TAH-BSO and surgical staging with optimal cytoreduction. Bilateral ovarian masses contained carcinosarcoma. There was metastatic disease in 1 of 4 PA nodes. The omentum, peritoneal biopsies and 21 pelvic nodes were negative. She received 8 cycles of carboplatin and paclitaxel with normalization of her CA-125 level after the sixth cycle. At the conclusion of chemotherapy, she had moderate neuropathy and was walker dependent.

Interval History: The patient had several vertebroplasties to treat osteoporotic fractures but experienced no functional improvement. After missing several oncology appointments, she presented 10 months after chemotherapy complaining of back and lower extremity pain and leg weakness.

Evaluation: *CT and PET* (***a,b***): 4.5 × 3.5 × 6-cm FDG-avid retroperitoneal mass displacing the aorta and IVC with probable invasion of L3 and psoas muscle; left hydronephrosis. *MRI* (*spine, brain*): No intracranial lesions or spinal cord impingement; *KPS*: 70; *Biopsy* (*FNA*): High-grade carcinoma.

Treatment Plan: Possible options were chemotherapy, palliative RT, definitive RT, and hospice care. The patient's chemotherapy tolerance had been poor, and the progression from NED to massive paraaortic disease in 10 months suggested that the tumor was not platinum sensitive. RT offered the best chance of palliation. She and the family wanted aggressive treatment and, after some discussion, it was decided to offer definitive RT.

EBRT (IMRT) (*c–e*): The CTV included uninvolved PA nodes 6 cm proximal and 3 cm distal to the GTV. Diagnostic images were fused with the planning CT to facilitate designation of the GTV, which was treated using integrated and sequential boosts. In the 4th week, repeat CT showed significant tumor regression, and the plan was adjusted to reduce the duodenal dose (***d***, ***e***).

Fractions 1–25 (***c***):

CTV (+7 mm): 45 Gy; GTV (+5 mm): 50 Gy

Fractions 26–30:

GTV (+7 mm): 10 Gy (total dose, 60 Gy)

Treatment was completed in 47 days.

Chemotherapy: Weekly cisplatin, discontinued after 1 cycle because of tinnitus.

Outcome: Rapid improvement in pain but minimal improvement in extremity weakness, the etiology of which remained unclear. At 4 months, NED by PET. At 10 months, new FDG-avid lesions in the left neck and thoracic inlet were biopsy positive for carcinoma (***f***). After 2 cycles of carboplatin, imaging showed further disease progression, and the patient was referred for RT. An aggressive "palliative" course was prescribed to treat the GTV to 45 Gy in 15 fractions (***g***). At 2.5 years after treatment of the neck (4 years after treatment of the PA nodes), NED without gastrointestinal complaints but wheelchair dependent.

Comments: This case demonstrates the challenges of determining when and how to treat with RT. This patient's disease did not disseminate rapidly as might have been expected. RT provided a long disease-free interval, but chemotherapy appeared to have little or no effect on the disease.

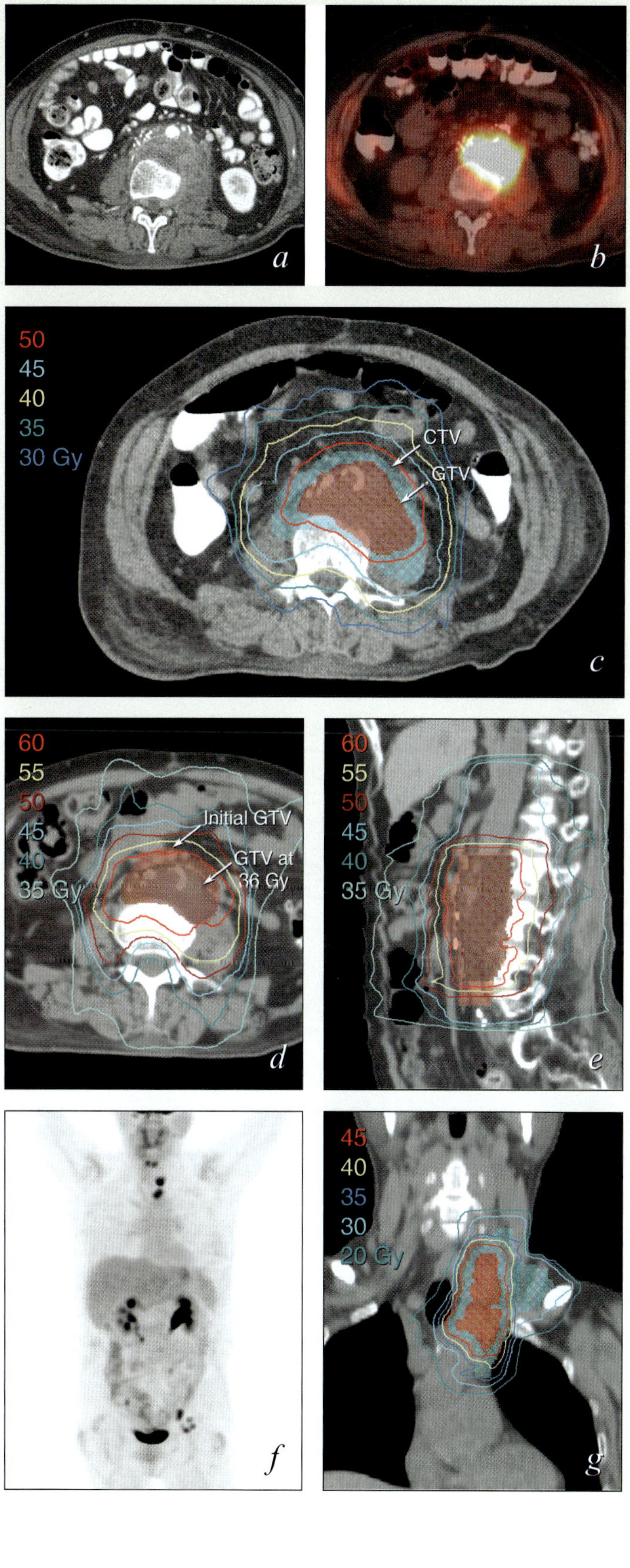

CS 14.6 • Clear Cell Carcinoma of the Ovary with Isolated Paraaortic Node Recurrence

History: A 48-year-old woman with stage IA clear cell carcinoma of the ovary had TAH-BSO followed by carboplatin and paclitaxel. She was referred 3 years later for evaluation of probable paraaortic recurrence.

Evaluation: *Pelvic exam*: NED. *KPS*: 90. *CT* (***a***): 3.6 × 1.8-cm node posterior to and anteriorly displacing the vena cava; the node was just inferior to the right renal artery. *PET*: FDG-avid node in the same location, otherwise NED. *CA-125*: Normal. *Biopsy* (*FNA*): Adenocarcinoma consistent with the original ovarian primary tumor.

Treatment Plan: Clear cell carcinomas tend to be resistant to chemotherapy, and it was thought that chemotherapy alone was unlikely to cure this recurrent cancer. However, several features suggested that a good outcome might be achieved with aggressive regional treatment: (1) a single nodal site, (2) no prior extraregional disease, (3) a long disease-free interval, and (4) clear cell histology. Although we have frequently treated smaller retrocaval nodes with RT alone, the proximity of the duodenum usually limits the safely deliverable dose to about 60 Gy. For a tumor of this size (>3 cm), the risk of local recurrence after 60 Gy may be as high as 30%–40%, significantly greater than for lesions <3 cm. After consultation with a vascular surgeon, the gynecologic oncologist concluded that the node was probably resectable. Resection would also provide an opportunity to search for other possible sites of microscopic disease. The final plan was for resection followed by RT with curative intent.

Surgery: Resection of a large retrocaval node leaving no gross residual disease. The operative bed was marked with clips.

Histologic Findings: A 3.5 × 2 × 2-cm lymph node was largely replaced by tumor. Five other nodes and random peritoneal biopsy specimens were negative for disease.

Radiation Therapy: *Setup*: Upper and lower cradle with arms above the head. Isocenter anterior to L2/L3 in the center of the operative bed.

IMRT plan (in 28 fractions; completed in 37 days) (***b***, ***c***): The paraaortic CTV (+7 mm) was treated to 49 Gy (175 cGy/fraction). Using an integrated boost, a HRCTV including the site of the original lesion and the operative bed (demarcated by surgical clips; *arrows* in ***b***, ***c***) was treated with a 7-mm margin to 53.2 Gy (190 cGy/fraction).

Note: Because this patient had extensive retrocaval disease, the entire vena cava was included in the CTV to a level 1–2 cm above the renal vein (***c***). We elected to extend the CTV approximately 6 cm proximal and 4 cm distal to the HRCTV to cover possible areas of microscopic disease in adjacent undissected nodes. However, the optimal CTV margin in such cases is not well established.

Chemotherapy: No chemotherapy was given during or after RT.

Outcome: At 4 months after RT, NED on PET. At 6 years after recurrence and 9 years after initial diagnosis, NED with negative review of systems.

Comments: Although the role of RT is controversial in ovarian cancer of all cell types, some patients with isolated locoregional recurrences can be cured with locoregional treatment. Coordination between members of the multidisciplinary team is important, and the risks and potential benefits of treatment should be carefully considered and discussed with the patient.

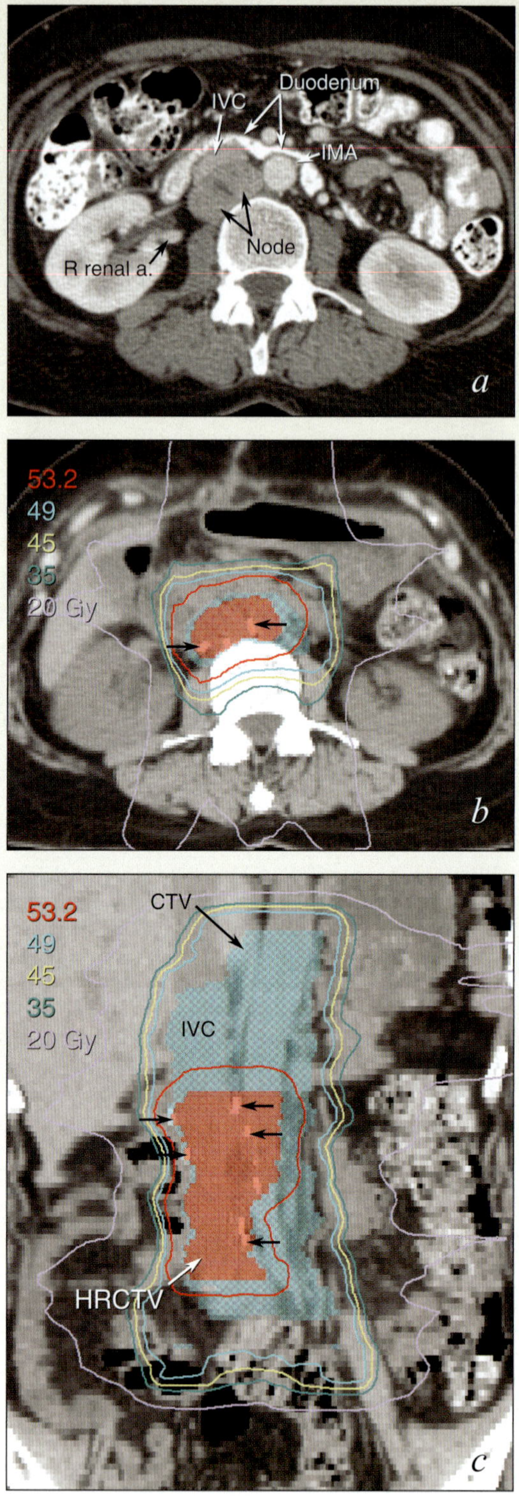

CS 14.7 • High-Grade Serous Ovarian Cancer Multiply Recurrent in Paraaortic Nodes

History: A 57-year-old woman underwent TAH-BSO and staging for a pelvic mass. Pathology showed high-grade serous carcinoma in both ovaries. One paraaortic node, 5 pelvic nodes, the omentum, and peritoneal biopsies were negative for metastasis; the cancer was classified as stage II because of adherence to the pelvic wall. The patient was treated with 6 cycles of carboplatin and paclitaxel.

Three years later, CT revealed paraaortic lymphadenopathy. One node was removed and showed recurrent adenocarcinoma. The patient was treated with 2 cycles of carboplatin and paclitaxel, after which she developed carboplatin sensitivity and was switched to weekly paclitaxel for 22 cycles.

Three years later, the patient recurrent paraaortic lymphadenopathy. Lymphadenectomy with "complete removal of nodes between the inferior mesenteric artery and renal vessels" showed poorly differentiated adenocarcinoma in 9 of 9 paraaortic nodes. The patient was treated with additional weekly paclitaxel and then enrolled in a trial of investigational immunotherapy. Less than 1 year after completion of paclitaxel, the patient had a third paraaortic recurrence and sought a second opinion regarding treatment.

Evaluation: *Exam*: NED. *KPS*: 90–100. *PET–CT*: Two FDG-avid nodes underlying the left renal vein (***a***, *black arrows*) and one in the deep aortocaval space (***b***, *arrow*); otherwise NED. *Biopsy*: Metastatic serous adenocarcinoma.

Treatment Plan: Although the cancer had responded to previous chemotherapy, the patient's tolerance was waning, and the short interval to the third recurrence suggested that the tumor was becoming more resistant to standard agents. Although serous cancer tends to be associated with a poorer prognosis than other histologic subtypes after salvage RT, the continued absence of peritoneal involvement, initial platinum sensitivity, and repeated recurrences confined to a single nodal region made this patient a relatively good candidate for local treatment. Definitive RT was recommended.

Radiation Therapy (*c,d*): The CTV extended from 4 cm above the renal vessels to the aortic bifurcation. In addition to the sites of known involvement, the deep aortocaval and left paraaortic spaces contained a number of small nodes that were not FDG avid; because of the history of extensive paraaortic node involvement, this entire region (designated the HRCTV) was considered high risk and was treated with an integrated boost. A sequential boost was used to bring the total dose to the 3 PET-positive nodes (GTV) to 62 Gy.

Fractions 1–27: CTV (+7 mm): 47 Gy (175 cGy/fraction)
HRCTV (+5 mm): 54 Gy (200 cGy/fraction)
Fractions 28–32: GTV + 5 mm: 8 Gy (200 cGy/fraction)
The duodenal $V_{55\,Gy}$ and $V_{60\,Gy}$ were 10 cc and 3 cc, respectively.

Outcome: At 3 months, NED by PET and exam. At 3 years (10 years after initial diagnosis), NED with no gastrointestinal complaints.

Comments: This patient had a third nodal recurrence despite an extensive lymphadenectomy. Both sites of recurrence were adjacent to surgical clips left during the lymphadenectomy (***b***, ***c***, *arrows*). Nodes in the deep aortocaval region and beneath the left renal vein can be difficult for the surgeon to reach but are common sites of metastasis from adnexal cancers. We scrutinize these areas carefully to rule out residual gross disease, even after a "complete" lymphadenectomy. Today, we would have slightly adjusted the plan to keep the duodenal $V_{60\,Gy}$ below 2 cc.

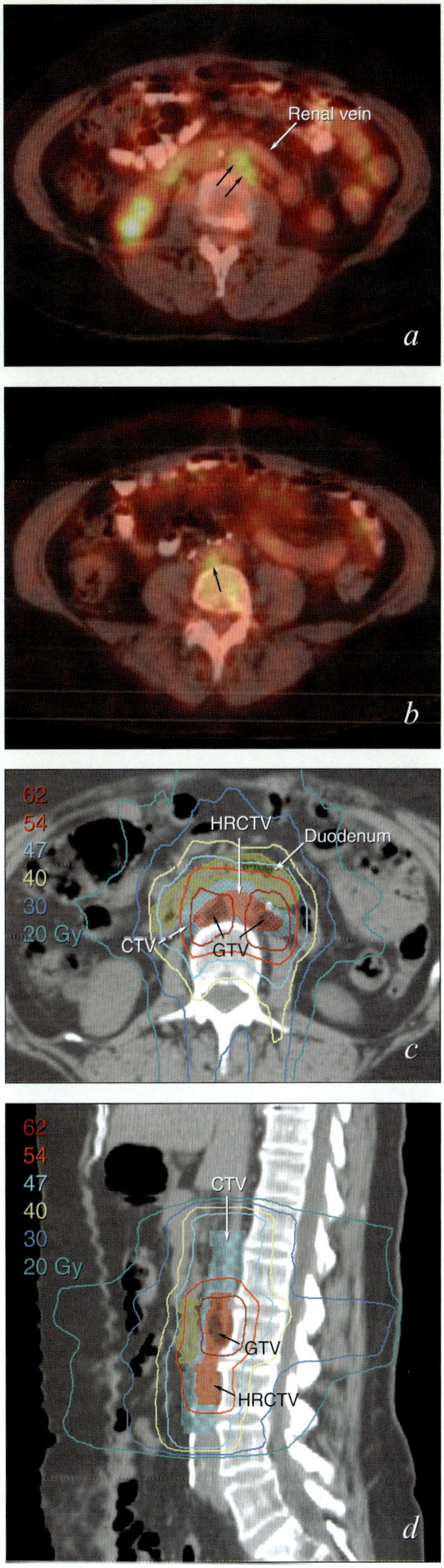

CS 14.8 • Isolated Inguinal Recurrence of Endometrioid Carcinoma of the Ovary

History: A 49-year-old woman with stage IA, grade 2 endometrioid adenocarcinoma of the ovary had TAH-BSO followed by carboplatin and cyclophosphamide. Eleven years later, an isolated groin recurrence was treated with resection and 6 cycles of carboplatin and paclitaxel. Three years later, the patient (then 63 years old) was referred for management of a second recurrence in the same site.

Evaluation: *Exam*: 5-cm fixed, indurated mass in the right groin. *KPS*: 90. *CT (chest, abdomen, pelvis)* (***a***): Heterogeneous, infiltrative 5 × 6-cm mass (*arrows*) involving the right groin and extending through the inguinal canal to the distal external iliac region. Otherwise NED. *CA-125*: 117 U/mL. *Biopsy*: Adenocarcinoma consistent with ovarian primary tumor.

Treatment Plan: Definitive chemo-RT with curative intent. Despite the large tumor, the presentation—a single first echelon nodal site, nonserous histology, and a long disease-free interval—was relatively favorable. The lesion, which extensively involved extranodal soft tissues and femoral vessels (***a***, *arrows*), was deemed unresectable. The cancer was still considered platinum sensitive but was probably not curable with chemotherapy alone. Chemo-RT followed by carboplatin and paclitaxel was recommended.

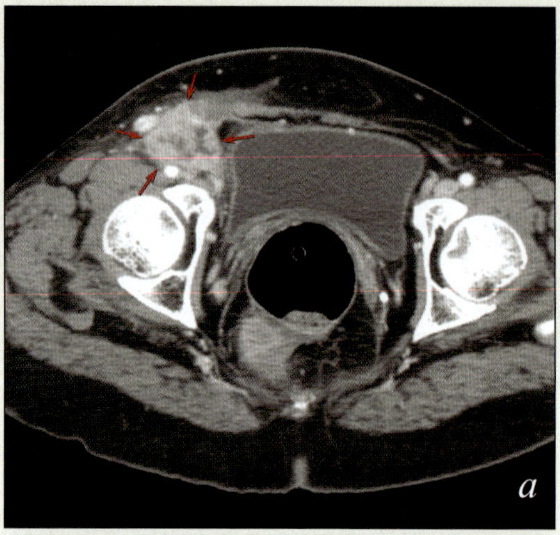

EBRT (*b, c*): *Setup*: Supine position, right hip abducted with bent knee in a custom cradle.

Plan: To optimize treatment of the gross lesion and minimize treatment planning steps, boosts were integrated within a single IMRT plan. A relatively tight 5-mm PTV margin was added to the GTV because the tumor was fixed, the setup was stable, and the GTV was integrated within a larger CTV. A "nested GTV" (GTV + 1–3 mm) was treated to 65 Gy; this enabled delivery of >60 Gy to the main tumor mass and most of the adjacent region of possible fatty infiltration without exceeding tolerance of the femoral head. The ipsilateral internal and external iliac nodes were included in the CTV.

Total RT doses (completed in 31 fractions over 43 days):

GTV (+1–3 mm) (nested internal GTV): 65 Gy (210 cGy/fraction)

GTV (+5 mm): 60.1 Gy (194 cGy/fraction)

CTV (+7 mm): 50 Gy (167 cGy/fraction)

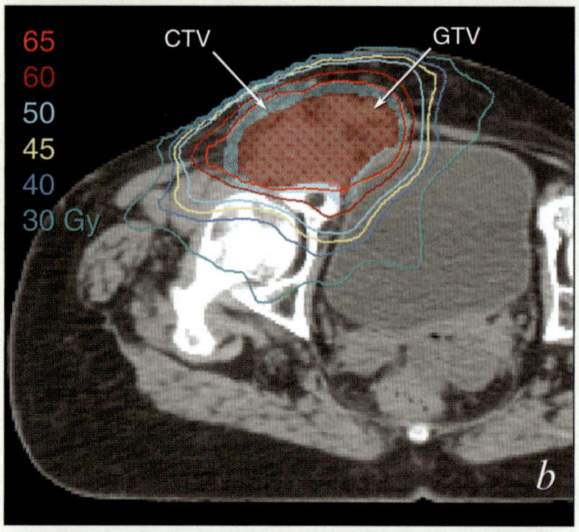

Chemotherapy: Weekly paclitaxel × 4. After chemo-RT, 4 cycles of carboplatin and paclitaxel at conventional doses.

Outcome: Rapid relief of pain. At 1 week after completion of RT, the CA-125 level had fallen to 16 U/dL. Patchy moist desquamation resolved within 2–3 weeks. At 7 years, the patient was continuously with NED with mild induration and edema in the groin but no pain or leg edema; the CA-125 level was 6 U/mL.

Comment: RT would also have been a reasonable treatment choice at the time of this patient's first recurrence. Although she could have been treated with a combination of photons and electrons, it would have been difficult to match the degree of femoral head sparing that was achieved with IMRT. Cisplatin is a more usual choice for concurrent chemotherapy, but weekly paclitaxel is effective in the treatment of ovarian cancer, is an active radiation sensitizer, and, because there was little bowel in the treatment field, was tolerated with few adverse effects.

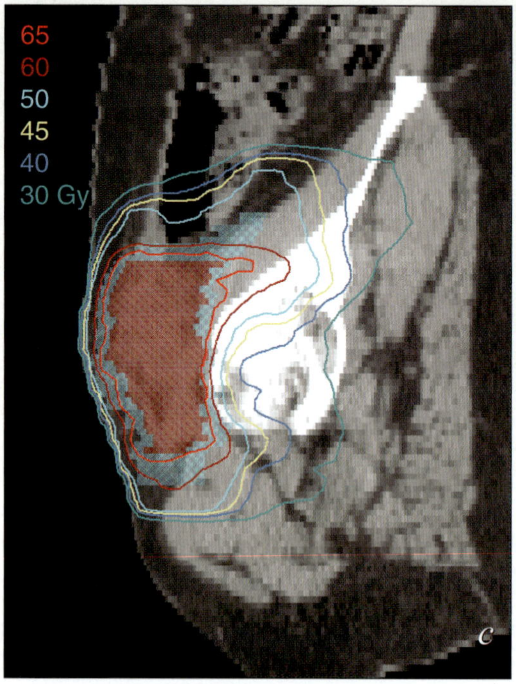

CHAPTER 15

Unknown Primary

INTRODUCTION

Most gynecologic cancers present with bleeding, pain, or other symptoms caused by an enlarging primary tumor. However, in some cases, patients are initially diagnosed when lymphadenopathy or extragenital masses are found to contain squamous carcinoma or mullerian adenocarcinoma suggestive of a gynecologic primary cancer. In rare cases, even an exhaustive search fails to reveal any primary source.

Although this is an uncommon problem, it is worthy of special consideration for several reasons:

- Many cases initially labeled as having an unknown primary have a source discovered after additional search (**Fig. 15.1**, **CS 12.8 and 12.9**). Failure to identify the source before radiotherapy is initiated can severely compromise the chance for cure.
- Even patients who have large pelvic masses or extensive lymphadenopathy are frequently curable with definitive chemoradiation (**CS 15.2–15.4**). For this reason, such patients should not be equated with the generally incurable patients who present with hematogenously disseminated disease from an unknown primary source.
- Because they do not develop symptoms of a primary lesion, these patients often have very bulky lymphadenopathy. For this reason, they provide good case studies for the management of patients with extensive inguinal or pelvic lymphadenopathy.

These are always challenging cases that require careful workup, multidisciplinary collaboration, and skillful technique.

PRETREATMENT EVALUATION

The primary goals of the pretreatment evaluation of patients who present with inguinal or pelvic cancers without an evident primary are to:

- Rule out a previously undetected primary source
- Evaluate the extent of locoregional involvement
- Rule out distant metastases that would preclude a definitive treatment approach
- Assess and treat secondary symptoms of tumor

Search for a Primary Source

Several features including the distribution of nodal disease (**Fig. 15.1**, Chapter 5, Table 5.1) and the type of carcinoma can suggest a direction for the initial evaluation. Squamous carcinomas are more likely to arise in the lower genital tract and müllerian adenocarcinomas in the cervix, endometrium, tubes, or ovaries. Testing for high-risk HPV types can be helpful in determining the potential source of poorly differentiated carcinomas or adenocarcinomas but cannot differentiate between squamous carcinomas of the anus, urethra, or lower genital tract, all of which can be sources of HPV-positive squamous lesions.[1] Extragenital pelvic cancer can also arise from endometriosis (**CS 15.5**).[2–4]

If the patient has a history of pelvic or vulvar surgery, an effort should be made to obtain histologic material from that surgery to determine whether a cancer was present. However, if a source is not found in the most obvious sites, patients should always have a thorough evaluation of all potential primary sites.

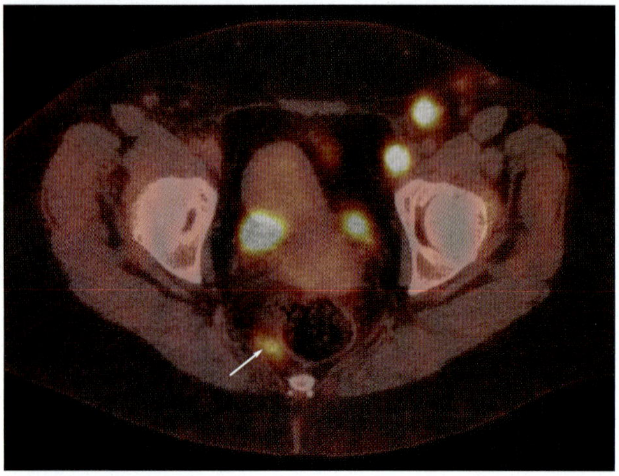

FIGURE 15.1 The pattern of nodal involvement can give important clues to the potential primary sites. This 42-year-old woman presented with bulky inguinal and external iliac lymphadenopathy; biopsy revealed squamous carcinoma positive for high-risk HPV. The patient was referred for treatment of lymphadenopathy from an unknown primary of probable gynecologic origin. However, PET–CT revealed an FDG-avid perirectal node (*arrow*). This pattern strongly suggested an anal primary lesion. Although the patient reportedly had negative findings for a proctosigmoidoscopy before referral, a repeat study revealed a small anal carcinoma just proximal to the dentate line.

Evaluation should begin with a careful pelvic examination including colposcopy of the cervix and vagina if no gross lesions are found. Endometrial and endocervical curettage should be obtained, and any suspicious lesions should be biopsied. In our experience, the vulva and vagina are the most common sites of initially undetected primary cancers (**CS 11.6, 12.8, and 12.9**). Small cancers of the anal canal can also be missed on initial examination (**Fig. 15.1**). In many cases, anesthesia is required to perform an optimal examination. Examination under anesthesia can be combined with cystoscopy to rule out primaries of the bladder or urethra and with proctoscopy to rule out primary cancers of the anus or rectum. If there is evidence of or a history of cervical intraepithelial neoplasia, a cervical cone biopsy may be indicated (**CS 15.1**).

Evaluation of Regional and Distant Disease Extent

Techniques for evaluation of regional disease extent are discussed in detail in Chapter 4. PET–CT is recommended in all cases to evaluate regional sites and to help to rule out distant metastases. CT with contrast can be helpful and can be fused with radiation planning CT scans to assist in target volume designation. If patients undergo treatment with lymphadenectomy, postoperative CT should always be obtained to rule out residual gross nodal disease. MRI is useful in evaluating soft tissue masses and the extent of soft tissue infiltration from large nodal masses.

Evaluation and Management of Secondary Symptoms

At diagnosis, most patients have pain that can be severe. Good pain control is important for patient comfort and also to achieve stable positioning for radiation treatment. Bulky lymphadenopathy or pelvic masses can also cause hydronephrosis, and bulky lymphadenopathy places patients at increased risk for venous thrombosis. Management of these symptoms is discussed in Chapter 7.

RISK ASSESSMENT

Very few data have been published concerning the outcome of patients presenting with regionally confined pelvic or inguinal carcinoma of unknown primary. In a study of 37 patients with soft tissue or nodal lesions presenting in the abdomen or pelvis, Kelly et al. reported better survival rates for patients with squamous carcinomas versus adenocarcinoma or other histologic types.[5]

MULTIDISCIPLINARY TREATMENT STRATEGY

The Role of Surgery

Adenocarcinoma Arising in Pelvic Soft Tissues

Adenocarcinoma of unknown primary can arise in the soft tissues of the pelvis, usually in the region of the pouch of Douglas or adjacent to the rectosigmoid. Endometrioid histology with associated endometriosis or a history of endometriosis suggests an origin in pelvic endometriosis.

For patients who have adenocarcinoma thought to be arising from endometriosis, some form of surgical evaluation, often by laparoscopic approach, may be recommended to rule out microscopic intraperitoneal disease. The decision whether to attempt surgical resection of gross disease may be influenced by the size of the tumor, proximity to critical structures, and likelihood of complete resectability. Large tumors that are intimately associated with the sigmoid can be difficult to control with definitive radiotherapy without causing serious bowel damage; if it can be accomplished, surgical resection of tumors in this region is probably beneficial although close or positive operative margins are frequent; for this reason postoperative radiotherapy is usually recommended if there is no evidence of peritoneal or distant metastases (**CS 15.5**).

Carcinoma Involving Lymph Nodes

As demonstrated in **CS 15.1–15.4**, even patients who have extensive lymphadenopathy can often be cured if locoregional control can be achieved. Although it is tempting to remove gross lymphadenopathy, the side effects of lymphadenectomy can easily outweigh the benefits. Because these cases usually present with very large nodal masses, resected nodes are nearly always found to have extracapsular disease extension, requiring postoperative radiation therapy doses nearly as high as those given for definitive treatment. Postoperative complications can delay radiation, potentially decreasing its effectiveness (CS 15.4). However, in many cases, optimal treatment of regionally extensive cancers requires skill in advanced techniques including IMRT, image guidance, and adaptive planning. If these are unavailable, the arguments for initial surgical treatment may be stronger.

In general, well-circumscribed, moderate-sized nodes adjacent to critical structures that might limit the ability to deliver a definitive radiation dose may be good candidates for surgical resection. However, partial debulking of unresectable tumors is usually not recommended because it does not increase the effectiveness of radiation therapy and increases the likelihood of lymphocyst, infection, lymphedema, and harmful treatment delays. See Chapter 3 for further discussion of this subject.

The Role of Chemotherapy

Because these cases nearly always present with large tumor masses or extensive regional disease, chemotherapy is usually recommended either as a concurrent treatment with radiation or as an adjuvant. The sequencing is guided by the established role of chemotherapy for primary cancers of similar histologic type. For example, squamous carcinomas that present with an unknown primary are treated with concurrent chemoradiation, using regimens (typically weekly cisplatin) that have been proven effective for squamous carcinomas of the cervix or vulva. Concurrent chemotherapy is also given with radiation to maximize the chance of local control of adenocarcinomas arising in endometriosis or lymph nodes; however, in these cases we have usually also recommended the addition of adjuvant chemotherapy (typically carboplatin and paclitaxel) as would be used for node-positive müllerian adenocarcinomas arising in the endometrium or ovary.

RADIATION THERAPY—TECHNICAL CONSIDERATIONS

The Target Volume

The target volume should include the involved nodal basin with a cephalad margin of at least 6 cm above the most proximal gross disease; larger cephalad margins may be indicated to prevent marginal recurrences in patients with extensive lymphadenopathy (CS 15.3). For patients with pelvic nodal disease, treatment of the bilateral pelvic nodes is usually recommended, although the evidence supporting this decision is admittedly weak. For patients who present with unilateral groin disease that has not extended beyond the distal iliac nodes, we typically treat unilaterally.

Routine treatment of potential primary sites is generally not practical because of the added morbidity of central treatment and because a moderate dose of 45 to 50 Gy is not sufficient if an existing primary lesion has been missed. However, if the tumor is close enough to require partial treatment of the vagina, we have sometimes included a vaginal ITV (**CS 15.2, 15.3 and 15.5**).

Definitive Treatment of Bulky Nodal or Soft Tissue Disease

After Surgical Resection

If lymphadenectomy or surgical resection has been performed, postoperative radiation therapy is recommended to a minimum dose of 45 to 50 Gy. However, patients who present with bulky lymphadenopathy nearly always have evidence of extranodal extension, requiring a minimum dose of 60 Gy in 30 fractions (CS 15.4). Postoperative imaging should always be obtained to confirm that all gross disease has been resected. Multidisciplinary management of bulky nodal disease is also discussed in Chapter 3.

Definitive Management

Because high radiation doses of at least 60 to 65 Gy are required to control grossly enlarged nodes, IMRT is strongly recommended. Treatment breaks should be avoided to maximize the effectiveness of the delivered dose of radiation. Judicious use of integrated boosts and adaptive planning can be particularly helpful in the management of these cases, as demonstrated in the case studies appended to this chapter.

In some cases, the tumor response can be very rapid (CS 15.2). For this reason, the tumor should be monitored with cone beam or planning CT at least every 2 to 3 weeks to determine the need for adaptive planning. If a somewhat hypofractionated integrated boost is used to accelerate the initial response of large tumors, a weekly assessment is recommended. However, every effort should be made to avoid breaks in treatment during adaptive planning (Chapter 7).

The use of very high fractional "stereotactic" treatments is not recommended because of the large treatment volumes typically needed to treat sites of gross and potential microscopic disease and because of the close proximity of multiple critical structures.

References

1. Clements A, Euscher E, Lacour R, et al. The presence of human papillomavirus or p16 in six cases of retroperitoneal carcinoma. *Obstet Gynecol.* 2010;116:1042–1046.
2. Heaps JM, Nieberg RK, Berek JS. Malignant neoplasms arising in endometriosis. *Obstet Gynecol.* 1990;75:1023–1028.
3. Modesitt SC, Tortolero-Luna G, Robinson JB, et al. Ovarian and extraovarian endometriosis-associated cancer. *Obstet Gynecol.* 2002;100:788–795.
4. Ulrich U, Rhiem K, Kaminski M, et al. Parametrial and rectovaginal adenocarcinoma arising from endometriosis. *Int J Gynecol Cancer.* 2005;15:1206–1209.
5. Kelly P, Das P, Varadhachary GR, et al. Role of definitive radiation therapy in carcinoma of unknown primary in the abdomen and pelvis. *Int J Radiat Oncol Biol Phys.* 2012;82:2012–2017.

Case Studies

The five case studies appended to this chapter were chosen to demonstrate a range of disease presentations and to emphasize the potential curability of these cancers. These cases also provide good examples of the management of bulky regional disease.

List of Case Studies for Chapter 15:

CS 15.1 Squamous carcinoma of the pelvis and PANs with unknown primary site

CS 15.2 Squamous carcinoma presenting as a large presacral mass with unknown primary

CS 15.3 Pelvic mass with unknown primary; PAN recurrence after pelvic RT

CS 15.4 Inguinopelvic lymphadenopathy in a patient with a history of intraepithelial neoplasia

CS 15.5 High-grade carcinoma, probably arising in endometriosis

Abbreviations Used in the Case Studies:

BSO	Bilateral salpingo-oophorectomy
CA-125	Cancer antigen 125
CBC	Complete blood count
CTV	Clinical target volume
CT	Computed tomography
DM	Distant metastases
DVT	Deep venous thrombosis
EBRT	External beam radiotherapy
ECE	Extracapsular extension
EUA	Examination under anesthesia
FDG	Fluorodeoxyglucose
FNA	Fine needle aspirate
GTV	Gross tumor volume
HPV	Human papilloma virus
HRCTV	High-risk clinical target volume
IMRT	Intensity-modulated radiation therapy
ITV	Internal target volume
KPS	Karnofsky performance status
LVSI	Lymph vascular space invasion
MRI	Magnetic resonance imaging
NED	No evidence of disease
PAN	Paraaortic node
PET	Positron emission tomography
RT	Radiotherapy
TAH	Total abdominal hysterectomy
VIN	Vulvar intraepithelial neoplasia

CS 15.1 • Squamous Carcinoma of the Pelvis and PANs with Unknown Primary Site

History: A 33-year-old woman noted left groin pain shortly after an uncomplicated pregnancy. Over 6 months, she also developed increasingly severe left flank pain. Imaging revealed a large soft tissue mass adjacent to and invading the psoas muscle; biopsy was positive for squamous carcinoma.

Evaluation (Before Chemotherapy): Pap results were negative but because of a distant history of cervical intraepithelial neoplasia, a cone biopsy was performed; the patient also had EUA, proctoscopy, and random biopsies of the endometrium, vagina, and anus with no evidence of invasive cancer or dysplasia. *PET (**a–c**) and CT:* Large hypermetabolic, partially necrotic mass adjacent to and invading the left psoas extending from L4–L5 and distally through the inguinal canal with scalloping of the adjacent iliac wing; separate 1.6-cm hypermetabolic PAN at L3–L4.

After this evaluation failed to reveal a primary source, her local oncologist recommended chemotherapy with carboplatin and paclitaxel. Despite initial symptomatic relief and partial response shown by CT, the patient began to note recurrence of her pain before each cycle. Three weeks after the third cycle, she sought a second opinion.

Evaluation (Before RT): *CT:* Tumor was slightly smaller than at diagnosis but unchanged since CT 6 weeks prior (just before cycle 3 of chemotherapy). No DM. *Pathology review:* Squamous carcinoma, HPV-16 positive.

Treatment Plan: With only a modest response and evidence of progression between cycles, chemotherapy was held to preserve bone marrow for chemoradiation. The regional disease was massive (***d***), but with no DM there was a chance of cure if local control could be achieved. Concurrent chemoradiation was recommended. The central pelvis was not treated, but the opposite contralateral iliac nodes were included in the CTV and the upper border was extended to T12 to provide margin on the PAN disease; the CTV also extended 4 cm distal to the groin disease. The GTV was designated using diagnostic PET and CTs fused with the planning CT. Repeat CTs during treatment showed progressive necrosis but no significant change in the size of the tumor mass.

EBRT (IMRT): *Set up:* Supine, custom cradles with arms above the head.

Fractions 1–26 (***e, f***):

Left regional CTV and GTV (+6 mm): 45.2 Gy (190 cGy/fraction)

Right iliac CTV (+6 mm): 43.2 Gy (180 cGy/fraction)

Internal nested GTV (excluding lumbosacral plexus and other critical structures): 49.2 Gy (205 cGy/fraction)

Fractions 27–34:

GTV (+6 mm): 16 Gy (200 cGy/fraction)

The final dose to the GTV was 63–66 Gy (***g, h***). *All treatment was completed in 43 days.*

Chemotherapy: Concurrent weekly cisplatin × 4; cisplatin was held for several weeks due to thrombocytopenia and neutropenia.

Outcome: At 4 months, NED by PET (***i, j***). Through 3 years, the patient had mild numbness in the left leg and CTs showed NED with stable changes consistent with post-treatment effect. At 3.5 years, sudden onset of left leg edema prompted imaging that showed a left pelvic DVT and hydronephrosis. Biopsy of tissue adjacent to S2 showed squamous carcinoma.

Comments: Persistant nodal disease typically causes symptoms within 2 years. This late recurrence, despite complete resolution on PET and sequential CTs was unusual.

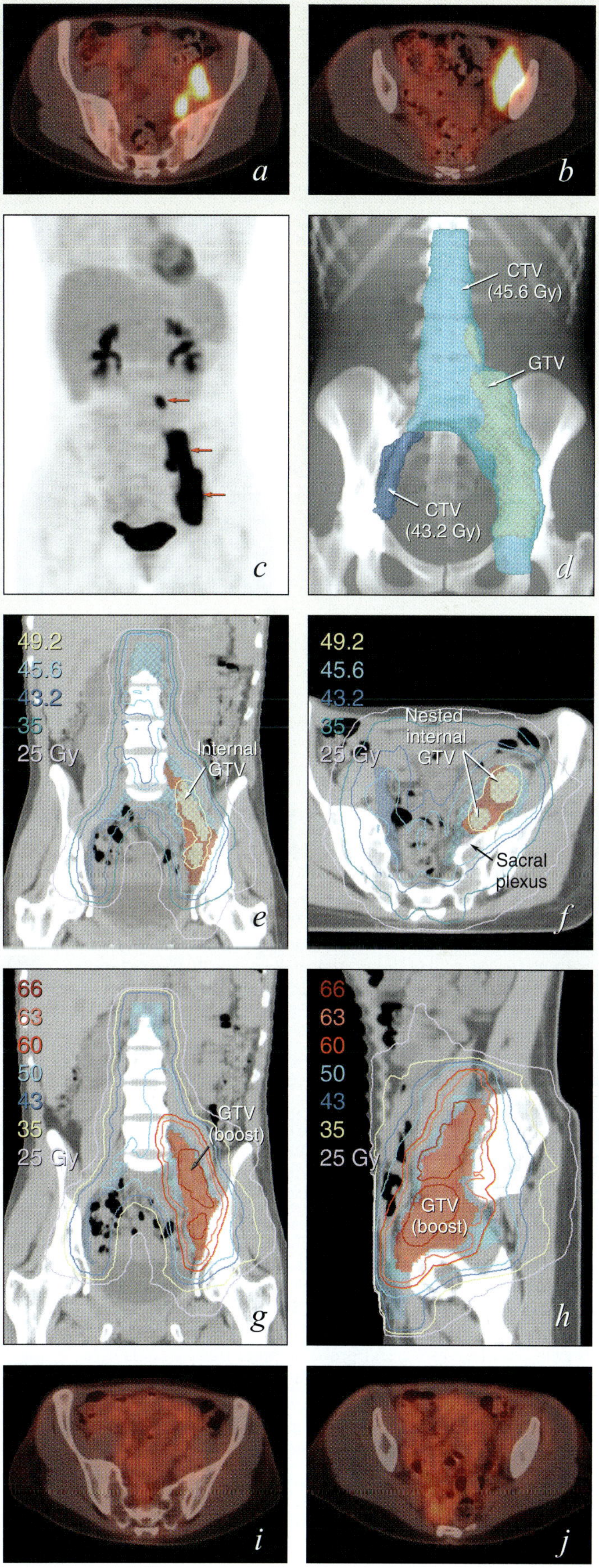

CS 15.2 • Squamous Carcinoma Presenting as a Large Presacral Mass with Unknown Primary

History: A 38-year-old woman with a 4-year history of severe menometrorrhagia and increasing constipation underwent TAH-BSO after MRI demonstrated uterine fibroids. A large, fixed posterior pelvic mass that was separate from the uterus was biopsied, showing poorly differentiated squamous carcinoma. The uterus, tubes, and ovaries contained no invasive cancer or dysplasia. The patient was referred for evaluation and treatment.

Evaluation: *Exam:* A 6-cm fixed mass in the right paravaginal and perirectal space with normal vaginal mucosa; there was a small wound abscess in the surgical incision (***b***). *KPS:* 90. *Colonoscopy:* External compression of the rectum beginning 4 cm from the anal verge; no mucosal lesions. *PET (**a**, **b**) and CT:* 6 × 7 cm FDG-avid mass in the lower right pelvis abutting the rectum; suspicious right external iliac node (***e***); no DM.

Treatment Plan: Despite an extensive workup, no primary site was found. Because the lesion was localized, concurrent chemoradiation with curative intent was recommended. Because of the central location of the tumor and distal extent, the pelvic and inguinal nodes were included in the CTV (***c***, ***d***). The PET scan was fused with the planning CT to assist GTV definition. Hypofractionated internal GTVs that avoided critical structures were used to create a high-dose gradient within the tumor (Chapters 5 and 6).

EBRT (IMRT): *Set up:* Supine, custom cradle.

Treatment was begun using a single IMRT plan with integrated boosts.

In 16 fractions (***e***, ***f***):

Pelvic and inguinal CTV (+7 mm): 26.7 Gy (167 cGy/fraction)

PET-positive GTV and vagina (+7 mm): 32 Gy (200 cGy/fraction)

PET-positive GTV (no margin): 35.2 Gy (220 cGy/fraction)

Internal GTV (PET-positive GTV – 5 mm): 37.3 Gy (233 cGy/fraction)

At the end of 2 weeks, the patient had complete resolution of pain and exam already revealed a dramatic reduction in the tumor diameter. Repeat CT was obtained that day, demonstrating a 50% response (***i***). An adapted plan using the new volumes without the internal GTV began on day 17. The final composite plan delivered 50.1 Gy to the nodal CTV and 60–68 Gy to the GTV (***g***–***h***). *Treatment was completed in 43 days.*

Chemotherapy: Concurrent weekly cisplatin × 6. Adjuvant carboplatin and paclitaxel × 3.

Outcome: At 1 month (after RT), NED by PET (***j***). At 2 years, NED by PET; two episodes of hemorrhagic cystitis were successfully treated with fulguration. At 10 years, NED receiving follow-up by her local physician.

Comments: In retrospect, it is impossible to accurately calculate the doses received by critical structures as they change position with tumor response. Today we use more conservative fractionation to treat such cases with integrated and sequential boosts and would follow tumor response with weekly cone beam CTs. More rapid, and probably more frequent, adaptive planning could also reduce exposure to critical structures. We do not recommend SBRT for such cases because of the close proximity of critical structures (Chapter 6).

See Figure 7.7 for additional images of this case.

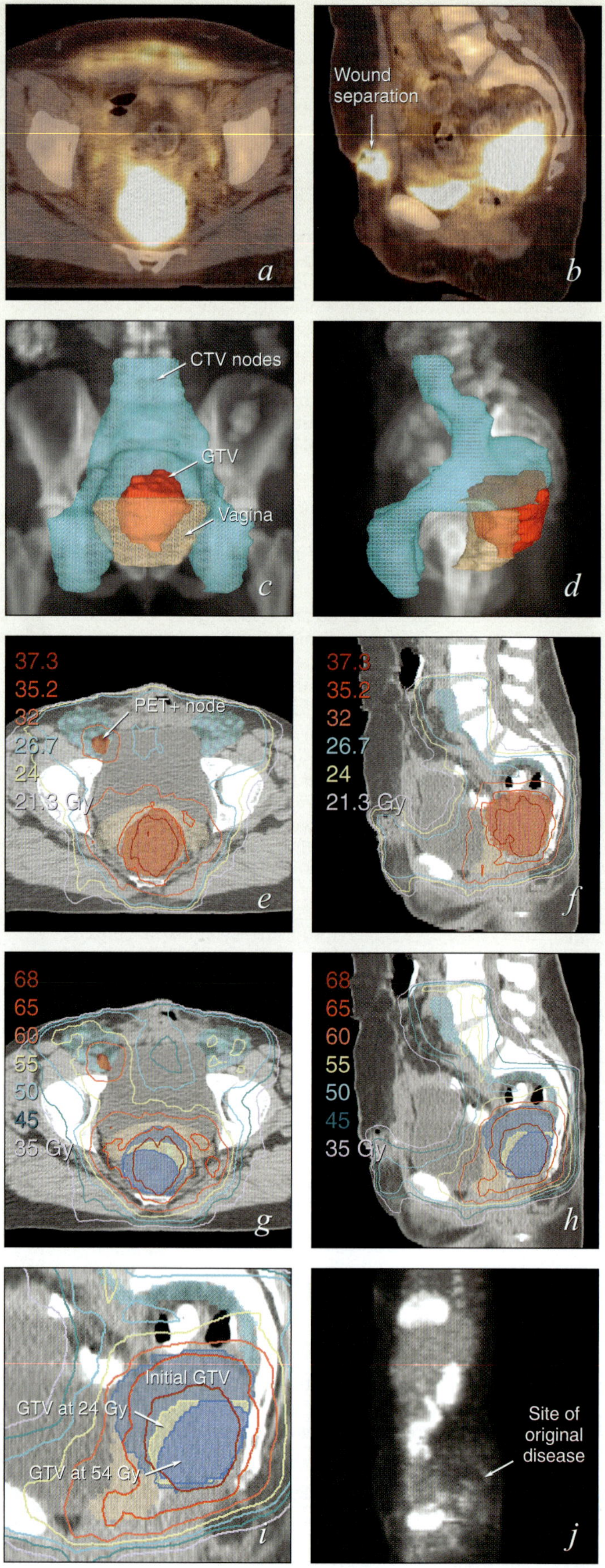

CS 15.3 • Pelvic Mass with Unknown Primary; Pan Recurrence After Pelvic RT

History: A 69-year-old woman with lower back pain and mildly elevated creatinine had CT showing a right pelvic mass and hydronephrosis. She was referred for evaluation after placement of a right nephrostomy tube. Forty years prior to this, the patient had hysterectomy for early cervical cancer.

Evaluation: *Exam:* A 4-cm fixed right pelvic wall mass; otherwise NED; *KPS: 90; Cystoscopy:* NED; *MRI (a, arrows), PET–CT (**b**):* 3.5 × 4-cm mass in the right obturator region inseparable from the obturator internus; *Biopsy (FNA):* Moderately differentiated squamous carcinoma positive for high-risk HPV; *Pap and vaginal biopsies:* Negative.

Treatment Plan: IMRT with concurrent chemoradiation was recommended. After some consideration, it was decided to include the vagina and contralateral nodes in the CTV. Because of the extensive obturator disease and several small 4–5-mm PET-negative nodes proximal to the lesion, the CTV extended to L3/4, 12 cm above the primary mass. The plan employed an integrated internal (nested) GTV and sequential boost. The tumor had not responded sufficiently to require interval adaptive planning, but the GTV was adjusted before the final boost plan to account for a reduction of approximately 25% in the tumor volume.

EBRT (IMRT): *Set up:* Supine, custom cradle.

Fractions 1–25 (***c***, ***d***):

Right pelvic, common iliac, and vaginal CTVs (+7 mm): 50 Gy (200 cGy/fraction)

Left iliac CTV: 45 Gy (180 cGy/fraction)

GTV + 0 mm margin: 53.75 Gy (215 cGy/fraction)

Fractions 26–32:

Boost GTV + 5 mm: 12.6 Gy (180 cGy/fraction)

Boost GTV + 2 mm: 14 Gy (200 cGy/fraction)

The total GTV dose was 65–68 Gy (***e***). *All treatment was completed in 46 days.*

Chemotherapy: Concurrent weekly cisplatin × 5.

Outcome: At 4 months, PET showed resolution of the pelvic mass but development of two new small FDG-avid nodes at the margin of the previous radiation fields (***f**, arrows*). FNA showed squamous carcinoma. A second course of concurrent chemoradiation was recommended. The isocenter was placed at the distal margin of the fields to minimize divergence into the pelvis and to maximize reproducibility (***g***). A small but suspicious left PAN (HRCTV, ***h***) was prescribed an intermediate radiation dose.

IMRT in 30 fractions (over 39 days):

PAN CTV (+7 mm; +5 mm distally): 50 Gy

HRCTV (+5 mm): 55 Gy

GTV (+5 mm): 60 Gy

Composite plan demonstrated a small region of overlap at the field margins (***i***).

At 6 months from second course and 2 years from initial RT, NED by PET (***j***) and exam. At 3 years from the initial course, NED in the care of her local physician.

Comments: After 40 years, this node was unlikely to have been a metastasis from the original cervical cancer. A proximal CTV margin should always be included to treat potential upstream lymphatic metastases, although the 12-cm margin used here is usually sufficient. Surgical dissection of the involved PANs was considered, but postoperative PAN treatment would still have been required.

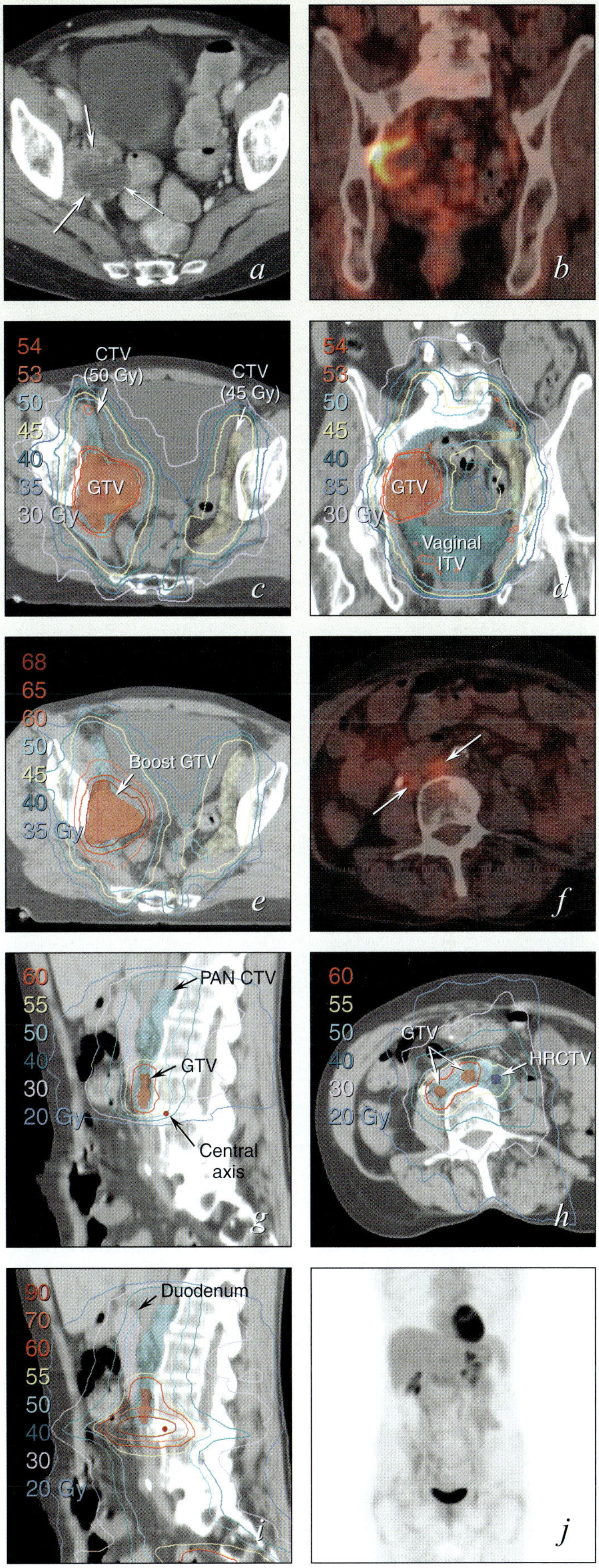

CS 15.4 • Inguinopelvic Lymphadenopathy In a Patient with a History of Intraepithelial Neoplasia

History: A 38-year-old woman on mild immunosuppressive therapy for systemic lupus had four resections of warty right labial and periclitoral lesions over 18 months. All specimens showed VIN without invasion or LVSI. Nine months after the last resection, an enlarged left inguinal node was noted on exam.

Evaluation: *Exam:* A 3-cm left inguinal mass; normal pelvic exam with postoperative sequelae in the vulva but no lesions suspicious for cancer or dysplasia. *PET–CT (**a**, **b**):* 4 × 2.5-cm nodal mass in the left common femoral region; 2.5-cm left external iliac node; 1.5-cm left obturator node; no other FDG-avid sites. *FNA of left groin:* Squamous carcinoma.

Treatment Plan: After multidisciplinary discussion, resection of the enlarged nodes followed by postoperative chemoradiation was recommended. The patient had resection of the left inguinal mass, retroperitoneal distal left pelvic node dissection, and cervical cone biopsy; EUA of the vulva and vagina and procto-sigmoidoscopy all were normal.

Pathology: The left inguinal node was replaced by squamous carcinoma with extensive necrosis and fibroadipose tissue infiltration; there were also metastases with associated ECE in 5 of 14 pelvic lymph nodes. The cervix had only mild dysplasia.

Postoperative Course: Ten days after surgery, a wound infection and lower extremity cellulitis required admission for antibiotics. Seven weeks after surgery, postoperative RT was delayed by admission for an infected lymphocyst (*arrows*, ***c***) draining purulent material, recurrent lower extremity cellulitis, and lymphedema. The patient improved after IV antibiotics and placement of a new pelvic drain. RT was finally started 56 days after surgery; the pelvic drain remained in place throughout.

Radiation Therapy: Given the extensive ECE and soft tissue infiltration, the surgical incision and drain sites were included in the CTV. Because a large number of pelvic nodes were involved, the contralateral pelvic nodes were treated.

EBRT (IMRT): *Set up:* Frog leg position, custom cradle.

Fractions 1–25 (***d***, ***e***):

Left nodal and operative bed CTV (+7 mm): 50 Gy (200 cGy/fraction)

Right pelvic CTV (+7 mm): 45 Gy (180 cGy/fraction)

Fractions 26–30: HRCTV (+7 mm): 12 Gy (200 cGy/fraction) (total dose 62 Gy, ***f***). *Treatment was completed in 46 days.*

Chemotherapy: Concurrent weekly cisplatin × 3; other cycles held because of infection problems.

Outcome: In the last week of RT, readmission for cellulitis and moist desquamation of the groin area. At 1 month, readmission for sepsis and cellulitis involving the left buttock. At 6 months, NED by CT and exam, with significant left leg edema but no other treatment-related complaints. At 3 years, NED by exam with no evidence of VIN or recurrent cancer; fluctuating leg edema.

Comments: The multidisciplinary management of extensive inguinopelvic lymphadenopathy is particularly challenging. The risk of wound complications, always high after resection of extensive nodal disease, was increased by this patient's immunosuppression. With extensive ECE, the RT dose was nearly as high as that required for gross disease. The need to treat the operative bed and drain sites substantially increased the RT volume, and delays could have affected RT effectiveness. However, although we are increasingly using definitive chemoradiation to treat bulky groin disease in patients who are receiving definitive vulvar RT, most surgeons consider combined treatment standard in this setting.

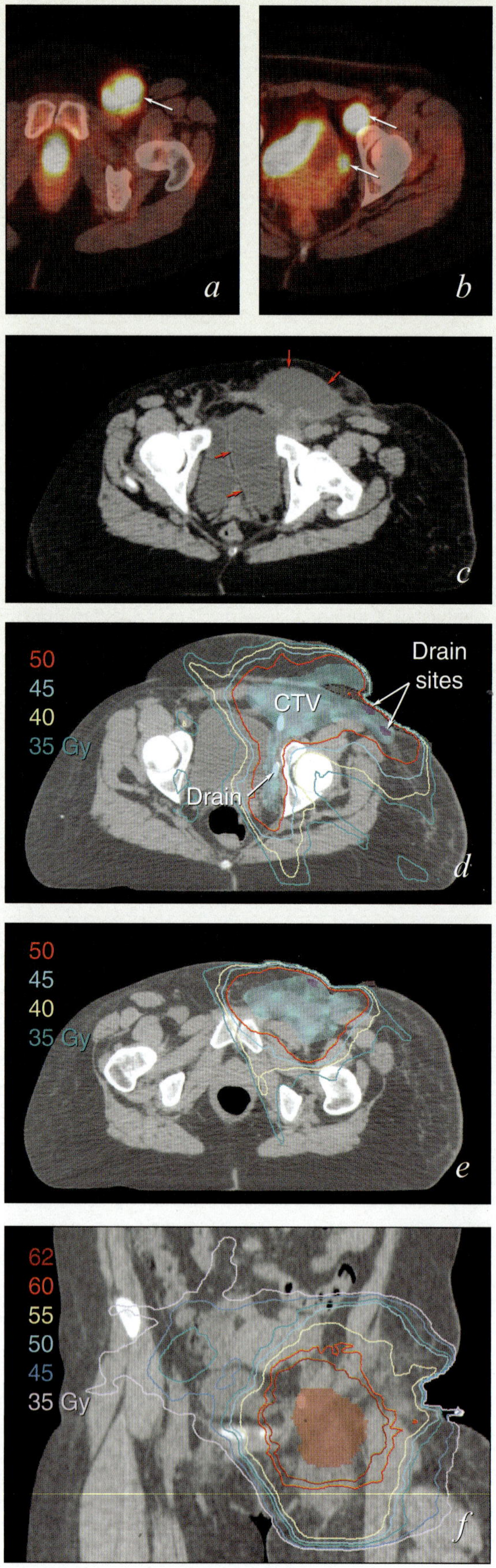

CS 15.5 • High-Grade Carcinoma, Probably Arising in Endometriosis

History: A 53-year-old woman was found to have a paravaginal mass on routine pelvic examination. Ten years previously, she had undergone hysterectomy for painful endometriosis. She was placed on hormone replacement therapy immediately after that surgery and believed that her ovaries had been removed, but efforts to obtain records and histologic material from that surgery were unsuccessful.

Evaluation: *Exam:* A 4-cm right adnexal mass; normal vaginal mucosa; *CT of chest, abdomen, and pelvis (**a**, **b**):* 3.8 × 3.9 × 3.7 cm right pelvic mass intimately associated with the sigmoid and right ureter; prominent right external iliac and common iliac nodes up to 7 mm in diameter; no DM. On the basis of the location, an ovarian primary was thought possible but unlikely. *Pelvic ultrasound:* 4-cm complex cystic and solid mass highly suspicious for malignancy; *CA-125:* 78.

Treatment Plan: Although the past history and imaging suggested that this was probably a cancer arising in endometriosis, an ovarian primary could not be ruled out. It was decided to proceed with surgical exploration. The patient underwent a resection of the right pelvic mass as well as pelvic and PAN dissection, omentectomy, and excision of a small cul-de-sac nodule. Although a gross total resection was accomplished, the tumor was adherent to the vaginal apex, sigmoid, and posterior bladder peritoneum and was encasing the ureter. Significant microscopic disease was thought to have been left behind, particularly in the paravaginal and periureteral tissues.

Pathology: High-grade carcinoma with extensive squamous differentiation and foci of attempted gland formation; 17 pelvic nodes, 9 PANs, the omentum, and cul-de-sac biopsy showed NED. There was no ovarian tissue, and the histologic findings were considered to be most consistent with carcinoma arising in endometriosis.

Postoperative Evaluation: MRI showed no evidence of residual disease; equivocal pelvic nodes had been excised.

Radiation Therapy: The CTV included the bilateral pelvic nodes and vaginal ITV; the operative bed was designated a HRCTV in an integrated boost. A slightly more restricted HRCTV, including the highest risk regions surrounding the right ureter, vagina, posterior bladder wall, and paravaginal space, received a sequential boost to bring the total dose to 60 Gy.

EBRT (IMRT): *Set up:* Supine, custom cradle.

Fractions 1–25 (***b***, ***c***):

Nodal CTV, vaginal ITV (+7 mm): 45 Gy (180 cGy/fraction)

HRCTV (+6 mm): 50 Gy (200 cGy/fraction).

Fractions 26–30 (***d***):

HRCTV (+6 mm): 10 Gy (200 cGy/fraction). *Treatment was completed in 39 days.*

Chemotherapy: Concurrent weekly cisplatin × 5; adjuvant carboplatin and paclitaxel × 4.

Outcome: At 4 months, NED by exam and CT and without complaints; at 2 years, followed at an outside facility with NED and CA-125 of 8.

Comments: Today, carcinomas arising in endometriosis are sometimes categorized as primary peritoneal cancers and are treated with chemotherapy alone. However, when disease is localized to a single pelvic site without peritoneal spread, pelvic RT is recommended to reduce the risk of operative bed recurrence.

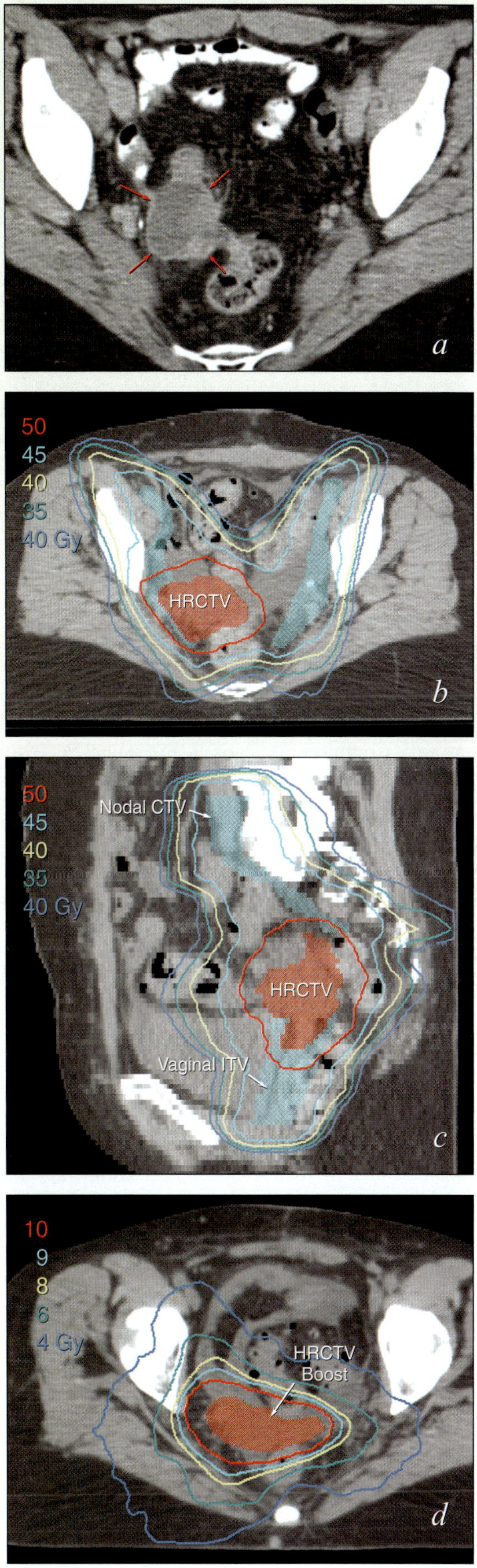

CHAPTER 16

Palliation

INTRODUCTION

Radiation therapy (RT) can be a highly effective tool for the treatment of symptoms caused by progressive gynecologic cancers. Common indications for palliative treatment of gynecologic cancers include the following:

- Pain caused by erosive lesions involving the primary tumor site or lymph nodes
- Vaginal bleeding
- Symptomatic systemic metastases

This chapter focuses on the first two of these indications. Palliative treatment of symptomatic systemic metastases is similar for gynecologic cancers and other cancers.

In most cases, the decision to recommend radiation therapy is based primarily on the location of the lesion and the associated symptoms rather than the histology of the tumor. Gynecologic carcinomas, with rare exceptions, are more likely to respond to radiation therapy than to systemic chemotherapy. As a result, radiation therapy is often the palliative treatment of choice in patients with incurable gynecologic cancers. In general, palliative treatment fields should cover the disease that is causing symptoms but do not include elective nodal regions. The use of smaller fields minimizes acute toxic effects and preserves marrow function to improve tolerance of future chemotherapy regimens.

Palliative radiation therapy is frequently given to patients who also require systemic chemotherapy for metastatic disease. Integration of these treatments requires consideration of many factors:

- *The severity of the symptom.*
- *The nature of the symptom.* Debilitating bleeding, pain, or neurologic compromise should be addressed first with radiation since radiation will produce the most rapid response in nearly all cases.
- *The likelihood of a response to chemotherapy.* In patients with less severe symptoms and highly chemosensitive disease, such as small cell carcinoma, initial chemotherapy is preferred since chemotherapy will address all sites of metastatic disease.
- *The overall extent of the patient's disease.* Systemic therapy may be a higher priority for patients with extensive metastatic disease. Often, a short break is recommended between the completion of radiation therapy and the start of chemotherapy. The delay in starting chemotherapy can be a concern for patients and physicians. The use of hypofractionated regimens can reduce this delay.

INDICATIONS FOR PALLIATIVE RADIATION THERAPY

Vaginal Masses

For patients with recurrence in the vagina as well as distant metastasis, palliative radiation therapy can reduce vaginal bleeding and pain. Treatment fields should cover the involved region of the vagina with a 2- to 3-cm margin. Because the vaginal apex can move 2 cm or more with bladder filling, it is useful to assess vaginal motion by performing simulation both when the patient has a full bladder and when the patient has an empty bladder so that treatment fields can be designed to ensure that the tumor remains in the treatment field without unnecessary irradiation of normal tissues. Intracavitary vaginal brachytherapy may be useful for palliative treatment of very superficial

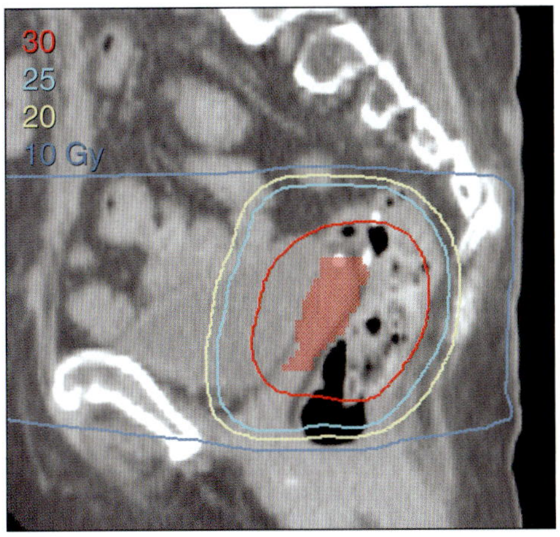

FIGURE 16.1 A 71-year-old woman presented with stage IIIC ovarian cancer and underwent three cycles of carboplatin and paclitaxel followed by interval optimal cytoreduction and three additional cycles of carboplatin and paclitaxel. Two years later, she developed vaginal bleeding and was found to have a recurrence at the vaginal apex. A computed tomography scan also revealed evidence of small-volume peritoneal disease. The patient was treated with platinum-based chemotherapy and biologically targeted treatment, but the vaginal lesion persisted and exhibited clinical evidence of progression. The patient was referred for radiation therapy. The vaginal apex was treated with 30 Gy in 10 fractions followed by a single pulsed-dose rate brachytherapy treatment to deliver 50 Gy (surface dose) to the vaginal apex. The patient tolerated treatment well. One year later, she developed progressive peritoneal disease. She ultimately died of disease 4½ years after completion of radiation therapy but did not experience symptoms of vaginal recurrence during this time.

lesions but generally does not deliver an adequate dose for lesions thicker than 5 mm. For patients who have small volume metastatic disease combined with vaginal recurrence, a short course of palliative external beam therapy with brachytherapy can provide high rates of local control (**Fig. 16.1**). In general, we do not recommend treatment of lymph nodes in patients with minimal metastatic disease and recurrence at the vaginal apex unless an adjacent node is causing pain or is large and thought likely to cause pain in the near future.

Cervical or Uterine Cancer with Metastasis at Presentation

Patients who present with metastatic cervical or uterine cancer frequently suffer from pain and bleeding from the primary cancer. If the patient has an estimated life expectancy of 6 months or more, it may be appropriate to deliver aggressive palliative radiation therapy to the cervix in hopes of providing durable local control in the pelvis. One regimen that we have used in patients with an initial presentation of metastatic cervical cancer is to treat the pelvis to 30 Gy in 10 fractions with concurrent cisplatin and then use brachytherapy to deliver an EqD2 of ~30 Gy to point A or to 90% of the high-risk clinical target volume. For patients who have massive disease or a short life expectancy, hypofractionated external beam RT can be very effective, with 50% to 100% of patients experiencing marked improvement in symptoms of bleeding and pain.[1] Kim et al. reported high rates of response with minimal toxicity with this approach.[2]

A variety of alternative dose and fractionation schemes have been reported for palliation of pelvic tumors. The Radiation Therapy Oncology Group reported an analysis of patients treated on a prospective study delivering 3.7-Gy fractions twice a day for 2 days (total of 14.8 Gy) repeated every 2 to 4 weeks up to a maximum of 44.4 Gy. Among 61 cervical cancer patients treated, 53% had an objective response to this regimen, and only 7% experienced late toxic effects.[3] Treatment with single large fractions can be effective for patients with a poor performance status and poor prognosis. A single 10-Gy fraction provides rapid palliation and can be repeated in a month for patients with persistent symptoms (**Fig. 16.2**). This regimen results in cessation or substantial reduction in bleeding in ~75% of patients and elimination or a substantial reduction in pain in ~50% of patients.[1] Our current practice for patients with a poor performance status, defined as a Karnofsky performance status score of 60 or less, is to deliver one 8- to 10-Gy treatment with a conformal plan that excludes as much bowel as possible. If the patient continues to have symptoms a month later, resimulation and treatment with an additional 8 to 10 Gy is considered. This treatment is generally well tolerated; however, retrospective studies of early MD Anderson experience demonstrated that the use of more than two treatments of 10 Gy had an unacceptable rate of major complications.[3]

For selected patients with limited oligometastatic disease, such as supraclavicular nodal metastases or solitary pulmonary nodules, a full course of definitive radiation therapy for cervical cancer with concurrent definitive treatment to the site of oligometastasis may be indicated (**CS 10.10**).

Pelvic Sidewall Recurrence

Erosion of disease from a pelvic node into adjacent bones or muscles can cause severe pain. The target volume in these cases is the gross tumor volume, which is often best evaluated on positron emission tomography or magnetic resonance imaging if computed tomography scans do not accurately distinguish the mass from muscles. For patients with a poor performance status, a single dose of 8 to 10 Gy can be highly effective. A conformal or intensity-modulated radiation therapy plan that targets the gross target volume can help to spare adjacent bowel (**Fig. 16.3**). For patients with a good performance status and a limited burden of metastatic disease, a higher effective dose may be indicated to achieve durable symptom control; the treatment technique, total dose, and fractionation should be selected to

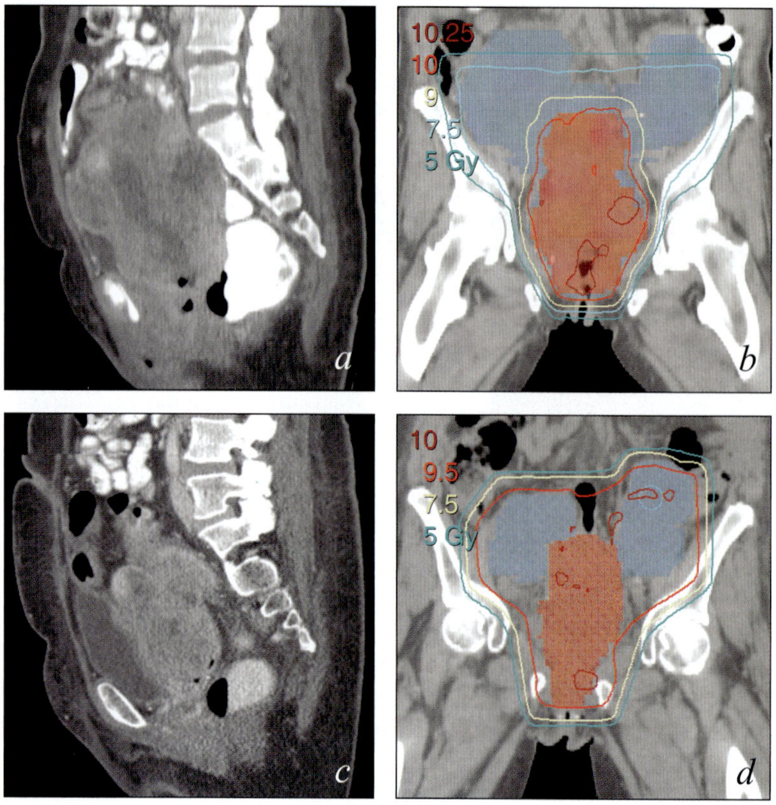

FIGURE 16.2 A 63-year-old woman with a 3-year history of postmenopausal bleeding sought medical attention when her bleeding increased. A pelvic mass was initially interpreted as uterine fibroids, but biopsy of a necrotic cervix eventually yielded a diagnosis of poorly differentiated adenocarcinoma. The patient was referred with massive bleeding and a hemoglobin of 4.9 g/dL. CT (*a*) demonstrated massive uterine and bilateral adnexal disease. Physical exam also demonstrated tumor extending to the distal one-third of the vagina. The patient was referred for emergent RT to control her bleeding and pain. The patient was treated with a single fraction of RT; using a 4-field, 3-D technique with field-in-field, the uterus, cervix, and vagina were treated to a dose of 10 Gy, and the distal adnexal masses received 7.5 Gy (*b*). To reduce the volume of bowel and bone marrow in the field, the proximal portions of the adnexa, which were largely cystic, were not treated. The patient had prompt resolution of her symptoms. She was begun on chemotherapy with carboplatin and paclitaxel. After two cycles, 2 months after RT, CT showed marked regression of her disease (*c*). One month after completing her sixth cycle of chemotherapy, the patient returned complaining of increased bleeding and discomfort. CT showed slight increase of her cervical disease and more marked increase in the adnexal masses. She was treated with a second single fraction of radiation therapy and again had prompt improvement in her symptoms (*d*). However, after 3 months, she developed abdominal pain and was found to have liver metastases; she died 12 months after her first RT and 6 months after the second.

maximize symptom relief without causing injury to adjacent critical structures.

Vulvar Cancer

Patients with vulvar cancer rarely present with metastatic disease because vulvar cancer tends cause symptoms that bring the disease to the patient's attention at a relatively early stage. However, when patients with vulvar cancer do present with metastasis, palliative treatment to the vulva may be recommended. Because most advanced tumors are superinfected with bacteria, a course of antibiotics can sometimes bring significant pain relief. Although we do not recommend neoadjuvant chemotherapy if the treatment intent is curative (Chapter 12), for patients with metastatic disease, a initial trial of chemotherapy may be indicated to reduce the local tumor burden before a course of palliative RT. If tolerated, a course of hypofractionated RT (e.g., 30 Gy in 10 fractions) can be given with concurrent weekly cisplatin with the goal of achieving effective palliation and durable local control.

Paraaortic and Psoas Metastases

Paraaortic nodal metastases that invade the psoas muscle can cause very severe pain, worsened by leg extension. Infiltration of paraaortic nodal disease into the space between the psoas and vertebral bodies, which is traversed by many nerves, also can cause very severe pain. These lesions can be very gratifying to treat since responses can dramatically improve the patient's quality of life. Palliative courses of radiation therapy should target the gross tumor volume and deliver an appropriate dose according to the disease extent and performance status.

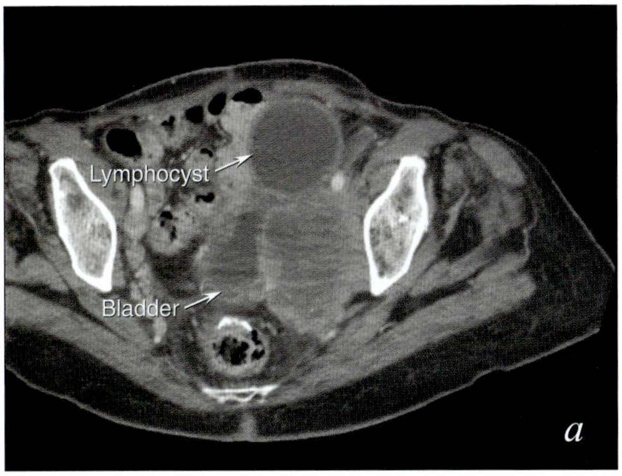

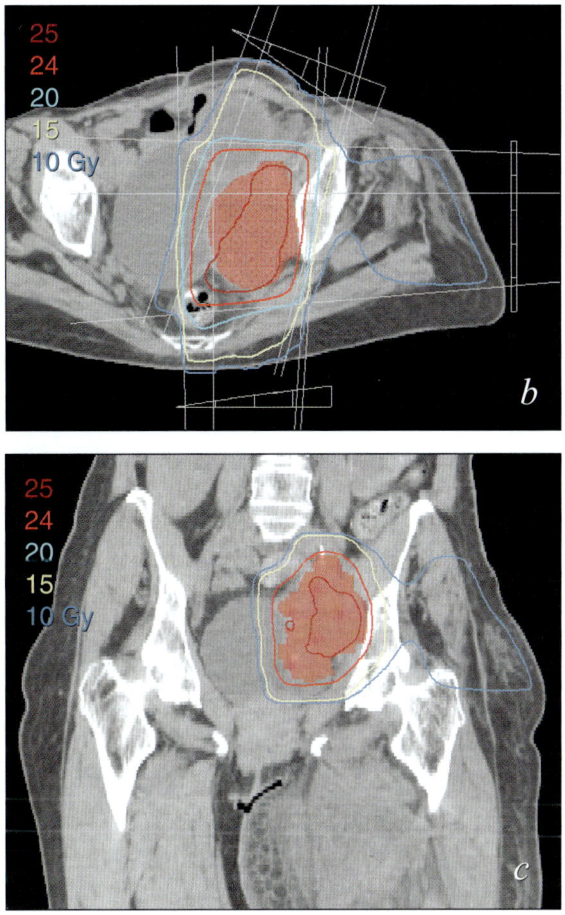

FIGURE 16.3 A 62-year-old woman presented with hematuria, pelvic pain, and a swollen left leg. Imaging demonstrated a large mass on the pelvic sidewall with liver metastasis *(a)*. Biopsy demonstrated a spindle cell neoplasm of müllerian origin. The patient was treated with palliative radiation therapy to the pelvic sidewall mass to 20 Gy in five fractions with a conformal three-beam treatment plan *(b, c)* followed by systemic therapy. She subsequently experienced a reduction in leg swelling and pain and went on to receive systemic therapy.

Skin Metastasis

Metastasis to the abdominal wall, often in surgical sites, or to the umbilicus, referred to as a "Sister Mary Joseph" nodule, can cause significant pain and bleeding. When disease is isolated to these sites, surgery followed by radiation therapy has a high likelihood of producing local control.[4] For patients with skin metastasis in the context of widespread disease, radiation therapy using appositional electron fields for small lesions or tangential fields for larger lesions can provide palliation.

Bone Metastasis

Metastasis to the bone from gynecologic cancers can be managed similarly to metastasis to the bone from other sites. In general, the target is the gross disease with a margin of 2 to 5 cm. The optimal fractionation scheme can be decided on the basis of the patient's performance status. A single fraction of 8 to 10 Gy[5] provides rapid palliation and is preferred over more protracted courses of radiation therapy for patients who have a large burden of disease or a poor performance status. Studies have shown that single fractions are as effective as longer courses of radiation therapy but may have slightly less durable benefits. For patients with oligometastatic disease in bones, definitive doses to these sites may sometimes be considered using standard fractionation or stereotactic approaches.

CONDITIONS FOR WHICH PALLIATIVE RADIATION THERAPY IS GENERALLY NOT INDICATED

Central Recurrence or Persistent Disease in a Previously Irradiated Site

The risk of central recurrence is highest during the first 3 years after definitive radiation therapy (Fig. 9.1).[6] When biopsy demonstrates isolated recurrent or persistent disease in the cervix, pelvic exenteration is the standard treatment.[5] For patients who are not candidates for exenteration or who decline exenteration, chemotherapy is the standard, but some authors have reported success with reirradiation using interstitial brachytherapy.[7]

For cases of nodal recurrence within the prior treatment field, the location of the recurrent disease relative to the initial treatment field should be carefully evaluated to ensure that the site of recurrence received the full dose in the initial treatment plan. Very often, recurrences lie just above the

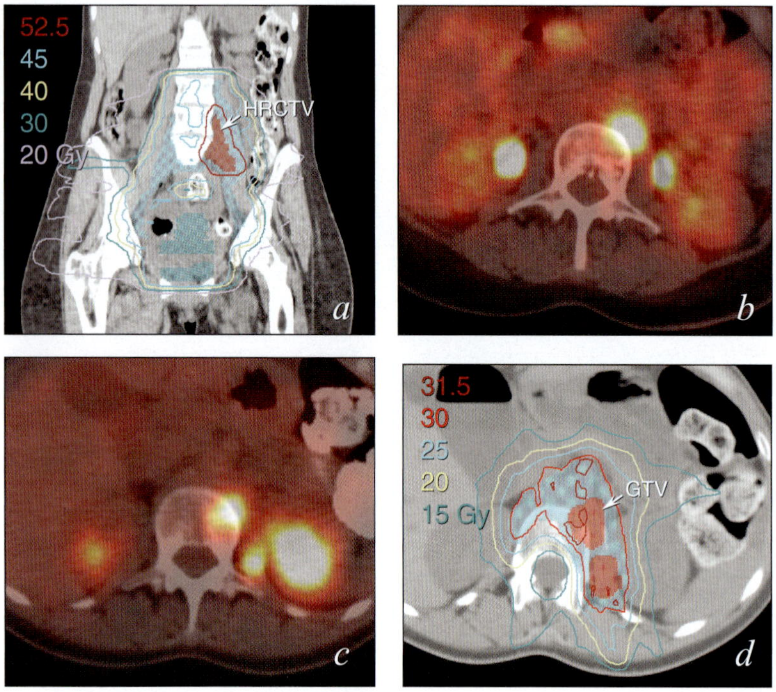

FIGURE 16.4 **A 46-year-old woman presented with severe pelvic pain, and imaging demonstrated a 7-cm mass in the psoas muscle.** A biopsy of the mass revealed squamous cell carcinoma. No primary tumor site was identified after directed biopsies and imaging. She received four cycles of carboplatin and Taxol, had a near-complete response, and was then referred for chemoradiation therapy (*a*). However, 1 year later, she developed a recurrence just above the prior treatment field in a paraaortic node adjacent to the duodenum and the L2 vertebral body (*b*). Because of concerns about risk of retreatment to the duodenum, she underwent resection of this mass followed by intraoperative radiation therapy. Unfortunately, the disease recurred again in the same site above L2 with erosion into the vertebral body (*c*). The patient was treated with palliative radiation therapy to treat her back pain to a total dose of 30 Gy in 10 fractions with an intensity-modulated radiation therapy plan (*d*). She experienced some improvement in her pain but died of disease 6 months after her last course of radiation. This case highlights the challenges of balancing the risk of toxicity of surgery and radiation against the critical need for disease control.

prior treatment field, especially if a lower upper border (L5/S1) was used for the pelvic field.[8] Common iliac nodes above L5/S1 can be read as pelvic nodes on diagnostic imaging sets, leading to the misperception that the recurrence lies within the prior treatment field. If the nodal site received less than the full dose, definitive radiation therapy can be considered. However, if the node lies within the prior treatment field, it is usually not possible to deliver an effective dose without causing major complications; however, in rare cases, if the recurrence is not close to critical structures, retreatment may be effective (**CS 13.5**).

Peritoneal Disease

Patients with advanced gynecologic cancers, especially ovarian cancer, develop extensive omental and peritoneal metastases, which cause highly morbid bowel obstructions. Unfortunately, metastasis to the omentum and peritoneum is inherently a diffuse process that frequently involves a significant portion of the peritoneal cavity. Large field abdominal RT is generally ineffective and has unacceptable morbidity. Bowel obstructions caused by infiltrative tumor can rarely be reversed with RT, which is not recommended in most cases.

Fistula

Patients with progressive local disease can develop a fistula between the vagina and bladder or rectum. Surgical diversion is required for symptom management and to prevent further complications. For rectal fistulas, a colostomy is indicated; vaginal fistulas necessitate a urostomy. In many of these cases, radiation has been used previously. In the absence of prior radiation therapy, the relative risks and benefits of radiation therapy should be carefully assessed. RT may reduce pain and bleeding. However, radiation therapy may also enlarge the fistula and worsen symptoms.

Concurrent Peritonitis

Intra-abdominal infections can occur in patients with advanced disease as a result of surgical complications or bowel perforation from tumor. The inflammation associated with peritonitis significantly increases the risk of radiation-related complications.[9] Therefore, radiation therapy in an active site of infection is to be avoided. The risk associated with radiation therapy is likely significantly lower once the infection has been successfully treated, but the history of peritonitis will continue to put the woman at risk for complications in the future.

References

1. van Lonkhuijzen L, Thomas G. Palliative radiotherapy for cervical carcinoma, a systematic review. *Radiother Oncol.* 2011; 98(3):287–291. doi: 10.1016/j.radonc.2011.01.009.
2. Kim DH, Lee JH, Ki YK, et al. Short-course palliative radiotherapy for uterine cervical cancer. *Radiat Oncol J.* 2013; 31(4):216–221. doi: 10.3857/roj.2013.31.4.216.
3. Spanos WJ Jr, Pajak TJ, Emami B, et al. Radiation palliation of cervical cancer. *J Natl Cancer Inst Monogr.* 1996;(21):127–130.
4. Grant JD, Garg AK, Gopal R, et al. Isolated port-site metastases after minimally invasive hysterectomy for endometrial cancer: outcomes of patients treated with radiotherapy. *Int J Gynecol Cancer.* 2015;25(5):869–874. doi: 10.1097/IGC.0000000000000424.
5. Westin SN, Rallapalli V, Fellman B, et al. Overall survival after pelvic exenteration for gynecologic malignancy. *Gynecol Oncol.* 2014;134(3):546–551. doi: 10.1016/j.ygyno.2014.06.034.
6. Eifel PJ, Jhingran A, Brown J, et al. Time course and outcome of central recurrence after radiation therapy for carcinoma of the cervix. *Int J Gynecol Cancer.* 2006;16(3):1106–1111. doi: 10.1111/j.1525-1438.2006.00544.x.
7. Lee LJ, Damato AL, Viswanathan AN. Clinical outcomes following 3D image-guided brachytherapy for vaginal recurrence of endometrial cancer. *Gynecol Oncol.* 2013;131(3): 586–592. doi: 10.1016/j.ygyno.2013.08.040.
8. Beadle BM, Jhingran A, Yom SS, et al. Patterns of regional recurrence after definitive radiotherapy for cervical cancer. *Int J Radiat Oncol Biol Phys.* 2010;76(5):1396–1403. doi: 10.1016/j.ijrobp.2009.04.009.
9. Eifel PJ, Jhingran A, Bodurka DC, et al. Correlation of smoking history and other patient characteristics with major complications of pelvic radiation therapy for cervical cancer. *J Clin Oncol.* 2002;20(17):3651–3657.

INDEX

Note: Page numbers followed by 'f' denote figures and 't' denote tables.

A

B

C

D

E

W

RRS1606